Heterocyclic Compounds from Marine Organisms

Heterocyclic Compounds from Marine Organisms

Editor

Asunción Barbero

MDPI • Basel • Beijing • Wuhan • Barcelona • Belgrade • Manchester • Tokyo • Cluj • Tianjin

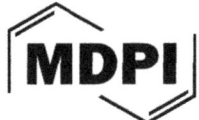

Editor
Asunción Barbero
Department of Organic
Chemistry, Faculty of Science,
Campus Miguel Delibes,
Valladolid, Spain

Editorial Office
MDPI
St. Alban-Anlage 66
4052 Basel, Switzerland

This is a reprint of articles from the Special Issue published online in the open access journal *Marine Drugs* (ISSN 1660-3397) (available at: https://www.mdpi.com/journal/marinedrugs/special_issues/Heterocyclic_Marine).

For citation purposes, cite each article independently as indicated on the article page online and as indicated below:

LastName, A.A.; LastName, B.B.; LastName, C.C. Article Title. *Journal Name* **Year**, *Volume Number*, Page Range.

ISBN 978-3-0365-5997-1 (Hbk)
ISBN 978-3-0365-5998-8 (PDF)

© 2022 by the authors. Articles in this book are Open Access and distributed under the Creative Commons Attribution (CC BY) license, which allows users to download, copy and build upon published articles, as long as the author and publisher are properly credited, which ensures maximum dissemination and a wider impact of our publications.

The book as a whole is distributed by MDPI under the terms and conditions of the Creative Commons license CC BY-NC-ND.

Contents

About the Editor vii

Preface to "Heterocyclic Compounds from Marine Organisms" ix

Pierre-Eric Campos, Gaëtan Herbette, Laetitia Fougère, Patricia Clerc, Florent Tintillier, Nicole J. de Voogd, Géraldine Le Goff, Jamal Ouazzani and Anne Gauvin-Bialecki
An Aminopyrimidone and Aminoimidazoles Alkaloids from the Rodrigues Calcareous Marine Sponge *Ernsta naturalis*
Reprinted from: *Mar. Drugs* **2022**, *20*, 637, doi:10.3390/md20100637 1

Lei Wang, Michael Marner, Ute Mettal, Yang Liu and Till F. Schäberle
Seven New Alkaloids Isolated from Marine Flavobacterium *Tenacibaculum discolor* sv11
Reprinted from: *Mar. Drugs* **2022**, *20*, 620, doi:10.3390/md20100620 19

Qi Wang, Chunhua Gao, Zhun Wei, Xiaowen Tang, Lixia Ji, Xiangchao Luo, Xiaoping Peng, Gang Li and Hongxiang Lou
A Series of New Pyrrole Alkaloids with ALR2 Inhibitory Activities from the Sponge *Stylissa massa*
Reprinted from: *Mar. Drugs* **2022**, *20*, 454, doi:10.3390/md20070454 31

Fuhang Song, Jiansen Hu, Xinwan Zhang, Wei Xu, Jinpeng Yang, Shaoyong Li and Xiuli Xu
Unique Cyclized Thiolopyrrolones from the Marine-Derived *Streptomyces* sp. BTBU20218885
Reprinted from: *Mar. Drugs* **2022**, *20*, 214, doi:10.3390/md20030214 41

Shun-Zhi Liu, Guang-Xin Xu, Feng-Ming He, Wei-Bo Zhang, Zhen Wu, Ming-Yu Li, Xi-Xiang Tang and Ying-Kun Qiu
New Sorbicillinoids with Tea Pathogenic Fungus Inhibitory Effect from Marine-Derived Fungus *Hypocrea jecorina* H8
Reprinted from: *Mar. Drugs* **2022**, *20*, 213, doi:10.3390/md20030213 51

Paula González-Andrés, Laura Fernández-Peña, Carlos Díez-Poza and Asunción Barbero
The Tetrahydrofuran Motif in Marine Lipids and Terpenes
Reprinted from: *Mar. Drugs* **2022**, *20*, 642, doi:10.3390/md20100642 63

Laura Fernández-Peña, Carlos Díez-Poza, Paula González-Andrés and Asunción Barbero
The Tetrahydrofuran Motif in Polyketide Marine Drugs
Reprinted from: *Mar. Drugs* **2022**, *20*, 120, doi:10.3390/md20020120 95

Jia-Xuan Yan, Qihao Wu, Eric J. N. Helfrich, Marc G. Chevrette, Doug R. Braun, Heino Heyman, Gene E. Ananiev, Scott R. Rajski, Cameron R. Currie, Jon Clardy and Tim S. Bugni
Bacillimidazoles A–F, Imidazolium-Containing Compounds Isolated from a Marine *Bacillus*
Reprinted from: *Mar. Drugs* **2022**, *20*, 43, doi:10.3390/md20010043 129

Junjie Yan, Weiwei Liu, Jiatong Cai, Yiming Wang, Dahong Li, Huiming Hua and Hao Cao
Advances in Phenazines over the Past Decade: Review of Their Pharmacological Activities, Mechanisms of Action, Biosynthetic Pathways and Synthetic Strategies
Reprinted from: *Mar. Drugs* **2021**, *19*, 610, doi:10.3390/md19110610 141

Kevin Seipp, Leander Geske and Till Opatz
Marine Pyrrole Alkaloids
Reprinted from: *Mar. Drugs* **2021**, *19*, 514, doi:10.3390/md19090514 169

Peihai Li, Mengqi Zhang, Haonan Li, Rongchun Wang, Hairong Hou, Xiaobin Li, Kechun Liu and Hao Chen
New Prenylated Indole Homodimeric and Pteridine Alkaloids from the Marine-Derived Fungus *Aspergillus austroafricanus* Y32-2
Reprinted from: *Mar. Drugs* **2021**, *19*, 98, doi:10.3390/md19020098 . . . . **249**

About the Editor

Asunción Barbero

Asunción Barbero studied Chemistry at the University of Valladolid and received her PhD degree at the same University, working with Prof. Pulido. She then conducted postdoctoral research as a Marie Curie fellow at the University of Cambridge under the supervision of Prof. Ian Fleming, working for two years on the use of silicon chemistry to control stereoselectivity in Organic Synthesis. She went back to Valladolid as Assistant Professor, where she was promoted to Associate Professor in 2001 and to full Professor in 2019. In 2013, she was appointed as Coordinator of the Grade of Chemistry of the University of Valladolid, and since 2018 she has served as the head of the Organic Chemistry department. She has been an Editorial Board member of *Marine Drugs* from 2019 to date. Prior to this Special Issue, she has edited two other Special Issues of *Marine Drugs* in 2020 and 2021.

The results of her research have been presented in several invited and plenary lectures at prestigious international conferences and are summarized in over 60 publications in highly qualified international journals and book chapters.

Her major research interests focus on the development of efficient and selective methodologies for the synthesis of heterocyclic compounds with potential biological properties.

Preface to "Heterocyclic Compounds from Marine Organisms"

Marine natural products have played an important role in the development of new bioactive compounds with a variety of interesting properties (antiviral, cytotoxic, antitumor, anti-inflammatory, antimicrobial, etc.). Within the molecules these marine organisms produce, the presence of heterocyclic subunits is quite frequent. The structural diversity of this group of marine compounds, together with their diverse biological activities, have attracted the attention of the scientific community. This Special Issue on "Heterocyclic Compounds from Marine Organisms" aimed to provide an overview of the most recent developments related to the isolation, characterization, synthesis or biosynthesis of marine compounds containing heterocyclic units or their analogs. The authors who contributed to this Special Issue are gratefully acknowledged. We hope that readers will be interested in this content.

Asunción Barbero
Editor

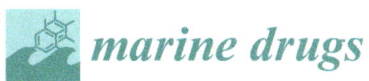

Article

An Aminopyrimidone and Aminoimidazoles Alkaloids from the Rodrigues Calcareous Marine Sponge *Ernsta naturalis*

Pierre-Eric Campos [1,2], Gaëtan Herbette [3], Laetitia Fougère [2], Patricia Clerc [1], Florent Tintillier [1], Nicole J. de Voogd [4,5], Géraldine Le Goff [6], Jamal Ouazzani [6] and Anne Gauvin-Bialecki [1,*]

[1] Laboratoire de Chimie et de Biotechnologie des Produits Naturels, Faculté des Sciences et Technologies, Université de La Réunion, 15 Avenue René Cassin, CS 92003, CEDEX 9, 97744 Saint-Denis, France
[2] Institut de Chimie Organique et Analytique, Université d'Orléans—CNRS—Pôle de Chimie, Rue de Chartres—UMR 6759, BP6759, CEDEX 2, 45067 Orléans, France
[3] CNRS, Aix-Marseille Université, Centrale Marseille, FSCM, Spectropole, Campus de St Jérôme-Service 511, 13397 Marseille, France
[4] Naturalis Biodiversity Center, Darwinweg 2, 2333 CR Leiden, The Netherlands
[5] Institute of Environmental Sciences, Leiden University, Einsteinweg 2, 2333 CC Leiden, The Netherlands
[6] CNRS, Institut de Chimie des Substances Naturelles, UPR 2301, Université Paris-Sud, Université Paris-Saclay, 1, Av. de la Terrasse, 91198 Gif-sur-Yvette, France
* Correspondence: anne.bialecki@univ-reunion.fr; Tel.: +33-262-262-93-81-97

Abstract: A chemical study of the CH_2Cl_2—MeOH (1:1) extract from the sponge *Ernsta naturalis* collected in Rodrigues (Mauritius) based on a molecular networking dereplication strategy highlighted one novel aminopyrimidone alkaloid compound, ernstine A (**1**), seven new aminoimidazole alkaloid compounds, phorbatopsins D–E (**2**, **3**), calcaridine C (**4**), naamines H–I (**5**, **7**), naamidines J–K (**6**, **8**), along with the known thymidine (**9**). Their structures were established by spectroscopic analysis (1D and 2D NMR spectra and HRESIMS data). To improve the investigation of this unstudied calcareous marine sponge, a metabolomic study by molecular networking was conducted. The isolated molecules are distributed in two clusters of interest. Naamine and naamidine derivatives are grouped together with ernstine in the first cluster of twenty-three molecules. Phorbatopsin derivatives and calcaridine C are grouped together in a cluster of twenty-one molecules. Interpretation of the MS/MS spectra of other compounds of these clusters with structural features close to the isolated ones allowed us to propose a structural hypothesis for 16 compounds, 5 known and 11 potentially new.

Keywords: *Ernsta naturalis*; marine sponge; aminoimidazolones alkaloids; aminopyrimidone alkaloid; molecular network

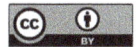

1. Introduction

Calcispongiae (Calcarea Bowerbank, 1864), commonly called calcareous sponges are much less studied chemically compared to another class of Porifera, the Demospongiae, due both to their relatively low number of representatives within the Porifera phylum and to their low biomass [1]. The result is an underexplored source of natural products while these sponges are prolific sources of bioactive alkaloids, especially 2-aminoimidazole alkaloids. The biological activities reported for this kind of alkaloids include antifungal [2], antimicrobial [3], cancer cell toxicity [4], or Mammalian and Protozoan DYRK and CLK kinases inhibitors [5]. Nowadays, more than sixty 2-aminoimidazole alkaloids have been isolated from Calcarea sponges, almost all belonging to the genus *Leucetta*. A few studies described the chemical composition of other calcareous sponges' genera such as *Clathrina* [6], *Leucosolenia* [7], *Leucascandra* [8,9], or *Pericharax* [10,11]. The genus *Ernsta* (Klautau, Azevedo and Cóndor-Luján, 2021) belongs to the order Clathrinida, and comprises 20 species, and despite a ubiquitous distribution, there is no report of chemical investigations of sponges belonging to this genus so far. The genus *Ernstia* was erected by Klautau et al. in 2013 after a thorough molecular evaluation and some species formerly belonging to the genus

Clathrina were placed under this newly erected genus. However, the genus name was already taken by a gastropod and in 2021, the new genus name *Ernsta* was proposed to replace *Ernstia* including *Ernstia naturalis*, thus presently known as *Ernsta naturalis* (Klautau et al., 2021) [12].

In our continuing search for bioactive metabolites from marine invertebrates, *Ernsta naturalis* (Van Soest and De Voogd, 2015, 2018) collected in Rodrigues (Indian Ocean) was investigated [13]. The organic crude extract of this animal exhibited moderate inhibitory activity against proteasome and tyrosinase. Our chemical investigation of this extract led to the isolation of a novel aminopyrimidone alkaloid compound, ernstine A (**1**), seven aminoimidazole alkaloid compounds, phorbatopsins D–E (**2**–**3**), calcaridine C (**4**), naamines H-I (**5**, **7**), naamidines J-K (**6**, **8**), together with the known thymidine (**9**). We report herein the purification and the structure elucidation by spectroscopic analysis including HRESIMS and 2D NMR for the new compounds (**1**–**8**) and comparison with published data for thymidine (**9**) [14]. In order to improve the investigation of this unstudied calcareous marine sponge, a metabolomic study by molecular networking (MN) was conducted. A molecular network is a computational strategy that may help visualization and interpretation of complex data from MS analysis, as crude extracts analysis, by organizing tandem mass spectrometry data through spectral similarities [15]. In MN, MS/MS data are represented in a graphical form, where an ion with an associated fragmentation spectrum is represented by a node and the links between two nodes indicate similarities between the two spectra. Consequently, only compounds with close fragmentation pathways will be linked together and will be grouped in clusters, highlighting families of compounds with the same skeletons. This representation can be particularly useful for the propagation of annotations from isolated compounds to other molecules of the crude extracts with close MS/MS data and so enhance the dereplication of the extract.

2. Results and Discussion

2.1. Characterization of New Compounds

The CH_2Cl_2-MeOH extract was first subjected to reverse-phase silica gel column chromatography to yield nine fractions. The fractions were subjected to SPE, repetitive reverse-phase semi-preparative, and analytical HPLC to yield nine compounds (**1**–**9**) (Figure 1). Eight were new: ernstine A (**1**), phorbatopsins D-E (**2**, **3**), calcaridine C (**4**), naamines H-I (**5**, **7**), naamidines J-K (**6**, **8**) described below and in addition, one other known compound was identified as thymidine (**9**) by comparison with published spectroscopic data.

Ernstine A (**1**) was obtained as a yellow solid. The molecular formula, $C_{19}H_{19}N_3O_3$, was established from HRESIMS molecular ion peak at *m/z* 338.1497 [M+H]$^+$. Analysis of the 1D and 2D ^{1}H, and ^{13}C NMR data for **1** (CD$_3$OD, Table 1) revealed resonances and correlations consistent with those of two para-substituted phenol, but not linked with an aminoimidazolone moiety, such as calcarine A, but linked with an aminopyrimidone moiety (Figure 2). The ^{1}H NMR spectrum of **1** recorded in CD$_3$OD showed the presence of two AA'BB' spin systems at δH 6.94 and 6.74 (each 2H, d, J = 8.8 Hz) and at δH 7.08 and 6.88 (each 2H, d, J = 8.8 Hz), one singlet at δH 3.78 (3H, s), one singlet at δH 3.73 (3H, s), and one singlet at δH 3.56 (2H, s). Analysis and comparison of HSQC and HMBC correlations pointed out one methylene C-7 (δH 3.56; δC 39.6), two oxymethyl carbons C-12, C-17 (δH 3.73, 3.78; δC 55.4, 55.4), eight aromatic methines C-9, C-9', C-10, C-10', C-14, C-14', C-15, C-15', (δH 2 × 6.94, 2 × 6.74, 2 × 7.08, 2 × 6.88; δC 2 × 129.9, 2 × 114.1, 2 × 132.2, 2 × 114.1) of four chemically equivalent spin-pairs indicating a symmetry in the aromatic moieties, four quaternary aromatic carbons C-8, C-11, C-13, C-16 (δC 130.4, 158.4, 126.5, 159.1), two quaternary sp^2 carbons due to the double bond C-5, C-6 (δC 115.9, 154.8), a guanidine-like carbon C-2 (δC 158.4) and one amide carbonyl group C-4 (δC 163.0). The COSY correlations between H-9 and H-10 in addition of the HMBC correlations between H-9 and C-7, C-9' and C-11 and between H-10 and C-8 and C-10' indicated a symmetry and the presence of a para-phenolic group linked to the methylene C-7 in C-8. The HMBC correlations between H-12 and C-11 confirmed the substitution of the aromatic moiety in C-11 by the methoxy group C-12. In the same way, the COSY correlations between H-14 and H-15 in addition to the HMBC correlations between H-14 and C-14′ and C-16, between H-15 and C-13, and C-15′ and between H-17 and C-16 also revealed the presence of symmetry and a second para-phenolic moiety substituted by the methoxy group C-17 in C-16. The connection of the different moieties is confirmed by the NOE correlation cross-peaks (Figure 2). The HMBC correlation between H-14 and C-5 allowed linking the second nonprotonated carbon of this moiety C-13 to the quaternary sp^2 carbon C-5. HMBC correlations between H-7 and C-2, C-4, C-5, and C-6, in addition to the molecular formula, $C_{19}H_{19}N_3O_3$ indicating 12 degrees of insaturations, revealed the presence of the aminopyrimidone moiety. This is the first report of an aminopyridine alkaloid from a calcareous sponge.

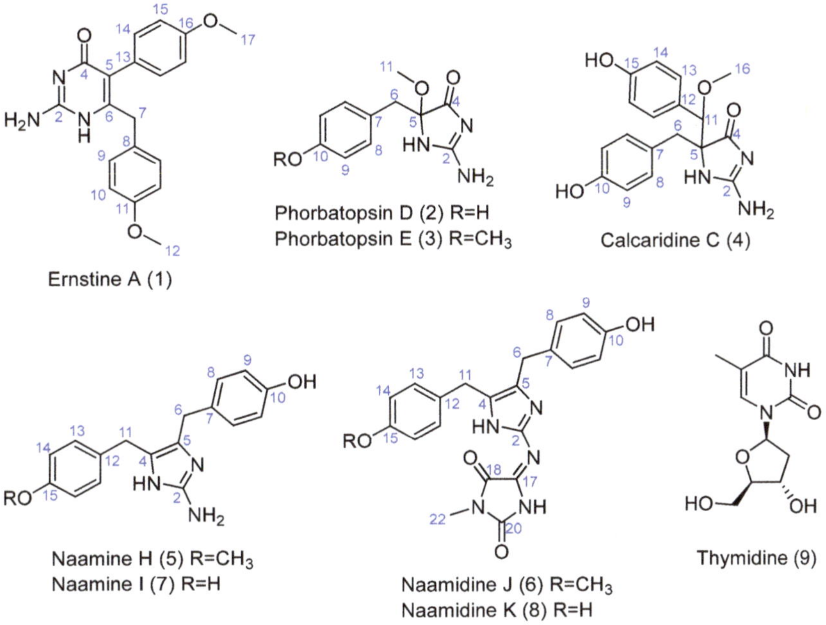

Figure 1. Chemical structures of compounds 1–9.

Table 1. The 1D and 2D NMR spectroscopic data (^{1}H, ^{13}C 600/150 MHz, CD$_3$OD) for ernstine A (**1**).

n°	δC, Type	δH (J in Hz)	COSY (^{1}H-^{1}H)	HMBC (^{1}H-^{13}C)	NOESY (^{1}H-^{1}H)
2	158.4, C	-	-	-	-
4	163.0, C	-	-	-	-
5	115.9, C	-	-	-	-
6	154.8, C	-	-	-	-
7	39.6, CH$_2$	3.56, 2H, s	-	2, 4, 5, 6, 8, 9, 9′	9, 9′, 14, 14′
8	130.4, C	-	-	-	-
9, 9′ *	129.9, CH	6.94, 2H, d (8.8)	10, 10′	7, 9, 9′, 11	7
10, 10′ *	114.1, CH	6.74, 2H, d (8.8)	9, 9′	8, 10, 10′	12
11	158.4, C	-	-	-	-
12	55.4, CH$_3$	3.73, 3H, s	-	11	10, 10′
13	126.5, C	-	-	-	-
14, 14′ *	132.2, CH	7.08, 2H, d (8.8)	15, 15′	5, 14, 14′, 16	7
15, 15′ *	114.2, CH	6.88, 2H, d (8.8)	14, 14′	13, 15, 15′	17
16	159.1, C	-	-	-	-
17	55.4, CH$_3$	3.78, 3H, s	-	16	15, 15′

* Chemically equivalent spin-pairs.

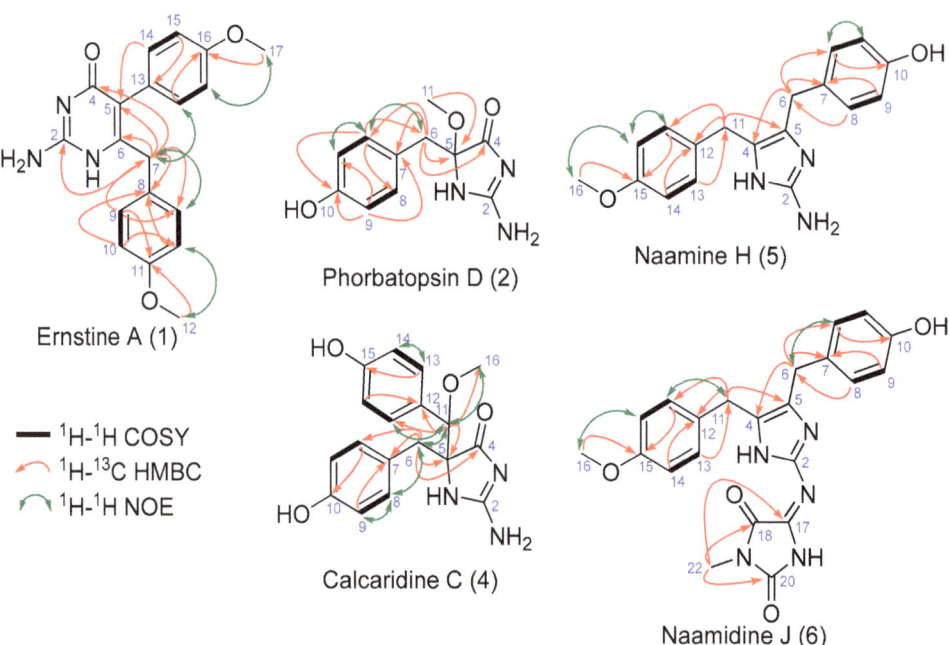

Figure 2. Key COSY, HMBC and NOE correlations for compounds **1**, **2**, **4**, **5** and **6**.

Phorbatopsin D (**2**) was obtained as a yellow solid. The molecular formula, $C_{11}H_{13}N_3O_3$, was established from HRESIMS molecular ion peak at *m/z* 236.1029 [M+H]$^+$. Analysis of the 1D and 2D ^{1}H, and ^{13}C NMR data for **2** (CD$_3$OD, Table 2) revealed resonances and correlations (Figure 2) consistent with those of a para-substituted phenol linked with an aminoimidazolone group, such as phorbatopsin B and C [16]. The ^{1}H NMR spectrum of **2** recorded in CD$_3$OD showed the presence of an AA'XX' spin system at δH 7.01 and 6.64 (each 2H, d, *J* = 8.4 Hz), one singlet at δH 3.17 (3H, s), and one AB spin system at δH 3.00 and 2.95 (each 1H, d, *J* = 13.7 Hz). Analysis of the HSQC and HMBC correlations and the comparison with the latter compounds pointed out one methylene C-6 (δH 3.00 and 2.95; δC 41.9), one oxymethyl C-11 (δH 3.17; δC 51.6), four aromatic methines C-8, C-8′, C-9, C-9′ (δH 2 × 7.01, 2 × 6.64; δC 2 × 132.4, 2 × 115.9) of two chemically equivalent spin-pairs indicating a symmetry in the aromatic moiety, two quaternary aromatic carbons C-7, C-10 (δC 125.7, 157.1), one quaternary carbon of hemiaminal C-5 (δC 95.2) and one amide carbonyl group C-4 (δC 188.3). Compound **2** was different from phorbatopsin C by the presence of the oxymethyl C-11 and the quaternary carbon of hemiaminal C-5 instead of one aminomethine. The COSY correlations between H-8 and H-9 in addition to the HMBC correlations between H-8 and C-6, C-8′ and C-10, and between H-9 and C-7 and C-9′ indicated a symmetry and the presence of a para-phenolic group linked to the methylene C-6 in C-7. The HMBC correlation between H-6 and C-4, C-5, C-7, and C-8 indicated the substitution of the methylene by the para-phenolic core and by the quaternary carbon of hemiaminal C-5. The HMBC correlation between H-11 and C-5 indicated the substitution of the quaternary carbon of hemiaminal C-5 by a methoxy group. The chemical shift of the amide carbonyl group C-4 (δC 188.0) of phorbatopsin D (**2**) was close to that of phorbatopsin C (δC 188.7) but 17.0 ppm higher than that of phorbatopsin B (δC 171.0) described by Nguyen et al. [16]; this difference could be explained by the annular tautomerism (as classified by Katritzky and Lagowski [17]) of the aminoimidazolone moiety. The chemical shift of C-4 in phorbatopsin D and phorbatopsin C corresponded to the C-4 of the tautomer **a** (Figure 3), whereas the chemical shift of C-4 in phorbatopsin B corresponds to the C-4 of the tautomer **b** [18,19]. Indeed, Krawczyk et al. [18], had demonstrated that for creatinines substituted at position 5 with an electron-withdrawing substituent, the amine tautomer **a** is preferred in a polar solvent. Compound **2** was named phorbatopsin D according to phorbatopsin B and C reported in 2012 [16].

Table 2. The 1D and 2D NMR spectroscopic data (^{1}H, ^{13}C 600/150 MHz, CD$_3$OD) for phorbatopsin D (**2**) and E (**3**).

	Phorbatopsin D (2)			Phorbatopsin E (3)		
n°	δC, Type	δH (J in Hz)	HMBC (^{1}H-^{13}C)	δC, Type	δH (J in Hz)	HMBC (^{1}H-^{13}C)
2	-	-	-	-	-	-
4	188.3, C	-	-	186.3, C	-	-
5	95.2, C	-	-	95.0, C	-	-
6	41.9, CH$_2$	2.95, 1H, d (13.7) 3.00, 1H, d (13.7)	4, 5, 7, 8, 8′	41.4, CH$_2$	3.01, 1H, d (13.6) 3.05, 1H, d (13.6)	4, 5, 7, 8, 8′
7	125.7, C	-	-	126.8, C	-	-
8, 8′ *	132.4, CH	7.01, 2H, d (8.4)	6, 8, 8′, 10	132.1, CH	7.11, 2H, d (8.5)	6, 8, 8′, 10
9, 9′ *	115.9, CH	6.64, 2H, d (8.4)	7, 9, 9′	114.3, CH	6.78, 2H, d (8.6)	7, 9, 9′, 10
10	157.1, C	-	-	160.1, C	-	-
11	51.6, CH$_3$	3.17, 3H, s	5	51.1, CH$_3$	3.19, 3H, s	5
12	-	-	-	55.2, CH$_3$	3.73, 3H, s	10

* chemically equivalent spin-pairs.

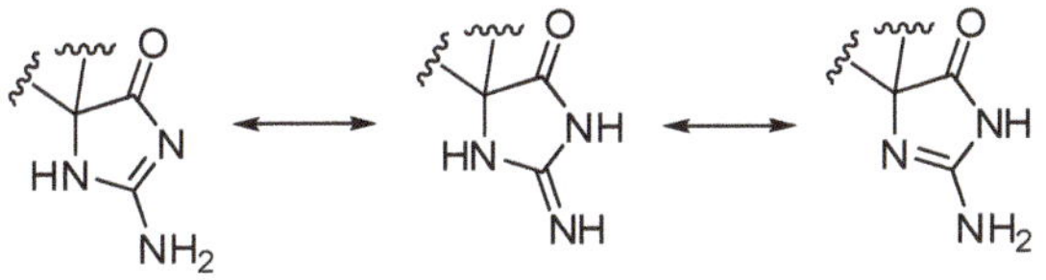

Figure 3. Three tautomeric forms (**a**–**c**) of the 5-substituted aminoimidazolone moiety.

Phorbatopsin E (**3**) was obtained as a yellow solid. The molecular formula, C$_{12}$H$_{15}$N$_3$O$_3$, was established from HRESIMS molecular ion peak at *m/z* 250.1188 [M+H]$^+$. Analysis of the 1D and 2D ^{1}H, and ^{13}C NMR data for **3** (CD$_3$OD, Table 2) revealed resonances and correlations consistent with those of a para-substituted phenol linked with an aminoimidazolone group, such as phorbatopsin D (**2**). Compound **3** was different from **2** by the presence of the oxymethyl C-12 (δH 3.73; δC 55.2) instead of an alcohol group. This is confirmed by the HMBC correlations between H-12 and C-10 and NOE correlations between H-12 and H-9/H-9′.

Calcaridine C (**4**) was obtained as a yellow solid. The molecular formula, C$_{18}$H$_{19}$N$_3$O$_4$, was established from HRESIMS molecular ion peak at *m/z* 342.1449 [M+H]$^+$. Analysis of the 1D and 2D ^{1}H, and ^{13}C NMR data for **4** (CD$_3$OD, Table 3) revealed resonances and correlations consistent with those of two para-substituted phenol linked with an aminoimidazolone moiety, such as calcarine A [3]. Compound **4** was different from calcaridine A by the presence of an alcohol group in C-15 instead of a methoxy group and the substitution of N-1 which was substituted by a proton instead of a methyl. Moreover, the chemical shift of the amide carbonyl group C-4 (δC 189.8) of calcaridine C (**4**) was 15.8 ppm higher than that of calcaridine A (δC 174.0) described by Edrada et al. [3], calcaridine C corresponded to the tautomer **a** (Figure 3) whereas calcaridine A corresponded to tautomer **b**. This difference in isomeric protonation states could be explained by differences in the isolation protocol, herein all the compounds had been isolated in acidic conditions (0.1% formic acid) while Edradra et al. had isolated calcaridine A without acid. Compound **4** was named calcaridine C according to calcaridine A reported in 2003 [3] and calcaridine B reported in 2018 [20].

Table 3. The 1D and 2D NMR spectroscopic data (^{1}H, ^{13}C 600/150 MHz, CD$_3$OD) for calcaridine C (4).

n°	δC, Type	δH (J in Hz)	COSY (^{1}H-^{1}H)	HMBC (^{1}H-^{13}C)
2	-	-	-	-
4	189.8, C	-	-	-
5	75.3, C	-	-	-
6	39.5, CH$_2$	2.35, 1H, d (13.8) 2.94, 1H, d (13.8)	6	4, 5, 7, 8, 8'
7	126.4, C	-	-	-
8, 8' *	132.2, CH	6.86, 2H, d (8.2)	9, 9'	6, 8, 8', 10
9, 9' *	115.9, CH	6.58, 2H, d (8.2)	8, 8'	7, 9, 9', 10
10	157.4, C	-	-	-
11	86.2, CH	4.35, 1H, s	-	5, 12, 13, 13', 16
12	128.3, C	-	-	-
13, 13' *	130.6, CH	7.25, 2H, d (8.3)	14, 14'	11, 13, 13', 15
14, 14' *	116.4, CH	6.86, 2H, d (8.3)	13, 13'	12, 14, 14', 15
15	159.0, C	-	-	-
16	57.1, CH$_3$	3.15, 3H, s	-	11

* Chemically equivalent spin-pairs.

Naamine H (5) was obtained as a yellow solid. The molecular formula, C$_{18}$H$_{19}$N$_3$O$_2$, was established from HRESIMS molecular ion peak at *m/z* 310.1544 [M+H]$^+$. Analysis of the 1D and 2D ^{1}H, and ^{13}C NMR data for 5 (CD$_3$OD, Table 4) showed that it was closely related to naamine A to G [4,21–27], namely resonances and correlations consistent with those of two para-substituted phenol linked with a 2-aminoimidazole group (Figure 2). Compound 5 was different from naamine A by the lack of a methyl group attached to the N-3 of the 2-aminoimidazole ring.

Table 4. The 1D and 2D NMR spectroscopic data (^{1}H, ^{13}C 600/150 MHz, CD$_3$OD) for Naamines H (5) and I (7).

	Naamine H (5)			Naamine I (7)		
n°	δC, Type	δH (J in Hz)	HMBC (^{1}H-^{13}C)	δC, Type	δH (J in Hz)	HMBC (^{1}H-^{13}C)
2	-	-	-	-	-	-
4	123.8, C	-	-	126.4, C	-	-
5	123.8, C	-	-	126.4, C	-	-
6	29.3, CH$_2$	3.73, 2H, s	4, 5, 7, 8, 8'	29.7, CH$_2$	3.80, 2H, s	4, 5, 7, 8, 8'
7	129.9, C	-	-	128.4, C	-	-
8, 8' *	129.8, CH	6.98, 2H, d (8.5)	6, 8, 8', 10	129.3, CH	6.95, 2H, d (8.3)	6, 8, 8', 9, 9', 10
9, 9' *	115.8, CH	6.70, 2H, d (8.5)	7, 9, 9'	115.6, CH	6.71, 2H, d (8.5)	7, 9, 9'
10	156.9, C	-	-	156.1, C	-	-
11	29.3, CH$_2$	3.76, 2H, s	4, 5, 12, 13, 13'	29.7, CH$_2$	3.80, 2H, s	4, 5, 12, 13, 13'
12	131.3, C	-	-	128.4, C	-	-
13, 13' *	129.8, CH	7.08, 2H, d (8.6)	11, 13, 13', 15	129.3, CH	6.95, 2H, d (8.3)	11, 13, 13', 15
14, 14' *	114.4, CH	6.84, 2H, d (8.7)	12, 14, 14'	115.6, CH	6.71, 2H, d (8.5)	12, 14, 14'
15	159.6, C	-	-	156.1, C	-	-
16	54.9, CH$_3$	3.76, 3H, s	-	-	-	-

* chemically equivalent spin-pairs.

Naamidine J (6) was obtained as a yellow solid. The molecular formula, C$_{22}$H$_{21}$N$_5$O$_4$, was established from HRESIMS molecular ion peak at *m/z* 420.1664 [M+H]$^+$. Analysis of the 1D and 2D ^{1}H, and ^{13}C NMR data for 6 (CD$_3$OD, Table 5) showed that it was closely related to naamine H (5) and to naamidines A to I [22,23,28,29]. Namely, as naamine H (5), resonances and correlations were consistent with those of two para-substituted phenol linked with a 2-aminoimidazole ring but herein this 2-aminoimidazole ring was also linked to a hydantoin ring. The substitution of the benzyl rings was the same as naamine H (5), namely, one alcohol function and one methoxy group and the substitution of the hydantoin ring was the same as naamidine A, by one methoxy group on nitrogen.

Table 5. The 1D and 2D NMR spectroscopic data (^{1}H, ^{13}C 600/150 MHz, CD$_3$OD) for naamidines J (**6**) and K (**7**).

	Naamidine J (6)			Naamidine K (8)		
n°	δC, Type	δH (J in Hz)	HMBC (^{1}H-^{13}C)	δC, Type	δH (J in Hz)	HMBC (^{1}H-^{13}C)
2	-	-	-	-	-	-
4	129.0, C	-	-	126.4, C	-	-
5	129.1, C	-	-	126.4, C	-	-
6	30.6, CH$_2$	3.88, 2H, s	4, 5, 7, 8, 8′	29.7, CH$_2$	3.80, 2H, s	4, 5, 7, 8, 8′
7	130.4, C	-	-	128.4, C	-	-
8, 8′ *	130.4 CH	6.97, 2H, d (8.2)	6, 8, 8′ 10	129.3, CH	6.93, 2H, d (8.5)	6, 8, 8′, 10
9, 9′ *	116.4, CH	6.69, 2H, d (8.2)	7, 9, 9′	115.6, CH	6.71, 2H, d (8.5)	7, 9, 9′
10	157.2, C	-	-	156.1, C	-	-
11	30.6, CH$_2$	3.85, 3H, s	5, 13, 13′	29.7, CH$_2$	3.80, 3H, s	4, 5, 13, 13′
12	131.7, C	-	-	128.4, C	-	-
13, 13′ *	130.4, CH	7.06, 2H, d (83)	11, 13, 13′, 15	129.3, CH	6.93, 2H, d (8.5)	11, 13, 13′ 15
14, 14′ *	115.1, CH	6.82, 2H, d (8.3)	14, 14′, 12	115.6, CH	6.71, 2H, d (8.5)	12, 14, 14′, 15
15	160.0, C	-	-	156.1, C	-	-
17	-	-	-	-	-	-
18	166.4, C	-	-	157.6, C	-	-
20	163.9, C	-	-	159.5, C	-	-
22	24.7, CH$_3$	3.04, 3H, s	18, 20	24.4, CH$_3$	3.06, 3H, s	18, 20
23	55.71, CH$_3$	3.75, 3H, s	15			

* Chemically equivalent spin-pairs.

Naamine I (**7**) and Naamidine K (**8**) were obtained as a yellow solid mixture. The molecular formula, C$_{17}$H$_{17}$N$_3$O$_2$, of naamine I was established from HRESIMS molecular ion peak at *m/z* 296.1389 [M+H]$^{+,}$ and the molecular formula, C$_{21}$H$_{19}$N$_5$O$_4$, of naamidine K was established from HRESIMS molecular ion peak at *m/z* 406.1502 [M+H]$^+$. Analysis of the 1D and 2D ^{1}H, and ^{13}C NMR data of the mixture of **7** and **8** (CD$_3$OD, Tables 4 and 5) showed that it was closely related to naamine H (**5**) and to naamidine J (**6**). They were only differing by the substitution of the benzyl rings by two hydroxyls instead of one hydroxyl and one methoxy group.

2.2. Dereplication of the Crude Extract

To obtain the first molecular fingerprint of the unstudied Rodrigues calcareous marine sponge *Ernsta naturalis*, the CH$_2$Cl$_2$-MeOH extract was profiled by HPLC-HRMS/MS. These data were subsequently processed by GNPS [30]. Beforehand, the mass spectra of the eight new molecules isolated and characterized by NMR were submitted to the library of the GNPS (Accession codes of the isolated compounds). These molecules could thus be reported directly in the molecular network of the extract. The molecular network (Figure 4) contains 167 nodes including 111 clustered molecules. The isolated molecules are distributed in two clusters of interest. Naamine and naamidine derivatives grouped together with ernstine A (**1**) in the first cluster 1 of twenty-three molecules (Figure 5). Phorbatopsin derivatives (**2**, **3**) and calcaridine C (**4**) grouped together in cluster 2 of twenty-one molecules (Figure 6).

Using the same approach, the cluster of phorbatopsin derivatives could be partially characterized. This cluster is divided into two parts. The first one contains two nodes identified as calcaridine C (**4**) with similar spectra but different retention times. Calcaridine C is characterized by the ions 107.0490 *m/z* [C$_7$H$_7$O]$^+$ and 137.0597 *m/z* [C$_8$H$_9$O$_2$]$^+$, characterized by the phenolic group. However, the fragmentation is distinguished by a loss of neutrality in C$_8$H$_{10}$O$_2$. This part of the cluster possesses many nodes with the same masses and similar spectra probably due to the presence of isomers. It complicates the interpretation of compound spectra, so no additional annotation was added in this part of the cluster. Finally, phorbatopsin D and E (**2**, **3**) were projected in the second part of the cluster where six other molecules could be proposed (Table 7). For these molecules, the losses of neutrals CO, CH_4O, and $C_2H_2N_2O$ due to fragmentation in the 2-aminoimidazolin-4-one cycle and the characteristic ions 107.0492 *m/z* $[C_7H_7O]^+$ and 121.0646 *m/z* $[C_8H_9O]^+$ which correspond to the phenolic group without and with a methoxy are found. Two known molecules with the same 2-aminoimidazolin-4-one moiety were proposed to be phorbatopsins A and C, along with three new compounds. Only one molecule with a different moiety has been proposed, leucettamine C, with a loss of $C_3H_6N_2O$ corresponding to a 2-imino-3-methyl-imidazolidin-4-one moiety.

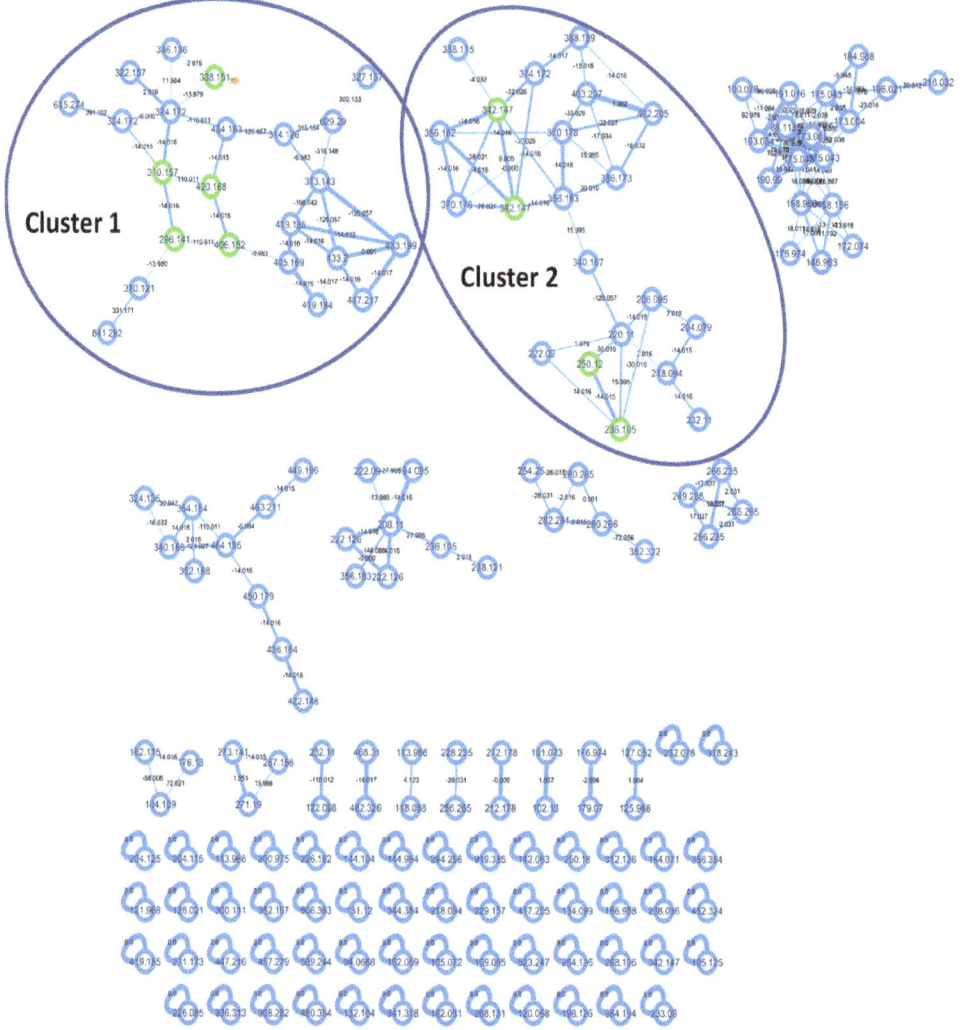

Figure 4. Molecular network of *Ernsta naturalis* crude extract. Isolated molecules are in green in the molecular network.

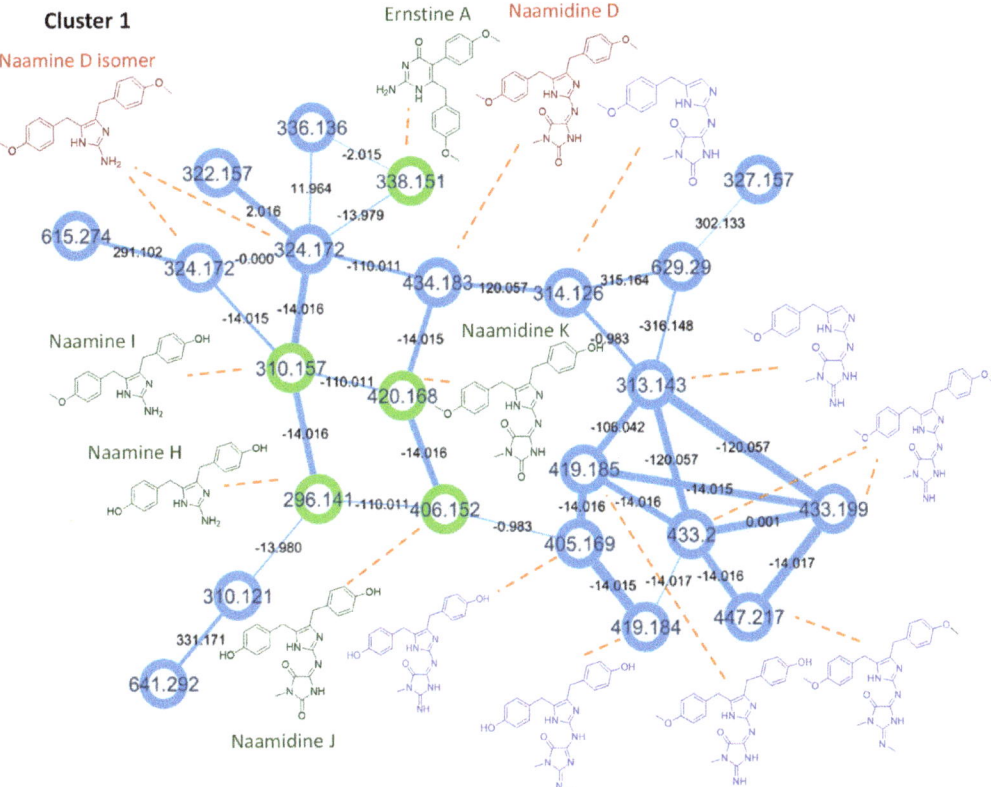

Figure 5. Cluster 1 of the molecular network of *Ernsta naturalis* crude extract. Isolated molecules are in green in the molecular network, the proposals of known molecules in red, and the proposals of new molecules in blue.

The naamidine derivatives cluster was characterized by the presence of neutral loss (C_7H_8O and C_6H_6O) which correspond to the methoxylated or hydroxylated phenolic group. In addition to the loss of neutral, characteristic ions were observed, as 160.0758 m/z [$C_{10}H_{10}NO$]$^+$ which determines the presence of the phenolic group with the 2-aminoimidazole moiety. Moreover, the presence of the loss of neutral ($C_3H_3NO_2$ or $C_3H_4N_2O$ or $C_4H_6N_2O$) corresponding to the fragmentation in the 3-methyl-imidazolidin-4-one ring helps to indicate whether the group corresponds to either 3-methylimidazolidine-2,4-dione (as naamidine), or 2-imino-3-methyl-imidazolidin-4-one or 2-methylimino-3-methyl-imidazolidin-2-one. With these elements, it is possible to propagate the annotations of cluster 1 by characterizing other nodes. Thus, structural hypotheses of nine additional molecules have been proposed (Table 6), in addition to the spectral confirmation of the five compounds already isolated and characterized by NMR. With this methodology, two nodes seem to correspond to naamine D isomers [23] and one node to naamidine D [22], two molecules isolated from the calcareous sponge Leucetta, eight other nodes seem to correspond to new molecules and for the last seven ones, the hypothesis was too uncertain to propose a structural hypothesis.

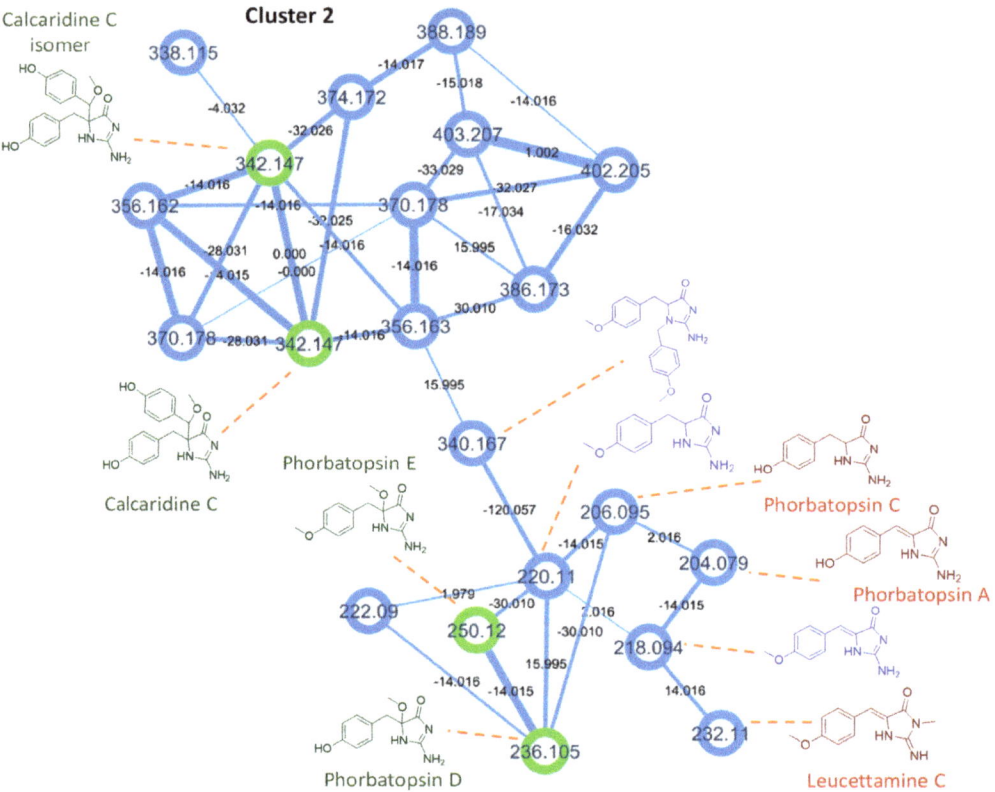

Figure 6. Cluster 2 of the molecular network of *Ernstia naturalis* crude extract. Isolated molecules are in green in the molecular network, the proposals of known molecules in red, and the proposals of new molecules in blue.

2.3. Biosynthetic Pathway

Even if a clear definition of biosynthetic origin of the 2-aminoimidazole alkaloids from the calcareous sponges has not been established at the present time, different hypotheses of biological pathway have been proposed but no experimental confirmation has been reported [31]. Crews had proposed a biosynthesis pathway including an intermediate with one phenyl ring coming from guanidine and *p*-hydroxyphenylpyruvic acid [31,32]. The presence in the crude extract of *Ernsta naturalis* of a compound with an ion peak in HRESIMS at *m/z* 220.1078 [M+H]$^+$ corresponding to the molecular formula of the intermediate *p*-methoxyphorbatopsin C, in addition to the presence of both aminoimidazole alkaloids with one phenyl ring and aminoimidazole alkaloids with two phenyl rings are in agreement with this proposal.

Table 6. Tentative identification of cluster A compounds from extract of the Rodrigues calcareous marine sponge *Ernsta naturalis* by LC-ESI-MS/MS in the positive ion mode. The presence of characteristic ion on the MS^2 spectra was indicated by a X in the table.

RT (min)	Neutral Loss MS^2					Ion Characteristic MS^2 C$_{10}$H$_{10}$N	m/z [M+H]+	Raw Formula	Error (ppm)	Molecule Tentative Identification (INCHI Key)	Confidence Level
	C$_6$H$_6$O	C$_7$H$_8$O	C$_3$H$_3$NO$_2$	C$_3$H$_4$N$_2$O	C$_4$H$_6$N$_2$O						
6.16	202.0975					X	296.1393	C$_{17}$H$_{18}$N$_3$O$_2$	0.3	Naamine H (KFOAYDULNDFMPQ-UHFFFAOYSA-N)	1
6.18	227.0925		321.1342			X	405.1664	C$_{21}$H$_{21}$N$_6$O$_3$	1.4	(BLKZRPHRHGCARC-UHFFFAOYSA-N)	3
6.2		205.0834	229.1081				313.1404	C$_{15}$H$_{17}$N$_6$O$_2$	1.2	(IIKZHJXIVNJXCB-UHFFFAOYSA-N)	3
6.52	227.0922			321.1337		X	419.1825	C$_{22}$H$_{23}$N$_6$O$_3$	0.3	(KSJXZPZLMWQEOL-UHFFFAOYSA-N)	3
6.92	216.1132	202.0974				X	310.1549	C$_{18}$H$_{20}$N$_3$O$_2$	0.3	Naamine I (QFSIYRFDLATYCH-UHFFFAOYSA-N)	1
6.94	241.1085	311.1247	335.1501			X	419.1825	C$_{22}$H$_{23}$N$_6$O$_3$	0.3	(AUUWFNXXXPZWIM-UHFFFAOYSA-N)	3
7.02		216.1128				X	324.1703	C$_{19}$H$_{22}$N$_3$O$_2$	1	Naamine D isomer (JIAXZLQLTAUEFZ-UHFFFAOYSA-N)	2
7.11	312.1089					X	406.1503	C$_{21}$H$_{20}$N$_5$O$_4$	1.6	Naamidine J (ZITLIVILDBHVPT-UHFFFAOYSA-N)	1
7.14		241.1084	349.1655				433.1981	C$_{23}$H$_{25}$N$_6$O$_3$	0.3	(CKFJLVUSNNSFGX-UHFFFAOYSA-N)	3
7.3		230.0921				X	338.1492	C$_{19}$H$_{20}$N$_3$O$_3$	2.2	Ernstine A (DDPTZQPAIVSDEH-UHFFFAOYSA-N)	1
7.39		206.0671	121.0508				314.1241	C$_{15}$H$_{16}$N$_5$O$_3$	2.1	(FJLZROPMRMSUSB-UHFFFAOYSA-N)	3
7.58		241.1078		349.1653			433.1972	C$_{23}$H$_{25}$N$_6$O$_3$	2.5	(CKFJLVUSNNSFGX-UHFFFAOYSA-N)	3
7.6							324.1703	C$_{19}$H$_{22}$N$_3$O$_2$	0.3	Naamine D isomer (JIAXZLQLTAUEFZ-UHFFFAOYSA-N)	4
7.87	339.1564				349.1655		447.2138	C$_{24}$H$_{27}$N$_6$O$_3$	0.2	(MZCUSFHZTJTHTHB-UHFFFAOYSA-N)	3
8.06	326.1246	312.1088	227.0926			X	420.1659	C$_{22}$H$_{22}$N$_5$O$_4$	1.7	Naamidine K (BIKAACVDYDVHU-UHFFFAOYSA-N)	1
9.1		326.1241	241.1080				434.1819	C$_{23}$H$_{24}$N$_5$O$_4$	0.8	Naamidine D (CXGRXOLKKUWCFJ-UHFFFAOYSA-N)	2

Table 7. Tentative identification of cluster B compounds from extract of the Rodrigues calcareous marine sponge *Ernsta naturalis* by LC-ESI-MS/MS in the positive ion mode. The presence of characteristic ion on the MS² spectra was indicated by a X in the table.

RT (min)	Neutral Loss MS²					Ion Characteristic MS²		m/z Measured [M+H]⁺	Raw Formula	Error (ppm)	Molecule Tentative Identification (INCHI Key)	Confidence Level
	CH_4O	CH_3NO	$C_2H_2N_2O$	$C_3H_6N_2O$	$C_4H_9O_2$	C_8H_9O	C_7H_7O					
1.25			136.0755				X	206.0929	$C_{10}H_{12}N_3O_2$	−2.5	Phorbatopsin C (MFHHWOMFRHLQSF-UHFFFAOYSA-N)	2
1.86	204.0767		166.0862			X	X	236.1031	$C_{11}H_{14}N_3O_3$	−0.6	Phorbatopsin D (IQLRXEDGGLMGEF-UHFFFAOYSA-N)	1
2.14		159.0553	132.0444				X	204.0766	$C_{10}H_{10}N_3O_2$	0.9	Phorbatopsin A (PZMLZQJKCWTTIV-YVMONPNESA-N)	2
4.05			150.0914			X		220.1078	$C_{11}H_{14}N_3O_2$	1	Methoxy phorbatopsin C (JQRQEDSHZOMVAE-UHFFFAOYSA-N)	2
5.6			180.1014			X		250.1181	$C_{12}H_{16}N_3O_3$	2.2	Phorbatopsin E (CECJNLRWMYCRSS-UHFFFAOYSA-N)	1
5.88		173.0708	146.0598			X		218.0920	$C_{11}H_{12}N_3O_2$	1.9	Methoxy phorbatopsin A (MDHOCGCTCYWXMY-TWGQIWQCSA-N)	2
6.07	218.0920				X		X	342.1463	$C_{18}H_{20}N_3O_4$	−1.5	Calcaridine C (SGBQZSSTVLPIET-UHFFFAOYSA-N)	1
6.26					X		X	342.1450	$C_{18}H_{20}N_3O_4$	−0.2	Calcaridine C isomer (SGBQZSSTVLPIET-UHFFFAOYSA-N)	2
7.13			270.1488			X		340.1656	$C_{19}H_{22}N_3O_3$	−0.1	(AUMUDBPKOINNCL-UHFFFAOYSA-N)	3
6.31				146.0601		X		232.1080	$C_{12}H_{14}N_3O_2$	0.2	Leucettamine C (GWKCHEJMMQELNU-YFHOESVSA-N)	2

3. Materials and Methods

3.1. General Experiment Procedures

Optical rotations were measured on a MCP 200 Anton Paar modular circular polarimeter at 25 °C (MeOH, c in g/100 mL). ^{1}H and ^{13}C NMR data were acquired with a Bruker Avance II+—600 MHz spectrometer equipped with a TCI Cryoprobe at 300 K with 2 mm o.d. Match NMR tubes. Chemical shifts were referenced using the corresponding solvent signals (δ_H 3.31 and δ_C 49.00 for CD$_3$OD). The spectra were processed using 1D and 2D NMR MNova software (Version No. 14.1.1-24571, Mestrelab Research S. L., Santiago de Compostela, Spain). HRESIMS spectra were recorded using a Waters SYNAPT G2 HDMS mass spectrometer (Waters, Guyancourt, France).

The sponge was lyophilized with Cosmos −80 °C CRYOTEC. MPLC separations were carried out on a Buchi Sepacore flash system C-605/C-615/C-660 and glass column (230 × 15 mm i.d.) packed with Acros Organics C18-RP, 23%C, silica gel (40−63 μm). Precoated TLC sheets of silica gel 60, Alugram SIL G/UV254 were used, and spots were visualized on the basis of the UV absorbance at 254 nm and by heating silica gel plates sprayed with formaldehyde−sulfuric acid or Dragendorff reagents. HPLC analyses were carried out using a Phenomenex Gemini C$_{18}$ (150 × 4.6 mm i.d., 3 μm) column and were performed on a Thermo Scientific Dionex Ultimate 3000 system equipped with a photodiode array detector and a Corona detector with Chromeleon software. Semi-preparative HPLC was carried out using a Phenomenex Geminin C$_{18}$ (250 × 10 mm i.d., 5 μm) column and was performed on a Thermo Scientific Dionex Ultimate 3000 system equipped with a photodiode array detector. All solvents were analytical or HPLC grade and were used without further purification.

3.2. Animal Material

The sponge *Ernsta naturalis* (phylum Porifera, class Calcarea, order Clathrinida, family Clathrinidae) was collected in October 2016 in Passe Balidirou, Rodrigues (19°40.098' S, 63°27.784' E at 12–15 m depth). One voucher specimen (RMNH Por. 11633) was deposited in the sponge collection of Naturalis Biodiversity Center, the Netherlands. Sponge samples were frozen immediately and kept at −20 °C until processed.

3.3. Extraction and Isolation

The frozen sponge (53.5 g, dry weight) was chopped into small pieces, lyophilized and extracted exhaustively by maceration with CH$_2$Cl$_2$-MeOH (1:1 *v:v*) (2 × 1.5 L, each 24 h) at room temperature. After evaporating the solvents under reduced pressure, a brown, oily residue (3.07 g) was obtained. The extract was then subjected to MPLC over C18-RP silica gel in a glass column (230 × 15 mm i.d.), eluting with a combination of water and MeOH of decreasing polarity (15 mL min^{-1}). Nine fractions were obtained: F0 eluted with H$_2$O-MeOH (95:5) over 5 min; F1 eluted with H$_2$O−MeOH (95:5) over 5 min; F2 eluted with H$_2$O-MeOH (75:25) over 5 min, F3 eluted with H$_2$O−MeOH (50:50) over 5 min, F4 eluted with H$_2$O-MeOH (25:75) over 5 min; F5 to F8 eluted with H$_2$O-MeOH (95:5) over 20 min.

Fraction F0 (1.21 g) was fractionated by C-18 SPE, eluted with a combination of water and MeOH of decreasing polarity and three subfractions were obtained (SF0–SF2).

Subfraction SF1 (57 mg) was subjected to semipreparative HPLC (Phenomenex Geminin C18 column, 250 × 10 mm i.d., 5 μm., 4.5 mL min^{-1} gradient elution with 5% ACN-H$_2$O (+0.1% formic acid) over 5 min, then 5% to 15% ACN-H$_2$O (+0.1% formic acid) over 30 min and 15% ACN-H$_2$O (+0.1% formic acid) over 10 min; UV 220, 280 nm) to provide pure compounds 2 (phorbatopsin D, 1.6 mg), 3 (phorbatopsin E, 2.7 mg), 4 (calcaridine C, 2.1 mg) and 9 (thymidine, 4.2 mg).

Fraction F2 (64 mg) was subjected to semipreparative HPLC (Phenomenex Geminin C18 column, 250 × 10 mm i.d., 5 μm., 4.5 mL min^{-1} gradient elution with 12% ACN-H$_2$O (+0.1% formic acid) over 5 min, then 12% to 35% ACN-H2O (+0.1% formic acid) over

35 min and 35% ACN-H$_2$O (+0.1% formic acid) over 5 min; UV 220, 280 nm) to obtain 11 subfractions (F2SF1-F2SF11). Pure compounds 5 (naamine H, 0.9 mg), 7 (naamidine J, 1.6 mg), and 1 (ernstine A, 1.1 mg) were obtained in the subfractions, F2SF7, F2SF11 and F2SF9, respectively.

Subfraction F2SF10 (3.1 mg) was subjected to semipreparative HPLC (Phenomenex Geminin C18 column, 250 × 10 mm i.d., 5 µm., 4.5 mL min^{-1} isocratic elution with 26% ACN-H$_2$O (+0.1% formic acid) over 20 min; UV 220, 280 nm) to provide one mixture of compound 6 and compound 8 (naamine I and naamidine K, 1.4 mg) and a pure compound 1 (ernstine A, 1.0 mg).

Ernstine A (**1**). Yellow oil, $[\alpha]_D^{25}$ 0.0 (*c 0.1*, MeOH); ^{1}H and ^{13}C NMR, see Table 1; HRESIMS *m/z* 338.1497 [M + H]$^+$ (calcd for C$_{19}$H$_{20}$N$_3$O$_3^+$, 338.1499).

Phorbatopsin D (**2**). Yellow oil, ^{1}H and ^{13}C NMR, see Table 2; HRESIMS *m/z* 236.1029 [M + H]$^+$ (calcd for C$_{11}$H$_{14}$N$_3$O$_3^+$, 236.1030).

Phorbatopsin E (**3**). Yellow oil, $[\alpha]_D^{25}$ 0.0 (*c 0.1*, MeOH); ^{1}H and ^{13}C NMR, see Table 2; HRESIMS *m/z* 250.1188 [M + H]$^+$ (calcd for C$_{12}$H$_{16}$N$_3$O$_3^+$, 250.1186).

Calcaridine C (**4**). Yellow oil, $[\alpha]_D^{25}$ 0.0 (*c 0.1*, MeOH); ^{1}H and ^{13}C NMR, see Table 3; HRESIMS *m/z* 342.1449 [M + H]$^+$ (calcd for C$_{18}$H$_{20}$N$_3$O$_4^+$, 342.1448).

Naamine H (**5**). Yellow oil, ^{1}H and ^{13}C NMR, see Table 4; HRESIMS *m/z* 310.1544 [M + H]$^+$ (calcd for C$_{18}$H$_{20}$N$_3$O$_2^+$, 310.1550).

Naamidine J (**6**). Yellow oil, $[\alpha]_D^{25}$ 0.0 (*c 0.1*, MeOH); ^{1}H and ^{13}C NMR, see Table 5; HRESIMS *m/z* 420.1664 [M + H]$^+$ (calcd for C$_{22}$H$_{22}$N$_5$O$_4^+$, 420.1666).

Naamine I (**7**). Yellow oil, ^{1}H and ^{13}C NMR, see Table 4; HRESIMS *m/z* 296.1389 [M + H]$^+$ (calcd for C$_{17}$H$_{18}$N$_3$O$_2^+$, 296.1394).

Naamidine K (**8**). Yellow oil, $[\alpha]_D^{25}$ 0.0 (*c 0.1*, MeOH); ^{1}H and ^{13}C NMR, see Table 5; HRESIMS *m/z* 406.1502 [M + H]$^+$ (calcd for C$_{21}$H$_{20}$N$_5$O$_4^+$, 406.1510).

3.4. UHPLC/HRMS/MS

Crude extract was analyzed on an Ultimate 3000 UHPLC system (Dionex, Germering, Germany) hyphenated with Impact II high resolution quadrupole time-of-flight (QqTOF) equipped with an electrospray ionization (ESI) source (Bruker Daltonics, Bremen, Germany). Separation of extract was achieved on a Luna C18 column (150 mm × 2.1 mm, 1.6 µm) with an injection volume of 2 µL. A binary solvent system was used as mobile phase, solvent A consisting of water with 0.1% (*v/v*) formic acid and solvent B consisting of acetonitrile with 0.1% (*v/v*) formic acid. The flow rate was 0.6 mL min^{-1}, and a gradient was applied: from 10% to 100% of B in 15min. The acquisition was carried out in ESI positive ionization mode with a range of 50–1200 Da. The capillary voltage was maintained at 3 kV, the gas flow to the nebulizer was set at 3.5 bars, the drying temperature was 200 °C, and the drying gas flow was 4 L min^{-1}. The collision-induced dissociated (CID) energy was applied from 20 to 40 eV.

Data were analyzed using Bruker Data Analysis 4.4 software. The data were processed using MetaboScape 4.0 (Bruker Daltonics, Bremen, Germany). A mgf file was submitted to the GNPS (Global Natural Product Social Networking) web-based platform for generating MS based molecular network [33]. The following parameters were applied to create the molecular network. The mass tolerance was 0.01 Da for precursor and fragment ions. Minimum score was 0.6 between two MS/MS spectra to be connected. The minimum number of common fragment ions between two MS/MS spectra was 3. The nearly identical MS/MS spectra were not merged into consensus MS/MS spectrum. A node was allowed to connect to a maximum of 10 nodes. A cluster can have a maximum of 100 nodes. The spectra in the network were then compared with GNPS spectral libraries [31]. Each MS^2 spectrum of the seven isolated compounds was assigned an individual accession number on the GNPS (Supplementary Materials). The molecular networking was visualized using Cytoscape (ver. 3.6.0). The obtained molecular network can be accessed at: https://gnps.ucsd.edu/ProteoSAFe/status.jsp?task=527472b15d4247dfad0534aa80f7ebfa, accessed on 8 October 2022.

4. Conclusions

In conclusion, one novel aminopyrimidone alkaloid compound, ernstine A (**1**), seven new aminoimidazole alkaloid compounds, phorbatopsins D-E (**2**, **3**), calcaridine C (**4**), naamines H–I (**5**, **7**), naamidines J–K (**6**, **8**) were isolated from a CH_2Cl_2-MeOH extract from *Ernsta naturalis* along with the known thymidine (**9**). To improve the investigation of this unstudied calcareous marine sponge, a metabolomic study by molecular networking was conducted. This strategy, based on the interpretation of MS/MS spectra of other compounds grouped in the same clusters than the isolated ones due to their structural feature similarities, allowed us to propose structural hypotheses for 16 compounds, 5 known and 11 potentially new.

Supplementary Materials: The following supporting information can be downloaded at: https://www.mdpi.com/article/10.3390/md20100637/s1, Figure S1: HRESIMS spectrum for ernstine A (1), Figure S2: ^{1}H NMR (600 MHz, CD$_3$OD) spectrum for ernstine A (1), Figure S3: ^{1}H-^{1}H COSY NMR (600 MHz) spectrum for ernstine A (1), Figure S4: ^{1}H-^{13}C HSQC NMR (600 MHz) spectrum for ernstine A (1), Figure S5: ^{1}H-^{13}C HMBC NMR (600 MHz) spectrum for ernstine A (1), Figure S6: ^{1}H-^{1}H NOESY NMR (600 MHz) spectrum for ernstine A (1), Figure S7: HRESIMS spectrum for phorbatopsin D (2), Figure S8: ^{1}H NMR (600 MHz, CD$_3$OD) spectrum for phorbatopsin D (2), Figure S9: ^{13}C NMR (125 MHz, CD$_3$OD) spectrum for phorbatopsin D (2), Figure S10: ^{1}H-^{13}C HSQC NMR (600 MHz) spectrum for phorbatopsin D (2), Figure S11: ^{1}H-^{13}C HMBC NMR (600 MHz) spectrum for phorbatopsin D (2), Figure S12: HRESIMS spectrum for phorbatopsin E (3), Figure S13: ^{1}H NMR (600 MHz, CD$_3$OD) spectrum for phorbatopsin E (3), Figure S14: ^{1}H-^{13}C HSQC NMR (600 MHz) spectrum for phorbatopsin E (3), Figure S15: ^{1}H-^{13}C HMBC NMR (600 MHz) spectrum for phorbatopsin E (3), Figure S16: ^{1}H-^{1}H NOESY NMR (600 MHz) spectrum for phorbatopsin E (3), Figure S17: HRESIMS spectrum for calcaridine C (4), Figure S18: ^{1}H NMR (600 MHz, CD$_3$OD) spectrum for calcaridine C (4), Figure S19: ^{13}C NMR (125 MHz, CD$_3$OD) spectrum for calcaridine C (4), Figure S20: ^{1}H-^{1}H COSY NMR (600 MHz) spectrum for calcaridine C (4), Figure S21: ^{1}H-^{13}C HSQC NMR (600 MHz) spectrum for calcaridine C (4), Figure S22: ^{1}H-^{13}C HMBC NMR (600 MHz) spectrum for calcaridine C (4), Figure S23: ^{1}H-^{1}H NOESY NMR (600 MHz) spectrum for calcaridine C (4), Figure S24: HRESIMS spectrum for naamine H (5), Figure S25: ^{1}H NMR (600 MHz, CD$_3$OD) spectrum for naamine H (5), Figure S26: ^{1}H-^{13}C HSQC NMR (600 MHz) spectrum for naamine H (5), Figure S27: ^{1}H-^{13}C HMBC NMR (600 MHz) spectrum for naamine H (5), Figure S28: ^{1}H-^{1}H NOESY NMR (600 MHz) spectrum for naamine H (5), Figure S29: HRESIMS spectrum for naamidine J (6), Figure S30: ^{1}H NMR (600 MHz, CD$_3$OD) spectrum for naamidine J (6), Figure S31: ^{13}C NMR (125 MHz, CD$_3$OD) spectrum for naamidine J (6), Figure S32: ^{1}H-^{1}H COSY NMR (600 MHz) spectrum for naamidine J (6), Figure S33: ^{1}H-^{13}C HSQC NMR (600 MHz) spectrum for naamidine J (6), Figure S34: ^{1}H-^{13}C HMBC NMR (600 MHz) spectrum for naamidine J (6), Figure S35: ^{1}H-^{1}H NOESY NMR (600 MHz) spectrum for naamidine J (6), Figure S36: HRESIMS spectrum for naamine I (7), Figure S37: HRESIMS spectrum for naamidine K (8), Figure S38: ^{1}H NMR (600 MHz, CD$_3$OD) spectrum for mixture of naamine I (7) and naamidine K (8), Figure S39: ^{1}H-^{13}C HSQC NMR (600 MHz) spectrum for mixture of naamine I (7) and naamidine K (8), Figure S40: ^{1}H-^{13}C HMBC NMR (600 MHz) spectrum for mixture of naamine I (7) and naamidine K (8), Figure S41: ^{1}H NMR (600 MHz, CD$_3$OD) spectrum for thymidine (9), Figure S42: ^{13}C NMR (125 MHz, CD$_3$OD) spectrum for thymidine (9), Figure S43: ^{1}H-^{1}H COSY NMR (600 MHz) spectrum for thymidine (9), Figure S44: ^{1}H-^{13}C HSQC NMR (600 MHz) spectrum for thymidine (9), Figure S45: ^{1}H-^{13}C HMBC NMR (600 MHz) spectrum for thymidine (9), Figure S46: MS/MS spectra of the isolated compounds were deposited in the GNPS spectral libraries under following identifier, Figure S47: MS/MS spectrum of ernstine A (1), Figure S48: MS/MS spectrum of Phorbatopsin D (2), Figure S49: MS/MS spectrum of Phorbatopsin E(3), Figure S50: MS/MS spectrum of Naamine H (5), Figure S51: MS/MS spectrum of Naamine I (7), Figure S52: MS/MS spectrum of Naamidine J (6), Figure S53: MS/MS spectrum of Naamidine K (8), Figure S54: MS/MS spectrum of Calcaridine C (4).

Author Contributions: A.G.-B., G.L.G. and J.O. designed the project, supervised the whole experiment, and prepared the manuscript. G.H., L.F., F.T., P.C. and P.-E.C. performed the chemical experiments (extraction, isolation, and structural identification of the compounds). P.-E.C. and L.F. wrote the first draft of the manuscript. A.G.-B. organized the sponge collection, and the sponge was identified by N.J.d.V. All authors have read and agreed to the published version of the manuscript.

Funding: This research was funded by the TASCMAR project, which is funded by the European Union under grant agreement number 634674.

Institutional Review Board Statement: Not applicable.

Informed Consent Statement: Not applicable.

Data Availability Statement: The MS/MS and NMR data presented in this study are openly available in Zenodo at https://doi.org/10.5281/zenodo.7152302. The obtained molecular network can be accessed at: https://gnps.ucsd.edu/ProteoSAFe/status.jsp?task=527472b15d4247dfad0534aa80f7ebfa.

Acknowledgments: The authors express their gratitude to the SALSA platform at ICOA for the access to Bruker Data Analysis 4.4 and MetaboScape 4.0 software and for the technical help for the retreatment of UPLC/HRMS/MS analysis.

Conflicts of Interest: The authors declare no conflict of interest.

References

1. Roué, M.; Quévrain, E.; Domart-Coulon, I.; Bourguet-Kondracki, M.-L. Assessing Calcareous Sponges and Their Associated Bacteria for the Discovery of New Bioactive Natural Products. *Nat. Prod. Rep.* **2012**, *29*, 739. [CrossRef]
2. Fu, X.; Schmitz, F.J.; Tanner, R.S.; Kelly-Borges, M. New Imidazole Alkaloids and Zinc Complexes from the Micronesian Sponge *Leucetta* cf. *Chagosensis*. *J. Nat. Prod.* **1998**, *61*, 384–386. [CrossRef] [PubMed]
3. Edrada, R.A.; Stessman, C.C.; Crews, P. Uniquely Modified Imidazole Alkaloids from a Calcareous *Leucetta* Sponge. *J. Nat. Prod.* **2003**, *66*, 939–942. [CrossRef]
4. Gross, H.; Kehraus, S.; König, G.M.; Woerheide, G.; Wright, A.D. New and Biologically Active Imidazole Alkaloids from Two Sponges of the Genus *Leucetta*. *J. Nat. Prod.* **2002**, *65*, 1190–1193. [CrossRef]
5. Loaëc, N.; Attanasio, E.; Villiers, B.; Durieu, E.; Tahtouh, T.; Cam, M.; Davis, R.A.; Alencar, A.; Roué, M.; Bourguet-Kondracki, M.-L.; et al. Marine-Derived 2-Aminoimidazolone Alkaloids. Leucettamine B-Related Polyandrocarpamines Inhibit Mammalian and Protozoan DYRK & CLK Kinases. *Mar. Drugs* **2017**, *15*, 316.
6. Ciminiello, P.; Fattorusso, E.; Magno, S.; Mangoni, A. Clathridine and Its Zinc Complex, Novel Metabolites from the Marine Sponge *Clathrina Clathrus*. *Tetrahedron* **1989**, *45*, 3873–3878. [CrossRef]
7. Ralifo, P.; Tenney, K.; Valeriote, F.A.; Crews, P. A Distinctive Structural Twist in the Aminoimidazole Alkaloids from a Calcareous Marine Sponge: Isolation and Characterization of Leucosolenamines A and B. *J. Nat. Prod.* **2007**, *70*, 33–38. [CrossRef]
8. D'Ambrosio, M.; Guerriero, A.; Pietra, F.; Debitus, C. Leucascandrolide A, a New Type of Macrolide: The First Powerfully Bioactive Metabolite of Calcareous Sponges (*Leucascandra caveolata*, a New Genus from the Coral Sea). *Helv. Chim. Acta* **1996**, *79*, 51–60. [CrossRef]
9. D'Ambrosio, M.; Tatò, M.; Pocsfalvi, G.; Debitus, C.; Pietra, F. Leucascandrolide B, a New 16-Membered, Extensively Methyl-Branched Polyoxygenated Macrolide from the Calcareous Sponge *Leucascandra caveolata* from Northeastern Waters of New Caledonia. *Helv. Chim. Acta* **1999**, *82*, 347–353. [CrossRef]
10. Ali, A.; Hassanean, H.A.; Elkhayat, E.S.; Edrada, R.A.; Ebel, R.; Proksch, P. Imidazole Alkaloids from the Indopacific Sponge *Pericharax heteroraphis*. *Bull. Pharm. Sci.* **2007**, *30*, 149. [CrossRef]
11. Gong, K.-K.; Tang, X.-L.; Liu, Y.-S.; Li, P.-L.; Li, G.-Q. Imidazole Alkaloids from the South China Sea Sponge *Pericharax heteroraphis* and Their Cytotoxic and Antiviral Activities. *Molecules* **2016**, *21*, 150. [CrossRef]
12. de Voogd, N.J.; Alvarez, B.; Boury-Esnault, N.; Carballo, J.L.; Cárdenas, P.; Díaz, M.-C.; Dohrmann, M.; Downey, R.; Hajdu, E.; Hooper, J.N.A.; et al. World Porifera Database. 2022. Available online: https://www.marinespecies.org/porifera (accessed on 5 September 2022).
13. Soest, R.W.M.; de Voogd, N.J. Calcareous Sponges of the Western Indian Ocean and Red Sea. *Zootaxa* **2018**, *4426*, 1–160. [CrossRef]
14. Xiao, Y.; Wang, Y.-L.; Gao, S.-X.; Sun, C.; Zhou, Z.-Y. Chemical Composition of *Hydrilla verticillata* (L. f.) Royle in Taihu Lake. *Chin. J. Chem.* **2007**, *25*, 661–665. [CrossRef]
15. Vincenti, F.; Montesano, C.; Di Ottavio, F.; Gregori, A.; Compagnone, D.; Sergi, M.; Dorrestein, P. Molecular Networking: A Useful Tool for the Identification of New Psychoactive Substances in Seizures by LC–HRMS. *Front. Chem.* **2020**, *8*, 572952. [CrossRef]
16. Nguyen, T.D.; Nguyen, X.C.; Longeon, A.; Keryhuel, A.; Le, M.H.; Kim, Y.H.; Chau, V.M.; Bourguet-Kondracki, M.-L. Antioxidant Benzylidene 2-Aminoimidazolones from the Mediterranean Sponge *Phorbas topsenti*. *Tetrahedron* **2012**, *68*, 9256–9259. [CrossRef]
17. Katritzky, A.R.; Lagowski, J.M. Prototropic Tautomerism of Heteroaromatic Compounds: I. General Discussion and Methods of Study. In *Advances in Heterocyclic Chemistry*; Elsevier: Amsterdam, The Netherlands, 1963; Volume 1, pp. 311–338.
18. Krawczyk, H.; Pietras, A.; Kraska, A. 1H and 13C NMR Spectra and Solution Structures of Novel Derivatives of 5-Substituted Creatinines. *Spectrochim. Acta Part A Mol. Biomol. Spectrosc.* **2007**, *66*, 9–16. [CrossRef]
19. Dai, J.; Jiménez, J.I.; Kelly, M.; Williams, P.G. Dictazoles: Potential Vinyl Cyclobutane Biosynthetic Precursors to the Dictazolines. *J. Org. Chem.* **2010**, *75*, 2399–2402. [CrossRef]
20. Tang, W.-Z.; Yang, Z.-Z.; Sun, F.; Wang, S.-P.; Yang, F.; Jiao, W.-H.; Lin, H.-W. (-)-Calcaridine B, a New Chiral Aminoimidazole-Containing Alkaloid from the Marine Sponge *Leucetta Chagosensis*. *J. Asian Nat. Prod. Res.* **2019**, *21*, 1123–1128. [CrossRef]

21. Carmely, S.; Kashman, Y. Naamines and Naamidines, Novel Imidazole Alkaloids from the Calcareous Sponge *Leucetta chagosensis*. *Tetrahedron Lett.* **1987**, *28*, 3003–3006. [CrossRef]
22. Carmely, S.; Ilan, M.; Kashman, Y. 2-Amino Imidazole Alkaloids from the Marine Sponge *Leucetta chagosensis*. *Tetrahedron* **1989**, *45*, 2193–2200. [CrossRef]
23. Chuck Dunbar, D.; Rimoldi, J.M.; Clark, A.M.; Kelly, M.; Hamann, M.T. Anti-Cryptococcal and Nitric Oxide Synthase Inhibitory Imidazole Alkaloids from the Calcareous Sponge *Leucetta cf chagosensis*. *Tetrahedron* **2000**, *56*, 8795–8798. [CrossRef]
24. Fu, X.; Barnes, J.R.; Do, T.; Schmitz, F.J. New Imidazole Alkaloids from the Sponge *Leucetta chagosensis*. *J. Nat. Prod.* **1997**, *60*, 497–498. [CrossRef]
25. Crews, P.; Clark, D.P.; Tenney, K. Variation in the Alkaloids among Indo-Pacific *Leucetta* Sponges. *J. Nat. Prod.* **2003**, *66*, 177–182. [CrossRef]
26. Hassan, W.; Edrada, R.; Ebel, R.; Wray, V.; Berg, A.; van Soest, R.; Wiryowidagdo, S.; Proksch, P. New Imidazole Alkaloids from the Indonesian Sponge *Leucetta chagosensis*. *J. Nat. Prod.* **2004**, *67*, 817–822. [CrossRef]
27. Carroll, A.R.; Bowden, B.F.; Coll, J.C. New Imidazole Alkaloids from the Sponge *Leucetta* Sp. and the Associated Predatory Nudibranch *Notodoris gardineri*. *Aust. J. Chem.* **1993**, *46*, 1229–1234. [CrossRef]
28. Mancini, I.; Guella, G.; Debitus, C.; Pietra, F. Novel Naamidine-Type Alkaloids and Mixed-Ligand Zinc(II) Complexes from a Calcareous Sponge, *Leucetta* Sp., of the Coral Sea. *Helv. Chim. Acta* **1995**, *78*, 1178–1184. [CrossRef]
29. Tsukamoto, S.; Kawabata, T.; Kato, H.; Ohta, T.; Rotinsulu, H.; Mangindaan, R.E.P.; van Soest, R.W.M.; Ukai, K.; Kobayashi, H.; Namikoshi, M. Naamidines H and I, Cytotoxic Imidazole Alkaloids from the Indonesian Marine Sponge *Leucetta chagosensis*. *J. Nat. Prod.* **2007**, *70*, 1658–1660. [CrossRef]
30. Nothias, L.-F.; Petras, D.; Schmid, R.; Dührkop, K.; Rainer, J.; Sarvepalli, A.; Protsyuk, I.; Ernst, M.; Tsugawa, H.; Fleischauer, M.; et al. Feature-Based Molecular Networking in the GNPS Analysis Environment. *Nat. Methods* **2020**, *17*, 905–908. [CrossRef]
31. Alvi, K.A.; Crews, P.; Loughhead, D.G. Structures and Total Synthesis of 2-Aminoimidazoles from a *Notodoris* Nudibranch. *J. Nat. Prod.* **1991**, *54*, 1509–1515. [CrossRef]
32. Koswatta, P.B.; Lovely, C.J. Structure and Synthesis of 2-Aminoimidazole Alkaloids from *Leucetta* and *Clathrina* Sponges. *Nat. Prod. Rep.* **2011**, *28*, 511–528. [CrossRef]
33. Wang, M.; Carver, J.J.; Phelan, V.V.; Sanchez, L.M.; Garg, N.; Peng, Y.; Nguyen, D.D.; Watrous, J.; Kapono, C.A.; Luzzatto-Knaan, T.; et al. Sharing and Community Curation of Mass Spectrometry Data with Global Natural Products Social Molecular Networking. *Nat. Biotechnol.* **2016**, *34*, 828–837. [CrossRef]

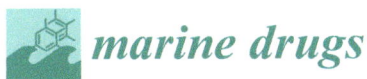

Article

Seven New Alkaloids Isolated from Marine Flavobacterium *Tenacibaculum discolor* sv11

Lei Wang [1,2], Michael Marner [2], Ute Mettal [1,2], Yang Liu [1,2,*] and Till F. Schäberle [1,2,3,*]

1. Institute for Insect Biotechnology, Justus-Liebig-University Giessen, 35392 Giessen, Germany
2. Fraunhofer Institute for Molecular Biology and Applied Ecology (IME), Branch for Bioresources, 35392 Giessen, Germany
3. German Center for Infection Research (DZIF), Partner Site Giessen-Marburg-Langen, 35392 Giessen, Germany
* Correspondence: liu.yang@agrar.uni-giessen.de (Y.L.); till.f.schaeberle@agrar.uni-giessen.de (T.F.S.); Tel.: +49-(0)641-97219-140 (T.F.S.)

Abstract: Marine flavobacterium *Tenacibaculum discolor* sv11 has been proven to be a promising producer of bioactive nitrogen-containing heterocycles. A chemical investigation of *T. discolor* sv11 revealed seven new heterocycles, including the six new imidazolium-containing alkaloids discolins C-H (**1–6**) and one pyridinium-containing alkaloid dispyridine A (**7**). The molecular structure of each compound was elucidated by analysis of NMR and HR-ESI-MS data. Furthermore, enzymatic decarboxylation of tryptophan and tyrosine to tryptamine and tyramine catalyzed by the decarboxylase DisA was investigated using in vivo and in vitro experiments. The antimicrobial activity of the isolated compounds (**1–7**) was evaluated. Discolin C and E (**1** and **3**) exhibited moderate activity against Gram-positive *Bacillus subtilis* DSM10, *Mycobacterium smegmatis* ATCC607, *Listeria monocytogenes* DSM20600 and *Staphylococcus aureus* ATCC25923, with MIC values ranging from 4 µg/mL to 32 µg/mL.

Keywords: Bacteroidetes; *Tenacibaculum*; nitrogen-containing heterocycles; imidazolium-containing alkaloids; pyridinium-containing alkaloid; antimicrobial activity

Citation: Wang, L.; Marner, M.; Mettal, U.; Liu, Y.; Schäberle, T.F. Seven New Alkaloids Isolated from Marine Flavobacterium *Tenacibaculum discolor* sv11. *Mar. Drugs* **2022**, *20*, 620. https://doi.org/10.3390/md20100620

Academic Editor: Asunción Barbero

Received: 4 September 2022
Accepted: 28 September 2022
Published: 30 September 2022

Publisher's Note: MDPI stays neutral with regard to jurisdictional claims in published maps and institutional affiliations.

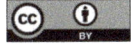

Copyright: © 2022 by the authors. Licensee MDPI, Basel, Switzerland. This article is an open access article distributed under the terms and conditions of the Creative Commons Attribution (CC BY) license (https://creativecommons.org/licenses/by/4.0/).

1. Introduction

Structurally diverse nitrogen-containing heterocycles, such as pyrroles, imidazoles, oxazoles, pyridines, and quinolones, are widely distributed in marine organisms and microorganisms. These naturally occurring secondary metabolites often exhibit significant pharmacological activities, including antibacterial, antifungal, antiparasitic, and anticancer activities [1–6]. Furthermore, these compounds are often amenable to further structural modifications [7–10]. Currently, marine-derived imidazole alkaloids are reported mainly to be isolated from sponges, while reports of marine bacteria as bioresource are relatively rare [2,6,11–14].

As a member of the family *Flavobacteriaceae* within the phylum *Bacteroidetes*, isolates of the genus *Tenacibaculum* have been mainly obtained from marine environments, such as sea water, tidal flat, and aquaculture systems, as well as marine organisms like bryozoan, sea anemone, oyster, sponge and green algae [15–22]. Bacteria of this genus are the etiological agent of an ulcerative disease known as tenacibaculosis, which affects a large number of marine fish species in the world [23]. Up to now, the natural products isolated from *Tenacibaculum* strains comprise only siderophores that showed beside their chelating activity also cytotoxicity [24–26], and phenethylamine-containing heterocycles. The latter include two imidazole alkaloids identified in our previous search for antimicrobial metabolites from marine flavobacteria. It was shown that they could be synthesized by decarboxylation of phenylalanine, catalyzed by the enzyme DisA [27]. Likewise, the tryptamine and phenethylamine moieties of imidazole alkaloids isolated from a marine sponge-associated *Bacillus* strain were proposed to be formed by an aromatic amino acid decarboxylase-dependent reaction [28]. In order to further expand the array of available nitrogen-containing heterocycles, the metabolome of *T. discolor* sv11 was further investigated. Herein, we present the isolation, structure elucidation and biological activity of new alkaloids from the bacterium, and link the enzymatic activity of DisA to their biosynthesis using both, in vivo and in vitro assays.

2. Results

In our continuous search for new bioactive molecules, the six new imidazolium-containing alkaloids discolins C–H (**1**–**6**) and one pyridinium-containing alkaloid dispyridine A (**7**) were isolated from the marine-derived bacterium *T. discolor* sv11 (Figure 1). The antimicrobial activity of these new compounds was investigated, among which, compounds **1** and **3** exhibited moderate activity against Gram-positive *Bacillus subtilis* DSM10, *Mycobacterium smegmatis* ATCC607, *Listeria monocytogenes* DSM20600 and *Staphylococcus aureus* ATCC25923. In vivo and in vitro experiments indicated that phenethylamine, tryptamine and tyramine residues of the new alkaloids are derived from an enzymatic decarboxylation.

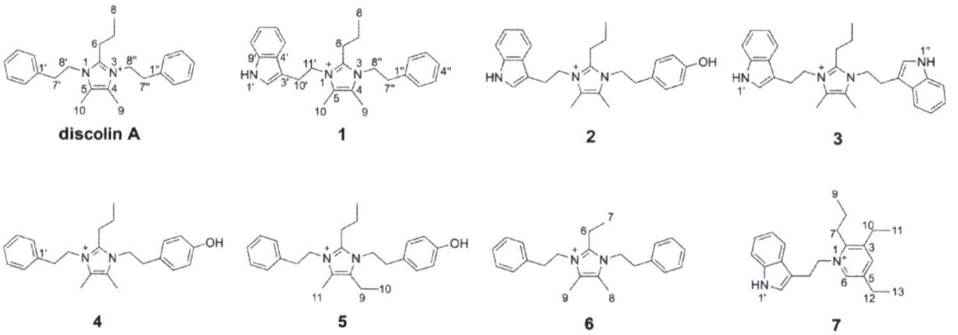

Figure 1. Discolin A and new compounds isolated from *T. discolor* sv11.

Compound **1** was obtained as a yellowish oil. The HR-ESI-MS spectrum of **1** showed a molecular formula of $C_{26}H_{32}N_3^+$ based on the prominent peak [M]$^+$ at *m/z* 386.2606 (calculated 386.2591, Figure S1). The analysis of ^{1}H NMR and HSQC spectra of **1** revealed three methyl groups at δ_H 0.80 (H-8), δ_H 2.15 (H-9) and δ_H 2.20 (H-10), six methylene groups at δ_H 1.34 (H-7), δ_H 2.41 (H-6), δ_H 2.80 (H-7''), δ_H 3.08 (H-10'), δ_H 4.22 (H-8'') and δ_H 4.30 (H-11'), as well as ten aromatic protons that resonated from δ_H 7.00 to δ_H 7.39 (Table 1). These NMR data exhibited a high similarity with the previously reported compound discolin A that was also isolated from *T. discolor* sv11 [27]. Therefore, a core structure of the 4,5-dimethyl-2-propyl imidazolium skeleton of **1** was elucidated based on the COSY spin system from H-6 to H-7 to H-8, as well as on HMBC correlations from both H-6 and H-7 to C-2, and from both, H-9 and H-10 to C-4 and C-5. The same phenylethyl moiety as present in discolin A was deducted from compound **1** based on the COSY spin system between H-7'' and H-8'', as well as between five benzene ring protons 7.16 (2H, H-2'' and H-6''), 7.28 (H-4'') and δ_H 7.32 (2H, H-3'' and H-5''), together with the core HMBC correlations from H-7'' to C-1'' and C-2'', and from H-8'' to C-1'' (Figure 2). The significant difference between compound **1** and discolin A are the HMBC correlations from a singlet aromatic proton resonating at δ_H 7.17 (H-2') to C-3', C-4' and C-9', from H-5' to C-3', C-4', C-7' and C-9' (Figure 2), as well as the COSY spin system from H-5' to H-6', to H-7' to H-8'. These results suggested an indole moiety instead of a phenyl residue in compound **1**. Together with the remaining COSY spin system between the two methylene groups H-10' and H-11' and the HMBC correlations from H-10' to C-2', C-3', C-4' and C-11', a 3-ethylindole moiety ($C_{10}H_{10}N$) was elucidated from compound **1**, which is further supported by the MS/MS fragment $[C_{10}H_{10}N]^+$ detected at *m/z* 144.0813 (calculated 144.0813, Figure S1). With the HMBC correlations from H-8'' to C-2 and C-4, and from H-11′ to C-2 and C-5, the above mentioned phenylethyl moiety and 3-ethylindole were supposed to be located at position 3 and 1 of the imidazolium skeleton (Figure 2). This assumption was proven by ^{1}H-^{15}N HMBC correlations from H-6, H-9, H-7″ and H-8″ to N-3 and from H-6, H-10, H-10′ and H-11′ to N-1 (Figure 2). The N-atom at position 1 was considered to be positively charged based on the detected chemical shift at δ_N 178.5, while N-3 was at δ_N 177.3 (Figures S7 and S8) [29–31]. An additional NMR measurement with added trifluoracetic acid (TFA) in DMSO-d_6 (ratio 1:3) was carried out to further prove this conclusion (Figures S9–S13). The methylene groups of H-8″ and H-7″ shifted to up-field with a deviation $\Delta\delta_{H-8″}$ value of 0.13 and $\Delta\delta_{H-7″}$ value of 0.10 ppm, while the deviation $\Delta\delta_{H-11′}$ and $\Delta\delta_{H-10′}$ values were 0.09 and 0.05 ppm, respectively. The addition of TFA lead to the protonation of the tertiary N-atom at position 3, which gives a higher influence on the chemical shift [32]. The detected different chemical shift deviations $\Delta\delta_{N-3}$ (155.1) and $\Delta\delta_{N-1}$ (154.1) further support this result (Figures S7, S8 and S13). Thus, the structure of compound **1** was elucidated as shown in Figure 1 and named discolin C.

Table 1. ^{1}H (700 MHz) and ^{13}C (175 MHz) NMR data of compounds **1–3** (DMSO-d_6, δ in ppm).

Position	1			2		3	
	δ_C, Type	δ_H, (J in Hz)	δ_H, (J in Hz) [a]	δ_C, Type	δ_H, (J in Hz)	δ_C, Type	δ_H, (J in Hz)
2	144.8, C			144.7, C		144.7, C	
4	125.5, C			125.5, C		125.5, C	
5	125.5, C			125.5, C		125.5, C	
6	23.8, CH$_2$	2.41, t (8.0)	2.20, m	23.8, CH$_2$	2.40, t (7.8)	23.7, CH$_2$	2.30, t (8.1)
7	20.6, CH$_2$	1.34, m	1.25, m	20.6, CH$_2$	1.34, m	20.5, CH$_2$	1.29, m
8	13.3, CH$_3$	0.80, t (7.3)	0.69, t (7.3)	13.3, CH$_3$	0.80, t (7.2)	13.2, CH$_3$	0.71, t (7.3)
9	7.9, CH$_3$	2.15, s	2.03, s	7.9, CH$_3$	2.13, s	8.0, CH$_3$	2.22, s
10	8.0, CH$_3$	2.20, s	2.10, s	8.0, CH$_3$	2.19, s	8.0, CH$_3$	2.22, s
1′ NH		11.11, s	10.80, s		11.02, s		11.03, s
2′	123.9, CH	7.17, s [b]	7.02, s [b]	123.8, CH	7.16, s	123.8, CH	7.16, s
3′	109.1, C			109.1, C		109.1, C	
4′	126.8, C			126.8, C		126.8, C	
5′	117.5, CH	7.39, d (7.3)	7.27, d (7.9)	117.5, CH	7.40, d (7.9)	117.5, CH	7.38, m
6′	118.6, CH	7.00, t (7.7)	6.93, d (7.5)	118.6, CH	7.00, t (7.4)	118.6, CH	7.01, t (7.5)
7′	121.2, CH	7.09, t (7.5)	7.02, m [b]	121.2, CH	7.09, t (7.4)	121.2, CH	7.09, t (7.5)
8′	111.6, CH	7.38, d (7.6)	7.32, d (8.1)	111.6, CH	7.38, d (8.0)	111.6, CH	7.38, m
9′	136.1, C			136.1, C		136.1, C	
10′	25.0, CH$_2$	3.08, t (7.0)	3.03, t (6.8)	25.0, CH$_2$	3.07, t (6.7)	24.9, CH	2.95, t (7.2)
11′	45.8, CH$_2$	4.30, t (7.0)	4.21, t (6.7)	45.7, CH$_2$	4.29, t (6.7)	45.6, CH	4.23, t (7.3)
1″ [c]	136.8, C			126.7, C			11.03, s
2″	128.9, CH	7.16, m [b]	7.02, m [b]	129.9, CH	6.91, d (7.9)	123.8, CH	7.16, s
3″	128.6, CH	7.32, t (7.3)	7.21, m	115.3, CH	6.70, d (8.0)	109.1, C	
4″	127.0, CH	7.28, m	7.17, m	156.5, C		126.8, C	
5″	128.6, CH	7.32, t (7.3)	7.21, m	115.3, CH	6.70, d (8.0)	117.5, CH	7.38, m
6″	128.9, CH	7.16, m [b]	7.02, m [b]	129.9, CH	6.91, d (7.9)	118.6, CH	7.01, t (7.5)
7″	35.0, CH$_2$	2.80, t (7.5)	2.70, t (7.3)	34.2, CH$_2$	2.69, t (6.9)	121.2, CH	7.09, t (7.5)
8″	45.8, CH$_2$	4.22, t (7.5)	4.09, t (7.2)	46.2, CH$_2$	4.14, t (6.9)	111.6, CH	7.38, m
9″						136.1, C	
10″						24.9, CH	2.95, t (7.2)
11″						45.6, CH	4.23, t (7.3)

[a] ^{1}H NMR data of compound **1** with TFA added. [b] Signals overlapped. [c] NH at 1″ for compound **3**.

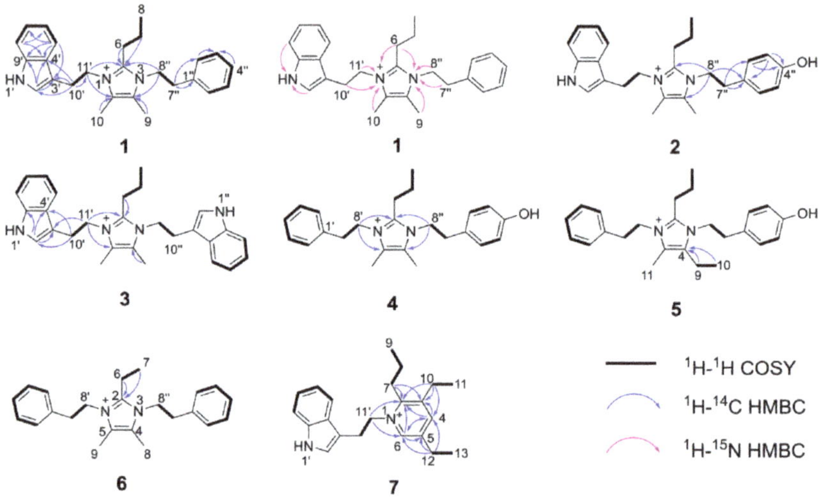

Figure 2. Key HMBC and ^{1}H-^{1}H COSY correlations of compounds 1–7.

Compound **2** was obtained as a yellowish oil. The molecular formula of **2** was determined to be $C_{26}H_{32}ON_3^+$ (m/z = 402.2543, [M]$^+$, calcd. 402.2540, Figure S14) based on the HR-ESI-MS spectrum. Comprehensive comparison of NMR data of compounds **1** and **2** revealed the high similarity except for the chemical shift of C-4″, which was shifted from 126.96 to 156.48, and one missing aromatic proton. Together with the detected 16 Da increase in the HR-ESI-MS spectrum of compound **2**, this suggested the presence of a 4-hydroxyphenylethyl moiety located at position 3 instead of a phenylethyl moiety (Table 1). This assumption was confirmed by the upfield chemical shifts of the benzene ring protons at δ_H 6.70 (2H, H-3″ and H-5″) and δ_H 6.91 (2H, H-2″ and H-6″), which showed similar behavior as the reported 4-hydroxyphenylethyl-containing compound N-Acetyltyramine [33]. This effect is explained by the fact that the hydroxyl group is an electron donor, which shields the protons of the benzene nucleus more strongly and leads to an upfield shift of the corresponding signals. Second, the hydroxyl group that appeared at C-4″ in compound **2** changes the spin system of this radical, and therefore influenced the shape of the proton multiplets of the benzene nucleus. Furthermore, the COSY spin system between H-2″ and H-3″, as well as the HMBC correlations from H-7″ to C-1″, C-2″, from H-3″ to C-1″, C-4″, and from H-8″ to C-2, C-4 and C-1″ proved the 4-hydroxyphenylethyl group in compound **2**. The detected MS/MS fragment at m/z 282.1963 ([$C_{18}H_{23}N_3$ + H]$^+$, calcd. 282.1965, Figure S14) of compound **2**, which lost the 4-hydroxyphenylethyl group (-C_8H_9O), strongly indicated the above mentioned assumption. Thus, the structure of compound **2** was elucidated as shown in Figure 1 and named discolin D.

Compound **3** was also obtained as a yellowish oil. The molecular formula of **3** was determined to be $C_{28}H_{33}N_4^+$ (m/z = 425.2702, [M]$^+$, calculated 425.2700, Figure S20) based on the HR-ESI-MS spectrum. The core scaffold of compound **3** shared the 4,5-dimethyl-2-propyl imidazolium skeleton with compound **1** as deduced from a comparison of both, 1D and 2D NMR data (Table 1), which also indicated compound **3** to be a symmetric structure. Integration of the proton signals in the ^{1}H NMR spectrum together with the COSY spin system of the aromatic protons and the HMBC correlations from H-2′ to C-3′, C-4′ and C-9′, from H-10′ to C-2′, C-4′ and C-11′, as well as from H-11′ to C-3′, C-10′, C-2, and C-5 proved that two identical 3-ethylindole moieties were connected to the central imidazolium ring as shown in Figure 2. Hence, compound **3** is a member of the discolin family and was named discolin E.

Compounds **4** and **5** were each obtained as a yellowish oil. The molecula formulae of compounds **4** and **5** were identified as $C_{24}H_{31}ON_2^+$ and $C_{25}H_{33}ON_2^+$, respectively, based on the HR-ESI-MS signals [M]$^+$ at *m/z* = 363.2442 (calculated 363.2431, compound **4**, Figure S26) and *m/z* = 377.2593 (calculated 377.2587, compound **5**, Figure S32), respectively. One phenylethyl moiety, one 4-hydroxyphenylethyl moiety and the 4,5-dimethyl-2-propyl imidazolium skeleton were disclosed as constituents of compound **4** by comparing the 1D and 2D NMR data with those of compounds **1** and **2** (Tables 1 and 2). The phenylethyl moiety and the 4-hydroxyphenylethyl moiety were assigned to be located at positions 1 and 3 of the imidazolium skeleton of compound **4**, based on the HMBC correlations from H-8′ to C-2 and C-5 and from H-8″ to C-2 and C-4 (Figure 2). In compound **5**, identical phenylethyl and 4-hydroxyphenylethyl moieties were assigned to be located at the same positions as in compound **4**. Comparing the 1D and 2D NMR data of compounds **4** and **5**, the only difference is one ethyl group present in compound **5**, while compound **4** carries a methyl group (Table 2). The presence of an ethyl group in compound **5** is corroborated by the COSY correlation between H-9 and H-10, and the HMBC correlations from both, H-9 and H-10 to C-4. In contrast, in compound **4**, the methyl group is directly connected to the unsaturated carbon C-4 (Figure 2), thus verifying the assumed structural relationship between compounds **4** and **5**. The 14 Da molecular weight difference between both compounds further supports their structural relationship. Thus, the structures of compounds **4** and **5** were elucidated as shown in Figure 1, and the names discolin F and discolin G were proposed, respectively.

Table 2. ^{1}H (700 MHz) and ^{13}C (175 MHz) NMR data of compounds **4–6** (DMSO-d_6, δ in ppm).

Position	4		5		6	
	$δ_C$, Type	$δ_H$, (*J* in Hz)	$δ_C$, Type [a]	$δ_H$, (*J* in Hz)	$δ_C$, Type	$δ_H$, (*J* in Hz)
2	144.8, C		144.8, C		146.0, C	
4	125.5, C		130.5, C		125.5, C	
5	125.6, C		125.7, C		125.5, C	
6	23.9, CH$_2$	2.53, t (7.9)	23.8, CH$_2$	2.55, m	16.1, CH$_2$	2.67, q (7.6)
7	20.7, CH$_2$	1.40, m	20.4, CH$_2$	1.43, m	11.8, CH$_3$	1.02, t (7.6)
8	13.4, CH$_3$	0.89, t (7.2)	13.1, CH$_3$	0.90, t (7.2)	7.9, CH$_3$	2.11, s
9	7.9, CH$_3$	2.10 or 2.11, s	15.1, CH$_2$	2.57, q (7.6)	7.9, CH$_3$	2.11, s
10	7.9, CH$_3$	2.10 or 2.11, s	13.3, CH$_3$	1.07, td (7.5, 1.9)		
11			7.6, CH$_3$	2.10, d (1.5)		
1′	136.9, C		136.8, C		136.9, C	
2′	129.0, CH	7.19, d (7.2)	128.7, CH	7.20 or 7.17, d (7.1)	129.0, CH	7.19, d (7.1)
3′	128.6, CH	7.33, t (7.3)	128.4, CH	7.33, m	128.6, CH	7.33, t (7.3)
4′	127.0, CH	7.28, t (7.2)	126.8, CH	7.29, m	127.0, CH	7.28, t (7.3)
5′	128.6, CH	7.33, t (7.3)	128.4, CH	7.33, m	128.6, CH	7.33, t (7.3)
6′	129.0, CH	7.19, d (7.2)	128.7, CH	7.20 or 7.17, d (7.1)	129.0, CH	7.19, d (7.1)
7′	35.0, CH$_2$	2.93, t (7.0)	35.2, CH$_2$	2.93, m	35.0, CH$_2$	2.95, t (7.3)
8′	46.0, CH$_2$	4.28, t (7.0)	45.6, CH$_2$	4.29, m	45.9, CH$_2$	4.28, t (7.3)
1″	126.5, C		126.4, C		136.9, C	
2″	129.9, CH	6.92, d (8.1)	129.6, CH	6.93 or 6.90, d (8.2)	129.0, CH	7.19, d (7.1)
3″	115.4, CH	6.70, d (8.1)	115.2, CH	6.71 or 6.70, d (8.4)	128.6, CH	7.33, t (7.3)
4″	156.8, C		156.7, C		127.0, CH	7.28, t (7.3)
5″	115.4, CH	6.70, d (8.1)	115.2, CH	6.71 or 6.70, d (8.4)	128.6, CH	7.33, t (7.3)
6″	129.9, CH	6.92, d (8.1)	129.6, CH	6.93 or 6.90, d (8.2)	129.0, CH	7.19, d (7.1)
7″	34.2, CH$_2$	2.81, t (6.8)	34.3, CH$_2$	2.81, m	35.0, CH$_2$	2.95, t (7.3)
8″	46.4, CH$_2$	4.21, t (6.9)	46.0, CH$_2$	4.21, m	45.9, CH$_2$	4.28, t (7.3)

[a] Deduced from HSQC and HMBC spectra.

Compound **6** was also obtained as a yellowish oil. The molecular formula of compound **6** was established as $C_{23}H_{29}N_2^+$ based on the prominent [M]$^+$ peak in HR-ESI-MS spectrum at m/z = 333.2329 (calculated 333.2325, Figure S37). Two identical phenylethyl moieties were deduced from the NMR spectra of compound **6** and connected at positions 1 and 3 of the core ring based on the HMBC correlations from H-8′ to C-2 and C-5, as well as from H-8″ to C-2 and C-4. The remaining signals of **6** were assigned to the 4,5-dimethyl-2-ethyl imidazolium scaffold, which showed an ethyl group rather than a propyl group at position 2. This difference was clarified by the COSY correlation between H-6 and H-7, as well as the HMBC correlations from both, H-6 and H-7 to C-2 (Figure 2). Therefore, compound **6** proved to be a representative of the discolin family and was named discolin H.

Compound **7** was isolated as a colorless powder. Its molecular formula was established as $C_{22}H_{29}N_2^+$ based on the prominent ion peak [M]$^+$ observed at m/z 321.2322 (calcd. 321.2325, Figure S43). Comprehensive analysis of 1D and 2D NMR data of compound **7** revealed one 3-ethylindole moiety as found in compounds **1–3**, as well as two ethyl groups and one propyl group (Table 3). The remaining two aromatic protons at δ_H 8.20 (H-4) and δ_H 8.40 (H-6) in the ^{1}H NMR spectrum and five aromatic carbons at δ_C 153.07 (C-2), δ_C 142.58 (C-3), δ_C 144.54 (C-4), δ_C 140.61 (C-5) and δ_C 142.62 (C-6) in the ^{13}C NMR spectrum were attributed to a pyridinium ring as apparent from comparison with the data of dispyridine, a pyridinium-containing alkaloid isolated previously [27]. The location of the 3-ethylindole moiety was determined from the HMBC correlations from H-11′ to C-2 and C-6, which also confirmed the location of the aromatic proton H-6 resonating at δ_H 8.40. The second aromatic proton resonating at δ_H 8.20 was attributed to position 4, based on the HMBC correlations from H-4 to C-2, C-3 and C-6. The propyl group and the two ethyl groups attached to the pyridinium ring were located at C-2, C-3 and C-5, as inferred from HMBC correlations from H-7 to C-2 and C-3, from H-10 to C-2, C-3 and C-4, and from H-12 to C-4, C-5 and C-6 (Figure 2). Therefore, compound **7** was found to be a new member of the dispyridine family and named dispyridine A.

Table 3. ^{1}H (700 MHz) and ^{13}C (175 MHz) NMR data of compound **7** (DMSO-d_6, δ in ppm).

Position	δ_C, Type	δ_H, (J in Hz)	Position	δ_C, Type	δ_H, (J in Hz)
2	153.1, C		1′ NH		11.06, s
3	142.6, C		2′	124.2, CH	7.13, s
4	144.5, CH	8.20, s	3′	108.3, C	
5	140.6, C		4′	126.8, C	
6	142.6, CH	8.40, s	5′	117.3, CH	7.25, d (7.9)
7	29.5, CH$_2$	2.83, t (8.2)	6′	118.6, CH	6.91, t (7.4)
8	21.8, CH$_2$	1.56, m	7′	121.2, CH	7.06, t (7.3)
9	13.8, CH$_3$	1.00, t (7.0)	8′	111.6, CH	7.35, d (8.1)
10	24.5, CH$_2$	2.73, q (7.5)	9′	136.0, C	
11	14.4, CH$_3$	1.13, t (7.5)	10′	26.5, CH$_2$	3.35, m ^{a}
12	24.5, CH$_2$	2.57, q (7.5)	11′	58.5, CH$_2$	4.78, t (6.5)
13	13.9, CH$_3$	1.01, t (7.5)			

^{a} Signal overlapped with H$_2$O.

Based on previous research, it was known that phenylalanine can be converted to phenethylamine by the catalytic action of the decarboxylase DisA. This molecule could serve as building block to yield different derivatives [27]. Hence, the newly isolated imidazolium-containing alkaloids (**1–6**) were also supposed to be produced via the same biosynthetic route, i.e., first an enzymatic decarboxylation of the aromatic-L-amino acid tryptophan or tyrosine yielding tryptamine or tyramine, respectively, followed by a non-enzymatic condensation to form the central imidazolium ring. To confirm this hypothesis, the candidate enzyme DisA from *T. discolor* sv11 was analyzed in vivo in a heterologous system. Therefore, the previously constructed transgenic host strain *E. coli* ROSETTA (disA) carrying the respective *disA* gene and *E. coli* ROSETTA (pRSF) (negative empty vector control) were cultivated in LB medium, whereby 2 mM tryptophan and tyrosine were added as substrates, respectively. After 24 h incubation, tryptamine and tyramine were only detected in the extract of *E. coli* ROSETTA (disA), while only the substrates, i.e., tryptophan and tyrosine were detected in the negative control (Figure 3). To further validate these results, a His-tagged version of DisA was purified using affinity chromatography and assayed in vitro. This confirmed that tryptamine and tyramine can be obtained from tryptophan and tyrosine by a DisA-dependent catalytic conversion (Figure 3).

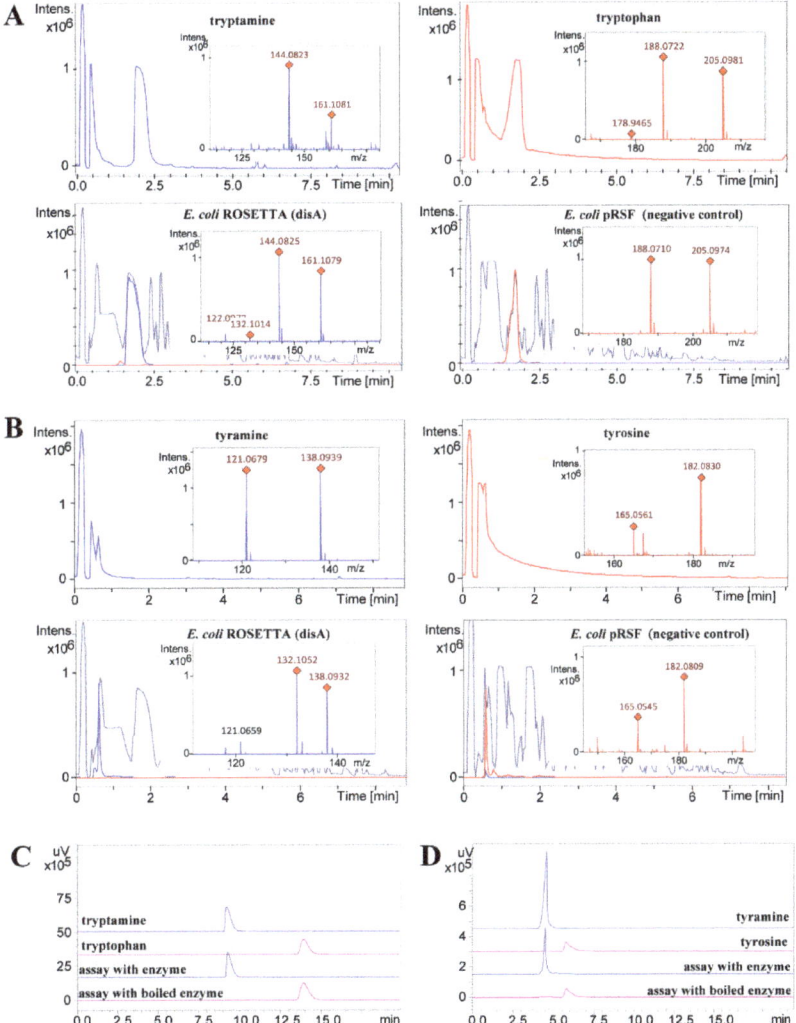

Figure 3. In vivo and in vitro decarboxylation of tryptophan and tyrosine catalyzed by DisA. (**A**) In vivo decarboxylation of tryptophan to tryptamine. Extracted ion chromatograms (EICs) of tryptophan ($C_{11}H_{13}N_2O_2$ 205.0977 [M + H]$^+$, in red) and tryptamine ($C_{10}H_{13}N_2$ 161.1079 [M + H]$^+$, in blue). (**B**) In vivo decarboxylation of tyrosine to tyramine. Extracted ion chromatograms (EIC) of tyrosine ($C_9H_{12}NO_3$ 182.0817 [M + H]$^+$, in red) and tyramine ($C_8H_{12}NO$ 138.0919 [M + H]$^+$, in blue). In A and B, the base peak chromatogram of the extracts is given in grey. (**C**) Comparative HPLC analysis of the in vitro decarboxylation of tryptophan. (**D**) Comparative HPLC analysis of the in vitro decarboxylation of tyrosine. In C and D, the UV absorbance at 254 nm is shown.

All isolated compounds **1–7** were investigated for their bioactivity against bacteria (*B. subtilis* DSM10, *M. smegmatis* ATCC607, *L. monocytogenes* DSM20600, *S. aureus* ATCC25923, and *E. coli* ATCC25922) and fungi (*Candida albicans* FH2173). As shown in Table 4, discolin C (**1**) showed activity against *M. smegmatis* ATCC607 and *B. subtilis* DSM10 with MIC values ranging from 4 µg/mL to 8 µg/mL and moderate to weak activity against *S. aureus* ATCC25923 and *L. monocytogenes* DSM20600 with MIC values ranging from 16 µg/mL to 32 µg/mL. Discolin E (**3**) exhibited activity against four tested Gram-positive bacteria with MIC values ranging from 4 µg/mL to 8 µg/mL and moderate activity against *C. albicans* FH2173 with an MIC value of 16 µg/mL. The other compounds (**2**, **4–7**) were inactive against all the tested microorganisms in the range tested.

Table 4. MIC values (µg/mL) for Compounds **1–7**.

Test organism	MIC (µg/mL, n = 3)									
	1	2	3	4	5	6	7	Rifampicin	Tetracycline	Gentamicin
B. subtilis DSM10	8	>32	8	>32	32	32	>32	<0.031	2–4	0.06
M. smegmatis ATCC607	4	>32	4	>32	>32	16	>32	8–16	0.25–0.5	4–8 [a]
L. monocytogenes DSM20600	32	>32	8	>32	>32	>32	>32	<0.031	0.5–1	<0.031
S. aureus ATCC25923	16	>32	8	>32	>32	32	>32	<0.031	0.25–0.5	0.06–0.125
E. coli ATCC25922	>32	>32	>32	>32	>32	>32	>32	4	2–4	0.06
C. albicans FH2173 [b]	>32	>32	16	>32	>32	>32	>32	Nystatin 1–2	Tebuconazole 0.25	Amphotericin B 0.5–1

[a] Isoniazid was used as positive control. [b] Nystatin, tebuconazole and amphotericin B were used as positive controls.

3. Conclusions and Discussion

In conclusion, seven new alkaloids were obtained from the crude extract of *T. discolor* sv11 after fermentation in LB medium. In vivo and in vitro experiments proved the decarboxylase DisA to catalyze the decarboxylation of the aromatic-*L*-amino acids phenylalanine, tryptophan and tyrosine to phenethylamine, tryptamine and tyramine, respectively. These molecules serve as substrates for the formation of the central imidazolium ring of discolins A–H through a non-enzymatic condensation. Hence, by combining an enzyme-catalyzed and a non-enzymatic reaction, the bacterium generates a mix of structurally related molecules. Besides the understanding of the biosynthetic mechanisms of the discolins, some insights into the structure–activity relationship of the antibacterial discolins A-H were also obtained [27]. Discolin A and discolin H feature the same molecular skeleton, except for the length of the carbon chain linked to C-2 of the central imidazolium ring. Both molecules showed the similar moderate bioactivity, which suggests that the substructure at position 2 can be altered without affecting the activity. The structural differences and changes in the bioactivity of discolins C-F and discolin A indicated that the substructures at position 1 and 3 of the central ring instead play an important role concerning antibacterial activity. Earlier evidence indicated that the activity of imidazolium salts is highly dependent upon the substituents on the nitrogen atoms of the imidazolium cation [34], which is in agreement with our observation. In summary, our finding, together with previous reports, clearly indicates that the genus *Tenacibaculum* exhibits a high potential to produce nitrogen-containing heterocycles with a unique structure and various biological activities. This includes positively charged imidazolium-containing natural products.

4. Materials and Methods

4.1. General Experimental Procedures

The 1D and 2D NMR spectra were recorded in DMSO-d_6 using a Bruker Avance Neo 700 MHz spectrometer equipped with a 5 mm CryoProbe Prodigy TCI (^{1}H,^{15}N,^{13}C Z-GRD) (Bruker, Ettlingen, Germany). The LC-HRMS data for new compounds were recorded on a micrOTOF-QII mass spectrometer (Bruker, Billerica, MA, USA) equipped with an ESI-source coupled to an Agilent Infinity 1290 UHPLC system using an ACQUITY UPLC BEH C18 Column, 130 Å, 1.7 µm, 2.1 mm × 100 mm (Waters, Eschborn, Germany) with an ACQUITY UPLC BEH C18 VanGuard Pre-column, 130 Å, 1.7 µm, 2.1 mm × 5 mm (Waters, Eschborn, Germany). HPLC was performed using a Shimadzu HPLC system (Shimadzu Deutschland GmbH, Duisburg, Germany) for analysis (EC 250/4.6 Nucleodur C18 Gravity-SB, 5 µm; Macherey-Nagel, Düren, Germany), and for semi-preparative purification (VP 250/10 Nucleodur C18 Gravity-SB, 5 µm; Macherey-Nagel, Düren, Germany). MPLC was performed on the Interchim Puriflash 4125 chromatography system (Interchim, Montluçon, France).

4.2. Extraction and Isolation

A fermentation (36 L) of *T. discolor* S11 was performed in 5 L flasks that contained 1.5 L of LB medium and were incubated at 30 °C and 140 rpm for 8 days, followed by an extraction using EtOAc (volume ratio 1:1) for three times, affording 11.9 g crude extract. Thirteen fractions (Fr. 1–13) were collected from reversed phase flash chromatography (Interchim Puriflash 4125 chromatography system with Puriflash C18-AQ30 µm F0120 column) with an elution gradient starting from 10% MeOH/H_2O to 100% MeOH over 1.5 h. Fr. 11 (973.8 mg) was further subjected to size exclusion chromatography on a Sephadex LH-20 column and eluted with 100% MeOH to give 10 subfractions (Frr. 11.1–11.10). Frr. 11.4 (229.4 mg) was further subjected to reversed phase flash chromatography (Interchim Puriflash 4125 chromatography system with Puriflash C18-HP30 µm F0025 Flash column) using an elution gradient from 10% MeOH/H_2O to 100% MeOH over 4 h to give 10 subfractions (Frrr. 11.4.1–11.4.10). Frrr. 11.4.6 was further purified by semi-preparative HPLC (0–1 min, 22% MeCN; 1–46 min, gradient increased from 22% to 37% MeCN) to yield compounds **1** (2.0 mg, t_R = 43 min) and **3** (0.6 mg, t_R = 45 min). Frrr. 11.4.5 was fractionated by semi-preparative HPLC (0–38.5 min, gradient increased from 10% to 46% MeOH) to give 6 subfractions (Frrrr. 11.4.5.1–11.4.5.6). Frrrr. 11.4.5.3 was again purified by semi-preparative HPLC (0–57 min, isocratic gradient with 29% MeOH) to yield compounds **2** (1.2 mg, t_R = 48.5 min), **4** (2.1 mg, t_R = 39 min) and **7** (1.5 mg, t_R = 44.4 min). Purification of Frrrr. 11.4.5.1 by semi-preparative HPLC (0–5 min, 5% MeCN; 5–50 min, gradient increased from 5% to 35% MeCN) yielded compound **5** (0.3 mg, t_R = 49.3 min). Compound **6** (0.3 mg, t_R = 51.2 min) was obtained from Frrrr. 11.4.5.6 by semi-preparative HPLC (0–5 min, 5% MeCN; 5–56 min, gradient increased from 5% to 39% MeCN).

Discolin C (**1**): yellowish oil; the ^{1}H NMR (DMSO-d_6, 700 MHz) and ^{13}C NMR (DMSO-d_6, 175 MHz) data are given in Table 1; HR-ESI-MS *m/z* 386.2606 [M]$^+$ (calculated for $C_{26}H_{32}N_3^+$, 386.2591, Figure S1).

Discolin D (**2**): yellowish oil; the ^{1}H NMR (DMSO-d_6, 700 MHz) and ^{13}C NMR (DMSO-d_6, 175 MHz) data are given in Table 1; HR-ESI-MS *m/z* 402.2543 [M]$^+$ (calculated for $C_{26}H_{32}ON_3^+$, 402.2540, Figure S14).

Discolin E (**3**): yellowish oil; the ^{1}H NMR (DMSO-d_6, 700 MHz) and ^{13}C NMR (DMSO-d_6, 175 MHz) data are given in Table 1; HR-ESI-MS *m/z* 425.2702 [M]$^+$ (calculated for $C_{28}H_{33}N_4^+$, 425.2700, Figure S20).

Discolin F (**4**): yellowish oil; the ^{1}H NMR (DMSO-d_6, 700 MHz) and ^{13}C NMR (DMSO-d_6, 175 MHz) data are given in Table 2; HR-ESI-MS *m/z* 363.2442 [M]$^+$ (calculated for $C_{24}H_{31}ON_2^+$, 363.2431, Figure S26).

Discolin G (**5**): yellowish oil; the ^{1}H NMR (DMSO-d_6, 700 MHz) and ^{13}C NMR (DMSO-d_6, 175 MHz) data are given in Table 2; HR-ESI-MS *m/z* 377.2593 [M]$^+$ (calculated for $C_{25}H_{33}ON_2^+$, 377.2587, Figure S32).

Discolin H (**6**): yellowish oil; the ^{1}H NMR (DMSO-d_6, 700 MHz) and ^{13}C NMR (DMSO-d_6, 175 MHz) data are given in Table 2; HR-ESI-MS *m/z* 333.2329 [M]$^+$ (calculated for $C_{23}H_{29}N_2^+$, 333.2325, Figure S37).

Dispyridine A (**7**): colorless powder; the ^{1}H NMR (DMSO-d_6, 700 MHz) and ^{13}C NMR (DMSO-d_6, 175 MHz) data are given in Table 3; HR-ESI-MS *m/z* 321.2322 [M]$^+$ (calculated for $C_{22}H_{29}N_2^+$, 321.2325, Figure S43).

4.3. Enzymatic Activity of Dis A

To investigate the enzymatic activity of Dis A in vivo, *E. coli* ROSETTA (disA) was cultured in 30 mL kanamycin-containing (50 µg mL^{-1}) LB medium at 30 °C overnight as pre-culture. A volume of 100 µL of this pre-culture was used to inoculate at 37 °C in two 300 mL Erlenmeyer flasks with 100 mL kanamycin-containing (50 µg mL^{-1}) LB medium; 0.1 mM IPTG was added into the medium when the cultures reached an OD$_{600}$ of 0.5 and were cultured at 30 °C for 3 h. Then, 2 mM tryptophan or tyrosine were added to the medium and cultured at 30 °C overnight. Next, 2 mL medium was harvested, dried *in vacuo*, re-dissolved in 200 µL DMSO and analyzed by UPLC-HRMS. The *E. coli* ROSETTA strain harboring the empty vector pRSF without the target *disA* gene was cultivated under the same conditions and analyzed by UPLC-HRMS as the negative control.

An in vitro enzymatic characterization was carried out after the purification of the His-tagged DisA. An inoculum of 15 mL of same pre-culture prepared for in vivo assay was used to inoculate 1.5 L kanamycin-containing (50 µg mL^{-1}) LB medium; 0.1 mM IPTG was added to the medium when the cultures reached an OD$_{600}$ of 0.5 and were cultured overnight. Cells were collected by centrifugation at 4 °C with 10,000 rpm and resuspended in lysis buffer (50 mM NaH$_2$PO$_4$, 300 mM NaCl and 10 mM imidazole; pH 8.0). The resulting suspensions were sonicated and centrifuged at 4 °C at maximum speed for 30 min. The supernatant was loaded onto a pre-equilibrated 750 µL Qiagen® Ni-NTA column. After washing with a 3 mL lysis buffer and 3 mL wash buffer (20 mM imidazole lysis buffer), the His-tagged protein DisA was eluted from the column using an elution buffer (250 mM imidazole lysis buffer) (Figure S49). The protein was resuspended into an imidazole-free buffer (50 mM NaH$_2$PO$_4$, 300 mM NaCl; pH 8.0) and concentrated using the Amicon® Ultra-15 centrifugation membrane column.

Enzymatic reactions were performed in 50 mM lysis buffer without imidazole (50 mM NaH$_2$PO$_4$, 300 mM NaCl, pH 8.0), containing 100 µM tryptophan (or 20 µM tyrosine) and 5 µM DisA in a total volume of 0.5 mL. After incubation at 30 °C overnight, the same volume of MeOH was added to quench the reactions. The reaction mixture was then centrifuged and the supernatant was dried and re-dissolved in 50 µL 50% MeOH and analyzed by analytical HPLC (0–16 min, 5% MeCN; 16–26 min, gradient increased from 5% to 100% MeCN).

4.4. Bioactivity Tests

Determination of the minimum inhibitory concentration (MIC) of purified compounds **1–7** was carried out by micro broth dilution assays in 96 well plates as described previously [27]. All compounds were dissolved in dimethyl sulfoxide (DMSO, Carl Roth GmbH + Co., Karlsruhe, Germany) with a concentration of 3.2 mg/mL and tested in triplicate. Dilution series (64–0.03 µg/mL) of rifampicin, tetracycline, and gentamicin (all Sigma-Aldrich, St. Louis, MS, USA) were prepared as positive controls for *B. subtilis* DSM10, *L. monocytogenes* DSM20600, *S. aureus* ATCC25923, and *E. coli* ATCC25922. Same dilution series of rifampicin, tetracycline, and isoniazid for *M. smegmatis* ATCC607. For fungi (*C. albicans* FH2173), tebuconazole (Cayman Chemical Company, Ann Arbor, MI, USA.), amphotericin B (Sigma-Aldrich, St. Louis, MS, USA) and nystatin (Sigma-Aldrich, St. Louis, MS, USA) were used as the positive control with same dilution series.

Supplementary Materials: The supporting information is available free of charge at: https://www.mdpi.com/article/10.3390/md20100620/s1, Figures S1–S48: HR-ESI-MS, HR-ESI-MS/MS and NMR spectra for compounds 1–7; Figure S49: SDS-PAGE gel of the purified His-tagged DisA (PDF).

Author Contributions: Conceptualization, L.W. and T.F.S.; methodology, L.W. and M.M.; data analysis, L.W., M.M., U.M. and Y.L.; writing—original draft preparation, L.W. and Y.L.; writing—review and editing, all authors; visualization, L.W.; supervision, project administration, and funding acquisition, T.F.S. All authors have read and agreed to the published version of the manuscript.

Funding: L.W. was funded by the China Scholarship Council (CSC NO. 201908080177). The Schäberle lab is part of the German Center of Infection Research (DZIF) and supported by the Hessen State Ministry of Higher Education, Research and the Arts (HMWK) via the LOEWE Center for Insect Biotechnology and Bioresources.

Acknowledgments: The authors would like to thank Heike Hausmann (Justus-Liebig-University Giessen, Germany) for measuring NMR spectra for structure elucidation.

Conflicts of Interest: The authors declare no conflict of interest.

References

1. Seipp, K.; Geske, L.; Opatz, T. Marine Pyrrole Alkaloids. *Mar. Drugs* **2021**, *19*, 514. [CrossRef] [PubMed]
2. Jin, Z. Muscarine, imidazole, oxazole and thiazole alkaloids. *Nat. Prod. Rep.* **2016**, *33*, 1268–1317. [CrossRef] [PubMed]
3. Chen, J.; Lv, S.; Liu, J.; Yu, Y.; Wang, H.; Zhang, H. An Overview of Bioactive 1, 3-Oxazole-Containing Alkaloids from Marine Organisms. *Pharmaceuticals* **2021**, *14*, 1274. [CrossRef] [PubMed]
4. O'Hagan, D. Pyrrole, pyrrolidine, pyridine, piperidine and tropane alkaloids. *Nat. Prod. Rep.* **2000**, *17*, 435–446. [CrossRef]
5. Ma, X.; Liang, X.; Huang, Z.H.; Qi, S.H. New alkaloids and isocoumarins from the marine gorgonian-derived fungus *Aspergillus* sp. SCSIO 41501. *Nat. Prod. Res.* **2000**, *34*, 1992–2000. [CrossRef]
6. Hassan, W.; Edrada, R.; Ebel, R.; Wray, V.; Berg, A.; Soest, R.V.; Wiryowidagdo, S.; Proksch, P. New imidazole alkaloids from the Indonesian sponge *Leucetta chagosensis*. *J. Nat. Prod.* **2004**, *67*, 817–822. [CrossRef]
7. Dyson, L.; Wright, A.D.; Young, K.A.; Sakoff, J.A.; McCluskey, A. Synthesis and anticancer activity of focused compound libraries form the natural product lead, oroidin. *Bioorg. Med. Chem.* **2014**, *22*, 1690–1699. [CrossRef]
8. Liu, L.P.; Zong, M.H.; Linhardt, R.J.; Lou, W.Y.; Li, N.; Huang, C.; Wu, H. Mechanistic insights into the effect of imidazolium ionic liquid on liquid production by *Geotrichum fermentas*. *Biotechnol. Biofuels* **2016**, *9*, 266. [CrossRef]
9. Johnson, N.A.; Southerland, M.R.; Youngs, W.J. Recent Developments in the Medicinal Applications of Silver-NHC Complexes and Imidazolium Salts. *Molecules* **2017**, *22*, 1263. [CrossRef]
10. Kirchhecker, S.; Antonietti, M.; Esposito, D. Hydrothermal decarboxylation of amino acid derived imidazolium zwitterions: A sustainable approach towards ionic liquids. *Green Chem.* **2014**, *16*, 3705–3709. [CrossRef]
11. Roué, M.; Domart-Coulon, I.; Ereskovsky, A.; Djediat, C.; Perez, T.; Bourguet-Kondracki, M.L. Cellular localization of clathridimine, an antimicrobial 2-aminoimidazole alkaloid produced by the Mediterranean calcareous sponge *Clathrina clathrus*. *J. Nat. Prod.* **2010**, *73*, 1277–1282. [CrossRef] [PubMed]
12. Bjørsvik, H.; Sandtorv, A. Synthesis of Imidazole Alkaloids Originated in Marine Sponges. In *Studies in Natural Products Chemistry*; Elsevier: Amsterdam, The Netherlands, 2014; Volume 42, pp. 33–57.
13. Dunbar, D.C.; Rimoldi, J.M.; Clark, A.M.; Kelly, M.; Hamann, M.T. Anti-cryptococcal and nitric oxide synthase inhibitory imidazole alkaloids from the calcareous sponge *Leucetta cf chagosensis*. *Tetrahedron* **2000**, *56*, 8795–8798. [CrossRef]
14. Gross, H.; Kehraus, S.; König, G.M.; Woerheide, G.; Wright, A.D. New and biologically active imidazole alkaloids from two sponges of the genus *Leucetta*. *J. Nat. Prod.* **2002**, *65*, 1190–1193. [CrossRef] [PubMed]
15. Bernardet, J.F. Family I. Flavobacteriaceae Reichenbach 1992. In *Bergey's Manual of Systematic Bacteriology*, 2nd ed.; Krieg, N.R., Staley, J.T., Brown, D.R., Hedlund, B.P., Paster, B.J., Ward, N.L., Ludwig, W., Whitman, W.B., Eds.; Springer: New York, NY, USA, 2011; Volume 4, pp. 106–111.
16. Frette, L.; Jørgensen, N.O.; Irming, H.; Kroer, N. *Tenacibaculum skagerrakense* sp. nov., a marine bacterium isolated from the pelagic zone in Skagerrak, Denmark. *Int. J. Syst. Evol. Microbiol.* **2004**, *54*, 519–524. [CrossRef]
17. Yoon, J.H.; Kang, S.J.; Jung, S.Y.; Oh, H.W.; Oh, T.K. *Gaetbulimicrobium brevivitae* gen. nov., sp. nov., a novel member of the family *Flavobacteriaceae* isolated from a tidal flat of the Yellow Sea in Korea. *Int. J. Syst. Evol. Microbiol.* **2006**, *56*, 115–119. [CrossRef]
18. Heindl, H.; Wiese, J.; Imhoff, J.F. *Tenacibaculum adriaticum* sp. nov., from a bryozoan in the Adriatic Sea. *Int. J. Syst. Evol. Microbiol.* **2008**, *58*, 542–547. [CrossRef]
19. Wang, J.T.; Chou, Y.J.; Chou, J.H.; Chen, C.A.; Chen, W.M. *Tenacibaculum aiptasiae* sp. nov., isolated from a sea anemone *Aiptasia pulchella*. *Int. J. Syst. Evol. Microbiol.* **2008**, *58*, 761–766. [CrossRef]
20. Lee, Y.S.; Baik, K.S.; Park, S.Y.; Kim, E.M.; Lee, D.H.; Kahng, H.Y.; Jeon, C.O.; Jung, J.S. *Tenacibaculum crassostreae* sp. nov., isolated from the Pacific oyster, *Crassostrea gigas*. *Int. J. Syst. Evol. Microbiol.* **2009**, *59*, 1609–1614. [CrossRef]
21. Pineiro-Vidal, M.; Riaza, A.; Santos, Y. *Tenacibaculum discolor* sp. nov. and *Tenacibaculum gallaicum* sp. nov., isolated from sole (*Solea senegalensis*) and turbot (*Psetta maxima*) culture systems. *Int. J. Syst. Evol. Microbiol.* **2008**, *58*, 21–25. [CrossRef]
22. Suzuki, M.; Nakagawa, Y.; Harayama, S.; Yamamoto, S. Phylogenetic analysis and taxonomic study of marine *Cytophaga*-like bacteria: Proposal for *Tenacibaculum* gen. nov. with *Tenacibaculum maritimum* comb. nov. and *Tenacibaculum ovolyticum* comb. nov., and description of *Tenacibaculum mesophilum* sp. nov. and *Tenacibaculum amylolyticum* sp. nov. *Int. J. Syst. Evol. Microbiol.* **2001**, *51*, 1639–1652.
23. Avendaño-Herrera, R.; Toranzo, A.E.; Magariños, B. Tenacibaculosis infection in marine fish caused by *Tenacibaculum maritimum*: A review. *Dis. Aquat. Organ.* **2006**, *71*, 255–266. [CrossRef] [PubMed]
24. Igarashi, Y.; Ge, Y.; Zhou, T.; Sharma, A.R.; Harunari, E.; Oku, N.; Trianto, A. Tenacibactins K–M, cytotoxic siderophores from a coral-associated gliding bacterium of the genus *Tenacibaculum*. *Beilstein. J. Org. Chem.* **2022**, *18*, 110–119. [CrossRef] [PubMed]

25. Jang, J.H.; Kanoh, K.; Adachi, K.; Matsuda, S.; Shizuri, Y. Tenacibactins a-d, hydroxamate siderophores from a marine-derived bacterium, *Tenacibaculum* sp. a4k-17. *J. Nat. Prod.* **2007**, *70*, 563–566. [CrossRef] [PubMed]
26. Fujita, M.J.; Nakano, K.; Sakai, R. Bisucaberin B, a Linear Hydroxamate Class Siderophore from the Marine Bacterium *Tenacibaculum mesophilum*. *Molecules* **2013**, *18*, 3917–3926. [CrossRef] [PubMed]
27. Wang, L.; Linares-Otoya, V.; Liu, Y.; Mettal, U.; Marner, M.; Armas Mantilla, L.; Willbold, S.; Kurtán, T.; Linares-Otoya, L.; Schäberle, T.F. Discovery and Biosynthesis of Antimicrobial Phenethylamine Alkaloids from the Marine Flavobacterium *Tenacibaculum discolor* sv11. *J. Nat. Prod.* **2022**, *85*, 1039–1051. [CrossRef]
28. Yan, J.X.; Wu, Q.; Helfrich, E.J.N.; Chevrette, M.G.; Braun, D.R.; Heyman, H.; Ananiev, G.E.; Rajski, S.R.; Currie, C.R.; Clardy, J.; et al. Bacillimidazoles A-F, Imidazolium-Containing Compounds Isolated from a Marine *Bacillus*. *Mar. Drugs* **2022**, *20*, 43. [CrossRef]
29. Silverstein, R.M.; Webster, F.X.; Kiemle, D.J.; Bryce, D.L. *Spectrometric Identification of Organic Compounds*, 8th ed.; John Wiley & Sons, Inc.: New York, NY, USA, 2015; pp. 299–305.
30. Zeng, Z.; Qasem, A.M.A.; Woodman, T.J.; Rowan, M.G.; Blagbrough, I.S. Impacts of Steric Compression, Protonation, and Intramolecular Hydrogen Bonding on the ^{15}N NMR Spectroscopy of Norditerpenoid Alkaloids and Their Piperidine-Ring Analogues. *ACS Omega* **2020**, *5*, 14116–14122. [CrossRef]
31. Wang, F.P.; Chen, D.L.; Deng, H.Y.; Chen, Q.H.; Liu, X.Y.; Jian, X.X. Further revisions on the diterpenoid alkaloids reported in a JNP paper (**2012**, *75*, 1145–1159). *Tetrahedron* **2014**, *70*, 2582–2590. [CrossRef]
32. Güntzel, P.; Schilling, K.; Hanio, S.; Schlauersbach, J.; Schollmayer, C.; Meinel, L.; Holzgrabe, U. Bioinspired Ion Pairs Transforming Papaverine into a Protic Ionic Liquid and Salts. *ACS Omega* **2020**, *5*, 19202–19209. [CrossRef]
33. Wu, L.X.; Xu, X.D.; Chen, X.; Miao, C.P.; Chen, Y.W.; Xu, L.H.; Zhao, L.X.; Li, Y.Q. Indole and tyramine alkaloids produced by an endophytic actinomycete associated with Artemisia annua. *Chem. Nat. Compd.* **2017**, *53*, 999–1001. [CrossRef]
34. Wright, B.D.; Deblock, M.C.; Wagers, P.O.; Duah, E.; Robishaw, N.K.; Shelton, K.L.; Southerland, M.R.; DeBord, M.A.; Kersten, K.M.; McDonald, L.J.; et al. Anti-tumor activity of lipophilic imidazolium salts on select NSCLC cell lines. *Med. Chem. Res.* **2015**, *24*, 2838–2861. [CrossRef] [PubMed]

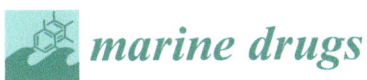

Article

A Series of New Pyrrole Alkaloids with ALR2 Inhibitory Activities from the Sponge *Stylissa massa*

Qi Wang [1,†], Chunhua Gao [1,†], Zhun Wei [1], Xiaowen Tang [1], Lixia Ji [1], Xiangchao Luo [2], Xiaoping Peng [1], Gang Li [1] and Hongxiang Lou [1,*]

[1] Department of Natural Medicinal Chemistry and Pharmacognosy, School of Pharmacy, Qingdao University, Qingdao 266021, China; wangqi@hmfl.ac.cn (Q.W.); gaochunhua@qdu.edu.cn (C.G.); biowei@qdu.edu.cn (Z.W.); xwtang1219@qdu.edu.cn (X.T.); lixiaji@qdu.edu.cn (L.J.); pengxiaoping@qdu.edu.cn (X.P.); gang.li@qdu.edu.cn (G.L.)

[2] Research Center for Marine Drugs, Department of Pharmacy, Ren Ji Hospital, School of Medicine, Shanghai Jiao Tong University, Shanghai, 200127, China; luoxiangchao@renji.com

* Correspondence: louhongxiang@sdu.edu.cn
† The authors contributed equally to this work.

Abstract: Twelve new and four known alkaloids including five different structural scaffolds were isolated from the sponge *Stylissa massa* collected in the South China Sea. Compound **1** is the first identified precursor metabolite of the classic 5/7/5 tricyclic skeleton with unesterified guanidine and carboxyl groups, compounds **2–5** and **13–15** belong to the spongiacidin-type pyrrole imidazole alkaloids (PIAs). Z- and E-configurations of the spongiacidin-type PIAs often appeared concomitantly and were distinguished by the chemical shift analysis of ^{13}C NMR spectra. The structures of all twelve new compounds were determined by NMR, MS, and ECD analysis combined with single-crystal data of compounds **1**, **5**, and **10**. In the aldose reductase (ALR2) inhibitory assay, six 5/7/5 tricyclic compounds (**2–5, 13–15**) displayed significant activities. Compounds **13** and **14**, as the representative members of spongiacidin-PIAs, demonstrated their ALR2-targeted activities in SPR experiments with K_D values of 12.5 and 6.9 µM, respectively.

Keywords: pyrrole-imidazole alkaloids; ALR2 inhibitory activities; sponge; *Stylissa massa*; spongiacidin

Citation: Wang, Q.; Gao, C.; Wei, Z.; Tang, X.; Ji, L.; Luo, X.; Peng, X.; Li, G.; Lou, H. A Series of New Pyrrole Alkaloids with ALR2 Inhibitory Activities from the Sponge *Stylissa massa*. *Mar. Drugs* **2022**, *20*, 454. https://doi.org/10.3390/md20070454

Academic Editor: Asunción Barbero

Received: 20 June 2022
Accepted: 8 July 2022
Published: 12 July 2022

Publisher's Note: MDPI stays neutral with regard to jurisdictional claims in published maps and institutional affiliations.

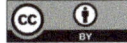

Copyright: © 2022 by the authors. Licensee MDPI, Basel, Switzerland. This article is an open access article distributed under the terms and conditions of the Creative Commons Attribution (CC BY) license (https://creativecommons.org/licenses/by/4.0/).

1. Introduction

Pyrrole-imidazole alkaloids (PIAs) and simple pyrrole alkaloids represent a specific structural class of compounds isolated from sponges including those from the genus *Agelas*, *Axinella*, *Hymeniacidon*, *Phakellia* and *Stylissa* [1–5]. PIAs can be divided into monomeric and polymeric groups. Like sceptrin[1], palau'amine [6], ageliferin [7], and stylissadine [8] represent members of polymeric PIAs. Biosynthesis of mono-PIAs originates from proline and lysine [9], evolving to form several skeletons such as oroidin [10], phakellin [11], ugibohlin [12], and spongiacidin types [13], which have 5/5 bicyclic, 5/6/5 tetracyclic, 5/6/5 tricyclic, and 5/7/5 tricyclic systems, respectively. Currently, although hundreds of PIAs have been discovered from sponges, the structural diversity of this alkaloid family, especially for the monomeric ones, is relatively conservative.

We collected the *Stylissa massa* sponge from the Xisha Islands (Paracel island) in the South China Sea. Targeted isolation for methanol extraction yielded twelve new and four known compounds. Five biosynthetic-related PIA skeletons including the 5/7 imidazole-acyclic compound **1**, 5/7/5 spongiacidins (**2–5**, and **13–15**), 5/6/5/5 phakellins (**6** and **16**), 5/7 bicyclic (**7–9**), and pyrrole single ring alkaloids (**10–12**) were obtained from *Stylissa massa*. Compound **1** is the first identified precursor metabolite of the classic 5/7/5 tricyclic skeleton with unesterified guanidine and carboxyl groups. Compounds **2a** and **2b** are a scalemic mixture with a hydroxyl group positioned at C-9. Compounds **3a** and **3b** are also scalemic mixture compounds with the E-configuration of $\Delta^{10,11}$ versus the

Z-configuration of **2**. Compound **4** has a hydroxide at C-9 with a double bond $\Delta^{9,10}$ at a different position, and the new compound **5** has an extra methyl group at 13-NH.

Guanidine compounds often exhibit effective diabetes related activities [14]. ALR2 is a key limiting enzyme of the glucose polyol metabolic pathway, which is the key target for the treatment of diabetes complications [15]. In the ALR2 enzyme activity assay in vitro, spongiacidin-type PIAs (compounds **2–5**, and **13–15**) presented superior inhibitory activities than the other skeletons at 20 μM. The IC$_{50}$ values ranged from 8.6 to 13.6 μM, respectively (Figure S23). The SPR experiments verified the interaction between ALR2 and compound **14**, with the K$_D$ value of 6.9 μM. In summary, spongiacidin-PIAs are efficient ALR2-targeted inhibitors with 5/7/5 tricyclic skeletons. Thus, the structural elucidation and the ALR2 inhibitory activities of these PIAs are concluded below (Figure 1).

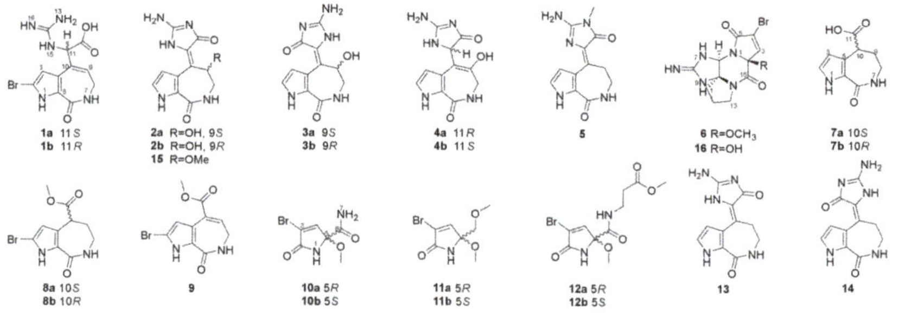

Figure 1. The structures of compounds **1–16**.

2. Results

Compound **1** was obtained as a colorless bulk crystal. Its molecular formula $C_{11}H_{12}BrN_5O_3$ was determined by HRESIMS with the ion peak at *m/z* 342.0197, and 344.0170 with the proportion of 1:1 (calcd. for [M + H]$^+$ *m/z* 342.0196, and 344.0176), with the unsaturation degree of 8. The ^{13}C NMR and DEPT spectra revealed 11 resonances (Table S1) including one methylene, three methines, and seven non-protonated carbons. The chemical shifts ranging from δ_C 104.3 to 133.6 ppm showed six olefinic carbons, which included two methines and four non-protonated carbons. In the low field of the ^{13}C NMR spectrum with the chemical shifts of δ_C 170.5, 162.1, and 156.4, there could be two carbonyl groups and one guanidyl group that exist in this molecule. The ^{1}H NMR and HSQC spectra (Table S2) showed the presence of two olefinic protons at δ_H 6.36 (1H, d, *J* = 2.3 Hz), and δ_H 6.04 (1H, t, *J* = 6.8 Hz), one methine proton at δ_H 5.21 (1H, d, *J* = 8.5 Hz), and one methylene proton at δ_H 3.42 (2H, m), and there were three additional heteroatomic protons at δ_H 12.71 (brs), δ_H 7.80 (1H, d, *J* = 8.3 Hz), and δ_H 7.79 (1H, q, *J* = 4.7 Hz). The ^{1}H-^{1}H COSY spectrum (Figure 2) revealed a pyrrole conjugate ring system and another spin system with the correlations between 1-NH and H-3, between 15-NH and H-11, between 7-NH and H$_2$-8, and between H$_2$-8 and H-9. Key HMBC correlations (Figure 2) of 1-NH/C-3, C-4, and C-5, H-3/C-2, and C-4, 7-NH/C-5, and C-9, H$_2$-8/C-6, C-9, and C-10, H-9/C-4, C-8, and C-10 determined the existence of a 5/7 bicyclic 2-bromo-6,7-dihydropyrrolo [2,3-*c*] azepin-8(1*H*)-one skeleton (Figure 2). The already existential bicyclic skeleton and four double bonds occupied six degrees of unsaturation, and the remaining two degrees pointed out that there was no other ring systems in compound **1**. The final planar structure of compound **1** was settled down by the HMBC correlations from H-11 to C-4, C-9, C-10, C-12, and C-14, together with the correlations from H-9 to C-11 as well as 15-NH to C-12. A suitable bulk single crystal of compound **1** was obtained to perform the X-ray diffraction experiment, which ensured the planar structure of **1** (Figure 3). The space group of **1** indicated that it was a scalemic mixture, and ECD calculation finally determined the absolute configurations of **1a** and **1b** isolated through chiral HPLC by comparison with each of their ECD spectra (Figures S1 and S2).

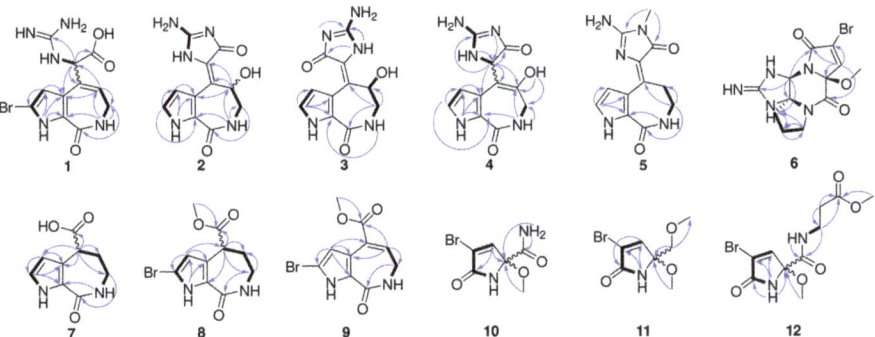

Figure 2. The key COSY (bolds), and HMBC (arrows) correlations of **1–12**.

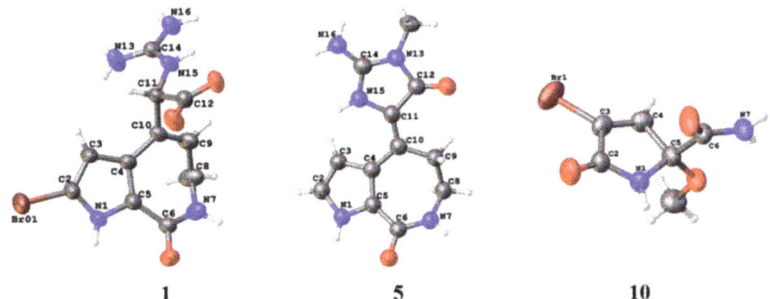

Figure 3. The X-ray structures of compounds **1**, **5**, and **10**.

Compound **2** was obtained as a yellow oil and its molecular formula was determined as $C_{11}H_{11}N_5O_3$ by the $[M + H]^+$ ion peak presented at m/z 262.0936 (calcd. $C_{11}H_{12}N_5O_3$ for m/z 262.0935) in the HRESIMS spectrum with nine unsaturation degrees. One more unsaturation degree and the similar chemical shifts of the carbons (Table S1) with **1** indicated that compound **2** may have a 5/7/5 tricyclic spongiacidin-PIA skeleton, close to the known compound **13**. The HMBC correlations (Figure 2) of 1-NH/C-3, and C-4, H-2/C-3, C-4, and C-5, H-3/C-2, C-4, and C-5, 7-NH/C-5, C-8, and C-9, H_2-8/C-6, C-9, and C-10, and H-9/C-2, C-4, C-10, and C-11, together with the COSY correlations of 1-NH/H-2/H-3, and 7-NH/H_2-8/H-9, constructed the classic 5/7/5 tricyclic structure with the hydroxyl group substituted at C-9, taking the chemical shift of C-9 (δ_C 62.8) into consideration. Thus, the planar structure of **2** was established.

The 1D and 2D NMR spectra as well as the HRESIMS spectrum indicated that compound **3** possessed the same planar structure with **2** (Figure 2). The Z- and E-configuration of double bond $\Delta^{10,11}$ in spongiacidin-type PIAs often concomitantly appeared and their differences can be attributed to the anisotropic effect of the carbonyl at C-12 [16]. Two configurations of known compounds **13** and **14** could be distinguished by the chemical shift values of H-3 and H_2-9, but the existence of 9-OH substituted in compounds **2** and **3** made it so that the judgement rule did not work [compound **2**: δ_H 6.45 (H-3), 5.80 (H-9); compound **3**: δ_H 6.43 (H-3), 5.83 (H-9)]. Through careful analysis of their ^{13}C NMR spectra, we found the double bonds of compounds **2** and **13** could be in the Z-configuration [16] because the signals for C-4, C-10, C-11, C-12, and C-14 were weak compared with the stronger signals for C-2, C-3, C-5, C-6, C-8, and C-9, while the carbon signals of compounds **3** and **14** were distributed on average comparatively (Figure 4). Known compound **15** co-isolated was also determined to be of a Z-configuration with the evidence of its carbon signal analysis in the ^{13}C NMR spectrum. Thus, the double bond of $\Delta^{10,11}$ in compound **2** was determined as the Z-configuration and compound **3** was the E-configuration. C-9's absolute configurations of compounds **2a**, **2b** and **3a**, **3b** were all identified based on the ECD calculations together with the chiral HPLC method (Figures S3–S6).

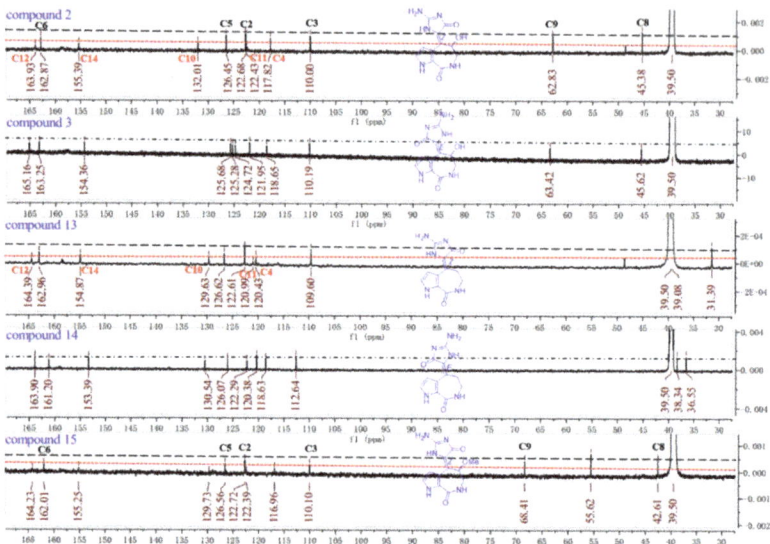

Figure 4. The comparison of the ^{13}C NMR spectra of compounds **2**, **3**, **13**, **14**, and **15** (125 MHz, DMSO-d_6).

Compound **4** is a molecule similar to compounds **2** and **3**, with the same molecular formula $C_{11}H_{11}N_5O_3$ by the [M + H]$^+$ ion peak presented at m/z 262.0931 (calcd. for m/z $C_{11}H_{12}N_5O_3$ 262.0935) in the HRESIMS spectrum. The key ^{1}H-^{1}H COSY correlations between 7-NH and H$_2$-8, and between H-11 and 15-NH uncovered the different structure of **4**, and its final planar structure was determined by the HMBC correlations from 1-NH to C-2, C-3, C-4, and C-5, from H-2 to C-3, C-4, and C-5, from H-3 to C-2, C-4, C-5, and C-10, from 7-NH to C-5, C-8, and C-9, from H-8 to C-6, C-9, and C-10, from H-11 to C-4, C-9, C-10, C-12, and C-14, from 15-NH to C-10, and from 9-OH to C-8, C-9, and C-10 (Figure 2). ECD calculation was also carried out to determine the absolute configurations of **4a** and **4b** (Figures S7 and S8).

Compound **5** was obtained as colorless bulk crystals. Its molecular formula was determined to be $C_{12}H_{13}N_5O_2$ by HRESIMS (m/z 260.1148, calcd. [M + H]$^+$ for m/z 260.1142), which required nine degrees of unsaturation. The 1D and 2D NMR data revealed its similarity with the known compound **13**, with the only difference at 13-NMe with the extra signals of δ_H 3.11 and δ_C 25.8 in the ^{1}H and ^{13}C NMR spectra (Tables S1 and S2). The HMBC correlations from 13-NMe to C-12 and C-14 further confirmed the planar structure of **5** (Figure 2). Fortunately, a suitable bulk crystal was obtained followed by X-ray diffraction (Figure 3), and the result showed that the previously proposed rule of distinguishing Z/E configurations of double bond $\Delta^{10,11}$ in 5/7/5 spongiacidin-type PIAs was trustworthy.

The molecular formula of compound **6**, obtained as a yellow oil, was determined to be $C_{12}H_{14}BrN_5O_3$, according to the HRESIMS results, which showed a protonated molecular ion at m/z 356.0357, 358.0329 (calcd. for [M + H]$^+$, m/z 356.0353, 358.0332). The analysis of the 1D and 2D NMR spectra (Tables S3 and S4) of **6** indicated that it had a very similar structure with the reported compound (**16**) obtained by organic synthesis [17], with the only difference of 2-OMe rather than 2-OH. The relative configuration of **6** was determined by DP4+ analysis, where the results showed that the only possibility was 2R*6R*10S*, and further ECD calculations confirmed the absolute configuration of **6** was 2S6S10R (Figures S9 and S10).

Compounds **7–9** were 5/7 bicyclic pyrrole alkaloids, in which compounds **8** and **9** were 2-bromo substituted ones. Their structures were confirmed by HRESIMS and NMR data (Tables S3 and S4). Compounds **7** and **8** were two pairs of scalemic mixture, and their absolute configurations were solved by the chiral HPLC and ECD calculation method (Figures S11–S14).

Compounds **10–12** were simple pyrrole alkaloids with the 2-carboxyl and 3-bromo characteristic, which were pairs of scalemic mixture. Their planar structures were determined by HRESIMS, NMR (Tables S3 and S4), and single crystal X-ray diffraction (Figure 3), and the absolute configurations were confirmed by chiral HPLC and ECD calculations (Figures S15–S20).

Five characteristic skeletons of the alkaloids (**1–12**) above-mentioned were isolated from the sponge *Stylissa massa*. Compound **1** was the first identified precursor metabolite of the classic 5/7/5 tricyclic skeleton with unesterified guanidine and carboxyl groups. Through the NMR data analysis of compounds **2**, **3**, **13**, **14**, and **15**, an experience rule to determine the Z/E configurations of double bond $\Delta^{10,11}$ was summarized based on the signal intensity in the ^{13}C NMR spectra (Figure 4).

Some guanidine compounds were reported to exhibit advantageous biological activities on diabetes [14], which indicated the following aldose reductase (ALR2) assay in vitro. We successfully obtained the protein AKR1B1 (ALR2) by genetic engineering methods (Figure S21) and compounds **1–16** were tested. Compounds **2–5** and **13–15**, representative of 5/7/5 tricyclic spogiacidin-type PIA compounds, displayed superior inhibitory activities compared with other compounds (Figure S22) with epalrestat as the positive control. Further concentration gradient experiments carried out to calculate their IC_{50} values showed results that ranged from 8.6 to 13.6 µM (Figure S23). The analysis of the structure–activity relationships indicated that 9-OH and 13-NMe may enhance the ALR2 inhibitory activities of this spongiacidin-alkaloid family. Compounds **13** and **14** with the basic 5/7/5 spongiacidin skeleton without stereoscopic configuration were isolated as the major metabolites in sponge *Stylissa massa*. In order to research the interaction mechanism between spongiacidin-skeleton compounds and ALR2, we carried out surface plasmon resonance (SPR) binding assays of compounds **13** and **14** under the Biacore T200 instrument, where the results showed the binding power (K_D value) between ALR2 and compound **13** was 12.5 µM (Figure S24), and **14** was 6.9 µM (Figures 5 and S25). Molecular docking using the GBVI/WSA ΔG rescoring method was applied to screen the best docking pose between ALR2 and compound **14**. The results showed that the pyrrole and imidazole ring systems were binding to the pocket of ALR2 by H–π and π–π conjugate bonds, respectively (Figure 5).

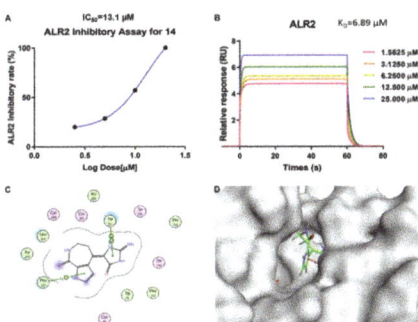

Figure 5. The ALR2 inhibitory activity for compound **14**. (**A**) Concentration dependent curve of the ALR2 inhibitory assay for **14**. (**B**) The result of the surface plasmon resonance (SPR) binding assay of **14** and ALR2 with a K_D value of 6.89 µM. (**C**) Ligand interactions between ALR2 and **14**. (**D**) The 3D binding model of compound **14** with ALR2, the surface of the protein is shown in grey, and the interaction bond is shown in the red dotted line.

3. Materials and Methods

3.1. General Experimental Procedures

Optical rotations were measured on a JASCO P-1020 digital polarimeter. UV and ECD spectra were obtained on a Jasco J-810 spectropolarimeter (Tokyo, Japan). The NMR spectra were measured by a Bruker AVANCE III 500 MHz spectrometer (Bruker company, Fällanden, Switzerland). The 2.50 ppm and 39.5 ppm resonances of DMSO-d_6 were used as internal references for the ^{1}H and ^{13}C NMR spectra, respectively. HRESIMS data were measured on Micromass Q-Tof Ultima Global GAA076LC (Waters, Milford, CT, USA) and Thermo Scientific LTQ Orbitrap Exploris 480 mass spectrometers (Waltham, MA, USA). X-ray data were obtained by a Rigaku Xtalab Synergy using Cu-Kα radiation (Tokyo, Japan). Semi-preparative HPLC utilized an ODS column (Agilent XDB C-18, 9.6 × 250 mm, 5 μm). Silica gel (200–400 mesh, Qingdao, China) was used for column chromatography, precoated silica gel plates (GF254, Qingdao, China) were used for TLC, and spots were visualized by heating SiO$_2$ plates sprayed with 10% H$_2$SO$_4$ in EtOH.

3.2. Sponge Material

The marine sponge *Stylissa massa* was collected from the Xisha Islands of the South China Sea in June 2013, and was frozen immediately after collection. The specimen was identified by Nicole J. de Voogd, National Museum of Natural History, Leiden, The Netherlands. The voucher specimen (No. XS-2013-07) was deposited at lab A1007, School of Pharmacy, Qingdao University, P. R. China.

3.3. Extraction and Isolation

Stylissa massa (8.0 kg, wet weight) was crushed and then extracted with MeOH four times (3 days each time) at room temperature. The combined solutions were concentrated in vacuo and the residue was subsequently desalted to yield the organic extract (191.0 g). The extract was subjected to silica gel vacuum liquid chromatography (VLC), eluting with a gradient of petroleum ether/EtOAc (from 10:1 to 0:1, *v:v*) and subsequently CH$_2$Cl$_2$/MeOH (from 10:1 to 0:1, *v:v*) to obtain 17 fractions (Fr.1–Fr.17). Fr.5 (0.5 g) was subjected to a silica gel CC (CH$_2$Cl$_2$/MeOH, 20:1, *v:v*) to give three fractions Fr.5-1–Fr.5-3. Fr.5-1 (200 mg) was then subjected to a silica gel CC (petroleum ether/EtOAc, from 5:1 to 1:1, *v:v*) to give five fractions Fr.5-1-1–Fr.5-1-5. Fr.5-1-2 was then purified by semi-preparative HPLC (ODS, 5 μm, 250 × 9.6 mm; MeOH/H$_2$O, 25:75, *v/v*; 2.0 mL/min, 33 min) to afford compound **12** (t_R = 21.8 min, 1.0 mg) and compound **11** (t_R = 24.3 min, 1.0 mg). Fr.7 (3.0 g) was subjected to an ODS CC (MeOH/H$_2$O, from 5:95 to 100:0, *v:v*) to give six fractions Fr.7-1–Fr.7-6. Fr.7-2 was then purified by semi-preparative HPLC (ODS, 5 μm, 250 × 9.6 mm; MeOH/H$_2$O, 20:80–60:40, *v/v*; 2.0 mL/min, 45 min) to afford compound **10** (t_R = 19.5 min, 3.0 mg). Fr.7-6 was purified by semi-preparative HPLC (ODS, 5 μm, 250 × 9.6 mm; MeOH/H$_2$O, 5:95–100:0, *v/v*; 2.0 mL/min, 48 min) to afford compound **8** (t_R = 40.3 min, 5.8 mg) and compound **9** (t_R = 45.0 min, 4.0 mg). Fr.8 (14.5 g) was subjected to a silica gel CC (CH$_2$Cl$_2$/MeOH, 50:1–1:1, *v:v*) to give nine fractions Fr.8-1–Fr.8-9. Fr.8-1 (5.0 g) was then subjected to a ODS CC (MeOH/H$_2$O, 50:1–1:1, *v:v*) to give five fractions Fr.8-1-1–Fr.8-1-5. Fr.8-1-3 was then purified by semi-preparative HPLC (ODS, 5 μm, 250 × 9.6 mm; MeOH/H$_2$O, 5:95–100:0, *v/v*; 2.0 mL/min, 35 min) to afford compound **16** (t_R = 19.2 min, 2.0 mg), compound **6** (t_R = 23.8 min, 3.7 mg) and compound **7** (t_R = 23.9 min, 3.0 mg). Fr.8-1-5 (4.0 g) was purified subjected to an ODS CC (MeOH/H$_2$O, from 5:95 to 100:0, *v:v*) to give six fractions Fr.8-1-5-1–Fr.8-1-5-6. Fr.8-1-5-4 (200 mg) was purified by semi-preparative HPLC (ODS, 5 μm, 250 × 9.6 mm; MeOH/H$_2$O, 5:95–100:0, *v/v*; 2.0 mL/min, 36 min) to afford compound **3** (t_R = 21.1 min, 2.6 mg), compound **5** (t_R = 26.1 min, 3.7 mg), and compound **13** (t_R = 24.7 min, 200 mg). Fr.15 (17.2 g) was subjected to a silica gel CC (CH$_2$Cl$_2$/MeOH, from 10:1 to 1:1, *v:v*) to give four fractions Fr.15-1–Fr.15-4. Fr.15-2 (1.1 g) was then subjected to an ODS CC (MeOH/H$_2$O, from 5:95 to 100:0, *v:v*) to give six fractions Fr.15-2-1–Fr.15-2-6. Fr.15-2-4 (300 mg) was then purified by semi-preparative HPLC (ODS, 5 μm, 250 × 9.6 mm; MeOH/H$_2$O, 10:90, *v/v*; 2.0 mL/min, 55 min) to afford compound **2** (t_R = 29.1 min, 16.0 mg), compound **15** (t_R = 44.3 min, 6.0 mg), and compound **14** (t_R = 47.5 min, 150 mg). Fr.17 (20.0 g) was subjected to an ODS CC (MeOH/H$_2$O, from 5:95 to 100:0, v:v) to give seven fractions Fr.17-1–Fr.17-7. Fr.17-3 (800 mg) was then subjected to a silica gel CC (CH$_2$Cl$_2$/MeOH, from 10:1 to 1:1, v:v) to give six fractions Fr.17-3-1–Fr.17-3-6. Fr.17-3-3 was then purified by semi-preparative HPLC (ODS, 5 μm, 250 × 9.6 mm; MeOH/H$_2$O, 5:90–100:0, v/v; 2.0 mL/min, 40 min) to afford compound **4** (t_R = 18.5 min, 6.8 mg). Fr.17-3-4 was then purified by semi-preparative HPLC (ODS, 5 μm, 250 × 9.6 mm; MeOH/H$_2$O, 5:90–100:0, v/v; 2.0 mL/min, 38min) to afford compound **1** (t_R = 21.2 min, 5.9 mg).

Compound **1**: Colorless crystals; UV (MeOH) λ_{max} 226 nm; ^{1}H and ^{13}C NMR (DMSO-d_6) data, see Tables S1 and S2; HRESIMS m/z 342.0184, 344.0162 ([M + H]$^+$ (calcd. for C$_{11}$H$_{13}$BrN$_5$O$_3$, 342.0184, 344.0165); compound **1a**: $[\alpha]_D^{20}$ −19.7 (c 0.1, MeOH), compound **1b**: $[\alpha]_D^{20}$ 27.3 (c 0.1, MeOH).

Compound **2**: Yellow oil; UV (MeOH) λ_{max} 354 nm; ^{1}H and ^{13}C NMR (DMSO-d_6) data, see Tables S1 and S2; HRESIMS m/z 262.0936 ([M + H]$^+$ (calcd. for C$_{11}$H$_{12}$N$_5$O$_3$, 262.0935); compound **2a**: $[\alpha]_D^{20}$ −40.3 (c 0.1, MeOH), compound **2b**: $[\alpha]_D^{20}$ 34.5 (c 0.1, MeOH).

Compound **3**: Yellow oil; UV (MeOH) λ_{max} 346 nm; ^{1}H and ^{13}C NMR (DMSO-d_6) data, see Tables S1 and S2; HRESIMS m/z 262.0933 ([M + H]$^+$ (calcd. for C$_{11}$H$_{12}$N$_5$O$_3$, 262.0935); compound **3a**: $[\alpha]_D^{20}$ −29.8 (c 0.1, MeOH), compound **3b**: $[\alpha]_D^{20}$ 36.3 (c 0.1, MeOH).

Compound **4**: Yellow oil; UV (MeOH) λ_{max} 346 nm; ^{1}H and ^{13}C NMR (DMSO-d_6) data, see Tables S1 and S2; HRESIMS m/z 262.0931 ([M + H]$^+$ (calcd. for C$_{11}$H$_{12}$N$_5$O$_3$, 262.0935); compound **4a**: $[\alpha]_D^{20}$ 30.1 (c 0.1, MeOH), compound **4b**: $[\alpha]_D^{20}$ −18.4 (c 0.1, MeOH).

Compound **5**: Colorless crystals; UV (MeOH) λ_{max} 354 nm; ^{1}H and ^{13}C NMR (DMSO-d_6) data, see Tables S1 and S2; HRESIMS m/z 260.1148 ([M + H]$^+$ (calcd. for C$_{12}$H$_{14}$N$_5$O$_2$, 260.1142).

Compound **6**: Yellow oil; UV (MeOH) λ_{max} 216 nm; ^{1}H and ^{13}C NMR (DMSO-d_6) data, see Tables S3 and S4; HRESIMS m/z 356.0357, 358.0353 ([M + H]$^+$ (calcd. for C$_{12}$H$_{15}$BrN$_5$O$_3$, 356.0353, 358.0332); $[\alpha]_D^{20}$ −19.5 (c 0.1, MeOH).

Compound **7**: Yellow oil; UV (MeOH) λ_{max} 216 nm; ^{1}H and ^{13}C NMR (DMSO-d_6) data, see Tables S3 and S4; HRESIMS m/z 195.0770 ([M + H]$^+$ (calcd. for C$_9$H$_{11}$N$_2$O$_3$, 195.0764); compound **7a**: $[\alpha]_D^{20}$ 27.7 (c 0.1, MeOH), compound **7b**: $[\alpha]_D^{20}$ −24.1 (c 0.1, MeOH).

Compound **8**: Yellow oil; UV (MeOH) λ_{max} 276 nm; ^{1}H and ^{13}C NMR (DMSO-d_6) data, see Tables S3 and S4; HRESIMS m/z 287.0025, 289.0003 ([M + H]$^+$ (calcd. for C$_{10}$H$_{12}$BrN$_2$O$_3$, 287.0026, 289.0005); compound **8a**: $[\alpha]_D^{20}$ 23.3 (c 0.1, MeOH), compound **8b**: $[\alpha]_D^{20}$ −20.8 (c 0.1, MeOH).

Compound **9**: Yellow oil; UV (MeOH) λ_{max} 250 nm; ^{1}H and ^{13}C NMR (DMSO-d_6) data, see Tables S3 and S4; HRESIMS m/z 284.9867, 286.9845 ([M + H]$^+$ (calcd. for C$_{10}$H$_{10}$BrN$_2$O$_3$, 284.9869, 286.9849).

Compound **10**: Colorless crystals; UV (MeOH) λ_{max} 240 nm; ^{1}H and ^{13}C NMR (DMSO-d_6) data, see Tables S3 and S4; HRESIMS m/z 234.9715, 236.9695 ([M + H]$^+$ (calcd. for C$_6$H$_8$BrN$_2$O$_3$, 234.9713, 236.9692); compound **10a**: $[\alpha]_D^{20}$ 26.8 (c 0.1, MeOH), compound **10b**: $[\alpha]_D^{20}$ −32.4 (c 0.1, MeOH).

Compound **11**: Yellow oil; UV (MeOH) λ_{max} 216 nm; ^{1}H and ^{13}C NMR (DMSO-d_6) data, see Tables S3 and S4; HRESIMS m/z 235.9920, 237.9899 ([M + H]$^+$ (calcd. for C$_7$H$_{11}$BrNO$_3$, 235.9920, 237.9899); compound **11a**: $[\alpha]_D^{20}$ 52.9 (c 0.1, MeOH), compound **11b**: $[\alpha]_D^{20}$ −46.5 (c 0.1, MeOH).

Compound **12**: Yellow oil; UV (MeOH) λ_{max} 212 nm; ^{1}H and ^{13}C NMR (DMSO-d_6) data, see Tables S3 and S4; HRESIMS m/z 321.0073, 323.0053 ([M + H]$^+$ (calcd. for C$_{10}$H$_{14}$BrN$_2$O$_5$, 321.0081, 323.0060); compound **12a**: $[\alpha]_D^{20}$ 20.0 (c 0.1, MeOH), compound **12b**: $[\alpha]_D^{20}$ −13.3 (c 0.1, MeOH).

Compound **13**: Yellow oil; UV (MeOH) λ_{max} 352 nm; C$_{11}$H$_{11}$N$_5$O$_2$; ^{1}H NMR (DMSO-d_6) data, δ_H 12.1 (brs, 1-NH), 8.04 (t, J = 4.3, 7-NH), 7.11 (t, J = 2.4, H-2), 6.54 (t, J = 2.4, H-3), 3.28 (m, H$_2$-8 and H$_2$-9); ^{13}C NMR (DMSO-d_6) data, δ_C 164.4, 163.0, 154.9, 129.6, 126.6, 122.6, 121.0, 120.4, 109.6, 39.1, and 31.4. [18]

Compound **14**: Yellow oil; UV (MeOH) λ$_{max}$ 352 nm; C$_{11}$H$_{11}$N$_5$O$_2$; ^{1}H NMR (DMSO-d_6) data, δ_H 11.9 (brs, 1-NH), 7.98 (t, J = 4.3, 7-NH), 6.91 (t, J = 2.3, H-2), 6.79 (t, J = 2.3, H-3), 3.26 (q, J = 4.5, H$_2$-8), 2.85 (q, J = 4.5, H$_2$-9); ^{13}C NMR (DMSO-d_6) data, δ_C 163.9, 161.2, 153.4, 130.5, 126.1, 122.3, 120.4, 118.6, 112.6, 38.3, and 36.6. [16]

Compound **15**: Yellow oil; UV (MeOH) λ$_{max}$ 360 nm; C$_{12}$H$_{13}$N$_5$O$_3$; ^{1}H NMR (DMSO-d_6) data, δ_H 12.0 (brs, 1-NH), 7.76 (dd, J = 6.5, 1.7, 7-NH), 7.09 (t, J = 2.8, H-2), 6.52 (m, H-3), 5.73 (d, J = 6.7, H-9), 3.57, 3.28 (m, H$_2$-8), 3.21 (s, 9-OMe); ^{13}C NMR (DMSO-d_6) data, δ_C 164.8, 162.6, 155.8, 130.3, 123.3, 122.9, 127.1, 123.3, 117.5, 110.6, 69.0, and 43.2. [19]

Compound **16**: Yellow oil; UV (MeOH) λ$_{max}$ 214 nm; C$_{12}$H$_{14}$BrN$_5$O$_3$; ^{1}H NMR (DMSO-d_6) data, δ_H 9.78 (brs, 9-NH), 9.44 (brs, 7-NH), 8.10 (brs, 16-NH$_2$), 7.68 (s, H-3), 5.74 (s, H-6), 3.47, 3.36 (m, H$_2$-13), 2.24 (m, H$_2$-11), 1.98 (m, H$_2$-12); ^{13}C NMR (DMSO-d_6) data, δ_C 163.6, 163.1, 156.5, 146.0, 118.4, 85.8, 81.4, 63.9, 44.8, 39.5, 19.7 [17].

3.4. Computational Section

Conformational analyses were carried out in the MMFF minimization force field by the Spartan 10 v1.2.4 software package (Microsoft, Redmond, WA, USA). The resulting conformers were optimized using DFT at the B3LYP/6-31+G(d,p) level in the gas phase by the GAUSSIAN 09 C.03 program (Gaussian, Inc. Wallingford, CT, USA). The optimized conformations, whose Boltzmann distributions of Gibbs free energies were more than 1.0 percent, were used for the ECD calculations using the TD-DFT method with the basis set RB3LYP/DGDZVP, or the NMR calculations using the GIAO method at the PCM/b3lyp/6-311+G(d,p) level.

3.5. Molecular Docking

The initial receptor structure was constructed based on the crystal structure of aldose reductase in complex with cofactor NADP+ and the inhibitor idd594 (PDB code: 1US0) from the Protein Data Bank [20]. All nonstandard groups (HETATM) were deleted except for the inhibitor and cofactor when preparing for the receptor structure. The Protonate 3D module in the Molecular Operating Environment (MOE) program was used to estimate the protonated state of titratable residues and add hydrogen atoms. Meanwhile, MOE was also used to construct the ligand structures (compound **14**). The subsequent molecular docking was performed with an induced fit protocol. During the process, the protein–cofactor complex was defined as the receptor and the position of the inhibitor idd594 was defined as the docking site. The triangle matcher placement with the London ΔG initial scoring methodology was set for conformational sampling and 100 poses were recorded, then the forcefield post-placement refinement with GBVI/WSA ΔG rescoring methodology was utilized to further screen the best docking pose. In addition, the MMFF94x force field was adopted for the whole process.

3.6. ALR2 Expression and Purification

For the AKR1B1 enzyme assay and SPR measurements, the protein was expressed and purified using the protocol related to the one reported previously [15]. The plasmid (pET28b, Novagen) containing the open reading frame of the human ALR2 gene was kindly provided by Atagenix, Wuhan, Hubei, China. The E. coli strain BL21 gold (DE3) (Novagen) was used to express the hexa-histidine tagged protein after induction with IPTG (Roth) for 16 h at 293 K. The pellet from a 4 L culture was resuspended in a buffer containing 20 mM Tris and 500 mM NaCl (pH 8.0) before being sonicated and centrifuged. A HiTrap chelating HP column (GE Healthcare) was loaded with the supernatant. After a short washing step with a low imidazole concentration, the fusion protein was eluted by applying a gradient of imidazole. The buffer was exchanged with 20mM Tris-HCl, 10 mM NaCl, 1mM EDTA, and the tag cleaved by thrombin (yuanyeBio-Technology Co. Ltd. Shanghai, China). A Hiprep DEAE FastFlow 16/10 column (GE Healthcare) was loaded with the remaining solution. A NaCl gradient was used to elute the ALR2 from the column.

3.7. ALR2 Enzyme Assay (In Vitro)

In the first step of the polyol pathway, glucose reduction is accompanied by the conversation of NADPH to NADP, where only NADPH has an obvious spectral absorption around 340 nm and NADP has none. Thus, the decrease in OD_{340}nm can represent the consumption of NADPH. Therefore, we detect the change of OD_{340}nm before and after reaction to screen the effective ARIs or evaluate the AR activity; assays with epalrestat were used as positive controls. Briefly, the incubation system contains 10 μL ALR2 enzyme (20 μg/mL), 80 μL DL-glyceraldehyde (0.16 mmol/L) as the substrate, 1.0 mmol/L NADPH·4Na as a coenzyme, and 0.1 mol/L PBS (pH = 6.2). The incubation mixture was minimized to a total volume of 100 μL and ongoing in a 96-well ultraviolet plate. Then, test wells were treated with the tested compounds for 10 min at 25 °C. Then, the absorbance was measured using FlexStation 3 Reader (Molecular Devices, San Francisco, CA, USA) at 340 nm. The absorbance of wells treated with PBS and NADPH was considered as 100% (OD_1) and the absorbance of wells treated with PBS and DL-glyceraldehyde was considered as 0% (OD_2); the inhibitory rate was calculated by the formula $OD_{compounds} - OD_2/OD_1 - OD_2$. IC_{50} represents the concentration that inhibits the ALR2 enzyme by 50%.

3.8. Surface Plasmon Resonance (SPR) Binding Assay

SPR binding analysis methodology can be used to study molecular interactions. Herein, SPR was applied to measure the interactions between compounds **13/14** and ALR2. Initially, ALR2 was prepared in 10 mM sodium acetate (pH 5.0) and then immobilized covalently by an amine-coupling reaction on a CM5 sensor chip. The remaining binding sites of the sensor chip were then blocked by ethanolamine. The addition of compound **13/14**, the flow-through analyte, to the chamber resulted in binding to the immobilized protein ligand, producing a small change in the refractive index at the gold surface. In this step, the compound was diluted in PBS-P$^+$ buffer to the desired concentration and was injected over the chip with a flow rate of 10 μL/min. All of the above buffers, solutions, and sensor chips were placed at room temperature before the run. The association time and dissociation time were both set at 60 s. Binding affinities were obtained from the ratio of rate constants to directly characterize the protein-molecular interactions. Data analysis was completed via the state model in T200 evaluation software (Cytiva Danaher, Marlborough, MA, USA).

4. Conclusions

In conclusion, a series of new pyrrole alkaloids including different structural scaffolds were isolated from the sponge *Stylissa massa* collected in the South China Sea, which enriched the structural diversity of this alkaloid family. Aldose reductase (ALR2), which participates in the glucose polyol metabolic pathway and cell inflammatory reaction, is an important target for the treatment of diabetes complications, and 5/7/5 tricyclic spongiacidin-PIAs isolated from sponge *Stylissa massa* provided a new skeleton targeted to ALR2 which have never been previously reported.

Supplementary Materials: The following supporting information can be downloaded at: https://www.mdpi.com/article/10.3390/md20070454/s1, Tables S1–S4: 1H (500 MHz) and 13C (125 MHz) NMR data for 1–14 acquired in DMSO-d6. Tables S5–S7: X-ray diffraction analysis of compounds 1, 5, and 10. Figures S1–S20: The chiral HPLC data and ECD spectra of compounds 1–12; Figures S21–S25: The ALR2 inhibitory activities of related compounds. Figures S26–S117: The spectroscopic data (including HRESIMS, 1H NMR, 13C NMR, and 2D NMR) of compounds 1–16.

Author Contributions: Q.W. and C.G. contributed equally to this work. They conducted the main experiments, analyzed the data, and wrote the manuscript; H.L. was the supervisor for this work and revised the manuscript. Z.W. expressed and purified the ALR2 protein. X.T. and X.L. finished the ECD calculations. L.J., X.P. and G.L. helped with the experimental procedures. All authors have read and agreed to the published version of the manuscript.

Funding: This research was funded by the National Natural Science Foundation of China (No. 41906030).

Institutional Review Board Statement: Not applicable.

Informed Consent Statement: Not applicable.

Data Availability Statement: The original contributions presented in the study are included in the article/Supplementary Materials; further inquiries can be directed to the corresponding author.

Conflicts of Interest: The authors declare no conflict of interest.

References

1. Walker, R.P.; Faulkner, D.J.; Vanengen, D.; Clardy, J. Sceptrin, an antimicrobial agent from the sponge *Agelas sceptrum*. *J. Am. Chem. Soc.* **1981**, *103*, 6772–6773. [CrossRef]
2. Urban, S.; Leone, P.D.; Carroll, A.R.; Fechner, G.A.; Smith, J.; Hooper, J.N.A.; Quinn, R.J. Axinellamines A-D, novel imidazo-azolo-imidazole alkaloids from the Australian marine sponge *Axinella* sp. *J. Org. Chem.* **1999**, *64*, 731–735. [CrossRef] [PubMed]
3. Kobayashi, J.; Inaba, K.; Tsuda, M. Tauroacidins A and B, new bromopyrrole alkaloids possessing a taurine residue from *Hymeniacidon* Sponge. *Tetrahedron* **1997**, *53*, 16679–16682. [CrossRef]
4. Al-Mourabit, A.; Zancanella, M.A.; Tilvi, S.; Romo, D. Biosynthesis, asymmetric synthesis, and pharmacology, including cellular targets of the pyrrole-2-aminoimidazole marine alkaloids. *Nat. Prod. Rep.* **2011**, *28*, 1229–1260. [CrossRef] [PubMed]
5. Miguel-Gordo, M.; Gegunde, S.; Jennings, L.K.; Genta-Jouve, G.; Calabro, K.; Alfonso, A.; Botana, L.M.; Thomas, O.P. Futunamine, a pyrrole-imidazole alkaloid from the sponge *Stylissa* aff. *carteri* collected off the Futuna Islands. *J. Nat. Prod.* **2020**, *83*, 2299–2304. [PubMed]
6. Kinnel, R.B.; Gehrken, H.P.; Scheuer, P.J. Palau'amine: A cytotoxic and immunosuppressive hexacyclic bisguanidine antibiotic from the sponge *Stylotella agminata*. *J. Am. Chem. Soc.* **1993**, *115*, 3376–3377. [CrossRef]
7. Kobayashi, J.; Tsuda, M.; Murayama, T.; Nakamura, H.; Ohizumi, Y.; Ishibashi, M.; Iwamura, M.; Ohta, T.; Nozoe, S. Ageliferins, potent actomyosin ATPase activators from the Okinawan marine sponge *Agelas* sp. *Tetrahedron* **1990**, *46*, 5579–5586. [CrossRef]
8. Buchanan, M.S.; Carroll, A.R.; Addepalli, R.; Avery, V.M.; Hooper, J.N.A.; Quinn, R.J. Natural products, stylissadines A and B, specific antagonists of the P2 × 7 Receptor, an important inflammatory target. *J. Org. Chem.* **2007**, *72*, 2309–2317. [CrossRef] [PubMed]
9. Mohanty, I.; Moore, S.G.; Yi, D.Q.; Biggs, J.S.; Gaul, D.A.; Garg, N.; Agarwal, V. Precursor-guided mining of marine sponge metabolomes lends insight into biosynthesis of pyrrole-imidazole alkaloids. *ACS Chem. Biol.* **2020**, *15*, 2185–2194. [CrossRef] [PubMed]
10. Genta-Jouve, G.; Cachet, N.; Holderith, S.; Oberhänsli, F.; Teyssié, J.L.; Jeffree, R.; Mourabit, A.A.; Thomas, O.P. New insight into marine alkaloid metabolic pathways: Revisiting oroidin biosynthesis. *Chem. Bio. Chem.* **2011**, *12*, 2298–2301. [CrossRef] [PubMed]
11. Sharma, G.M.; Burkholder, P.R. Structure of dibromophakellin, a new bromine-containing alkaloid from the marine sponge *Phakellia flabellata*. *Chem. Comm.* **1971**, *3*, 151–152. [CrossRef]
12. Goetz, G.H.; Harrigan, G.G.; Likos, J. Ugibohlin: A new dibromo-seco-isophakellin from *Axinella carteri*. *J. Nat. Prod.* **2001**, *64*, 1581–1582. [CrossRef] [PubMed]
13. Inaba, K.; Sato, H.; Tsuda, M.; Kobayashi, J. Spongiacidins A-D, new bromopyrrole alkaloids from *Hymeniacidon* sponge. *J. Nat. Prod.* **1998**, *61*, 693–695. [CrossRef] [PubMed]
14. Molinaro, A.; Bel Lassen, P.; Henricsson, M.; Wu, H.; Adriouch, S.; Belda, E.; Chakaroun, R.; Nielsen, T.; Bergh, P.O.; Rouault, C.; et al. Imidazole propionate is increased in diabetes and associated with dietary patterns and altered microbial ecology. *Nat. Comm.* **2020**, *11*, 5881. [CrossRef] [PubMed]
15. Maccari, R.; Ottanà, R. Targeting aldose reductase for the treatment of diabetes complications and inflammatory diseases: New insights and future directions. *J. Med. Chem.* **2015**, *58*, 2047–2067. [CrossRef] [PubMed]
16. Williams, D.H.; Faulkner, D.J. Isomers and tautomers of hymenialdisine and debromohymenialdisine. *Nat. Prod. Lett.* **1996**, *9*, 57–64. [CrossRef]
17. Foley, L.H.; Büchi, G. Biomimetic synthesis of dibromophakellin. *J. Am. Chem. Soc.* **1982**, *104*, 1776–1777. [CrossRef]
18. Schmitz, F.J.; Gunasekera, S.P.; Lakshmi, V.; Tillekeratne, L.M.V. Marine natural products: Pyrrololactams from several sponges. *J. Nat. Prod.* **1985**, *48*, 47–53. [CrossRef] [PubMed]
19. Horne, D.A.; Yakushijin, K. Preparation of Debromohymenialdisine and Analogs. Patent WO2001005794A2, 25 January 2001.
20. Human Aldose Reductase in complex with NADP+ and the inhibitor IDD594 at 0.66 Angstrom. Available online: https://www.rcsb.org/structure/1US0 (accessed on 7 July 2022).

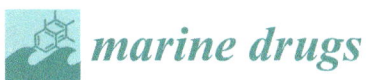

Communication

Unique Cyclized Thiolopyrrolones from the Marine-Derived *Streptomyces* sp. BTBU20218885

Fuhang Song [1,†], Jiansen Hu [2,†], Xinwan Zhang [3], Wei Xu [3], Jinpeng Yang [3], Shaoyong Li [4] and Xiuli Xu [3,*]

1. School of Light Industry, Beijing Technology and Business University, Beijing 100048, China; songfuhang@btbu.edu.cn
2. Laboratory of RNA Biology, Institute of Biophysics, Chinese Academy of Sciences, Beijing 100101, China; jiansenhu@ibp.ac.cn
3. School of Ocean Sciences, China University of Geosciences, Beijing 100083, China; zhangxinwan@cugb.edu.cn (X.Z.); xuwei1110@cugb.edu.cn (W.X.); yangjinpeng@cugb.edu.cn (J.Y.)
4. School of Pharmacy, Tianjin Medical University, Tianjin 300070, China; lishaoyong@tmu.edu.cn
* Correspondence: xuxl@cugb.edu.cn
† These authors contributed equally to this work.

Abstract: Two new cyclized thiolopyrrolone derivatives, namely, thiolopyrrolone A (**1**) and 2,2-dioxidothiolutin (**2**), together with the known compound, thiolutin (**3**) were identified from a marine-derived *Streptomyces* sp. BTBU20218885, which was isolated from a mud sample collected from the coastal region of Xiamen, China. Their chemical structures were determined using spectroscopic data, including HRESIMS, 1D and 2D NMR techniques. **1** possessed a unique unsymmetrical sulfur-containing thiolopyrrolone structure. All the compounds were tested for bioactivities against *Staphylococcus aureus*, *Escherichia coli*, Bacille Calmette–Guérin (BCG), *Mycobacterium tuberculosis*, and *Candida albicans*. **1** displayed antibacterial activities against BCG, *M. tuberculosis*, and *S. aureus* with minimum inhibitory concentration (MIC) values of 10, 10, and 100 µg/mL, respectively. Thiolutin (**3**) showed antibacterial activities against *E. coli*, BCG, *M. tuberculosis*, and *S. aureus* with MIC values of 6.25, 0.3125, 0.625, and 3.125 µg/mL, respectively.

Keywords: marine-derived *Streptomyces*; thiolopyrrolone; antibacterial; *M. tuberculosis*

Citation: Song, F.; Hu, J.; Zhang, X.; Xu, W.; Yang, J.; Li, S.; Xu, X. Unique Cyclized Thiolopyrrolones from the Marine-Derived *Streptomyces* sp. BTBU20218885. *Mar. Drugs* **2022**, *20*, 214. https://doi.org/10.3390/md20030214

Academic Editor: Asunción Barbero

Received: 15 February 2022
Accepted: 16 March 2022
Published: 18 March 2022

Publisher's Note: MDPI stays neutral with regard to jurisdictional claims in published maps and institutional affiliations.

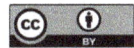

Copyright: © 2022 by the authors. Licensee MDPI, Basel, Switzerland. This article is an open access article distributed under the terms and conditions of the Creative Commons Attribution (CC BY) license (https://creativecommons.org/licenses/by/4.0/).

1. Introduction

Infectious diseases caused by infectious microorganisms continue to threaten human health. Moreover, the development of drug resistance by *Candida albicans*, *Staphylococcus aureus*, *Escherichia coli*, and *Mycobacterium tuberculosi* is becoming more and more serious in hospitals and the community [1–4]. There is an urgent need to develop new drugs to fight against these pathogens.

Streptomyces belongs to actinomycetes which are highly diverse Gram-positive bacteria with high guanine and cytosine content in their DNA. Actinomycetes are well known as an important resource for screening new antibiotics [5], representing 45% of the bioactive secondary metabolites originating from microorganisms [6]. Moreover, *Streptomyces* are the key source of many of the world's antibiotics in clinics [7,8]. With the detailed investigation on marine microorganisms, marine-derived actinomycetes have proven to be an inexhaustible source for bioactive secondary metabolites [9]. A number of new bioactive compounds were characterized from marine-derived *Streptomyces*, such as isoquinolinequinones [10], terpenoid derivatives [11,12], angucycline derivatives [13–15], glycosylated aromatic polyketides [16], bicyclic peptides [17], depsipeptides [18], benzodiazepines [19], and piericidin derivatives [20].

In the course of our screening of antibacterial secondary metabolites from marine-derived actinomycetes [21–24], the EtOAc extract of *Streptomyces* sp. BTBU20218885, isolated from a mud sample collected from the coastal area of Xiamen, Fujian Province, China, showed antibacterial activity against Bacille Calmette–Guérin (BCG), the live attenuated vaccine form of *Mycobacterium bovis*, with minimum inhibitory concentration (MIC) of 20 µg/mL. A chemical investigation of this *Streptomyces* strain resulted in the isolation of two new cyclized thiopyrrolone derivatives, namely, thiopyrrolone A (**1**) and 2,2-dioxido thiolutin (**2**), together with the known compound, thiolutin (**3**) (Figure 1). Details of fermentation, isolation, structural elucidation, and antibacterial activities are reported here.

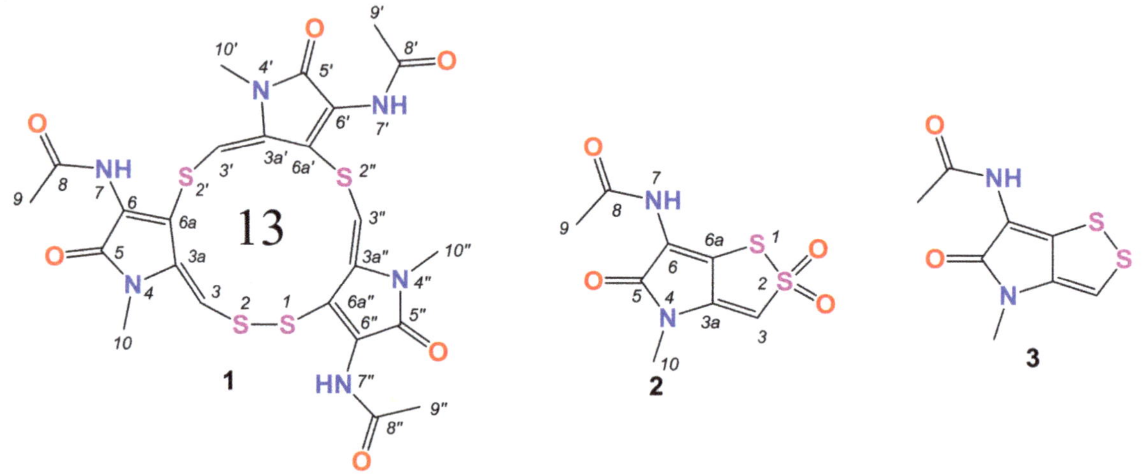

Figure 1. Chemical structures of **1**–**3**.

2. Results

2.1. Structure Elucidation

Compound **1** was isolated as a light-yellow amorphous powder. The molecular formula of **1** was deduced to be $C_{24}H_{24}N_6O_6S_4$ by the high-resolution electrospray ionization mass spectroscopy (HRESIMS) measurement (m/z [M+H]$^+$ 621.0712, calcd for $C_{24}H_{25}N_6O_6S_4$, 621.0713), accounting for sixteen degrees of unsaturation (Figure S1). The ^{1}H NMR spectrum (Table 1, Figure S2) showed the presence of three exchangeable singlets (δ_H 10.27, s, 7-NH; 10.21, s, 7'-NH; 10.17, s, 7''-NH), three olefinic protons (δ_H 6.58, s, H-3; 6.36, s, H-3'; 6.54, s, H-3''), three N-Me groups (δ_H 3.19, s, Me-10; 3.47, s, Me-10'; 3.40, s, Me-10''), as well as three methyl singlets for acetyl groups (δ_H 2.07, s, Me-9 and Me-9''; 2.06, s, Me-9'). The ^{13}C NMR spectrum (Figure S3), in association with the heteronuclear single quantum correlation (HSQC) spectrum (Figure S4), indicated 24 carbon signals (Table 1), including six methyls (δ_C 29.9, C-10; δ_C 29.2, C-10'/C-10''; δ_C 22.9, C-9; δ_C 22.8, C-9'/C-9''), three sp^2 methines (δ_C 111.9, C-3; δ_C 112.5, C-3'; δ_C 112.8, C-3''), six amide carbonyls (δ_C 164.0/163.7/163.8, C-5/C-5'/C-5''; δ_C 168.4/168.3/167.9, C-8/C-8'/C-8''), and nine sp^2 quaternary carbons (δ_C 137.1/131.9/133.8, 3a/3a'/3a''; δ_C 130.7/129.8/132.7, 6/6'/6''; δ_C 124.6/124.6/126.4, 6a/6a'/6a''). The amide carbonyls and olefinic carbons accounted for twelve degrees of unsaturation, which indicated compound **1** was a tetracyclic molecule. Comparison of the NMR data with those of the known compound thiolutin (**3**, Table 1) [25] revealed that **1** was an analogue of thiolutin with a pseudo trimer structure. Furthermore, the heteronuclear multiple bond correlation (HMBC) correlations (Figures 2, S5 and S6) from H$_3$-9 and H-7-NH to C-8, H$_3$-9' and H-7'-NH to C-8', and H$_3$-9'' and H-7''-NH to C-8'' revealed the presence of three acetamides. The HMBC correlations from H$_3$-10 to C-3a and C-5, H$_3$-10' to C-3a' and C-5', H$_3$-10'' to C-3a'' and C-5'' confirmed the presence of three N-Me amides. The moieties of 1,5-dihydro-2H-pyrrol-2-one were determined by HMBC correlations from H-3 to C-3a and C-6a, H-7-NH to C-6 and C-6a, H-3' to C-3a' and C-6a', H-7'-NH to C-6' and C-6a', H-3'' to C-3a'' and C-6a'', H-7''-NH to C-6'' and C-6a''. The monosulfur bonds between C-6a and C-3', C-6a' to C-3'' were revealed by the HMBC correlations from H-3′ to C-6a, and H-3″ to C-6a′. The absence of HMBC correlation from H-3 to C-6a″, together with molecular formula of **1**, indicated that the C-6a and C-3 were linked through a disulfur bond. Thus, the structure of **1** was established (Figure 1) and named thiolopyrrolone A.

Table 1. ^{1}H (500 MHz) and ^{13}C NMR (125 MHz) data of **1–3** (DMSO-d_6).

Position	1		2		3	
	δ_C	δ_H (J in Hz)	δ_C	δ_H (J in Hz)	δ_C	δ_H (J in Hz)
3/3′/3″	111.9/112.5/112.8	6.58/6.36/6.54, s	109.6	7.56, s	111.0	7.34, s
3a/3a′/3a″	137.1/131.9/133.8		145.5		136.0	
5/5′/5″	164.0/163.7/163.8		164.3		166.1	
6/6′/6″	130.7/129.8/132.7		114.1		114.8	
6a/6a′/6a″	124.6/124.6/126.4		123.1		132.4	
8/8′/8″	168.4/168.3/167.9		170.5		168.8	
9/9′/9″	22.9/22.8/22.8	2.07/2.06/2.07, s	22.6	2.10, s	22.4	2.02, s
10/10′/10″	29.9/29.2/29.2	3.19/3.47/3.40, s	27.9	3.10, s	27.5	3.25, s
7/7′/7″-NH		10.27/10.21/10.17, s	-			9.99, s

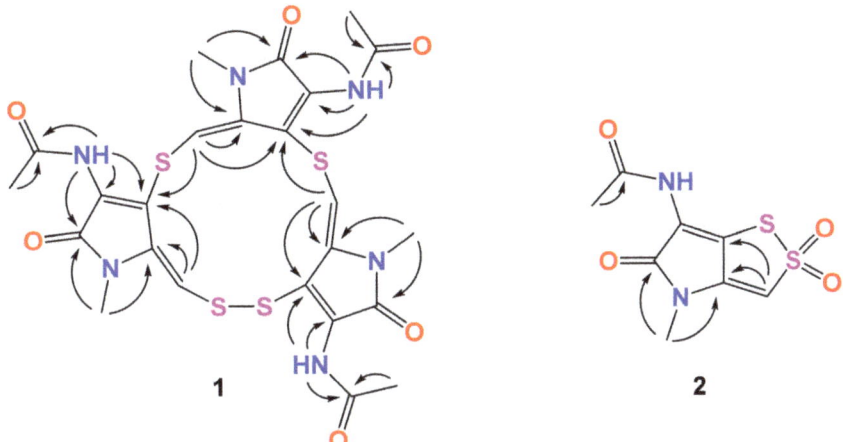

Figure 2. Key HMBC (arrows) correlations in **1** and **2**.

Compound **2** was isolated as a yellow amorphous powder. The molecular formula of **2** was deduced to be $C_8H_8N_2O_4S_2$ by the HRESIMS measurement (m/z [M + H]$^+$ 260.9996, calcd for $C_8H_9N_2O_4S_2$, 260.9998), accounting for six degrees of unsaturation (Figure S7). The ^{1}H ^{13}C and HSQC spectra (Figures S8–S10) displayed similar signals to those of **3**, including one sp^2 methine (δ_H 7.56, s, H-3; δ_C 109.6, C-3), one N-Me group (δ_H 3.10, s, H$_3$-10; δ_C 27.9, C-10), and one methyl singlet for acetyl group (δ_H 2.10, s, H$_3$-9; δ_C 22.6, C-9), two amide carbonyls (δ_C 164.3, C-5; δ_C 170.5, C-8), and three sp^2 quaternary carbons (δ_C 145.5, C-3; δ_C 114.1, C-6, δ_C 123.1, C-6a). The HMBC spectrum (Figure S11) showed correlations from H$_3$-9 to C-8, H$_3$-10 to C-3a and C-5, H-3 to C-3a and C-6a (Figure 2). Together with the molecular formula calculated by HRESIMS, there are two more oxygen atoms in compound **2**. So there are four possible structures for **2** as shown in Figure 3. The two oxygen atoms for sulfoxides formed *cis* and *trans* conformations, but the optical rotation did not reveal any solid data because of the decomposition of **2**. So, both of the conformations were subjected to quantum chemical calculation. By comparing the experimental and calculated ultraviolet spectra of **2a–2d** (Figure 4), the structures of **2b2** and **2d** are consistent with those of experimental data. In order to confirm the structure of **2**, the ^{13}C NMR data of the four possible structures were also calculated by density functional theory (DFT). The data were evaluated based on the statistical parameters including correlation coefficient (R^2) between experimental and calculated ^{13}C NMR spectroscopic data with a linear regression, the maximum error (MaxErr), and mean absolute error (MAE). Comparison of all these parameters for calculated ^{13}C chemical shifts of the four possible isomers with experimental data revealed the best fit was **2d** (Table 2). Thus, the structure of **2** was determined and named 2,2-dioxidothiolutin.

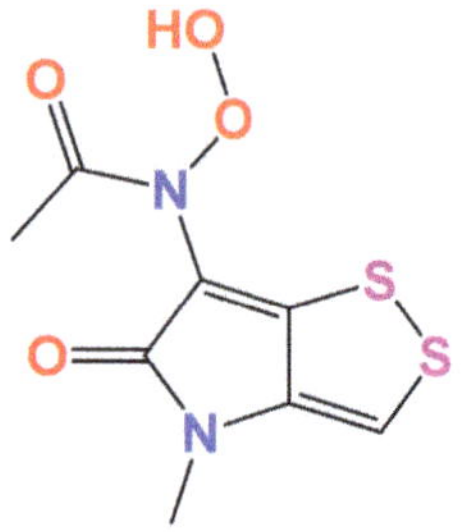

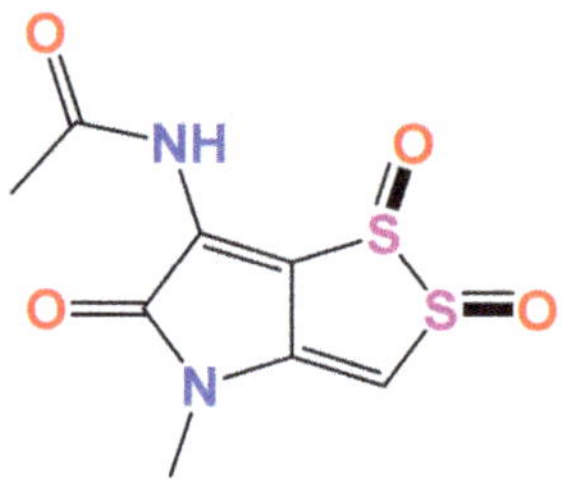

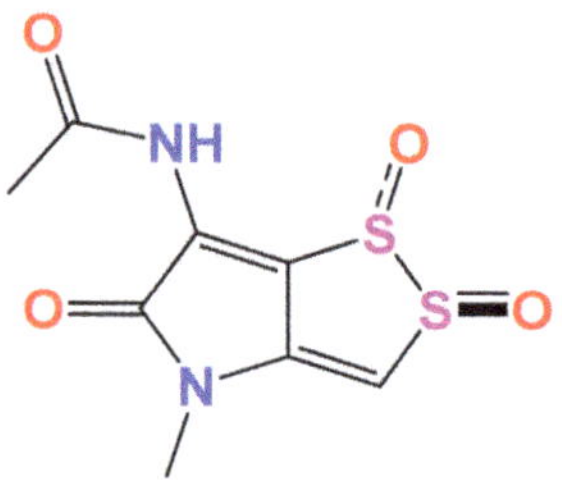

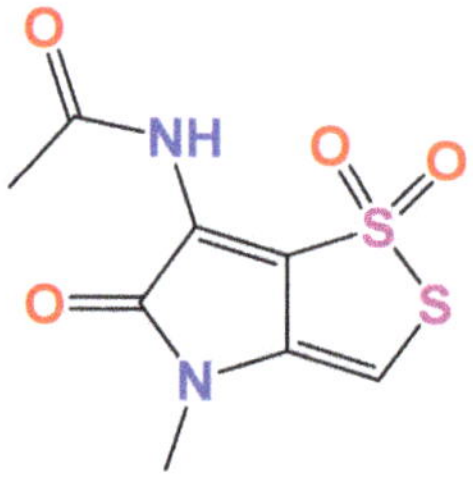

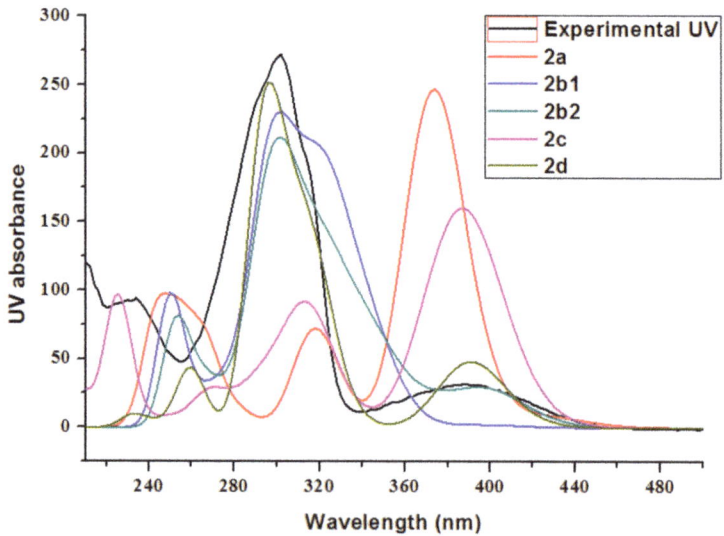

Figure 3. Four possible structures of **2** for calculating ^{13}C NMR data in DMSO-d_6.

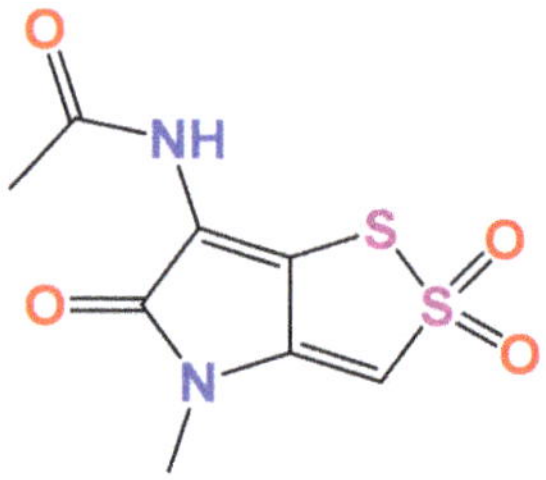

Figure 4. Calculated UV spectra for **2a–2d** and UV spectrum for compound **2**.

Table 2. Comparison of calculated (TMS as a reference standard) and experimental ^{13}C data for **2**.

Position	2a	2b1	2b2	2c	2d	2
3	115.2	110.2	111.8	107.4	103.9	109.6
3a	129.4	147.5	140.2	121.2	140.2	145.5
5	162.1	160.5	159.0	159.6	159.2	164.3
6	112.9	130.4	127.9	131.1	121.1	114.1
6a	138.1	135.9	131.3	124.5	129.5	123.1
8	167.3	164.1	163.5	163.4	163.9	170.5
9	21.3	23.1	22.8	23.0	22.6	22.6
10	27.6	27.4	26.8	26.4	27.3	27.9
R^2	0.9723	0.9776	0.9812	0.9534	0.9898	
MAE	5.6	5.4	5.4	7.3	4.6	
MaxErr	16.1	16.3	13.8	24.3	7.0	

Compound **3** was isolated as a yellow amorphous powder. The molecular formula of **3** was deduced to be $C_8H_8N_2O_2S_2$ by the HRESIMS measurement (m/z [M + H]$^+$ 229.0100, calcd for $C_8H_9N_2O_2S_2$, 229.0100), accounting for six degrees of unsaturation (Figure S12). The ^{1}H ^{13}C and HSQC spectra (Figures S13–S15) displayed almost the same signals as those of reported thiolutin 3 [21]. In the HMBC spectrum (Figure S16), the correlations from H$_3$-10 (δ_H 3.25) to C-3a (δ_C 136.0) and C-5 (δ_C 166.1), H-3 to C-3a and C-6a (δ_C 132.4), H-7-NH to C-6 (δ_C 114.8) and C-6a determined the chemical shifts of C-3, C-6, and C-6a. Thus, the chemical shifts for C-3a and C-6a should be swapped [21].

2.2. Biological Activity

These compounds were evaluated for their antimicrobial activities against *C. albicans* ATCC 10231, *S. aureus* ATCC 25923, *Mycobacterium bovis* (BCG Pasteur 1173P2), *M. tuberculosis* H37Rv (ATCC27294), and *E. coli* ATCC 25923. Compound **1** exhibited antibacterial activities against BCG, *M. tuberculosis*, and *S. aureus* with MIC values of 10, 10, and 100 μg/mL, respectively. Thiolutin (**3**) showed antibacterial activities against *E. coli*, BCG, *M. tuberculosis*, and *S. aureus* with MIC values of 6.25, 0.3125, 0.625, and 3.125 μg/mL, respectively (Table 3).

Table 3. Antibacterial activities of compounds **1–3** (MIC, μg/mL).

Number	C. albicans	S. aureus	BCG	M. tuberculosis	E. coli
1	>200	100	10	10	>100
2	>200	50	-	-	>200
3	>200	3.125	0.3125	0.625	6.25
Control	1 [a]	1 [b]	0.05 [c]	0.025 [c]	1 [d]

[a] Rapamycin, [b] vancomycin, [c] isoniazid, [d] ciprofloxacin.

3. Materials and Methods

3.1. General Experimental Procedures

NMR spectra were obtained on a Bruker Avance 500 spectrometer with residual solvent peaks as references (DMSO-d_6: δ_H 2.50, δ_C 39.52). High-resolution ESIMS measurements were obtained on an Accurate-Mass-Q-TOF LC/MS 6520 instrument (Santa Clara, CA, USA) in the positive ion mode. HPLC was performed using an Agilent 1200 Series separation module equipped with an Agilent 1200 Series diode array, Agilent 1200 Series fraction collector, and Agilent ZORBAX SB-C18 column (250 × 9.4 mm, 5 μm).

3.2. Microbial Material, Fermentation, Extraction, and Purification

Strain *Streptomyces sp.* BTBU20218885 was isolated from a mud sample collected from the intertidal zone, Xiamen, China, and grown on an ISP2 (yeast extract 0.4%, malt extract 1%, dextrose 0.4%, agar 2%; pH 7.2) agar plate at 28 °C. Colony characteristics of BTBU20218885 are shown in Figure S17. The genomic DNA of BTBU20218885 was extracted using a TINAamp Bacteria DNA Kit. PCR amplification of 16S rDNA was carried out by using universal primers (27f:5′-GAGAGTTTGATCCTGGCTCAG-3′; 1492r: 5′-CTACGGCTACCTTGTTACGA-3′). PCR amplification of the 16S rDNA was performed on TaKaRa PCR Thermal Cycler with the initial denaturation at 94 °C for 5 min, 30 cycles of denaturation (94 °C, 1 min), annealing (55 °C, 1 min), and elongation (72 °C, 1 min 15 s), and a final elongation at 72 °C for 10 min, in a 25 µL system (0.4 µL 20 µM of each primer, 2.5 µL 10× buffer, 2.5 µL 2.5 nM dNTP, 2 U rTap polymerase, and 1 µL DNA template). BTBU20218885 was identified as *Streptomyces* sp. by comparing the 16S rDNA sequence with the GenBank database using the BLAST program. A neighbor-joining (NJ) tree (Figure S18) was constructed using the software package Mega version 5 [26]. The strain was assigned the accession number BTBU20218885 in the culture collection at Beijing Technology and Business University, Beijing. The strain BTBU20218885 was inoculated on an ISP2 agar plate and cultured for 7 days. A 250 mL Erlenmeyer flask containing 40 mL of ISP2 medium was inoculated with BTBU20218885 and incubated at 28 °C (160 rpm) for 36 h. Aliquots (9 mL) of the seed cultures were aseptically transferred to 20 × 1 L Erlenmeyer flasks, each containing 300 mL of MPG media (glucose 1.0%, millet meal 2.0%, cotton seed gluten meal 2.0%, and MOPS 2.0%; pH 7.0), and the flasks were incubated at 28 °C, 160 rpm for 7 days. The culture broths were combined and centrifuged to yield a supernatant and a mycelial cake. The supernatant was extracted by equal volume of ethyl acetate (EtOAc, ×3 times), and the combined EtOAc extracts were evaporated to dryness in vacuo to give a dark residue. The residue was sequentially triturated with hexane, CH_2Cl_2, and MeOH to afford, after concentration in vacuo, hexane, CH_2Cl_2, and MeOH soluble fractions and precipitate. The precipitate was further purified by HPLC (Agilent ZORBAX SB-C18, 250 × 9.4 mm, 5 µm column, 3.0 mL/min, elution with 30% to 100% acetonitrile/H_2O (0–20 min) to yield **1** (3.5 mg), **3** (2.6 mg), and **2** (13.2 mg).

Thiolopyrrolone A (**1**): Light-yellow amorphous powder; ^1H and ^{13}C NMR data, Table 1; HRESIMS *m/z* 621.0712 [M + H]$^+$ (calcd for $C_{24}H_{25}N_6O_6S_4$, 621.0713).

2,2-Dioxidothiolutin (**2**): Yellow amorphous powder; ^1H and ^{13}C NMR data, Table 1; HRESIMS *m/z* 260.9996 [M + H]$^+$ (calcd for $C_8H_9N_2O_4S_2$, 260.9998).

3.3. Biological Activity

Compounds **1–3** were evaluated for their antimicrobial activities in 96-well plates according to the Antimicrobial Susceptibility Testing Standards outlined by the Clinical and Laboratory Standards Institute Document M07-A7 (CLSI) and our previous report [27–29]. The MIC was defined as the minimum concentration of the compound that prevented visible growth of the microbes.

3.4. Computational Methods

A random conformational search of starting geometries in Discovery studio 4.0 was used to produce low-energy conformers within a 10 kcal/mol energy, which were subsequently optimized using the DFT method at mPW1PW91/6-31g(2d,p) level with GAUSSIAN 09 [30]. The optimized conformers were further checked by frequency calculation at the same level of theory, and resulted in no imaginary frequencies. The time-dependent density functional theory (TDDFT) calculations of their low-energy conformations within 0–2.5 kcal/mol were performed to simulate their UV–vis spectra at the same level. Similarly, their ^{13}C NMR calculations were also carried out by GIAO method at the same level [31]. Solvent effect of dimethylsulfoxide was taken into account in the above calculations by using the polarizable continuum model (PCM).

Their theoretical UV–vis spectra based on Boltzmann statistics were generated in the program SpecDis 1.63 [32] by applying Gaussian band shape with a 0.40 eV exponential half-width from dipole-length rotational strengths. Statistical parameters were used to quantify the agreement between experimental and calculated data, including the correlation coefficient (R^2) between experimental and calculated ^{13}C NMR spectroscopic data with a linear regression, the mean absolute error (MAE), and the maximum error (MaxErr) [33].

The correlation coefficient (R^2) was determined from a plot of δ_{calc} (x axis) against δ_{exp} (y axis) for each particular compound. The mean absolute error (MAE) was defined as $\frac{1}{n}\sum_{i=1}^{n}\left|\delta_{calc,\,i}-\delta_{exp,\,i}\right|$. The maximum error (MaxErr) was defined as $\max|\delta_{calc}-\delta_{exp}|$.

4. Conclusions

In summary, chemical studies on the marine-derived *Streptomyces* sp. BTBU20218885 resulted in the characterization of three cyclized thiolopyrrolones, including a unique unsymmetrical thiolopyrrolone (**1**), 2,2-dioxidothiolutin (**2**), and the previously reported thiolutin (**3**). Dithiolopyrrolones are a class of structurally intriguing natural products with broad antibacterial spectrum [34]. Most of the analogues are characterized by a unique bicyclic pyrrolinonodithiole, with the differences in the substitution groups on *N*-4 and *N*-7 positions of the holothin core [35,36]; however, thiolopyrrolone A is the first sample of analogues with a macrocyclic skeleton. Compound **1** exhibited antibacterial activities against BCG, *M. tuberculosis*, and *S. aureus* with MIC values of 10, 10, and 100 µg/mL, respectively. Thiolutin (**3**) displayed potential antibacterial activities against *E. coli*, BCG, *M. tuberculosis*, and *S. aureus* with MIC values of 6.25, 0.3125, 0.625, and 3.125 µg/mL, respectively.

Supplementary Materials: The following are available online at https://www.mdpi.com/article/10.3390/md20030214/s1: Figures S1–S16: HRESIMS, 1D, and 2D NMR for compounds **1–3**; Figure S17: Colony characteristics of BTBU20211089; Figure S18: Neighbor-joining phylogenetic tree of strain BTBU20211089.

Author Contributions: Data curation, F.S.; funding acquisition, F.S.; investigation, F.S., J.H., X.Z., W.X., J.Y. and S.L.; supervision, X.X.; writing—original draft, F.S. and X.X.; writing—review and editing, F.S., J.H., X.Z. and X.X. All authors have read and agreed to the published version of the manuscript.

Funding: This work was funded by grants from the National Natural Science Foundation of China (81973204), the Key Lab of Marine Bioactive Substance and Modern Analytical Technique, SOA (MBSMAT-2019-06), and Research Foundation for Advanced Talents of Beijing Technology and Business University (19008021176).

Institutional Review Board Statement: Not applicable.

Informed Consent Statement: Not applicable.

Data Availability Statement: Data are contained within the text.

Conflicts of Interest: The authors declare no conflict of interest.

References

1. Dhasarathan, P.; AlSalhi, M.S.; Devanesan, S.; Subbiah, J.; Ranjitsingh, A.J.A.; Binsalah, M.; Alfuraydi, A.A. Drug resistance in *Candida albicans* isolates and related changes in the structural domain of Mdr1 protein. *J. Infect. Public Health* **2021**, *14*, 1848–1853. [CrossRef]
2. Miklasińska-Majdanik, M. Mechanisms of Resistance to Macrolide Antibiotics among *Staphylococcus aureus*. *Antibiotics* **2021**, *10*, 1406. [CrossRef] [PubMed]
3. Poirel, L.; Madec, J.-Y.; Lupo, A.; Schink, A.-K.; Kieffer, N.; Nordmann, P.; Schwarz, S.; Aarestrup, F.M.; Schwarz, S.; Shen, J.; et al. Antimicrobial resistance in *Escherichia coli*. *Microbiol. Spectr.* **2018**, *6*, ARBA-0026-2017. [CrossRef] [PubMed]
4. Chizimu, J.Y.; Solo, E.S.; Bwalya, P.; Tanomsridachchai, W.; Chambaro, H.; Shawa, M.; Kapalamula, T.F.; Lungu, P.; Fukushima, Y.; Mukonka, V.; et al. Whole-Genome Sequencing Reveals Recent Transmission of Multidrug-Resistant Mycobacterium tuberculosis CAS1-Kili Strains in Lusaka, Zambia. *Antibiotics* **2022**, *11*, 29. [CrossRef] [PubMed]
5. Barka, E.A.; Vatsa, P.; Sanchez, L.; Gaveau-Vaillant, N.; Jacquard, C.; Klenk, H.P.; Clément, C.; Ouhdouch, Y.; van Wezel, G.P. Taxonomy, physiology, and natural products of actinobacteria. *Microbiol. Mol. Biol. Rev.* **2016**, *80*, 1–43. [CrossRef]
6. Berdy, J. Thoughts and facts about antibiotics: Where we are now and where we are heading. *J. Antibiot.* **2012**, *65*, 385–395. [CrossRef] [PubMed]
7. Mast, Y.; Stegmann, E. Actinomycetes: The antibiotics producers. *Antibiotics* **2019**, *8*, 105. [CrossRef]
8. Takahashi, Y.; Nakashima, T. Actinomycetes, an inexhaustible source of naturally occurring antibiotics. *Antibiotics* **2018**, *7*, 45. [CrossRef]

9. Subramani, R.; Aalbersberg, W. Marine actinomycetes: An ongoing source of novel bioactive metabolites. *Microbiol. Res.* **2012**, *167*, 571–580. [CrossRef]
10. Shaaban, M.; Shaaban, K.A.; Kelter, G.; Fiebig, H.H.; Laatsch, H. Mansouramycins E–G, cytotoxic isoquinolinequinones from marine *Streptomycetes*. *Mar. Drugs* **2021**, *19*, 715. [CrossRef]
11. Shen, X.; Wang, X.; Huang, T.; Deng, Z.; Lin, S. Naphthoquinone-based meroterpenoids from marine-derived *Streptomyces* sp. B9173. *Biomolecules* **2020**, *10*, 1187. [CrossRef] [PubMed]
12. Wu, J.; Zhu, Y.; Zhang, M.; Li, H.; Sun, P. Micaryolanes A and B, two new caryolane-type sesquiterpenoids from marine *Streptomyces* sp. AH25. *Chem. Biodivers.* **2020**, *17*, e2000769. [CrossRef] [PubMed]
13. Chang, Y.; Xing, L.; Sun, C.; Liang, S.; Liu, T.; Zhang, X.; Zhu, T.; Pfeifer, B.A.; Che, Q.; Zhang, G.; et al. Monacycliones G–K and ent-gephyromycin A, angucycline derivatives from the marine-derived *Streptomyces* sp. HDN15129. *J. Nat. Prod.* **2020**, *83*, 2749–2755. [CrossRef] [PubMed]
14. Liu, M.; Yang, Y.-J.; Gong, G.; Li, Z.; Zhang, L.; Guo, L.; Xu, B.; Zhang, S.M.; Xie, Z.P. Angucycline and angucyclinone derivatives from the marine-derived *Streptomyces* sp. *Chirality* **2022**, *34*, 421–427. [CrossRef]
15. Guo, L.; Yang, Q.; Wang, G.; Zhang, S.; Liu, M.; Pan, X.; Pescitelli, G.; Xie, Z. Ring D-modified and highly reduced angucyclinones from marine dediment-derived *Streptomyces* sp. *Front. Chem.* **2021**, *9*, 756962. [CrossRef]
16. Cho, E.; Kwon, O.-S.; Chung, B.; Lee, J.; Sun, J.; Shin, J.; Oh, K.B. Antibacterial activity of chromomycins from a marine-derived *Streptomyces microflavus*. *Mar. Drugs* **2020**, *18*, 522. [CrossRef]
17. Karim, M.R.U.; In, Y.; Zhou, T.; Harunari, E.; Oku, N.; Igarashi, Y. Nyuzenamides A and B: Bicyclic peptides with antifungal and cytotoxic activity from a marine-derived *Streptomyces* sp. *Org. Lett.* **2021**, *23*, 2109–2113. [CrossRef]
18. Guo, Z.; Ma, S.; Khan, S.; Zhu, H.; Zhang, B.; Zhang, S.; Jiao, R. Zhaoshumycins A and B, two unprecedented antimycin-type depsipeptides produced by the marine-derived *Streptomyces* sp. ITBB-ZKa6. *Mar. Drugs* **2021**, *19*, 624. [CrossRef]
19. Çetinel Aksoy, S.; Küçüksolak, M.; Uze, A.; Bedir, E. Benzodiazepine derivatives from marine-derived *Streptomyces cacaoi* 14CM034. *Rec. Nat. Prod.* **2021**, *15*, 602–607. [CrossRef]
20. Peng, J.; Zhang, Q.; Jiang, X.; Ma, L.; Long, T.; Cheng, Z.; Zhang, C.; Zhu, Y. New piericidin derivatives from the marine-derived *Streptomyces* sp. SCSIO 40063 with cytotoxic activity. *Nat. Prod. Res.* **2021**. [CrossRef]
21. Xu, X.; Han, J.; Lin, R.; Polyak, S.W.; Song, F. Two new piperazine-triones from a marine-derived *Streptomycetes* sp. strain SMS636. *Mar. Drugs* **2019**, *17*, 186. [CrossRef] [PubMed]
22. Zhang, X.; He, H.; Ma, R.; Ji, Z.; Wei, Q.; Dai, H.; Zhang, L.; Song, F. Madurastatin B3, a rare aziridine derivative from actinomycete *Nocardiopsis* sp. LS150010 with potent anti-tuberculosis activity. *J. Ind. Microbiol. Biotechnol.* **2017**, *44*, 589–594. [CrossRef] [PubMed]
23. Chen, C.; Chen, X.; Ren, B.; Guo, H.; Abdel-Mageed, W.M.; Liu, X.; Song, F.; Zhang, L. Characterization of *Streptomyces* sp. LS462 with high productivity of echinomycin, a potent antituberculosis and synergistic antifungal antibiotic. *J. Ind. Microbiol. Biotechnol.* **2021**, *48*, kuab079. [CrossRef] [PubMed]
24. Song, F.; Yang, N.; Khalil, Z.G.; Salim, A.A.; Han, J.; Bernhardt, P.V.; Lin, R.; Xu, X.; Capon, R.J. Bhimamycin J, a rare benzo[f]isoindole-dione alkaloid from the marine-derived actinomycete *Streptomyces* sp. MS180069. *Chem. Biodivers.* **2021**, *18*, e2100674. [CrossRef] [PubMed]
25. Lamari, L.; Zitouni, A.; Dob, T.; Sabaou, N.; Lebrihi, A.; Germain, P.; Seguin, E.; Tillequin, F. New dithiolopyrrolone antibiotics from *Saccharothrix* sp. SA 233. II. Physicochemical properties and structure elucidation. *J. Antibiot.* **2002**, *55*, 702–706. [CrossRef]
26. Thompson, J.D.; Higgins, D.G.; Gibson, T.J. Clustal-W-Improving the sensitivity of progressive multiple sequence alignment through sequence weighting, position-specific gap penalties and weight matrix choice. *Nucleic Acids Res.* **1994**, *22*, 4673–4680. [CrossRef]
27. Clinical and Laboratory Standards Institute. *Methods for Dilution Antimicrobial Susceptibility Tests for Bacteria That Grow Aerobically*, 7th ed.; Approved standard; Clinical and Laboratory Standards Institute: Wayne, PA, USA, 2008.
28. Han, J.; Yang, N.; Wei, S.; Jia, J.; Lin, R.; Li, J.; Bi, H.; Song, F.; Xu, X. Dimeric hexylitaconic acids from the marine-derived fungus *Aspergillus welwitschiae* CUGBMF180262. *Nat. Prod. Res.* **2022**, *36*, 578–585. [CrossRef]
29. Wang, Q.; Song, F.; Xiao, X.; Huang, P.; Li, L.; Monte, A.; Abdel-Mageed, W.M.; Wang, J.; Guo, H.; He, W.; et al. Abyssomicins from the South China Sea deep-sea sediment *Verrucosispora* sp.: Natural thioether Michael addition adducts as antitubercular prodrugs. *Angew. Chem. Int. Ed. Engl.* **2013**, *52*, 1231–1234. [CrossRef]
30. Frisch, M.J.; Trucks, G.W.; Schlegel, H.B.; Scuseria, G.E.; Robb, M.A.; Cheeseman, J.R.; Scalmani, G.; Barone, V.; Mennucci, B.; Petersson, G.A.; et al. *Gaussian 09, Revision E.01*; Gaussian, Inc.: Wallingford, CT, USA, 2009.
31. Wolinski, K.; Hilton, J.F.; Pulay, P. Efficient Implementation of the Gauge-Independent Atomic Orbital Method for NMR chemical shift calculations. *J. Am. Chem. Soc.* **1990**, *112*, 8251–8260. [CrossRef]
32. Bruhn, T.; Schaumlöffel, A.; Hemberger, Y.; Bringmann, G. SpecDis: Quantifying the comparison of calculated and experimental electronic circular dichroism spectra. *Chirality* **2013**, *25*, 243–249. [CrossRef]
33. Tran, T.D.; Pham, N.B.; Quinn, R.J. Structure determination of pentacyclic pyridoacridine alkaloids from the Australian marine organisms *Ancorina geodides* and *Cnemidocarpa stolonifera*. *Eur. J. Org. Chem.* **2014**, *2014*, 4805–4816. [CrossRef]
34. Li, B.; Wever, W.J.; Walsh, C.T.; Bowers, A.A. Dithiolopyrrolones: Biosynthesis, synthesis, and activity of a unique class of disulfide-containing antibiotics. *Nat. Prod. Rep.* **2014**, *31*, 905–923. [CrossRef] [PubMed]

35. Qin, Z.; Huang, S.; Yu, Y.; Deng, H. Dithiolopyrrolone Natural Products: Isolation, Synthesis and Biosynthesis. *Mar. Drugs* **2013**, *11*, 3970–3997. [CrossRef] [PubMed]
36. Huang, S.; Tong, M.H.; Qin, Z.; Deng, Z.; Deng, H.; Yu, Y. Identification and characterization of the biosynthetic gene cluster of thiolutin, a tumor angiogenesis inhibitor, in *Saccharothrix algeriensis* NRRL B–24137. *Anticancer Agents Med. Chem.* **2015**, *15*, 277–284. [CrossRef]

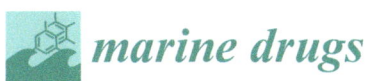

Article

New Sorbicillinoids with Tea Pathogenic Fungus Inhibitory Effect from Marine-Derived Fungus *Hypocrea jecorina* H8

Shun-Zhi Liu [1,†], Guang-Xin Xu [2,†], Feng-Ming He [1], Wei-Bo Zhang [3], Zhen Wu [1], Ming-Yu Li [1], Xi-Xiang Tang [2,*] and Ying-Kun Qiu [1,*]

1. State Key Laboratory of Cellular Stress Biology, School of Pharmaceutical Sciences, Xiamen University, South Xiang-An Road, Xiamen 361102, China; lsz@xmu.edu.cn (S.-Z.L.); fengminghe@stu.xmu.edu.cn (F.-M.H.); limingyu@xmu.edu.cn (M.-Y.L.)
2. Key Laboratory of Marine Biogenetic Resources, Third Institute of Oceanography State, Ministry of Natural Resources, Da-Xue Road, Xiamen 361005, China; xuguangxin@tio.org.cn (G.-X.X.); wuzhen@xmu.edu.cn (Z.W.)
3. State Key Laboratory of Marine Life, Ocean University of China, Yu-Shan Road, Qingdao 266100, China; 21200631103@stu.ouc.edu.cn
* Correspondence: tangxixiang@tio.org.cn (X.-X.T.); qyk@xmu.edu.cn (Y.-K.Q.); Tel./Fax: +86-592-2189868 (Y.-K.Q.)
† These authors contributed equally to this work.

Abstract: Four new dimeric sorbicillinoids (**1–3** and **5**) and a new monomeric sorbicillinoid (**4**) as well as six known analogs (**6–11**) were purified from the fungal strain *Hypocrea jecorina* H8, which was obtained from mangrove sediment, and showed potent inhibitory activity against the tea pathogenic fungus *Pestalotiopsis theae* (*P. theae*). The planar structures of **1–5** were assigned by analyses of their UV, IR, HR-ESI-MS, and NMR spectroscopic data. All the compounds were evaluated for growth inhibition of tea pathogenic fungus *P. theae*. Compounds **5**, **6**, **8**, **9**, and **10** exhibited more potent inhibitory activities compared with the positive control hexaconazole with an ED_{50} of 24.25 ± 1.57 µg/mL. The ED_{50} values of compounds **5**, **6**, **8**, **9**, and **10** were 9.13 ± 1.25, 2.04 ± 1.24, 18.22 ± 1.29, 1.83 ± 1.37, and 4.68 ± 1.44 µg/mL, respectively. Additionally, the effects of these compounds on zebrafish embryo development were also evaluated. Except for compounds **5** and **8**, which imparted toxic effects on zebrafish even at 0.625 µM, the other isolated compounds did not exhibit significant toxicity to zebrafish eggs, embryos, or larvae. Taken together, sorbicillinoid derivatives (**6**, **9**, and **10**) from *H. jecorina* H8 displayed low toxicity and high anti-tea pathogenic fungus potential.

Keywords: *Hypocrea jecorina* H8; trichodermolide C, D; tea pathogenic fungus inhibitory effect; toxicity assessment

Citation: Liu, S.-Z.; Xu, G.-X.; He, F.-M.; Zhang, W.-B.; Wu, Z.; Li, M.-Y.; Tang, X.-X.; Qiu, Y.-K. New Sorbicillinoids with Tea Pathogenic Fungus Inhibitory Effect from Marine-Derived Fungus *Hypocrea jecorina* H8. *Mar. Drugs* 2022, 20, 213. https://doi.org/10.3390/md20030213

Academic Editors: Orazio Taglialatela-Scafati and Asunción Barbero

Received: 4 January 2022
Accepted: 12 March 2022
Published: 17 March 2022

Publisher's Note: MDPI stays neutral with regard to jurisdictional claims in published maps and institutional affiliations.

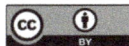

Copyright: © 2022 by the authors. Licensee MDPI, Basel, Switzerland. This article is an open access article distributed under the terms and conditions of the Creative Commons Attribution (CC BY) license (https:// creativecommons.org/licenses/by/ 4.0/).

1. Introduction

The influence of bioactive compounds from natural sources on human life has challenged scientists to research new environmental contexts and the associated biological diversity [1]. The ocean, as the largest frontier in biological exploration, represents one of the most favorable reservoirs of organisms producing secondary metabolites with biological activities [2]. The deep sea is an extreme environment; in this respect, its associated micro-organisms have great potential to produce natural products with novel biological properties [3].

The tea plant (*Camellia sinensis* L.) is an important commercial crop all over the world. However, the tea plant suffers from biotic stresses of some pathogenic fungi [4,5], which often exhibits severe damage of the blade tissue and discoloration of the leaves, common symptoms, including blight (*Exobasidium vexans* Massee), brown blight (*Colletotrichum camelliae* Massee), and red rust (*Cephaleuros parasiticus* Karst). These pathogenic fungi greatly reduce the quality of tea and damage human health [6–8].

As part of our continuing exploration for structurally novel and biologically interesting secondary metabolites from marine microorganisms, the fungal strain *Hypocrea jecorina* H8 (*H. jecorina* H8) was isolated from mangrove sediments and showed potent inhibitory activity against tea pathogenic fungus *P. theae*.

Chemical investigation of *H. jecorina* H8 from rice medium led to the isolation of 11 compounds, including five sorbicillinoids (**1–5**) and six known sorbicillinoid analogs. Some of these compounds exhibited significant inhibitory activity against tea pathogenic fungus *P. theae*. and low toxicity to zebrafish. Herein, we report the isolation, structural determination, as well as antifungal activity of these isolated compounds.

2. Results

2.1. Structural Elucidation of New Compounds

A series of column chromatography (CC) methods were used during the isolation of *H. jecorina* H8. As a result, 11 compounds were isolated, including five new compounds, trichodermolide C (**1**), trichodermolide D (**2**), 7,7′,9′-hydroxy-trichodimerol (**3**), 1-(2,4-dihydroxy-3,5-dimethylphenyl)-3,4,5-trihydroxyhexan-1-one (**4**), and isobisvertinol A (**5**). At the same time, by comparing NMR spectral data with those published in literatures, the six known compounds were determined to be 2′,3′-dihydrosorbicillin (**6**) [9], 6-demethylsorbicillin (**7**) [10], sorbicillin (**8**) [9], (2*E*,4*E*)-1-(2,4-dihydroxy-3,5-dimethylphenyl)-6-hydroxyhexa-2,4-dien-1-one (**9**), trichodimerol (**10**), and bisvertinol (**11**) [11] (Figure 1).

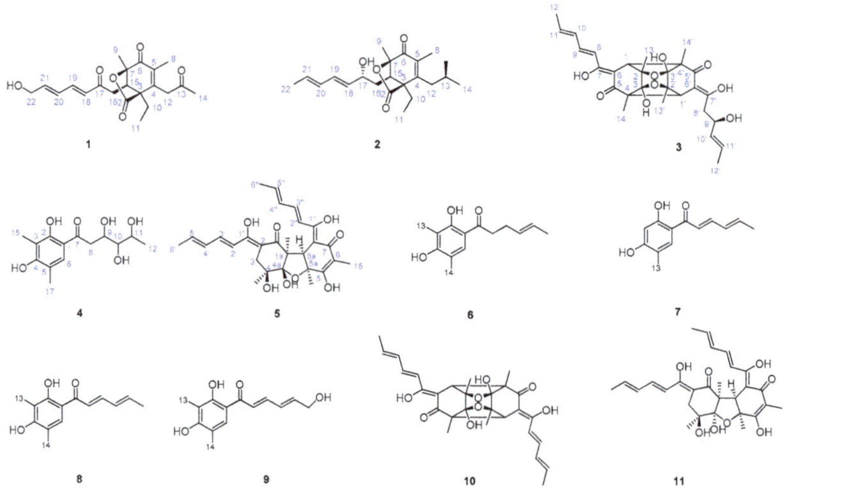

Figure 1. Structures of compounds **1–11** isolated from an extract of *Hypocrea jecorina* H8; the relative configuration of **5** is reported in this article.

Compound **1** was obtained as yellow amorphous powder. The molecular formula of **1** was established as $C_{21}H_{26}O_6$ based on the HR-ESI-MS peak at *m/z* 375.1798 [M + H]$^+$ (calcd for 375.1729 $C_{21}H_{27}O_6{}^+$), requiring nine degrees of unsaturation. The IR spectrum of **1** indicated the presence conjugated lactone carbonyl signal of at 1691 cm^{-1} [6]. In high chemical shifts region of ^{1}H NMR, four olefinic protons were observed at δ_H 6.20 (d, 15.4 Hz, H-20), 6.35 (dt, 15.2, 4.8 Hz, H-21), 6.43 (dd, 15.4, 10.2 Hz, H-18), and 7.25 (dd, 15.2, 10.8 Hz, H-19) (Table 1).

Table 1. ^{1}H NMR (600 Hz) and ^{13}C NMR (150 Hz) data of **1–2** (CDCl$_3$) and **4** (DMSO-d_6).

NO.	1		Trichodermolide B	2		4	
	δ_H (J in Hz)	δ_C	δ_C	δ_H (J in Hz)	δ_C	δ_H (J in Hz)	δ_C
2		174.9	174.7		176.4		113.6
3		55.7	55.9		56.2		159.9
4		149.2	150.9		152.1		111.7
5		134.4	133.9		133.8		160.3
6		191.3	191.2		191.9	7.34	118.4
7		86.8	86.5		87.1		125.1
8	1.77 s	11.6	11.9	1.87 s	12.1	2.89 dd (16.9, 13.7) 2.31 dd (16.9, 2.7)	192.1
9	1.48 s	16.4	16.5	1.56 s	17.3	4.64 dt (13.7, 2.6)	39.8
10	1.30 dq (13.7, 7.2) 2.08 dq (13.8, 7.2)	20.5	20.5	2.21 dq (14.2, 7.3) 1.75 s	20.9	3.09 td (8.5, 1.5)	77.1
11	0.95 t (7.2)	8.4	8.6	0.97 t (7.2)	8.6	3.88 dq (13.6, 6.0)	76.8
12	3.55 d (18.2) 3.63 d (18.2)	44.5	44.7	2.60 dd (13.7, 9.6) 2.39 brd (13.6)	39.2	1.19 d (6.0)	65.9
13		204	205.0	4.10 m	67.1	2.04 s	21.5
14	2.27 s	30.3	30.5	1.29 t (7.2)	24.1	2.12 s	9.2
15	3.55 t (5.3)	49.9	50.0	2.97 dd (6.4, 4.4)	51.3		16.7
16	2.43 dd (18.5, 5.2) 3.13 dd (18.5, 5.2)	35.2	35.0	1.52 m 1.37 m	32.3		
17		196.5	197.2	4.17 m	71.1		
18	6.43 br dd (15.4, 10.2)	127.9	127.6	6.16 dd (15.2, 10.5)	132.1		
19	7.25 dd (15.2, 10.8)	143.0	143.9	5.44 dd (15.2, 7.2)	131.9		
20	6.20 d (15.4)	128.8	130.6	5.75 dq (14.3, 6.8)	131.7		
21	6.35 dt (15.2, 4.8)	143.2	141.9	5.99 dd (15.2, 10.7)	130.0		
22	4.32 d (4.2)	62.7	19.1	1.76 br d (6.6)	18.2		

Their corresponding olefinic carbon signals were found in the sp^2 region of the ^{13}C NMR spectrum at δ_C 128.8 (C-20), 143.2 (C-21), 127.9 (C-18), and 143.0 (C-19). The sp^3 low chemical shifts region of the ^{1}H NMR spectrum displayed four notable methyl proton signals at δ_H 1.48 (9-CH$_3$), 1.77 (8-CH$_3$), 2.27(14-CH$_3$) linked to quaternary carbons, and δ_H 0.95 (t, 7.2 Hz, 11-CH$_3$) linked to a secondary carbon.

The ^{13}C NMR data showed four carbonyl signals at δ_C 204.0 (C-13), 196.5 (C-17), 191.3 (C-6), and 174.9 (C-2) attributing to a ketone carbonyl, two conjugated ketone carbonyl, and ester carbonyl, respectively. In addition, the ^{13}C NMR spectrum and DEPT data of **1** showed the presence of 21 carbons, sorted into four methyls, four methylenes, five methines (four olefinic carbons), and eight quaternary carbons (four carbonyl carbons and two olefinic carbons).

The above spectroscopic data showed high similarities to those of trichodermolide B, a known compound isolated from *Trichoderma reesei* (HN-2016-018) [12], except for the presence of signal for a hydroxyl group, a signal for methylene group at C-22 (δ_H 4.32, δ_C 62.7) and the lack of signal for a methyl group (δ_C 19.1). Thus, **1** was deduced to be a hydroxylated derivative of trichodermolide B at C-22, validated by the COSY correlations of δ_H 6.35 (H-21) with δ_H 4.32 (H2-22) (Figure 2a).

The two double bonds in sorbyl side chain for **1** were assigned both as *E* configuration based on their coupling constants ($J_{H-18/H-19}$ = 15.2 Hz, $J_{H-20/H-21}$ = 15.4 Hz) and the NOESY correlation between H-18/H-20. For the bridged bicycle lactone ring system, it was only possible if the CH$_3$-9 and CH$_2$-10 were oriented equatorially. In addition, the ^{1}H NMR chemical shifts of H-15 (δ_H 3.37 for trichodermolide B compared to δ_H 3.55 for **1**), H-16 (δ_H 2.54, 2.99 for trichodermolide B compared to δ_H 2.43, 3.13 for **1**), CH$_3$-9 (δ_H 1.37 for trichodermolide B compared to δ_H 1.48 for **1**), and CH$_2$-10 (δ_H 1.25, 2.03 for trichodermolide B compared to δ_H 1.30, 2.08 for **1**) suggested the same relative configurations of C-3, C-15, and C-7 in **1** as that in trichodermolide B [12].

Therefore, the relative configuration of **1** was assumed as 3*S**,15*R**,7*R**. The ECD curve of **1** showed a negative Cotton effect around 220 nm and a positive Cotton effect around 270 nm, respectively. These were the same as trichodermolide B (Figure S41: Calculated and experimental ECD spectra of trichodermolide B). The absolute configuration of **1** was assigned as 3*S*,15*R*,7*R* (Figure 3a). As a result, the structure of **1** was determined and named as trichodermolide C (Figure 1).

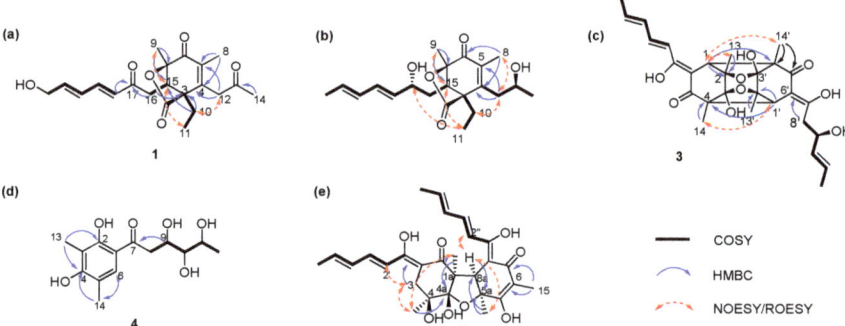

Figure 2. Key ^{1}H–^{1}H COSY, HMBC, and NOESY correlations of compounds **1–5**. (**a**) Key COSY, HMBC, and NOESY correlations of compounds **1**; (**b**) Key COSY, HMBC, and NOESY correlations of compounds **2**; (**c**) Key COSY, HMBC, and NOESY correlations of compounds **3**; (**d**) Key COSY, HMBC correlations of compounds **4**; (**e**) Key COSY, HMBC, and NOESY correlations of compounds **5**.

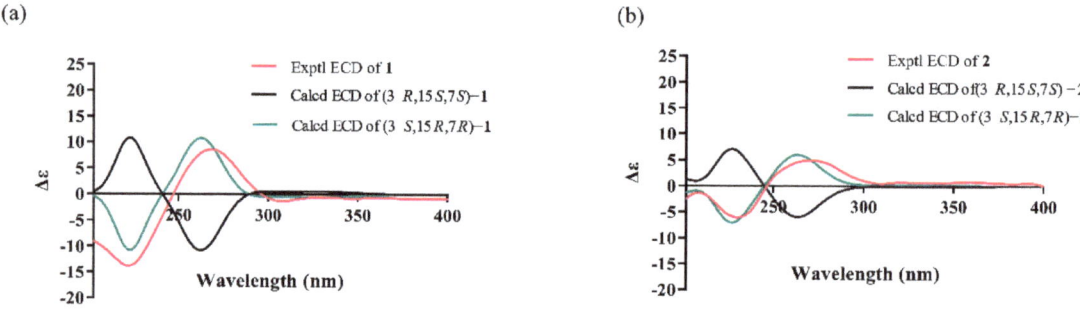

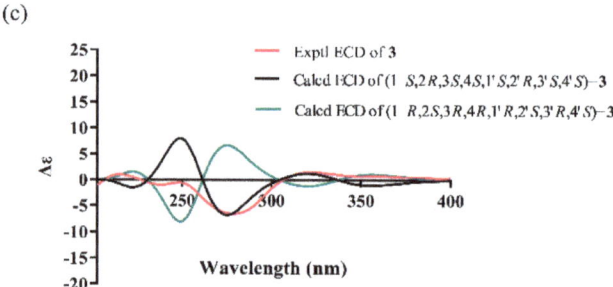

Figure 3. Calculated and experimental ECD spectra of compounds **1**, **2**, and **3**. (**a**) ECD spectra for compound **1**; (**b**) ECD spectra for compound **2**; (**c**): ECD spectra for compound **3**.

Compound **2** was also obtained as yellow amorphous powder. The molecular formula was deduced to be $C_{21}H_{30}O_5$ by interpretation of the HR-ESI-MS peak at *m/z* 363.2162 [M + H]$^+$ (calcd for 363.2093 $C_{21}H_{31}O_5{}^+$), implying seven degrees of unsaturation. Compound **2** presented ^{1}H and ^{13}C NMR signals similar to those of compounds **1**, especially those on the bridged bicyclic ring moiety. The structural differences in the side chains could be revealed by the DEPT spectra, in which two carbonyl signals vanished and two oxygenated methine signals emerged, together with the signal different from the oxygenated methylene (C-22) to methyl.

The corresponding ^{1}H NMR signals in **2** were found at δ_H 4.17 (H-17), 4.10 (H-13), and 1.76 (CH$_3$-22), respectively. Thus, compound **2** is considered to be a reduction product of compound **1**. On the aids of ^{1}H-^{1}H COSY spectrum, two continuous connected spin systems revealed the presence of two side chain as: CH$_3$-CH=CH-CH=CH-CH(O-)-CH$_2$- and -CH$_2$-CH(O)-CH$_2$-. The key HMBC correlations from δ_H 2.60 (CH$_2$-12) to δ_C 133.8 (C-5), 152.1 (C-4), 51.3 (C-3) and from δ_H 1.87 (CH$_3$-8) to δ_C 191.9 (C-6), C-4, C-5 allowed the elucidation of structure for compound **2**.

The E configurations among the two double bonds in the side chains of **2** could be confirmed by the large coupling constant ($J_{H-18/H-19} = J_{H-20/H-21}$ = 15.2 Hz). The relative configurations of three stereocenters, C-3, C-15, and C-7 of **2** were confirmed by comparison of its ^{1}H NMR data with compound **1**. The NOESY correlations between H-15 and CH$_3$-11, H-17/CH$_3$-11, and CH$_3$-8/CH$_2$-12 established the relative configuration of **2**. Therefore, the relative configuration of **2** was assumed as 3S*,15R*,7R*. The calculated ECD curve of 3S,15R,7R-**2** was consistent with the experimental data (Figure 3b), and hence the absolute configuration of **2** was assigned as 3S,15R,7R.

Compound **3** was obtained as a yellow amorphous powder. The results from the HR-ESI-MS peak at m/z 537.2090 [M + Na]$^+$ (calcd for 537.2100 C$_{28}$H$_{34}$O$_9$Na$^+$) suggested that the molecular formula of **3** was C$_{28}$H$_{34}$O$_9$, thus, implying twelve degrees of unsaturation. The ^{1}H and ^{13}C NMR data of **3** showed 30 protons and 28 carbons signals, and these carbon signals were classified into twelve quaternary carbons (four ethylenic bonds), two carbonyls, six ethylenic bonds, one oxygenated methines, two methines without an oxygen link, one methylene, and six methyls.

Comparison of the NMR data of **3** with those of **10**, a known metabolite isolated from a strain of the same genus [6], indicated that **3** possessed an identical trichodimerol [13] skeleton to **10**. Although compound **10** afforded only 14 signals because of a symmetric structure, some ^{13}C signals of compound 3 split, suggesting an asymmetric structure (Table 2). The major difference were found at the signals due to C-8′, C-10′ moiety, suggesting a hydration at C-8′/C-9′ double bond in compound **3**. In ^{13}C NMR and DEPT, the double bond signals of C-8′ and C-9′ in **10** turn to a methylene (δ_C 40.9, C-8′) and an oxygen-linked methine (δ_C 80.7, C-9′) in **3**. The conclusion was confirmed by the COSY correlation from δ_H 2.38 (H-8′) to δ_H 4.31 (H-9′), and to δ_H 5.67 (H-10′). In the HMBC spectrum of **3**, the correlations from H-8′ to C-7′, C-9′ were also found.

The NOESY correlations between δ_H 1.41 (CH$_3$-14) and δ_H 3.31 (H-1′) indicated the same orientation of these signals. In addition, the protons δ_H 1.41 (CH$_3$-14′) and δ_H 2.94 (H-1) were simultaneously correlated with δ_H 1.35 (CH$_3$-13), reflecting that these signals locate at the same orientation. (Figure 2c). The absolute configuration of **3** was established as 1S,2R,3S, 4S, 1′S,2′R, 3′S, 4′S by comparison on experimental and calculated ECD spectra (Figure 3c).

Compound **4** was isolated as a colorless amorphous powder. The molecular formula of C$_{14}$H$_{20}$O$_6$, which gave five unsaturation degrees, was established by the positive HR-ESI-MS ion peak at m/z 285.1342 [M + H]$^+$ (calcd for 285.1338 C$_{14}$H$_{21}$O$_6^+$). The UV maximum absorption bands at λmax (log ε): 216 (3.66) nm were assigned to a conjugated carbonyl, which was confirmed by the ^{13}C NMR data at δ_C 192.1 (C-1′). In the ^{1}H NMR, three methyl peaks at δ_H 1.19 (d, 6.0 Hz, CH$_3$-12), 2.04 (s, CH$_3$-13), and 2.12 (s, CH$_3$-14) were assigned. One olefinic proton was also observed at 7.34 (H-6).

Table 2. ^{1}H NMR (600 Hz) and ^{13}C NMR (150 Hz) data of **3**, **5** (CDCl$_3$) and ^{13}C NMR data of Compounds **10** and **11**.

No.	3		10	No.	5		11
	δ_H (J in Hz)	δ_C	δ_C		δ_H (J in Hz)	δ_C	δ_C
1	2.94, s	58.3	57.5	1		191.8	194.3
1'	3.31, s	52.3	57.5	2		100.7	101.9
2,2'		78.3	78.9	3	2.58 br d (14.1) 2.73 m	35.9	35.4
3,3'		108.7	104.1	4		73.9	72.7
4		59.0	58.8	5		168.7	168.8
4'		59.0	58.8	6		103.9	105.6
5,5'		199.0	198.0	7		191.7	191.6
6'		104.0	102.8	8		106.1	106.2
6		103.8	102.8	1'		179.7	178.0
7		172.5	175.9	2'	6.40 br d (14.9)	120.3	121.4
7'		175.2	175.9	3'	7.25 br s	139.0	137.8
8	6.18 d (14.7)	118.6	118.5	4'	6.21 m	130.8	131.4
8'	2.38 dd (16.9, 3.5) 2.54 dd (16.9,13.6)	40.9	118.5	5'	6.10 br d (7.0)	131.1	131.7
9	7.35 dd (14.8,10.9)	143.0	143.6	6'	1.86 br d (6.4)	18.8	18.9
9'	4.31 ddd (13.5, 7.1,3.2)	80.7	143.6	1"		168.8	167.3
10	6.31 dd (15.4, 11.0)	130.8	130.9	2"	6.27 m	120.2	121.3
10'	5.67 dq (15.2,6.6)	131.8	130.9	3"	6.29 m	140.3	140.1
11	6.22 dd (13.6,6.6)	140.1	140.5	4"	6.23 br s	131.8	131.4
11'	5.49 ddd (15.3,7.0,1.6)	127.2	140.5	5"	6.18 m	137.0	136.6
12	1.91 brd (6.6)	18.9	18.8	6"	1.86 br d (6.4)	18.9	19.1
12'	1.68 brd (6.4)	17.8	18.8	1a		58.4	59.1
13	1.43 s	21.5	21.3	1a-CH$_3$	1.34 s	19.2	19.9
13'	1.35 s	20.7	21.3	4a		110.2	108.4
14	1.41 s	18.2	18.9	4-CH$_3$	1.29, s	22.4	22.8
14'	1.41 s	18.4	18.9	5a		79.6	78.8
				5a-CH$_3$	1.48 br s	25.6	25.8
				6-CH$_3$	1.53, s 1.86 br d (6.4)	6.8	7.3
				8a	3.63, s	53.6	53.6

In the ^{13}C NMR, except for the carbonyl, six sp^2 carbons at δ_C 160.3 (C-4), 159.9 (C-2), 125.1 (C-6), 118.4 (C-5), 113.6 (C-1), and 111.7 (C-3) and three oxygenated methines at δ_C 77.1 (C-3'), 76.8 (C-3'), and 65.9 (C-5') were assigned, respectively. The benzene ring signals in compound **4** closely resembled those of the known compound 2′,3′-dihydrosorbicillin (**6**) [14]; however, they were different regarding the side chain. The COSY correlation data suggested the side chain of **4** was -CH$_2$-CH(OH)-CH(OH)-CH(OH)-CH$_3$. In addition, the HMBC correlation from δ_H 2.89 (CH$_2$-8) to δ_C 192.1 (C-7) indicated that the carbonyl was at C-7. Comprehensive HSQC, COSY, and HMBC established the structure of **4** (Figure 1).

Compound **5** was obtained as a white amorphous powder with positive HR-ESI-MS ion peaks at m/z 499.2312 [M + H]$^+$ indicating 12 degrees of unsaturation. According to the HR-ESI-MS data, compound **5** and **11** shared the same molecular formula (Figure S42). The NMR data of **5** had similar features compared to those of **11**, which suggests that they are stereoisomers. The planar structure of **5** was determined by the COSY and HMBC data. The main differences of NMR signals were attributable to C-1, C-4, and C-4a, with the ^{13}C NMR deference of [δ_C 191.8 (C-1), 73.9 (C-4), and 110.2 (C-4a) in **5** vs. δ_C 194.3 (C-1), 72.7 (C-4), and 108.4 (C-4a) in **11**].

Thus, compounds **5** and **11** should be epimers around either C-4 or C-4a. In the NOESY spectrum, key cross peaks were observed between δ_H 3.63 (H-8a) and δ_H 1.34 (CH$_3$-1a) and δ_H 1.48 (CH$_3$-5a) (Figure 2e), indicating that the methyls CH$_3$-1a and CH$_3$-5a were at the same side with H-8a. Furthermore, NOESY were observed between CH$_3$-1a and δ_H 1.29 (CH$_3$-4). These results indicated that the relative configuration of C-4 was same as that of **11**. Therefore, we concluded that **5** is a stereoisomer of **11** on C-4a. The relative configuration of **5** was defined as shown in Figure 1.

2.2. Evaluation of Antifungal Activity

Compounds **1** to **11** were evaluated for antifungal activities by a paper disc inhibition assay. Compounds **5**, **6**, **8**, **9**, and **10** possessed significant activities against the tea pathogenic fungus *P. theae* (Table 3). The ED$_{50}$ values of **5**, **6**, **8**, **9**, and **10** were 9.13 ± 1.25, 2.04 ± 1.91, 18.22 ± 1.29, 1.83 ± 1.37, and 4.68 ± 1.44 µg/mL, respectively. Compared to positive control hexaconazole (24.25 ± 1.57 µg/mL), compounds **5**, **6**, **8**, **9**, and **10** exhibited more potent antifungal activity. Particularly, new compound **5** had nearly 3-fold more, and known compound **9** had a 13-fold stronger anti-tea pathogenic fungus effect.

Table 3. Antifungal activities of **5**, **6**, **8**, **9**, and **10** (ED$_{50}$, µg/mL).

Compd.	*Pestalotiopsis theae*	Compd.	*Pestalotiopsis theae*
1	>100	8	18.22 ± 1.29
2	>100	9	1.83 ± 1.37
3	>100	10	4.68 ± 1.44
4	>100	11	>100
5	9.13 ± 1.25	hexaconazole *	24.25 ± 1.57
6	2.04 ± 1.91	DMSO	None
7	>100		

* hexaconazole serves as positive control.

2.3. Evaluation of Toxicity

The zebrafish is a small teleost that is becoming increasingly popular in many biomedical and environmental studies [15]. This model has shown sensitivity to a broad variety of contaminants (such as endocrine disruptors and organic pollutants), indicating their suitability as a biological method for environmental monitoring in risk assessment.

We evaluated the toxicity of compounds **5**, **6**, **8**, **9**, and **10** in a zebrafish model (Figure 4). Figure 4a showed that these compounds, except compound **8**, killed zebrafish embryo less than 50% when treated with a concentration of 10 µM. When the treatment time was prolonged to 72 h (Figure 4b), the mortality rate of zebrafish embryo caused by compound **8** at 0.625 µM increased to nearly 60%, whereas the effects of compounds **5**, **6**, **9**, and **10** did not change greatly.

In addition, the impact on the malformation of zebrafish by these compounds was observed using a Leica stereomicroscope. Figure 4c showed graphically under the same treatment that compounds **5** and **8** had greater effects than other compounds on the mortality rate and malformation of zebrafish both at a concentration of 0.625 µM for 24 h and at a concentration of 10 µM for 72 h. In summary, our data demonstrated that compounds **6**, **9**, and **10** were of low toxicity and could be used against tea pathogenic fungi agents and deserve further optimization.

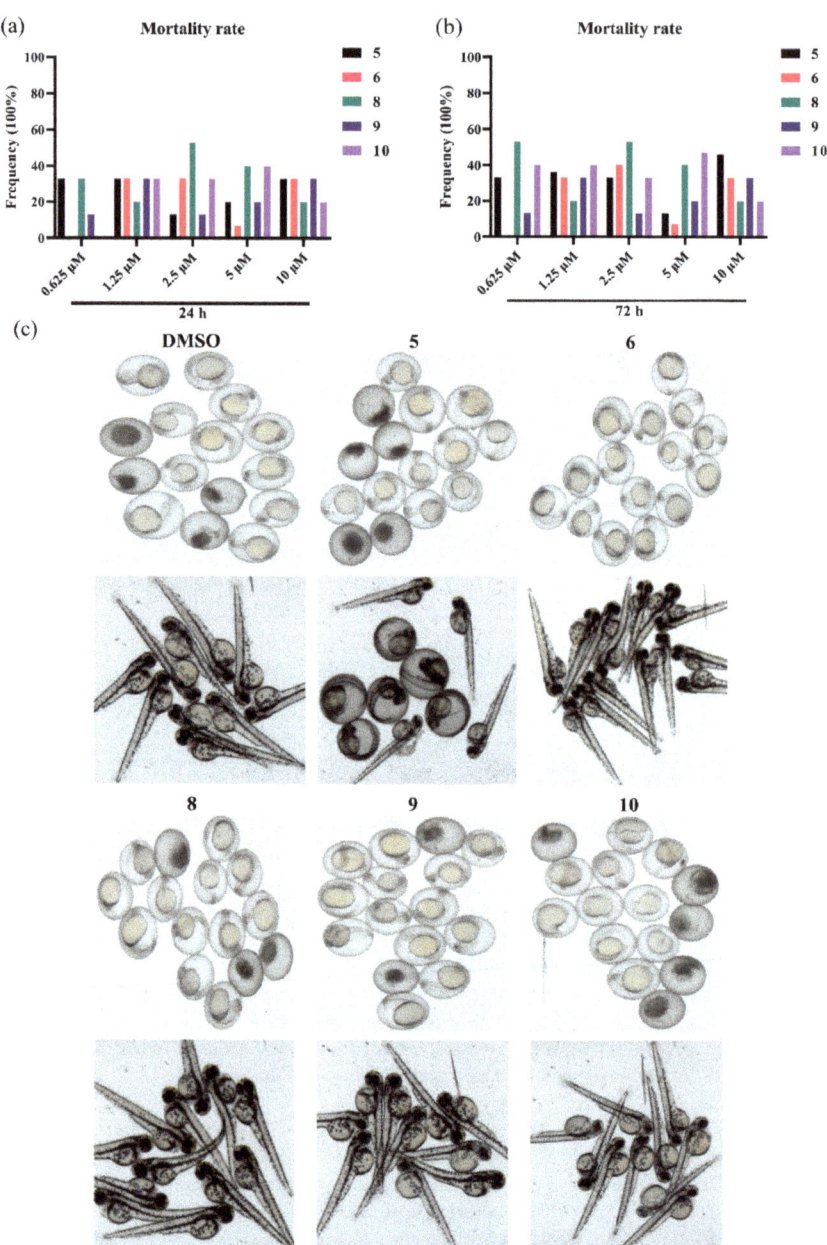

Figure 4. Embryotoxicity and developmental toxicity assay; 15 zebrafish embryos per condition were exposed to compounds at the concentrations of 10, 5, 2.5, 1.25, and 0.625 µM, and 0.1% DMSO was used as blank control. (**a**) The mortality rate of 24 embryo treated with compounds; (**b**) The mortality rate of 72 embryo treated with compounds; (**c**) The impact on the malformation of zebrafish treated with compounds) The statistics of 24 and 72 h mortality rate; © Morphology of 24 h embryo or 72 h zebrafish larvae treated with compounds or control.

3. Discussion

During the analyses of natural products from the ethyl acetate (EtOAc) extract of antibacteria from special growing environment, we discovered five new sorbicillinoids (**1–5**) together with six known analogs (**6–11**). These compounds were obtained from the marine-derived *H. jecorina* (H8) from the mangrove sediments collected from Zhangjiangkou Mangrove National Nature Reserve, China.

Chemically, the configurations and absolute of these compounds were described by their NOESY and CD spectra, respectively. All the isolated compounds of anti-tea pathogenic fungus *Pestalotiopsis theae* activities were evaluated. Compounds **5**, **6**, **8**, **9**, and **10** had stronger inhibitory effects against the fungi assays compared with hexaconazole.

However, the security of the antifungal regents is an important factor for use in agricultural applications. Although it showed potent activity, compound **5** exhibited strong anti-proliferative effects on the embryonic development of zebrafish, and compound **8** killed zebrafish embryos more than 50% at both a concentration of 0.625 µM for 24 h and a concentration of 10 µM for 72 h, thus, indicating high toxicity. Compounds **6**, **9**, and **10** showed much lower toxicity to zebrafish. In summary, sorbicillinoid derivatives (**6**, **9**, and **10**) from *H. jecorina* H8 had low toxicity and potent potency against tea pathogenic fungus.

4. Materials and Methods

4.1. General Experimental Procedures

An electrospray ionization source (ESI)-equipped Q-Exactive Mass spectrometer (Thermo Fisher Scientific Corporation, Waltham, MA, USA) was used to analyse the HR-ESI-MS data. A Shimadzu UV-260 spectrometer (Shimadzu Corporation, Tokyo, Japan) and a Perkin–Elmer 683 infrared spectrometer (PerkinElmer, Inc., Waltham, MA, USA) were used to obtain the UV and IR spectra, respectively. A JASCO P-200 polarimeter (JASCO Corporation, Tokyo, Japan) with a 5 cm cell was applied to measure the optical rotation value. The NMR spectra with TMS as the internal standard were taken on a Brucker Avance III 600 FT NMR spectrometer (Bruker Corporation, Billerica, MA, USA).

Column chromatography was performed with silica gel (Yantai Chemical Industry Research Institute, Shandong, China), Cosmosil 75 C18-MS-II (75 µm, Nacalai Tesqye corporation, Kyoto, Japan), and Spehadex LH-20 (GE Healthcare, Danderyd, Sweden). Semi-preparative HPLC was conducted on an Aglient HPLC (Agilent Technologies Inc., Santa Clara, CA, USA) system equipped with a diode array detector via a preparative Cosmosil ODS column. The HR-ESI-MS spectra were measured using a thermo Q-Exactive Mass spectrometer (Thermo Fisher Scientific Corporation).

4.2. Eletronic Circular Dichroism (ECD) Calculations

The circular dichroism (CD) spectra were recorded on a MOS-500 dichroism spectrometer. The conformational analyses were conducted with MOE 2018 using MMFF94. All calculations were conducted with Gaussian 09 using various functionals (b3lyp/6-31+g(d) and cam-b3lyp/6-31+g(d)). The overall theoretical ECD data were weighted by Boltzmann distribution, and the ECD spectra were produced by SpecDis 1.70 software [6,16].

4.3. Fungus Carbohydrate Fermentation

H. jecorina (H8) was isolated from the mangrove sediments collected from Zhangjiangkou Mangrove National Nature Reserve, Fujian province, China. The strain was identified as *Hypocrea jecorina* on the basis of the internal transcribed spaces (ITS) sequence. The ITS region of the fungus was a 636 bp DNA sequence (GenBank accession number OL376355), which had 99% identity to *Hypocrea jecorina*. The fungal strain has been preserved at Third Institute of Oceanography, China. *P. theae* (ITS GenBank accession number HQ832793) was isolated from foliar lesions of the tea leaf, and its pathogenicity to tea leaves was verified both in vitro and in vivo.

4.4. Extraction and Isolation

The fungus H8 was cultivated on rice-artificial sea water medium, incubated at 28 °C for 20 days in a standing position. After 20 days of fermentation, the solid cultures were dispersed in water (H$_2$O) and extracted with EtOAc (1:1, *v/v*) three times. The EtOAc extract was concentrated under reduced pressure at 40 °C to afford 22.0 g residue. The residue (21 g) was subjected to silica gel CC with petroleum ether (PE)-EtOAc (*v/v*) (20:1; 10:1; 5:1; 2:1; 1:1; 0:1) and chloroform (CDCl$_3$)-methanol (MeOH) (*v/v*) (100:1; 50:1; 20:1; 10:1; 5:1; 100% MeOH) to yield nine fractions (Fr. 1–9).

Fr. 2 (400 mg) was subjected to octadecylsilyl (ODS) chromatography and eluted with MeOH-H$_2$O (80–100%) to give 10 subfractions (Fr. 2A–2J). Then, Fr. 2G was purified using preparative reversed-phase HPLC C18 column (pre. Rp-C18) and isocratic eluted with MeOH-H$_2$O (85%) to obtain compound **6** (50 mg). Fr.3 (500 mg) was subjected to CC over ODS gel eluting with to MeOH-H$_2$O (70–100%) to obtain four subfractions (Fr. 3A-Fr.3D). Subfraction Fr.3C was purified by Prep. Rp-C18 using MeOH-H$_2$O (74%) elution to obtain **7** (11.9 mg). Fraction Fr.4 (496 mg) was subjected to CC over Sephadex LH-20 (MeOH) to yield six subfractions (Fr.4A–Fr.4F).

Compounds **1** (1.3 mg), **3** (1.1 mg), **10** (4.4 mg), and **8** (10 mg) were separated from subfraction Fr.4C by Prep. Rp-C18 (MeOH-H$_2$O, 80%). Fraction Fr.5 was purified by CC on Sephadex LH-20 (MeOH) to yield four subfractions (Fr.5A–Fr.5D), and then fraction Fr.5B was purified by Prep. Rp-C18 isocratic eluted with MeOH-H$_2$O (80:20) to provide **2** (5.5 mg). Fr. 5C was also purified by Prep. Rp-C18 isocratic eluted with MeOH-H$_2$O (52:48) to obtain compound **4** (1.0 mg). Compounds **5** (9.3 mg), **9** (20 mg), and **11** (25 mg) were separated from subfraction Fr.5D by Prep. Rp-C18 (MeOH-H$_2$O, 80%).

4.5. Structrural Elucidation of the New Compounds **1–5**

Trichodermolide C (**1**): yellow amorphous powder; HR-ESI-MS *m/z* 375.1798 [M + H]$^+$ (calcd. for 375.1729 C$_{21}$H$_{27}$O$_6$$^+$) and 397.1609 [M + Na]$^+$ (calcd. for 397.1627 C$_{21}$H$_{26}$O$_6$Na$^+$) in the positive mode; $[\alpha]_D^{30}$ = +54° (*c* = 0.5, MeOH). IR (KBr) (νmax): 3385, 1646, and 1436 cm^{-1}. ^{1}H NMR and ^{13}C NMR data are listed in Table 1.

Trichodermolide D (**2**): yellow amorphous powder; HR-ESI-MS *m/z* 363.2162 [M + H]$^+$ (calcd. for 363.2093 C$_{21}$H$_{31}$O$_5$$^+$) and 389.1972 [M + Na]$^+$ (calcd. for 385.1991 C$_{21}$H$_{30}$O$_5$Na$^+$) in the positive mode; $[\alpha]_D^{30}$ = +105° (*c* = 0.5, MeOH). IR (KBr) (νmax): 3406, 2927, 1560, and 1430 cm^{-1}. ^{1}H NMR and ^{13}C NMR data are listed in Table 1.

7, 7′, 9′-Hydroxy-trichodimerol (**3**) isolated as a yellow amorphous powder; HR-ESI-MS *m/z* 51.2265 (calcd. for 515.2281 C$_{28}$H$_{35}$O$_9$$^+$) and 537.2090 [M + Na]$^+$ (calcd. for 537.2100 C$_{28}$H$_{34}$O$_9$Na$^+$) in the positive mode; $[\alpha]_D^{30}$ = −35° (*c* = 0.5, MeOH), IR (KBr) νmax: 3406, 1570, and 1430 cm^{-1}. UV (MeOH) λmax (log ε): 286 (4.39) and 359 (4.46) nm. ^{1}H NMR and ^{13}C NMR data are listed in Table 2.

1-(2,4-Dihydroxy-3,5-dimethylphenyl)-3,4,5-trihydroxyhexan-1-one (**4**): colorless amorphous powder; HR-ESI-MS *m/z* 285.1342 [M + H]$^+$ (calcd. for 285.1338 C$_{14}$H$_{21}$O$_6$$^+$) in the positive mode; $[\alpha]_D^{30}$ = +6° (*c* = 0.05, MeOH), IR (KBr) (νmax): 3416, 2927, 1601, 1367, 1188, and 1075 cm^{-1}. UV (MeOH) λmax (log ε): 216 (3.66), 285 (3.72), and 329 (3.41) nm. ^{1}H NMR and ^{13}C NMR data are listed in Table 1.

Isobisvertinol A (**5**): white amorphous powder; HR-ESI-MS *m/z* 499.2312 [M + H]$^+$ (calcd. for 499.2326 C$_{28}$H$_{35}$O$_8$$^+$) in the positive mode, and 497.2194 [M − H]$^-$ (calcd. for 497.2181 C$_{28}$H$_{33}$O$_8$$^-$) in the negative mode; $[\alpha]_D^{30}$ = −46.2° (*c* = 0.5, MeOH), IR (KBr) (νmax): 3416, 1570, and 1430 cm^{-1}. UV (MeOH) λmax (log ε): 278 (3.44) and 374 (3.52) nm. ^{1}H NMR and ^{13}C NMR data are listed in Table 2.

4.6. Antifungal Activity Assay

Initial evaluations of the antifungal activity of the purified compounds were conducted against tea pathogenic fungus *P. theae* in six-well microplates as described by Xia Yan with certain modifications [17]. The final concentrations of each compound in the wells were 80, 40, 20, 10, 5, and 2.5 μg/mL (two-fold dilutions). DMSO and hexaconazole were used as a blank control and positive control, respectively. The ED$_{50}$ (μg/mL) values were calculated statistically using Probit analyses.

4.7. Toxicity Evaluation

Wild-type (AB strain) zebra fish (Danio rerio) were used in this test. Compounds **5**, **6**, **8**, **9**, and **10** were dissolved in DMSO (10 mM) and stored at −20 °C. Toxicity evaluations were analyzed regarding the anti-proliferative effects on embryos according to the literature [18]. In brief, 15 zebrafish embryos per condition were exposed to compounds at the concentrations of 10, 5, 2.5, 1.25, and 0.625 μM, and 0.1% DMSO was used as the vehicle control. A Leica stereomicroscope was used to observe the embryos every 24 h.

Supplementary Materials: The following are available online at https://www.mdpi.com/article/10.3390/md20030213/s1, Figures S1–S8: Spectra of **1**, Figures S9–S16: Sepctra of **2**, Figures S17–S25: Spectra of **3**, Figures S26–S32: Spectra of **4**, Spectra of **3**, Figures S33–S40: Spectra of **5**, Figure S41: ECD spectra of trichodermolide B, Figure S42: HR-ESI-MS spectra of 11. ECD calculation of **1**–**3**.

Author Contributions: X.-X.T. and G.-X.X. identified the fungus and performed the antifungal activity assay. W.-B.Z. performed the toxicity evaluation. S.-Z.L. and F.-M.H. isolated the compounds. Z.W. was responsible for the structural elucidation. Y.-K.Q. and M.-Y.L. supervised the project. All authors have read and agreed to the published version of the manuscript.

Funding: The project was supported by Key Laboratory of Marine Biotechnology of Fujian Province (2021MB02 to ML) and Asian Countries Maritime Cooperation Fund (99950410). The project was also supported by National Survey of Traditional Chinese Medicine Resources (Grant No. (2019)39) and Deep Sea Habitats Discovery Project (DY-XZ-04).

Conflicts of Interest: The authors have no conflict of interest to declare. The founding sponsors had no role in the design of the study; in the collection, analyses, or interpretation of data; in the writing of the manuscript, and in the decision to publish the results.

References

1. Chen, S.; Cai, R.; Liu, Z.; Cui, H.; She, Z. Secondary metabolites from mangrove-associated fungi: Source, chemistry and bioactivities. *Nat. Prod. Rep.* **2021**, *10*, 1–36. [CrossRef] [PubMed]
2. Rateb, M.E.; Ebel, R. Secondary metabolites of fungi from marine habitats. *Nat. Prod. Rep.* **2011**, *28*, 290–344. [CrossRef] [PubMed]
3. Niu, S.W.; Tang, X.X.; Fan, Z.W.; Xia, J.M.; Xie, C.L.; Yang, X.W. Fusarisolins A–E, Polyketides from the Marine-Derived Fungus Fusarium solani H918. *Mar. Drugs* **2019**, *17*, 408–411. [CrossRef] [PubMed]
4. Guo, M.; Pan, Y.M.; Dai, Y.L.; Gao, Z.M. First Report of Brown Blight Disease Caused by Colletotrichum gloeosporioides on Camellia sinensis in Anhui Province, China. *Plant Dis.* **2014**, *98*, 284. [CrossRef] [PubMed]
5. Li, J.; Sun, K.; Ma, Q.P.; Chen, J.; Wang, L.; Yang, D.J.; Chen, X.; Li, X.H. Colletotrichum gloeosporioides-Contaminated Tea Infusion Blocks Lipids Reduction and Induces Kidney Damage in Mice. *Front. Microbiol.* **2017**, *8*, 2089–2097. [CrossRef] [PubMed]
6. Tang, X.X.; Yan, X.; Fu, W.H.; Yi, L.Q.; Tang, B.W.; Yu, L.B.; Fang, M.J.; Wu, Z.; Qu, Y.K. New beta-Lactone with Tea Pathogenic Fungus Inhibitory Effect from Marine-Derived Fungus MCCC3A00957. *J. Agric. Food Chem.* **2019**, *67*, 2877–2885. [CrossRef] [PubMed]
7. Ponmurugan, P.; Baby, U.I.; Rajkumar, R. Growth, photosynthetic and biochemical responses of tea cultivars infected with various diseases. *Photosynthetica* **2007**, *45*, 143–146. [CrossRef]
8. Sanjay, R.; Ponmurugan, P.; Baby, U.I. Evaluation of fungicides and biocontrol agents against grey blight disease of tea in the field. *Crop Prot.* **2008**, *27*, 689–694. [CrossRef]
9. Lan, W.J.; Zhao, Y.; Xie, Z.L.; Liang, L.Z.; Shao, W.Y.; Zhu, L.P.; Yang, D.P.; Zhu, X.F.; Li, H.J. Novel sorbicillin analogues from the marine fungus Trichoderma sp. associated with the seastar Acanthaster planci. *Nat. Prod. Commun.* **2012**, *7*, 1337–1340. [CrossRef] [PubMed]
10. Du, L.; Zhu, T.; Li, L.; Cai, S.; Zhao, B.; Gu, Q. Cytotoxic sorbicillinoids and bisorbicillinoids from a marine-derived fungus Trichoderma sp. *Chem. Pharm. Bull.* **2009**, *57*, 220–223. [CrossRef] [PubMed]
11. Koyama, N.; Ohshiro, T.; Tomoda, H.; Omura, S. Fungal isobisvertinol, a new inhibitor of lipid droplet accumulation in mouse macrophages. *Org. Lett.* **2007**, *9*, 425–428. [CrossRef] [PubMed]
12. Rehman, S.U.; Yang, L.J.; Zhang, Y.H.; Wu, J.S.; Shi, T.; Haider, W.; Shao, C.L.; Wang, C.Y. Sorbicillinoid Derivatives From Sponge-Derived Fungus Trichoderma reesei (HN-2016-018). *Front. Microbiol.* **2020**, *11*, 1334. [CrossRef] [PubMed]
13. Shi, Z.Z.; Liu, X.H.; Li, X.N.; Ji, N.Y. Antifungal and Antimicroalgal Trichothecene Sesquiterpenes from the Marine Algicolous Fungus Trichoderma brevicompactum A-DL-9-2. *J. Agric. Food Chem.* **2020**, *68*, 15440–15448. [CrossRef] [PubMed]

14. Zhang, P.; Deng, Y.; Lin, X.; Chen, B.; Li, J.; Liu, H.; Chen, S.; Liu, L. Anti-inflammatory Mono- and Dimeric Sorbicillinoids from the Marine-Derived Fungus Trichoderma reesei 4670. *J. Nat. Prod.* **2019**, *82*, 947–957. [CrossRef] [PubMed]
15. Vieira, L.R.; Hissa, D.C.; de Souza, T.M.; Sa, C.A.; Evaristo, J.A.M.; Nogueira, F.C.S.; Carvalho, A.F.U.; Farias, D.F. Proteomics analysis of zebrafish larvae exposed to 3,4-dichloroaniline using the fish embryo acute toxicity test. *Environ. Toxicol.* **2020**, *35*, 849–860. [CrossRef] [PubMed]
16. Yang, L.H.; Ou-Yang, H.; Yan, X.; Tang, B.W.; Fang, M.J.; Wu, Z.; Chen, J.W.; Qiu, Y.K. Open-Ring Butenolides from a Marine-Derived Anti-Neuroinflammatory Fungus Aspergillus terreus Y10. *Mar. Drugs* **2018**, *16*, 428. [CrossRef] [PubMed]
17. Kundu, A.; Saha, S.; Walia, S.; Shakil, N.A.; Kumar, J.; Annapurna, K. Cadinene sesquiterpenes from Eupatorium adenophorum and their antifungal activity. *J. Environ. Sci. Health B* **2013**, *48*, 516–522. [CrossRef] [PubMed]
18. Liu, S.-Z.; Yan, X.; Tang, X.-X.; Lin, J.-G.; Qiu, Y.-K. New Bis-Alkenoic Acid Derivatives from a Marine-Derived Fungus Fusarium solani H915. *Mar. Drugs* **2018**, *16*, 7–12. [CrossRef] [PubMed]

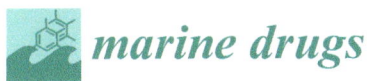

Review

The Tetrahydrofuran Motif in Marine Lipids and Terpenes

Paula González-Andrés [1], Laura Fernández-Peña [1], Carlos Díez-Poza [2,*] and Asunción Barbero [1,*]

[1] Department of Organic Chemistry, Campus Miguel Delibes, University of Valladolid, 47011 Valladolid, Spain
[2] Departamento de Química Orgánica y Química Inorgánica, Facultad de Farmacia e Instituto de Investigación Química Andrés M. del Río (IQAR), Universidad de Alcalá, Ctra. Madrid-Barcelona, 28871 Madrid, Spain
* Correspondence: carlos.diezp@uah.es (C.D.-P.); asuncion.barbero@uva.es (A.B.)

Abstract: Heterocycles are particularly common moieties within marine natural products. Specifically, tetrahydrofuranyl rings are present in a variety of compounds which present complex structures and interesting biological activities. Focusing on terpenoids, a high number of tetrahydrofuran-containing metabolites have been isolated during the last decades. They show promising biological activities, making them potential leads for novel antibiotics, antikinetoplastid drugs, amoebicidal substances, or anticancer drugs. Thus, they have attracted the attention of the synthetics community and numerous approaches to their total syntheses have appeared. Here, we offer the reader an overview of marine-derived terpenoids and related compounds, their isolation, structure determination, and a special focus on their total syntheses and biological profiles.

Keywords: marine natural products; oxygen heterocycles; tetrahydrofuran; total synthesis; biological activity; terpenes; fatty acids

1. Introduction

Marine organisms are a source of intriguing and fascinating compounds. These living beings have continuously evolved over time, since they are part of the oldest habitat on earth. Being also the largest ecosystem, the ocean has the potential to offer innumerable compounds with interesting biological activities yet to be discovered [1]. This is supported by the fact that hundreds of new molecules are reported within the scientific community every year [2–4].

Usually, the isolation of pure active compounds is a time-consuming and expensive process, due to the need of efficient extraction processes and sequential purification steps. Moreover, large amounts of raw materials have to be collected to finally isolate fairly low quantities of the desired compounds.

Fortunately, the great contribution of chemists in the field of total synthesis and asymmetric catalysis over the last decades has had countless benefits. On one hand, even though nuclear magnetic resonance (NMR) techniques are very powerful tools, in some cases, the characterization of complex molecules can be difficult, leading to misassignments [5]. Fortunately, total synthesis has emerged as a—somewhat—costly but effective tool for the determination of the absolute configuration of marine metabolites. On the other hand, synthesis provides access to sufficient quantities of the desired compounds for further extensive biological studies.

Within the marine-derived metabolites, terpenes represent one of the most significant families. They are a large and diverse group of compounds that usually present valuable pharmacological properties. Various reviews summarize the discovery of a high number of these metabolites in recent years from different sources, namely sponges [6,7], fungi [8–10], and corals [11,12], among others [13,14].

Other common structural motifs present in marine drugs are heterocycles. Within them, five-, six-, and seven-membered oxygenated heterocycles are frequently found in such bioactive compounds. The six-membered tetrahydropyrans, the most abundant, are

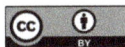

common targets of study [15,16]. The corresponding seven-membered oxepanes, and their appearance in relevant bioactive marine compounds, were reviewed by our group [17]. Regarding tetrahydrofurans, Fernandes and coworkers recently reviewed the most iconic examples of total synthesis of 2,3,5-trisubstituted tetrahydrofuran-containing natural products [18,19]. We have also recently summarized the synthesis and biological properties of marine-derived tetrahydrofuran-containing compounds, focusing on the polyketide family [20].

Continuing our series, here we give an overview of tetrahydrofuran-containing marine drugs, focusing on the terpene family and related compounds. We searched SciFinder for tetrahydrofuran-containing compounds with biological activity, focusing on the period 2000–2022. Our search was refined to compounds of the terpenoid family of compounds of marine origin, finding 81 compounds (Table 1). The main source (see Figure 1) was algae (32 compounds), followed by sponges (19 compounds), fungi (15 compounds), lampreys (6), bacteria (5), and corals (4). Excluding nonterpenoid lipids, we found 55 terpenoid compounds (see Figure 2), most of them being triterpenes (23) followed by meroterpenes (14), monoterpenes (9), diterpenes (5) and, finally, sesquiterpenes (4).

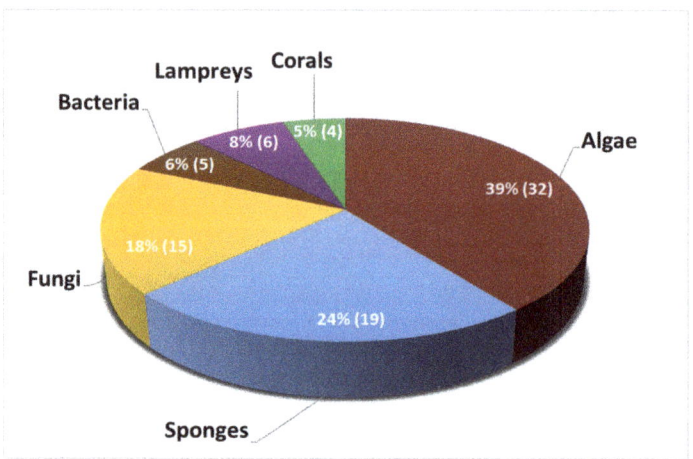

Figure 1. Distribution of the number of metabolites from this review, according to their marine source (color code coincides with that of Table 1).

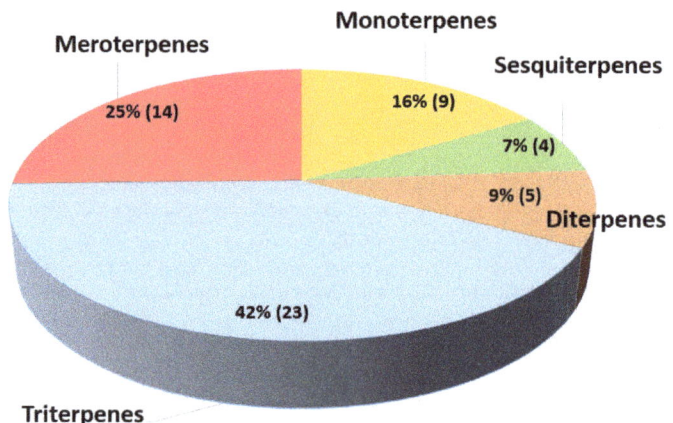

Figure 2. Distribution of compounds from this review according to terpenoid type.

Table 1. Overview of compounds from this review, their sources, classes, and species (background color code coincides with that of Figure 1).

Marine Source	Compound Class	Marine Species	Compound Name
Lampreys	Fatty acids	*Petromyzon marinus* L.	(+)-Petromyroxol (−)-Petromyroxol (+)-PMA (−)-PMA (+)-PMB (−)-PMB
Corals	Diterpenes	*Eunicea mammosa*	Uprolides D–E
	Substituted THF	*Sinularia* sp.	Sinularones E–F
Algae	C19 lipid diols	*Notheia anomala*	*Trans*-oxylipid *Cis*-oxylipid
	Monoterpenes	*Plocamium cartilagineum*	Furoplocamioids A–C
		Pantoneura plocamioides	Pantofuranoids A–F
	Sesquiterpenes	*Laurencia nipponica* Yamada	(−)-Kumausallene (+)-*Trans*-Kumausyne
	Triterpenes	*Laurencia intricata*	Intricatetraol
		Laurencia omaezakiana	Omaezakianol
		Laurencia viridis	Longilenes Laurokanols A–E Yucatecone Thyrsenols A–B Saiyacenols A–C
		Laurencia obtusa	Teurilene
		Laurencia thyrsifera	Thyrsiferol
Sponges	Fatty acids	*Xestospongia muta*	Mutafurans A–G
		Xestospongia testudinaria	Mutafuran H
		Aspergillus sp. LS78	Aspericacid A–B
	Diterpenes	*Dendrillamembranosa*	(+)-Darwinolide
	Triterpenes	*Rhabdastrella* sp.	Rhabdastins H–I
	Meroterpenes	New Caledonian	Alisiaquinones A–C Alisiaquinol
	Substituted THF	*Pachastrissa/Jaspis* sp.	Jaspines A-B
Fungi	Meroterpenes	*Alternaria alternata*	Tricycloalterfurenes A–D
		Stemphylium sp.	Tricycloalterfurenes E–G
	Substituted THF	*Myrothecium* sp. BZO-L062	(−)-1*S*-Myrothecol (−)-1*R*-Myrothecol Methoxy-myrothecol
		Astrosphaeriella nypae BCC-5335	Astronypyrone Astronyquinone Astronyurea
		Emericella variecolor	(+)-Varitriol (−)-Varitriol
Bacteria	Sesquiterpenes	*Streptomyces* sp. CMB-M0423	Heronapyrroles C–D
	Meroterpenes	*Streptomyces* sp. AJS-327 and CNQ-253	Marinoterpins A–C

We want to offer the reader an overview of the most recent tetrahydrofuran-containing terpenoids and related compounds of marine origin, their natural source of isolation, biological properties, and synthetic strategies towards them. We have also included classic examples, as their structure and activity are closely related to the more recently isolated metabolites and help to understand structure–activity relationships. We start with some examples of fatty acids with interesting biological profiles, and then move to the broad family of terpenoid compounds (monoterpenes, sesquiterpenes, diterpenes, triterpenes, and meroterpenoids). At the end, we also highlight other small THF-containing compounds that show interesting biological activities or were recently isolated and, thus, have potential to be shown in the near future.

2. Lipids

2.1. Lipid Alcohols

C19 Lipid Diols

Diastereomeric *trans*-oxylipids **1**, and *cis*-oxylipid **2** (Figure 3), were isolated in 1980 [21] and 1998 [22], respectively, from the brown alga *Notheia anomala*. Their structure and relative stereochemistry were assigned by 1D and 2D NMR spectral data and confirmed by single-crystal X-ray analysis. Their absolute configuration was determined by the Horeau method in the case of compound **1**, and by the advanced Mosher method for compound **2**. Both of them display in vitro antihelmintic activity, inhibiting larval development in parasitic nematodes. The *trans*-isomer **1** showed LD_{50} values against *Haemonchus contortus* (1.8 ppm) and *Trichostrongylus colubriformis* (9.9 ppm), comparable to those of the commercial nematocides levamisole and closantel. Synthetic routes for these oxylipids were recently reviewed [18].

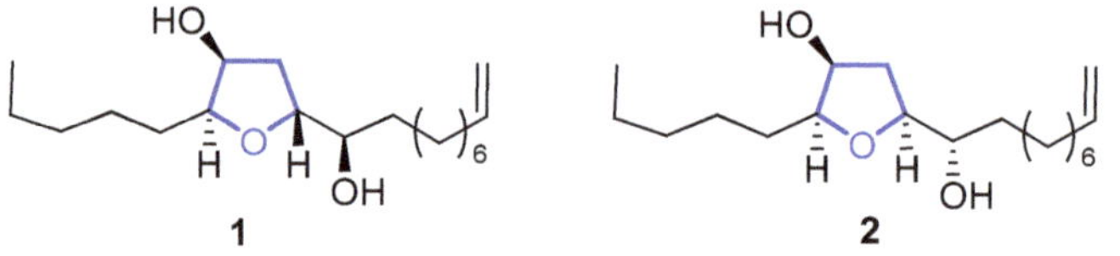

Figure 3. Structure of *trans*-oxylipid **1** and *cis*-oxylipid **2**.

An elegant example of the stereodivergent synthesis of both isomers was developed by Kim et al. [23]. They developed an intramolecular amide enolate alkylation, where the C3-hydroxy protecting group selection permits the formation of the desired isomer (Scheme 1). Thus, starting from PMB-protected bromoamide **3**, reaction with LiHMDS afforded only the *cis*-product **4**. The preferent formation of the *cis*-isomer was due to the chelating ability of the PMB group. Therefore, when using a nonchelating group such as TIPS (compound **5**), the reaction with KHMDS predominantly yielded the *trans*-THF **6**. Further reaction of **4** and **6** with $CH_2=CH(CH_2)_7MgBr$ and reduction with L-selectride afforded **7** and **8** in good yields (76% and 53% over two steps, respectively). Deprotection of **7** with DDQ, and **8** with TBAF, respectively, gave *cis*-oxylipid **2** in 82% yield and the *trans*-isomer **1** in 94% yield.

2.2. Fatty Acids

2.2.1. Petromyroxols

In 2015, Li reported the isolation of (+)- and (−)-petromyroxols (**9**) [24]. They are oxylipids isolated from water conditioned with larval sea lamprey *Petromyzon marinus* L. Interestingly, these molecules are the first tetrahydrofuran acetogenindiols isolated from a vertebrate animal (Figure 4). The absolute configuration of each enantiomer was determined by a combination of Mosher ester analysis and comparison with related natural and synthetic products. The **(+)-9** shows a potent olfactory response of 0.01 to 1 μM in the sea lamprey, while the (−)-isomer has a softer effect. Synthetic routes towards them were recently reviewed [18].

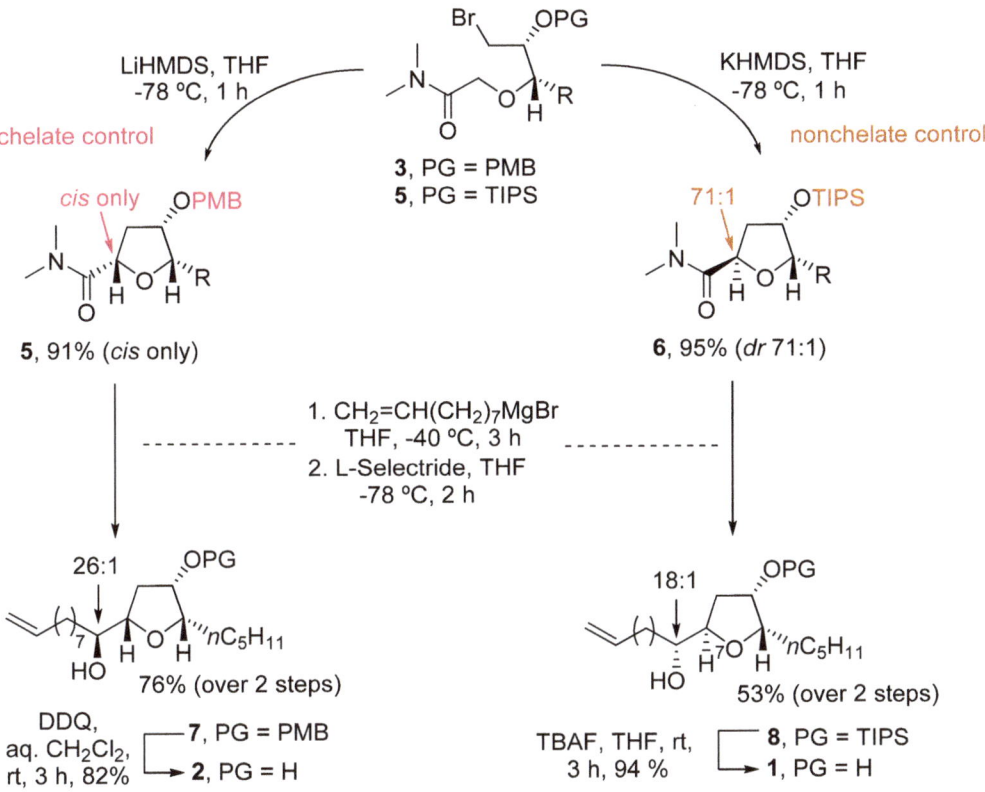

Scheme 1. Stereodivergent synthesis of *trans-* and *cis-*oxylipids **1** and **2** by Kim.

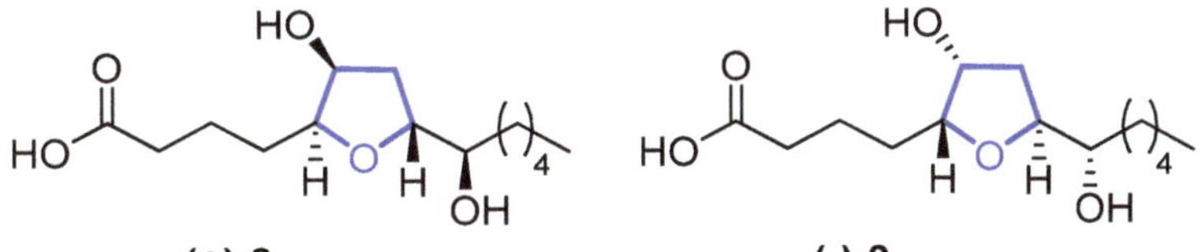

Figure 4. Structures of (+)-and (−)-petromyroxol **9**.

A recent example of the synthesis of **(+)-9**, along with all possible diastereoisomers, was presented in 2020 by Ramana and coworkers [25]. The synthetic route started from the commercial THF compound **10** (Scheme 2). The alkyl chain was installed by reaction with the appropriate cuprate. Subsequent benzyl protection of **11** afforded **12**, which after reaction with allyltrimethylsilane, yielded the desired diastereomer (7:2 ratio) of the allylated THF **13**. After protection with a para-nitrobenzoate (PNB) group under Mitsunobu conditions, compound **14** was subjected to oxidative olefin cleavage with $OsO_4/NaIO_4$ and subsequent Wittig olefination to obtain a-b-unsaturated ester **15**. Hydrogenation with Pearlman catalyst (20% $Pd(OH)_2/C$) afforded **16** in 89% yield, where the benzyl group, the double bond, and the nitro group were all reduced. Finally, hydrolysis of both ester groups with KOH in methanol afforded the desired (+)-petromyroxol in 77% yield.

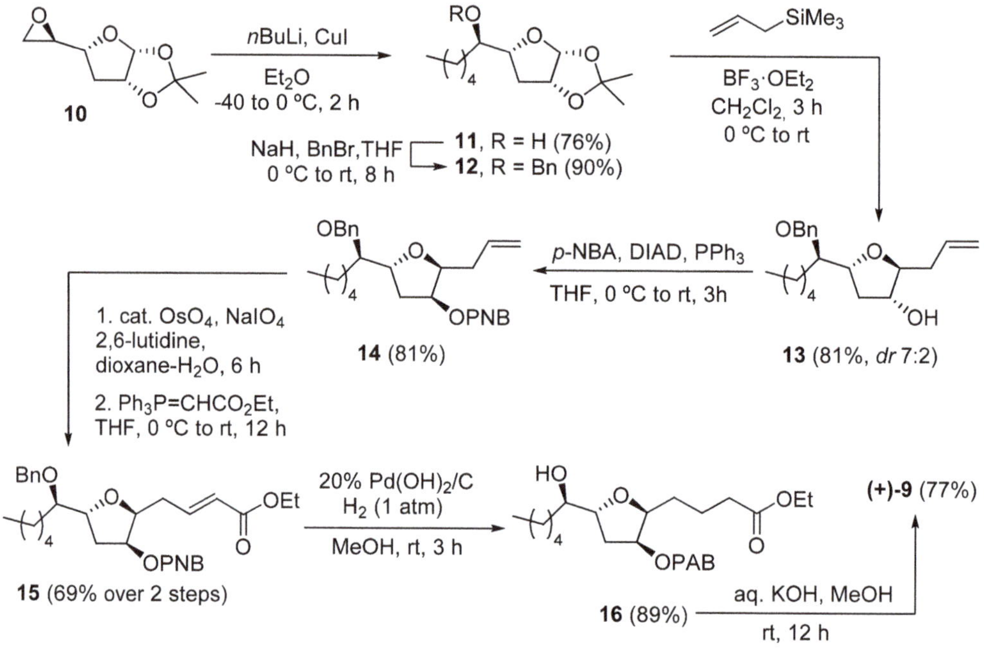

Scheme 2. Synthesis of (+)-petromyroxol by Ramana and coworkers.

2.2.2. PMA

Petromyric acids A and B (PMA and PMB) are dehydroxylated tetrahydrofuranyl fatty acids that were isolated from larval washing extracts from the sea lamprey *Petromyzon marinus* in 2018 [26]. From the washing extract, four fatty acids related to the acetogenin family were identified: (+)-PMA (**(+)-17**), (−)-PMA (**(−)-17**), (+)-PMB (**(+)-18**), and (−)-PMB (**(−)-18**) (Figure 5). Their chemical structure was elucidated by NMR spectroscopy and confirmed by chemical synthesis and X-ray crystallography.

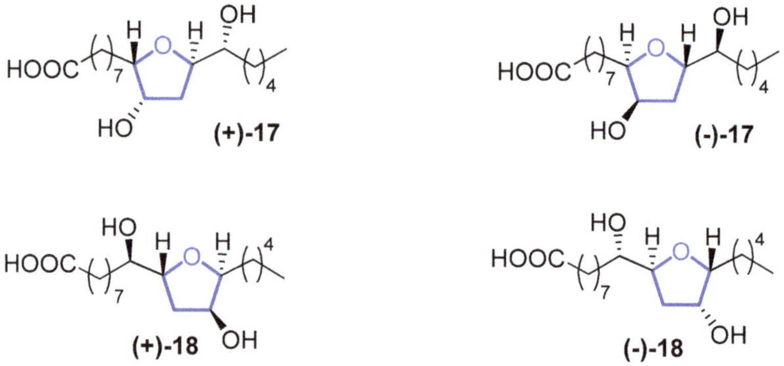

Figure 5. Structure of (+)-PMA (**(+)-17**), (−)-PMA (**(−)-17**), (+)-PMB (**(+)-18**), and (−)-PMB (**(−)-18**).

Sea lampreys are anadromous fishes that migrate, using their olfactory cues to orientate, from the ocean to freshwater to find a suitable spawning stream. When approaching river mouths, the decision of which stream is optimal to spawn in is taken using their olfactory system to detect a pheromone emitted from larval sea lampreys. When investigating larval washing extracts, four fatty acids were identified, but only **(+)-17** has proven to be the pheromone that guides lamprey adults. However, its enantiomer, (−)-17, does not produce the same behavioral effect. Fatty acid analogues have been reported to be pheromones in insects, but this is the first identification in fish. The sea lamprey is a destructive invader in the Laurentian Great Lakes, while in Europe, its population has decreased precipitously, so (+)-17 can be used for the control and conservation of their populations.

Although they have a high potential for application, to the best of our knowledge, no total synthesis has been reported so far for these compounds.

2.2.3. Mutafurans

Mutafurans A–G (**19–25**) are brominated ene-ynetetrahydrofurans (Figure 6) that were isolated by Molinski in 2007 from the marine sponge *Xextospongia muta* [27]. Later, Liu reported the isolation of mutafuran H (**26**), a brominated ene-tetrahydrofuran isolated from sponge *Xextospongia testudinaria* within other sterols and brominated compounds [28]. Their structure and absolute configuration were determined by 1D and 2D magnetic resonance, mass spectrometry, and circular dichroism.

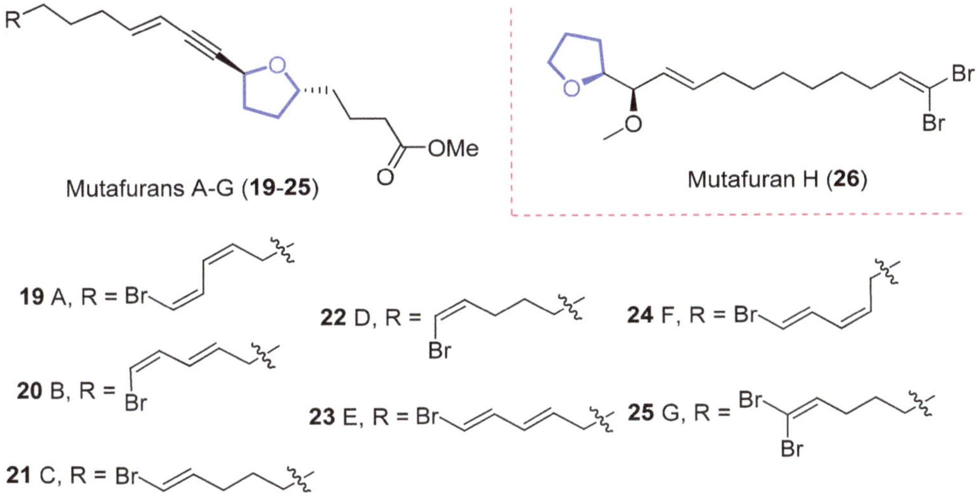

Figure 6. Structure of mutafurans A–G and the yne-lacking mutafuran H.

Mutafurans A–D showed moderate antifungal activity against the fungus *Cryptococcus neoformans var. grubii*, but were inactive against *Candida albicans* (ATCC14503 and 96–489) and *Candida glabrata* [27]. Furthermore, mutafuran H showed biological activity against *Artemia salina* larvae (LC$_{50}$ = 2.6 µM) and a significant acetylcholinesterase inhibitory activity (IC$_{50}$ = 0.64 µM) [28]. No synthetic approach has been reported to date.

2.2.4. Aspericacids

Aspericacids A (**27**) and B (**28**) were isolated in 2020 by Ding and He from the sponge-associated *Aspergillus* sp. LS78 [29]. Both compounds bear a 2,5-disubstituted tetrahydrofuran ring coupled with an unsaturated fatty acid (Figure 7). Their structure was determined by HRESIMS and 1D and 2D NMR spectroscopy, while their absolute configuration was established relying on electronic circular dichroism (ECD). Compound **27** presents a moderate inhibitory activity against *Candida albicans* and *Cryptococcus neoformans* with a MIC value of 50 µg/mL, although **28** has a weaker activity, MIC = 128 µg/mL. No synthetic approach has been reported to date.

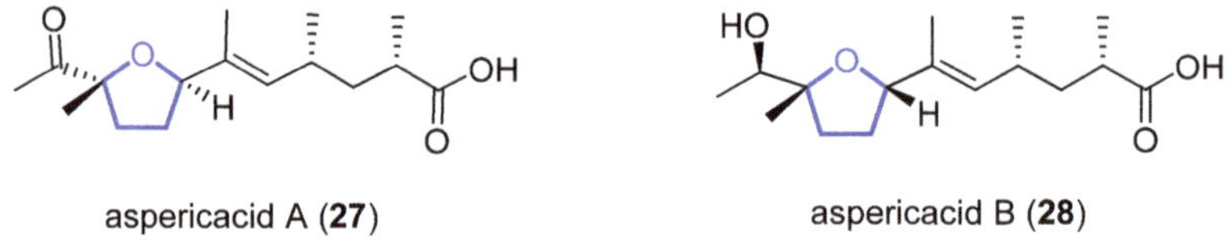

aspericacid A (**27**)

aspericacid B (**28**)

Figure 7. Structure of aspericacids A **27** and B **28**.

3. Terpenes

3.1. Monoterpenes

3.1.1. Pantofuranoids

Pantofuranoids A–F (**29–34**) are monoterpenes that were isolated in 1996 from the Antarctic red alga *Pantoneura plocamioides* [30]. They are the first monoterpenes found to contain a tetrahydrofuran moiety, and their common framework (Figure 8) suggests that they all come from the same terpene precursor.

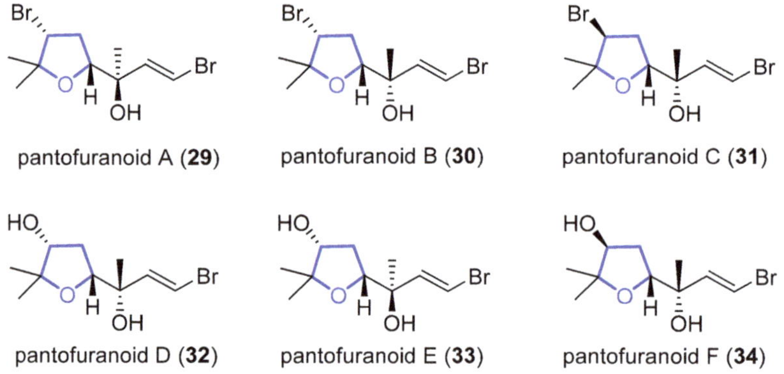

pantofuranoid A (**29**)

pantofuranoid B (**30**)

pantofuranoid C (**31**)

pantofuranoid D (**32**)

pantofuranoid E (**33**)

pantofuranoid F (**34**)

Figure 8. Proposed structure of pantofuranoids.

In 2006, Toste reported the enantioselective total synthesis of (−)-**33**, in which the key step is a vanadium-catalyzed sequential resolution/oxidative cyclization [31]. Using an in situ generated vanadium(V)–oxo complex with chiral tridentate Schiff base ligand **35** as catalyst, racemic homoallylic alcohol **36** was readily converted into 2,4-*cis*-substituted THF **37** (Scheme 3). The observed stereochemistry can be explained through a chair-like transition state in which coordination of the pseudo-equatorial ester group to the vanadium complex determines the selectivity of the *syn*-epoxidation step. Then, compound **37** was further elaborated to (−)-**33** in 6 steps and 29% overall yield from **37**.

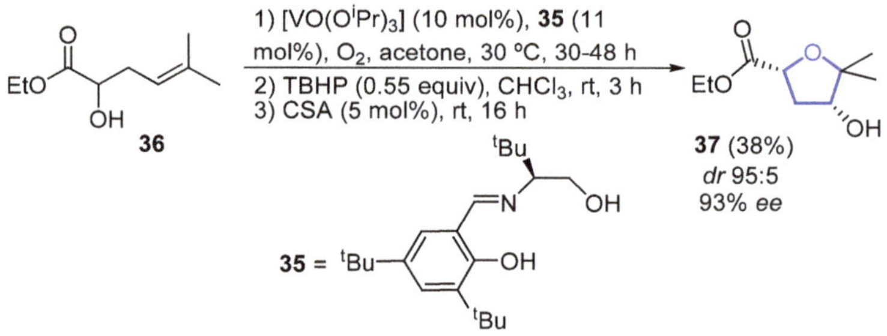

Scheme 3. Vanadium-catalyzed synthesis of the tetrahydrofuranyl core of (−)-pantofuranoid E by Toste.

3.1.2. Furoplocamioids

Furoplocamioids A–C **38–40** (Figure 9) are monoterpenes that were isolated in 2001 from the red marine alga *Plocamium cartilagineum* [32]. They bear an unusual polyhalogenated tetrahydrofuranyl ring. Their structural similarity to pantofuranoids suggests a close relationship between the species that produce them. This is an interesting fact, since *Plocamium cartilagineum* and *Pantoneura plocamioides* are classified in different orders, Gigartinales and Ceramiales. Therefore, a taxonomic revision could be required. Later, the Darias group determined the C7 relative stereochemistry by comparison with the NMR spectra of similar reported terpenes [33]. González-Coloma and coworkers found that **38** and **40** show antifeedant effects against *Leptinotarsa decemlineata*. It was shown that **40** was also an efficient aphid repellent (against *Mizuspersicae* and *Ropalosiphumpadi*) and selective insect cell toxicant. In addition, both compounds showed low mammalian toxicity and phytotoxic effects [34].

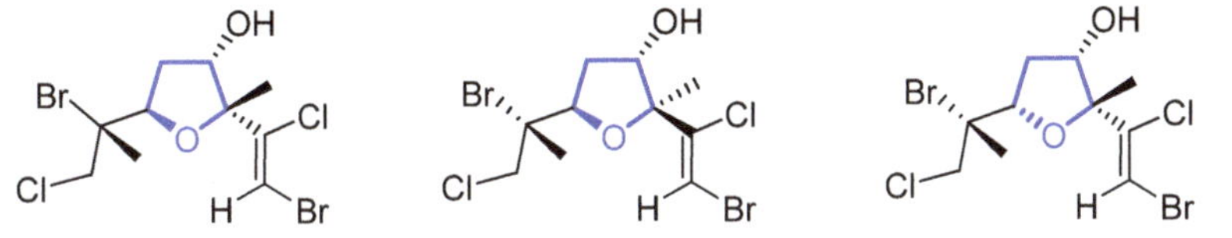

furoplocamioid A (**38**)   furoplocamioid B (**39**)   furoplocamioid C (**40**)

Figure 9. Structure of furoplocamioids A–C (**38–40**).

3.2. Sesquiterpenes
3.2.1. Heronapyrrols

Heronapyrrols A–C are pyrroloterpenes that were isolated in 2010 from a marine *Streptomyces* sp. CMB-M0423 [35]. They present bioactivity against Gram-positive bacteria *Staphylococcus aureus* ATCC 9144 and *Bacillus subtilis* ATCC 6633 but no mammalian cytotoxicity. Heronapyrrol C (**41**), apart from the characteristic and unusual 2-nitropyrrol moiety of this family, presents a *bis*-tetrahydrofuran core. Later, Capon and Stark first synthesized and then isolated heronapyrrol D (**42**) (Figure 10) from the same marine-derived microbe [36]. Heronapyrrol D displays bioactivity against Gram-positive bacteria *Staphylococcus aureus* ATCC 25923 (IC_{50} = 1.8 µM), *Staphylococcus epidermidis* ATCC 12228 (IC_{50} = 0.9 µM), and *Bacillus subtilis* ATCC 6633 (IC_{50} = 1.8 µM). However, it is inactive against the Gram-negative bacteria *Pseudomonas aeruginosa* ATCC 10145 and *Escherichia coli* ATCC 25922.

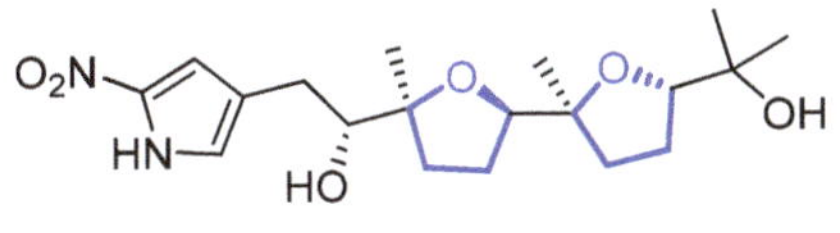

heronapyrrol C (**41**)

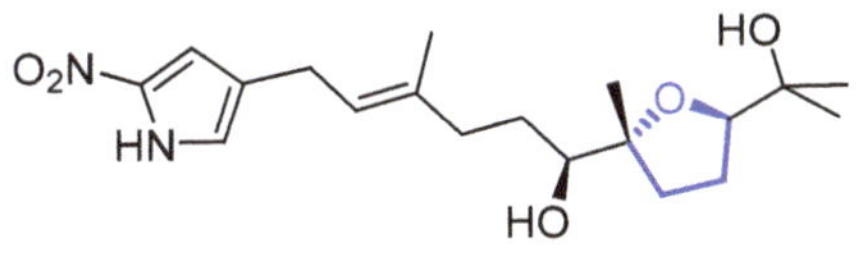

heronapyrrol D (**42**)

Figure 10. Structure of (+)-heronapyrrol C (**41**) and (+)-heronapyrrol D (**42**).

To determine the relative and absolute stereochemistry of (+)-41, Stark and coworkers proposed and synthesized the most likely stereostructure of its enantiomer (−)-41, based on a biomimetic polyepoxide cyclization [37]. The same authors also reported the preparation of a bioisosteric carboxylate analog of (−)-41 [38].

The first total synthesis of (+)-41 was reported in 2014 by Brimble and coworkers, who used as key steps to introduce the five stereogenic centers a Julia–Kocienski coupling, a Shi epoxidation, and a catalytic epoxide-opening reaction [39]. The same year, the first total synthesis of (+)-42 was achieved by Capon and Stark using a similar approach [36]. In 2016, Brimble and Furkert reviewed the isolation and synthesis of this family of compounds [40].

Later on, the same authors reported another total synthesis for both (+)-41 and (+)-42 [41]. Shi epoxidation of diol 43, followed by CSA-catalyzed epoxide opening and cyclization, produces diastereomerically pure 44 in 75% yield over two steps. A further eight steps, with 31% yield over them, produces intermediate 45, which deprotection gives (+)-heronapyrrol D (42). Epoxidation of 42 with a Shi ketone catalyst, followed by CSA-catalyzed epoxide opening, produced enantiomerically pure (+)-heronapyrrol C (41) in 75% yield (Scheme 4).

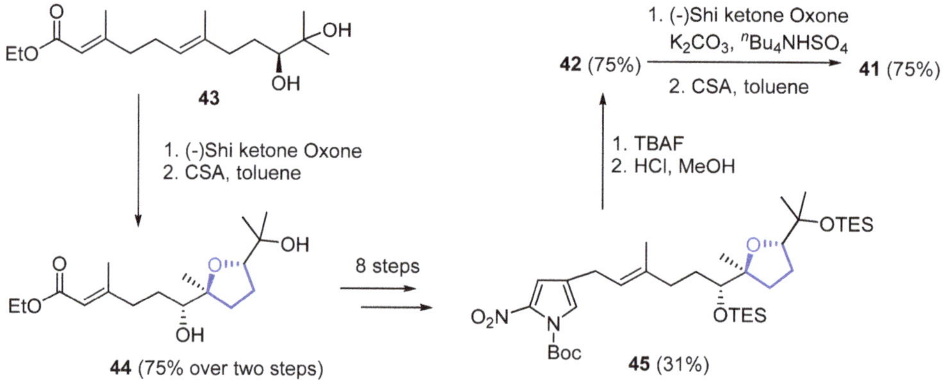

Scheme 4. Synthesis of (+)-heronapyrrol C (41) and (+)-heronapyrrol D (42).

Other synthetic approaches towards the 2-nitropyrrole system have been investigated by Brimble and Furkert, finding that Sonogashira coupling of 4-iodo-2-nitropyrrole with the appropriate alkyne was more effective than an approach relying on Stille coupling [42].

3.2.2. Kumausallene and Kumausyne

(−)-Kumausallene (46) was isolated in 1983 from the marine red alga *Laurencia nipponica* Yamada [43]. This compound belongs to a family of non-isoprenoid sesquiterpenes that contain a 2,6-dioxa-bicyclo [3.3.0]octane core with an *exo*-cyclic bromoallene (Figure 11).

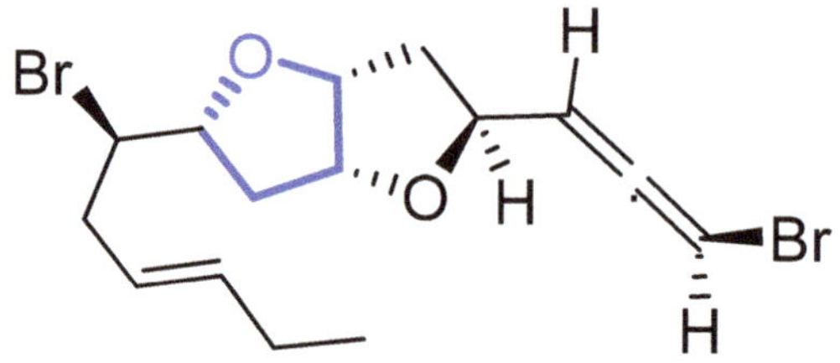

Figure 11. Structure of kumausallene.

In 1993, the first total synthesis of (±)-**46** was reported by Overman, who chose a hexahydrobenzofuranone **47** (obtained by a Prins cyclization–pinacol rearrangement from **48**) as the key intermediate for the construction of the *bis*-tetrahydrofuran unit (Scheme 5). Further transformation of **47** into bicyclic lactone **49** (within three further steps) and final methanolisis and tandem cyclization of the corresponding hydroxyester provided, in good yield, the desired dioxabicyclo [3.3.0]octane **50** [44].

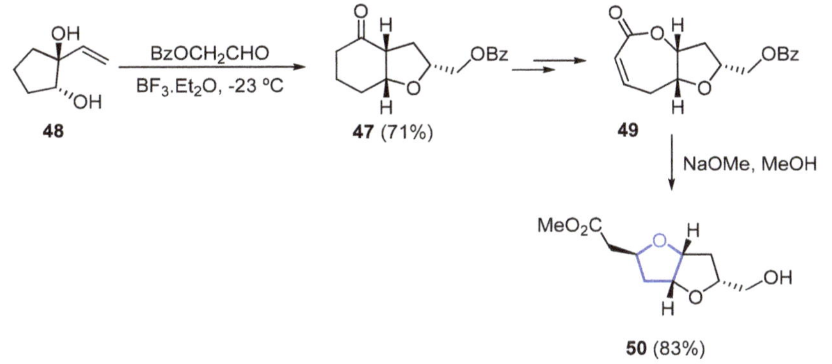

Scheme 5. Synthesis of the dioxabicyclo [3.3.0]octane unit of (±)-kumausallene (**46**) by Overman.

In 2011, a synthetic approach for (−)-**46** by Tang employed a desymmetrization strategy for the formation of the 2,5-*cis*-substituted THF ring [45]. C_2-symmetric diol **51** is desymmetrized by a palladium-catalyzed cascade reaction to form lactone **52** in 87% yield (Scheme 6). The total synthesis comprised just 12 steps from commercial acetylacetone. In 2015, Ramana et al. published a different formal total synthesis of (−)-**46** based on a chiral pool approach [46].

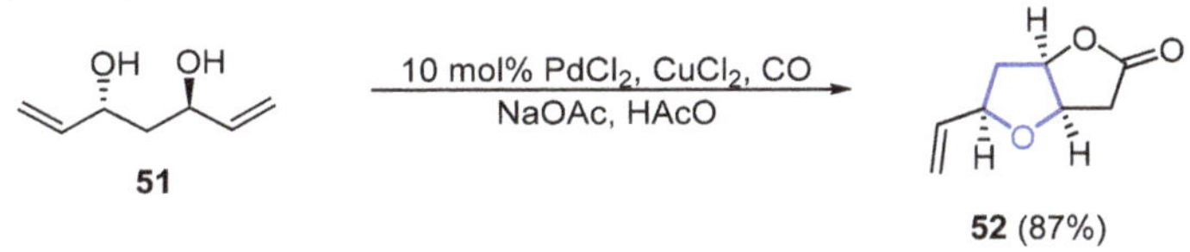

Scheme 6. Synthesis of the tetrahydrofuranyl ring of (−)-**46** through desymmetrization by Tang.

(+)-*Trans*-Kumausyne (**53**) (Figure 12) is a halogenated non-isoprenoid sesquiterpene isolated in 1983 from red alga *Laurencia nipponica* Yamada [47]. Its first total synthesis was achieved in 1991 by Overman and coworkers [48]. A review covering the synthetic approaches towards kumausallene and kumausyne, and other natural products containing a 2,3,5-trisubstituted tetrahydrofuran moiety, was published by Fernandes in 2020 [18].

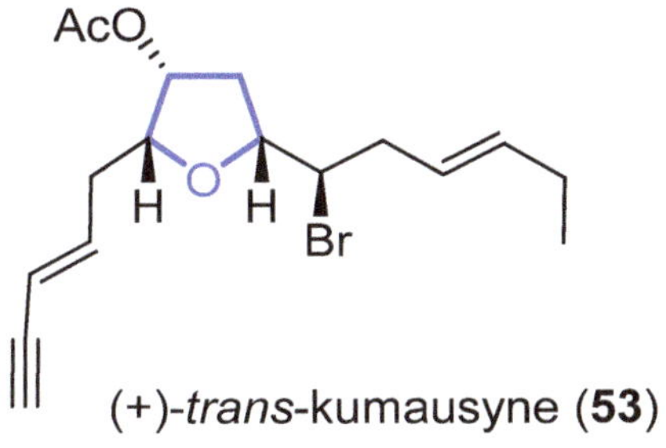

Figure 12. Structure of (+)-*trans*-Kumausyne (**53**).

3.3. Diterpenes

3.3.1. Darwinolide

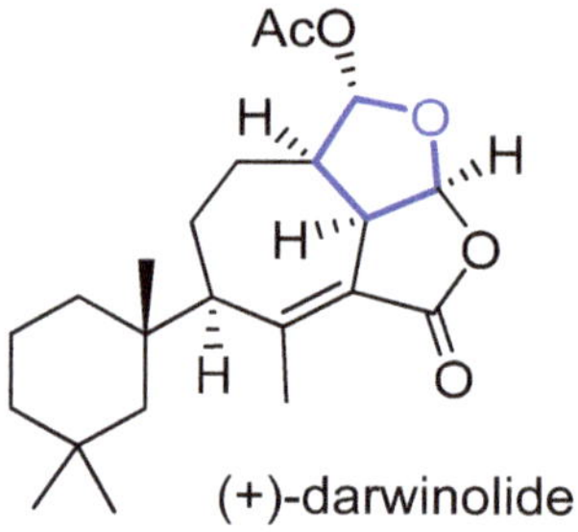

(+)-Darwinolide (**54**) (Figure 13) is a diterpene isolated in 2016 by Baker from the Antarctic Dendroceratid sponge *Dendrilla membranosa* [49]. It presents fourfold selectivity against a biofilm phase of methicillin-resistant *Staphylococcus aureus* (IC$_{50}$ of 33.2μM), compared to the planktonic phase (with the higher MIC of 132.9 μM). This interesting property and its low mammalian cytotoxicity (IC$_{50}$ of 73.4 mM) against a J774 macrophage cell line turn darwinolide into a possible scaffold for antibiofilm-specific antibiotics. Additionally, it was found to have modest activity (11.2 μM) against *L. donovani*-infected macrophages [50].

Figure 13. Structure of (+)-darwinolide ((+)-**54**).

Its total synthesis was reported in 2019 by Christmann [51]. The required tetrahydrofuranyl ring is installed starting from the commercially available anhydride **55**, which is converted to the 2,5-dimethoxylated tetrahydrofuran **56** in four steps. A sequence of oxidation (with o-iodoxybenzoic acid), saponification, and Criegee oxidation with Pb(OAc)$_4$ is then used to convert **56** into **57** in 61% yield over three steps (Scheme 7). A further 14 linear steps are needed to complete the total synthesis of **54**, with an overall yield of 1.4%.

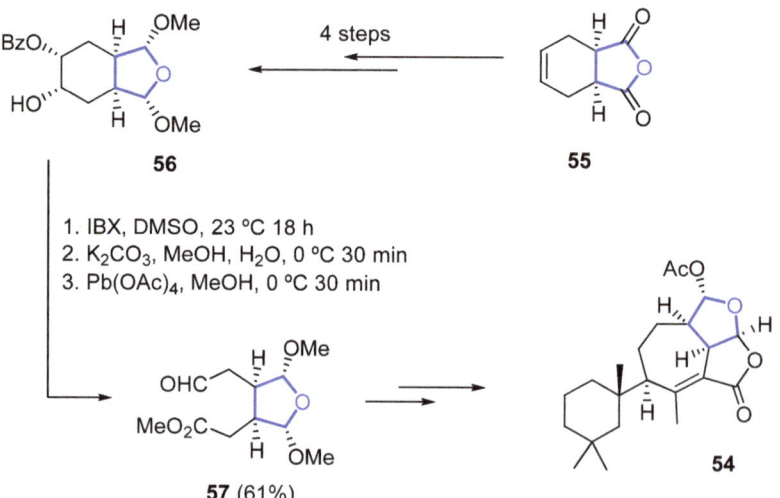

Scheme 7. Synthesis of the key THF-containing intermediate in Christmann's total synthesis of darwinolide.

3.3.2. Uprolides

Cembranolides are a family of compounds related to cembrene, which is a 14-membered macrocyclic diterpene with multiple (*E*)-double bonds. Among them, uprolides are a subfamily of compounds named after the University of Puerto Rico. Uprolides A–G were isolated in 1995 by Rodríguez and coworkers from the Caribbean gorgonian *Eunicea Mammosa* and their structure was assigned by spectroscopic methods and chemical interconversion [52,53]. They are the first natural cembranolides from a Caribbean gorgonian that bear a double bond at C6 or C8. While uprolides A–C show an epoxy moiety, uprolides D–G seemed to contain a tetrahydrofuran moiety instead. Uprolides D (**58**), D acetate (**59**), D diacetate (**60**), and E acetate (**61**) (Figure 14) present a moderate cytotoxicity against HeLa cells ((IC_{50} = 2.5 to 5.1 µg/ml). Moreover, **59** shows cytotoxicity against the following human tumor cell lines: CCRF-CEM T-cell leukemia (IC_{50} = 7.0 µg/mL), HCT-116 colon cancer (IC_{50} = 7.0 µg/mL), and MCF-7 breast adenocarcinoma (IC_{50} = 0.6 µg/mL).

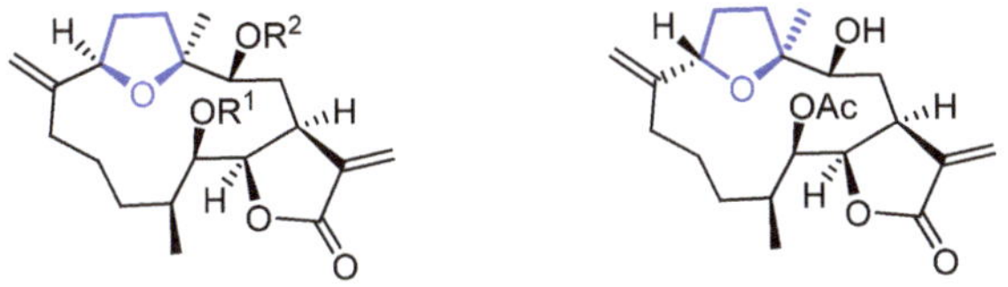

Uprolide D   **58** $R^1 = R^2 = H$
Uprolide D acetate **59** $R^1 = Ac, R^2 = H$
Uprolide D diacetate **60** $R^1 = R^2 = Ac$

Uprolide E acetate **61**

Figure 14. Structure of tetrahydrofuran-containing members of the uprolide family.

Later structural revisions determined the presence of a tetrahydropyran ring, instead of the previously proposed tetrahydrofuran, in uprolides F diacetate and G acetate, hypotheses that were confirmed by asymmetric total synthesis of these natural products [54–57].

In 2007, a synthetic approach to obtain the macrocyclic core of **58** was proposed by Ramana [58]. The formation of the macrocyclic core is produced by ring-closing metathesis (RCAM) using a Grubbs' first-generation catalyst. The RCAM of acetate **62** produces 13-membered macrocyclic **63** in 67% yield (Scheme 8). The macrocyclic core of uprolide E could not be synthesized using the same methodology.

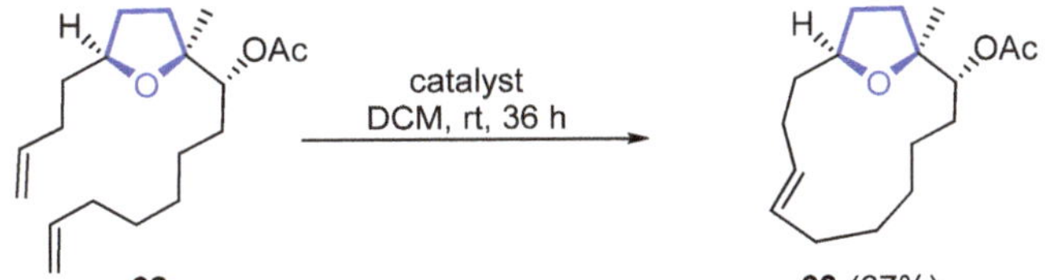

Scheme 8. Synthesis of macrocyclic core of uprolide D by Ramana.

Marshall developed a synthetic route for C1/C14 *bis*-epimer of **58** in which the macrocyclization is produced by an intramolecuar Barbier reaction [59]. Some years later, other members of the uprolide family, which lack the tetrahydrofuran ring, have been isolated from the gorgonian octocoral *Eunicea succinea* [60].

3.4. Triterpenes
3.4.1. Intricatetraol

Intricatetraol (**64**) is a halogenated triterpenoid with a C_2 symmetry that was isolated in 1993 from the red alga *Laurencia intricata* (Figure 15). Suzuki and coworkers observed that a crude fraction of the extract showed cytotoxic activity against P388 leukemia cells with an IC_{50} value of 12.5 µg/mL. Nevertheless, pure intricatetraol was no longer active after chromatography. At first, its stereostructure was proposed as being based on its hypothetical biogenesis [61]. In 2006, Morimoto confirmed this assignment by synthesizing a degradation product of intricatetraol through a two-directional synthesis [62].

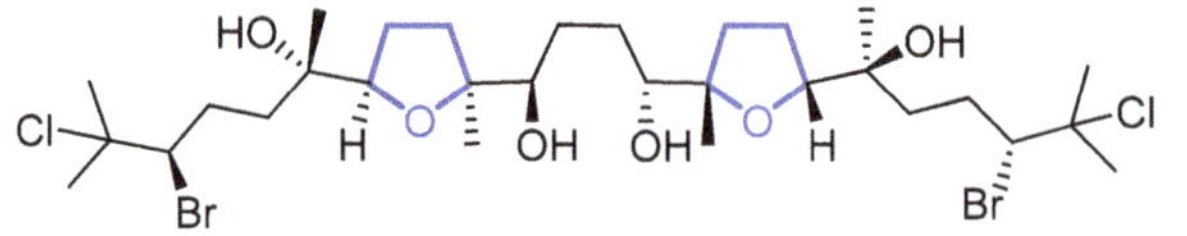

intricatetraol **64**

Figure 15. Structure of (+)-intricatetraol **64**.

One year later, Morimoto completed the asymmetric total synthesis of **(+)-64** and, thus, determined its absolute configuration [63]. The tetrahydrofuran ring **65** was stereospecifically constructed by treatment of diepoxyalcohol **66** with lithium hydroxide aqueous solution. A further 10 steps (with an accumulated yield of 30%) were needed to obtain intermediate **67**, which was then dimerized to afford **68** by olefin metathesis with a second-generation Grubbs catalyst. Final diimide reduction of intermediate **68** produced **(+)-64** (Scheme 9).

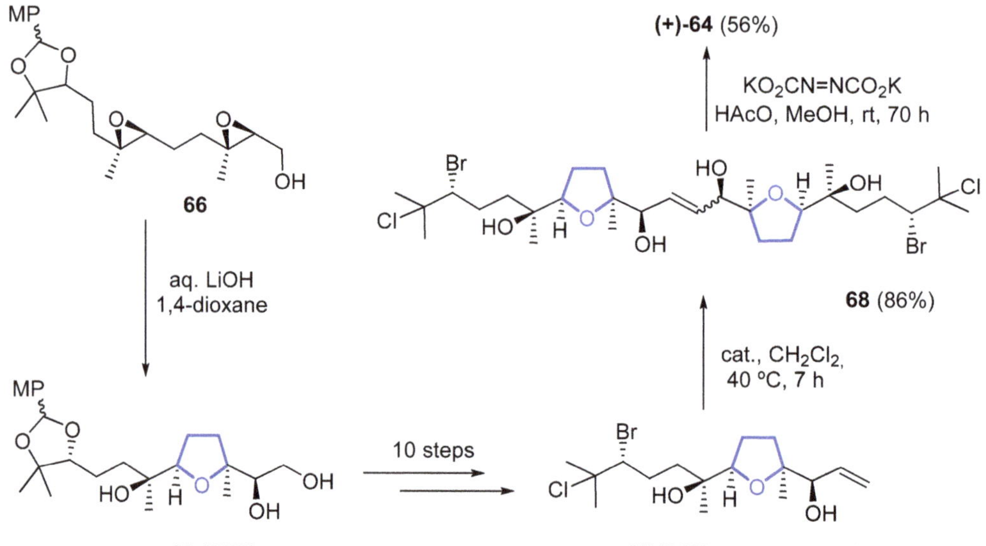

Scheme 9. Synthesis of (+)-intricatetraol (**(+)-64**).

3.4.2. Omaezakianol

Omaezakianol **(69)** (Figure 16) is a squalene-derived triterpene polyether that was isolated in 2008 from the red alga *Laurencia omaezakiana* by Morimoto and coworkers [64]. The same group rapidly reported its first asymmetric total synthesis and, therefore, stablished its absolute configuration [65]. Key steps were olefin cross-metathesis and an epoxide-opening cascade.

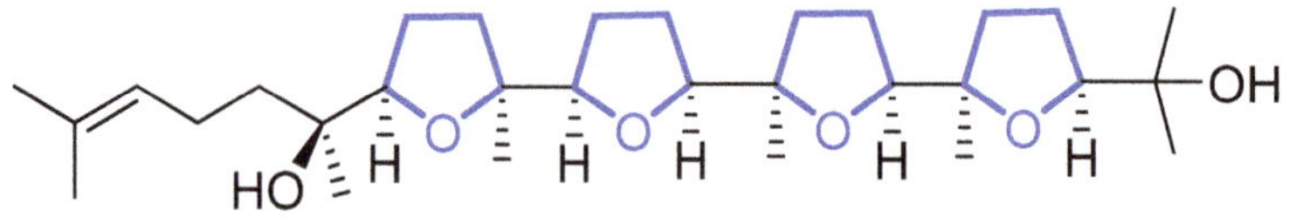

omaezakianol **69**

Figure 16. Structure of (+)-omaezakianol (**69**).

In 2010, Corey reported a short total synthesis via a biomimetic epoxide-initiated cationic cascade reaction [66]. Compound **70** was treated with camphorsulfonic acid (CSA) to induce the epoxide-opening cascade cyclization, producing **71**. Reduction of **71**, with sodium in acetone under reflux, formed the terminal double bond with opening of the THF ring, affording **69** in 76% yield (Scheme 10). Thus, the synthesis was accomplished in just six steps from squalene.

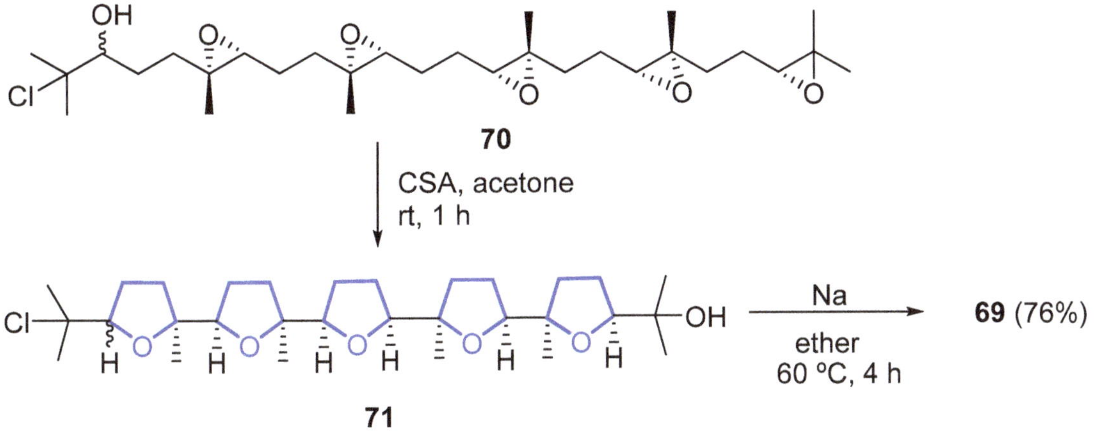

Scheme 10. Synthesis of (+)-omaezakianol **69** by Corey via an epoxide-initiated cationic cascade.

Another biomimetic epoxide-opening cascade for the synthesis of **(+)-69** was reported in 2013 by Morimoto and coworkers [67]. The cascade, which mimics the direct hydrolysis mechanism of epoxide hydrolases, begins with 5-*exo* cyclization of the terminal epoxide triggered by Brønsted acid catalysis. Intermediate **72** then undergoes an epoxide-opening cascade reaction with TfOH to afford **(+)-69** in 33% yield (Scheme 11).

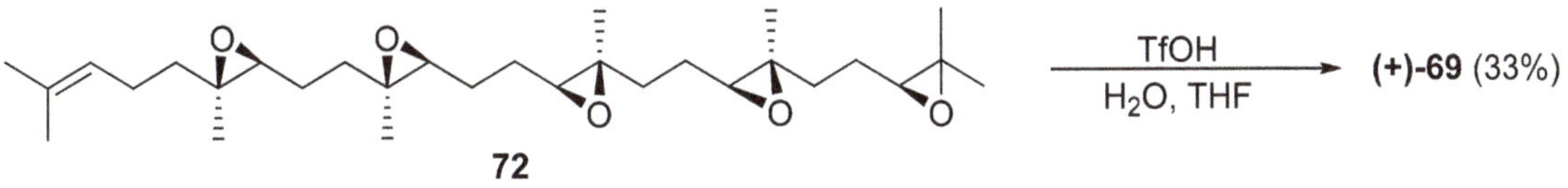

Scheme 11. Synthesis of (+)-omaezakianol (**(+)-69**) by a biomimetic epoxide-opening cascade.

3.4.3. Longilenes

Longilenes are triterpene polyethers that were first isolated from the wood of *Eurycoma longifolia* in the form of (−)-longilene peroxide ((−)-**73**) [68,69]. In 2001, Morimoto accomplished its total synthesis [70] and determined its absolute configuration. The same author also developed a biomimetic synthesis of the C9–C16 fragment of oxasqualenoids in an enantioselective manner [71]. This chiral building block could be used as an advanced intermediate for the synthesis of different polyethers, such as teurilene, longilene peroxide, or glabrescol.

In 2018, Fernández and Daranas reported the isolation of other members of the family, namely (+)-longilene peroxide (**(+)-73**), longilene (**74**), and the derivative (+)-prelongilene (**(+)-75**), from the red seaweed *Laurencia viridis* [72]. These compounds present Ser/Thr protein phosphatase 2A inhibitory activity (Figure 17). To date, no synthetic approaches have been reported.

(-)-longilene peroxide (**(-)-73**)

(+)-longilene peroxide (**(+)-73**)

longilene (**74**)

(+)-prelongilene (**(+)-75**)

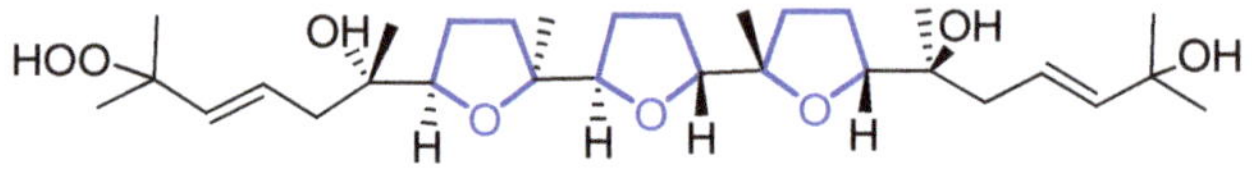

Figure 17. Structure of (−)-longilene peroxide (**(−)-73**), (+)-longilene peroxide (**(+)-73**), longilene (**74**), and the derivative (+)-prelongilene (**(+)-75**).

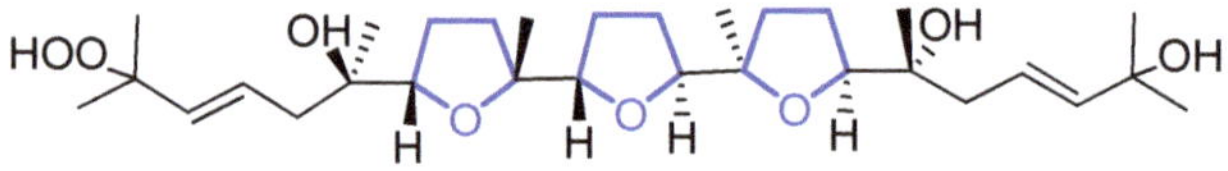

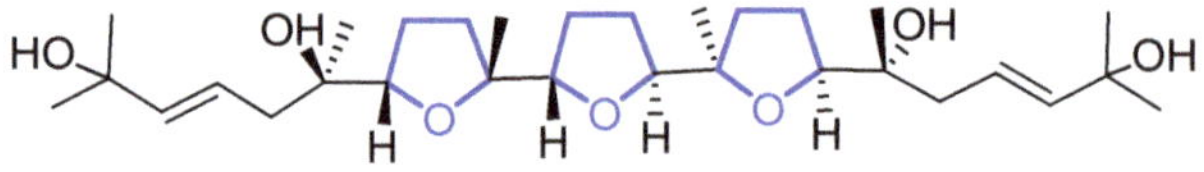

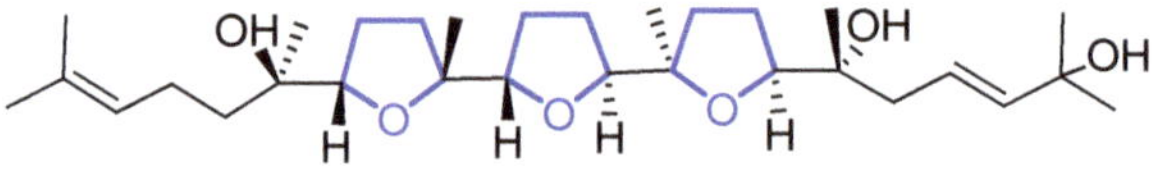

3.4.4. Laurokanols and Yucatecone

In 2021, laurokanols A–E (**76–80**) and yucatecone (**81**) (Figure 18), polyether triterpenes, were isolated from the red alga *Laurencia viridis* [73]. Laurokanols have an unprecedented tricyclic core with an [6,6]-spiroketal system. Yucatecone is the first compound of this series with an *R* configuration at the C14 position. A biogenetic model, supported by DFT calculations, was then postulated for the biogenesis of yucatecone.

Laurokanol A **76**: R^1 = Me, R^2 = H
Laurokanol B **77**: R^1 = CH_2Cl, R^2 = OH
Laurokanol C **78**: R^1 = OH, R^2 = CH_2Cl
Laurokanol D **79**: R^1 = OH, R^2 = CH_2Br

Laurokanol E (**80**)

Yucatecone (**81**)

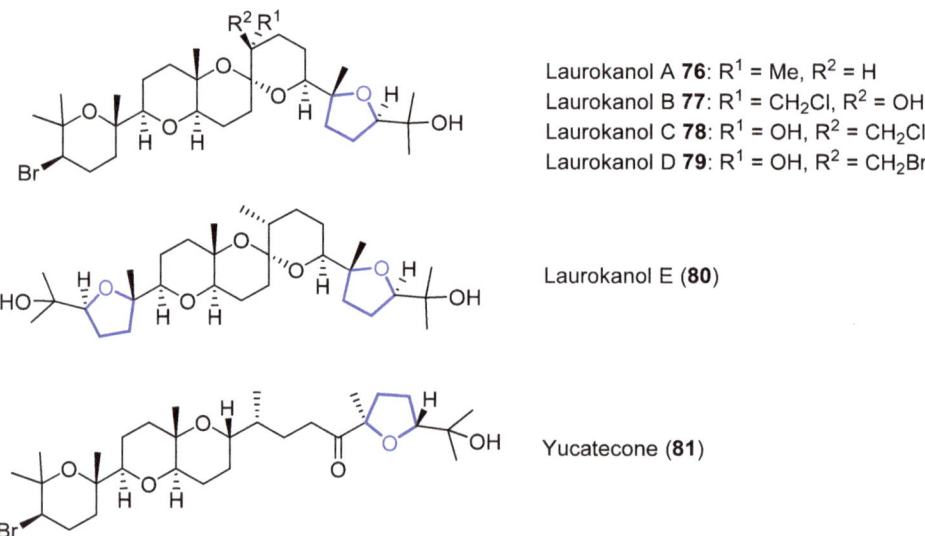

Figure 18. Structures of laurokanols A–E (**76–80**) and yucatecone (**81**).

3.4.5. Thyrsenol

Thyrsenol A (**82**) and B (**83**) (Figure 19) are polyether squalene derivatives that were isolated by Norte and coworkers in 1997 from the red alga *Laurencia viridis* [74]. Although both compounds show high activity against murine lymphoid neoplasm P-388 cells, compound **83** induced significantly higher inhibitory effects [75]. Other related compounds, such as thyrsiferol derivatives and dehydrovenustatriol, were found to be even more active. Therefore, it was postulated that the presence of a flexible chain around C14 to C19, and its configuration, are of particular importance for the bioactivity of these compounds. Later, Fernández and coworkers also found **83** to have protein phosphatase PP2A inhibitory activity [76]. The activity was comparable to that of dehydrothyrsiferol and thysiferyl-23-acetate, concluding that a hydroxyl group at C15 or C16 is a key factor for their intrinsic activity. In 2011, the isolation of other derivatives has been reported [77].

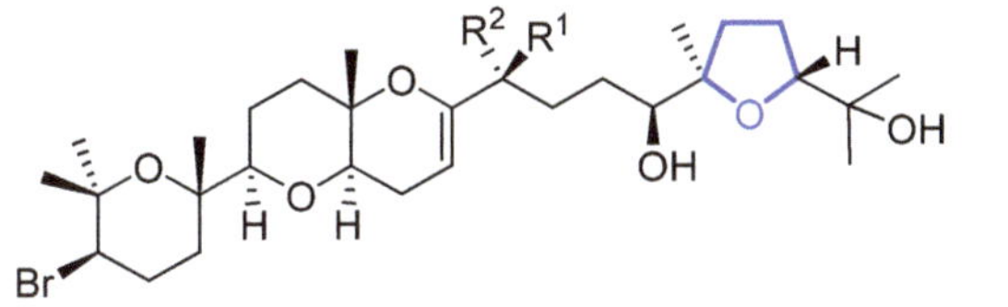

Thyrsenol A (**82**): R^1 = OH, R^2 = CH_2OH
Thyrsenol B (**83**): R^1 = CH_2OH, R^2 = OH

Figure 19. Structure of thyrsenol A (**82**) and B (**83**).

3.4.6. Saiyacenol

Saiyacenols A (**84**) and B (**85**) (Figure 20) are triterpene polyethers that were isolated in 2012 from the red alga *Laurencia viridis*. Both inhibit cell proliferation of various human tumor cell lines (MM144 (human multiple myeloma), HeLa (human cervical carcinoma), CADO-ES1 (human Ewing's sarcoma), and show the best inhibitory activity against Jurkat (human T-cell acute leukemia) [78]. In 2015, saiyacenol C (**86**), and two hydroxylated derivatives **87** and **88**, were isolated from the same alga [79]. Although saiyacenols showed no activity toward a range of bacteria and fungal strains, compounds **85** and **86** avoid *Navicula* cf. *salinicola* and *Cylindrotheca* sp. growth, while compounds **87** and **88** were also active against germination of *Gayralia oxysperma*.

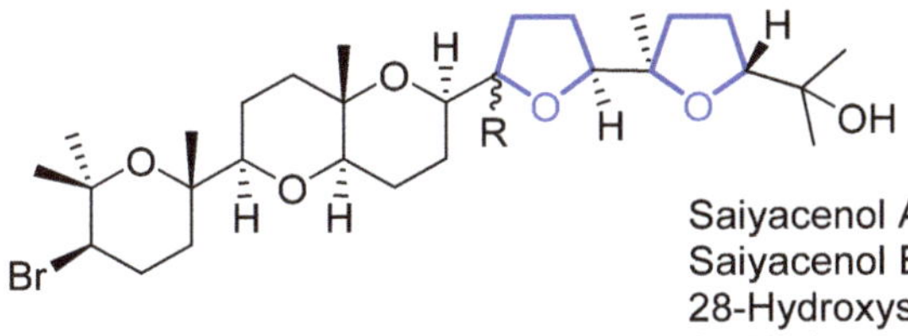

Saiyacenol A (**84**): R = CH_3; 15S*
Saiyacenol B (**85**): R = CH_3; 15R*
28-Hydroxysaiyacenol A (**87**): R = CH_2OH; 15S*
28-Hydroxysaiyacenol B (**88**): R = CH_2OH; 15R*

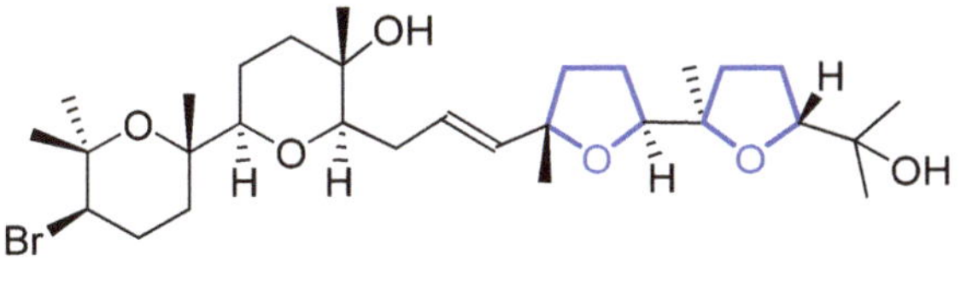

Saiyacenol C (**86**)

Figure 20. Structure of saiyacenols A–C (**84**–**86**) and their hydroxylated derivatives **87** and **88**.

More recently, Piñero and Fernández evaluated a range of natural and semisynthetic terpenoid polyethers against protozoan parasites of the *Trypanosoma* and *Leishmania* genera [80]. Both **84** and **85** have anti-protozoal activity against *Leishmania amazonensis* (IC$_{50}$ = 12.96 and 10.32 µM, respectively). Interestingly, saiyacenol A **84** was also effective against the highly resistant *Trypanosoma cruzi* (IC$_{50}$ = 13.75 ± 2.28 µM). The semisynthetic 28-iodosaiyacenol B showed a high value (IC$_{50}$ = 5.40 ± 0.13 µM) against *Leishmania amazonensis* and no toxicity to murine macrophage J774.A1. This turns it into a possible scaffold for antikinetoplastid drugs, as the data are comparable to those of the reference drug miltefosine (IC$_{50}$ = 6.48).

Very recently, Nishikawa and Morimoto reported the asymmetric total synthesis of saiyacenol A, along with that of the related Aplysiol B [81]. In their research, an epoxide-opening cascade was used to form both THF rings in the same step (Scheme 12). Thus, from advanced precursor **89**, treatment with CSA provoked two sequential 5-*exo* openings to form the oxygenated rings in *bis*-tetrahydrofuran **90**. The last step consisted of cross-methathesis with the ruthenium catalyst **91** and later bromoetherification with BDSB. Preliminary cytotoxicity was tested against P388, HT-29, and HeLa tumor cell lines, showing values of 5.4, 85, and >100 µM, respectively.

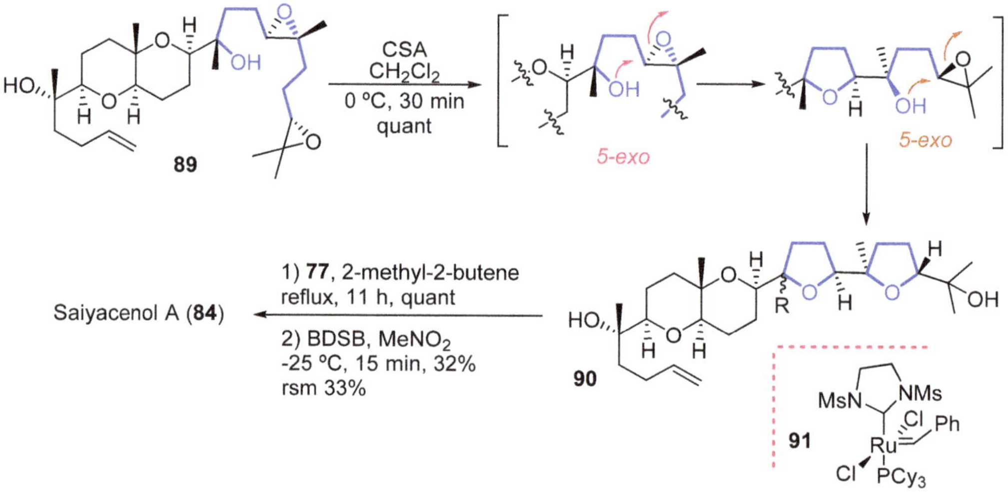

Scheme 12. Synthesis of saiyacenol A by Nishikawa and Morimoto.

3.4.7. Teurilene

Teurilene (**92**) (Figure 21) is a triterpene polyether that was isolated in 1985 from the red alga *Laurencia obtusa* by Kurosawa and coworkers [82]. It has three linked 2,5-disubstituted THF rings and, even though it has eight stereogenic centres, it is an achiral compound due to its *meso*-symmetry (C$_s$). Compound **92** has a remarkable cytotoxic activity against KB cells (IC$_{50}$ = 7.0 µg mL^{-1}) [69]. Synthetic approaches and routes up to 2014 are commented on in a previous review [83].

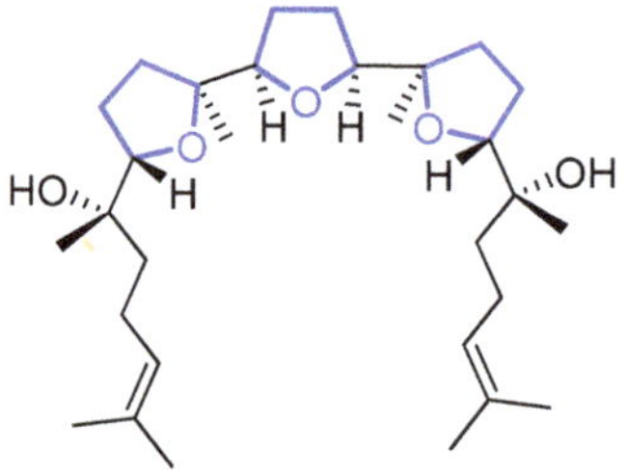

Figure 21. Structure of teurilene **92**.

3.4.8. Thyrsiferol

Thyrsiferol (**93**) is a polyoxygenated triterpenoid ether that was isolated in 1978 from the red alga *Laurencia thyrsifera* [84]. Its absolute stereochemistry (Figure 22) was determined in 1986 when venustatriol was isolated, since the latter could be crystallized and characterized by X-ray diffraction [85]. During the next two decades, a plethora of thyrsiferol derivatives have been isolated. Their biological profiles (cytotoxic, anti-viral, anti-tumor) have attracted much attention and several syntheses were published and reviewed in 2008 [86].

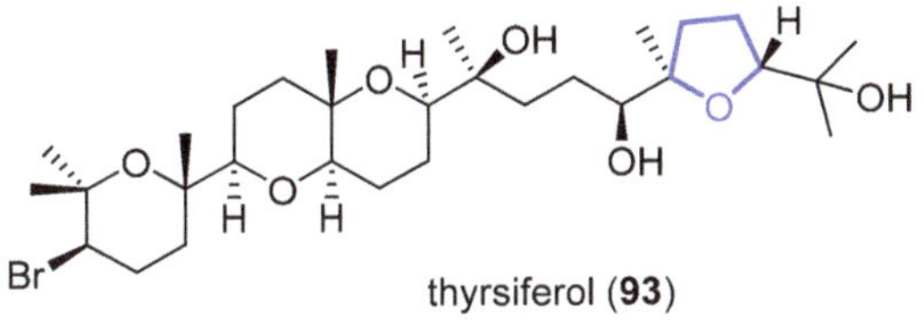

Figure 22. Structure of thyrsiferol (**93**).

Thyrsiferol has later been found to inhibit hypoxia-induced hypoxia-inducible factor-1 (HIF-1) activation in T47D human breast tumor cells, as well as to inhibit a mitochondrial ETC complex I and show tumor cell line-selective time-dependent inhibition of cell viability/proliferation [77]. In addition, Piñero and Fernández recently reported it to be active against *Acanthamoeba castellanii* trophozoites (IC_{50} = 13.97 µM). Its derivative, 22-hydroxydehydrotyrsiferol, was similarly active (IC_{50} = 17.00 µM) and both were not toxic against murine macrophages, which makes them potential leads for the discovery of novel amoebicidal substances [87].

3.4.9. Rhabdastins

The first members of this family, Rhabdastins A–G, were first isolated in 2010 by Iwagawa from the sponge *Rhabdastrella globostellata* [88]. They belong to the group of isomalabaricane triterpenes. In 2021, the tetrahydrofuran-containing rhabdastins H (**94**) and I (**95**) (Figure 23) were isolated from the sponge *Rhabdastrella* sp. [89]. They are the first marine isomalabaricanes that present a tetrahydrofuran unit in their structure. Both compounds show antiproliferative effect against K562 (IC_{50} 11.7 and 9.8 µM, respectively) and Molt4 (IC_{50} 16.5 and 11.0 µM) leukemic cells.

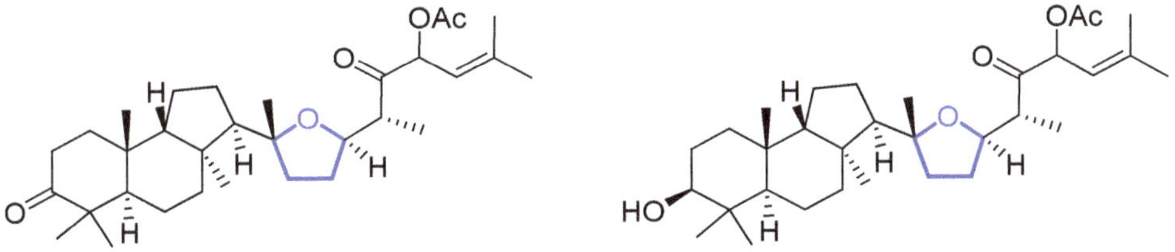

Figure 23. Structure of rhabdastins H (**94**) and I (**95**).

3.5. Meroterpenes

3.5.1. Alisiaquinones and Alisiaquinol

Alisiaquinones A–C (**96–98**) and alisiaquinol (**99**) (Figure 24) are meroterpenes that were isolated in 2008 from a New Caledonian deep-water sponge [90]. They display mild antimalarial activity, but the high level of toxicity (100% and 80% mortality, respectively) shown in in vivo assays limited their interest as antimalarial agents. Nevertheless, their structure can be an inspiration for the development of related structures towards novel antimalarial drugs.

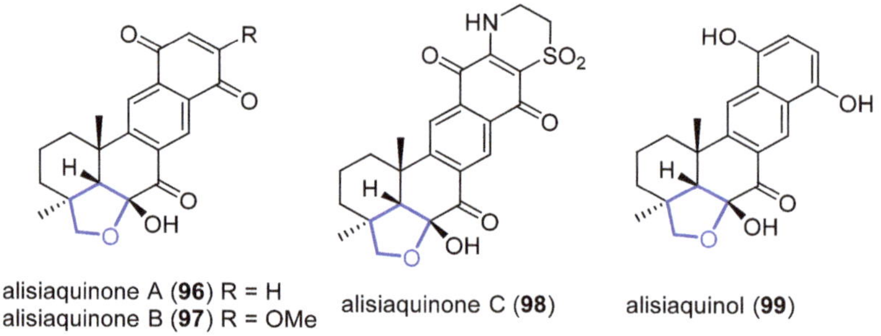

alisiaquinone A (**96**) R = H
alisiaquinone B (**97**) R = OMe
alisiaquinone C (**98**)
alisiaquinol (**99**)

Figure 24. Structure of alisiaquinones A–C (**96**–**98**) and alisiaquinol (**99**).

3.5.2. Tricycloalterfurenes

Tricycloalterfurenes A–D (**100**–**103**) were isolated in 2017 from the culture extract of an *Alternaria alternata* strain (k21-1) isolated from the surface of the marine red alga *Lomentaria hakodatensis* [91]. These meroterpenes present activity against three phytoplankton (*Chattonella marina*, *Heterosigma akashiwo*, and *Prorocentrum donghaiense*) and one marine zooplankton (*Artemia salina*). The higher activity of tricycloalterfurene A (64, 37, 46%, respectively, against the phytoplankton species) indicates that hydroxylation at C2 or C3 negatively influences the activity against these organisms. Later, Oh and Shin reported the isolation, from a marine-derived *Stemphylium* sp. fungus, of tricycloalterfurenes E–G (**104**–**106**) [92]. Very recently, Fraga proposed some structural revisions [93]. Regarding tricycloalterfurenes A–C, the correct configuration of the hydroxyl group would be *4R* (Figure 25), comparing the NMR data with that of guignardone T [94]. With respect to trycicloalterfurene D, the correct configuration was proposed to be 6-β-OH (*6R*), also by NMR data comparison to similar systems [95]. To date, no synthetic approaches have been reported.

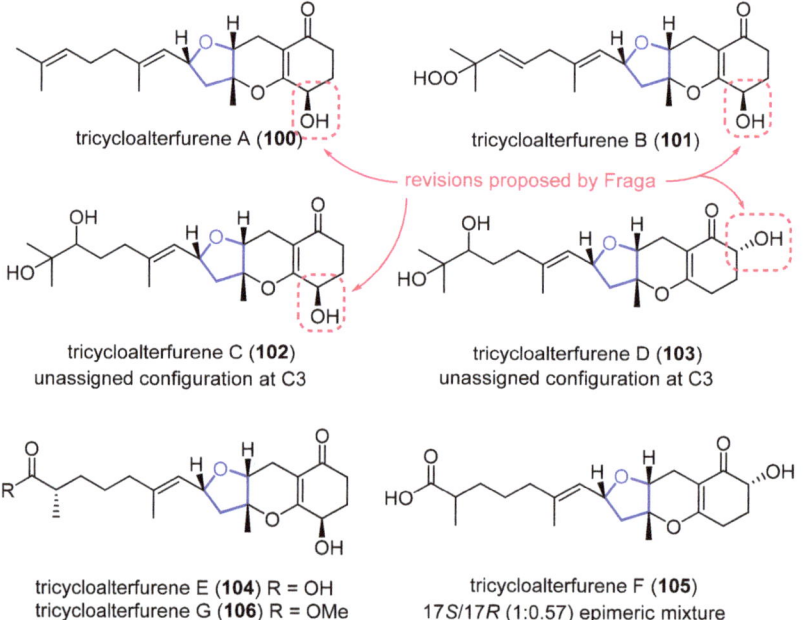

tricycloalterfurene A (**100**)

tricycloalterfurene B (**101**)

revisions proposed by Fraga

tricycloalterfurene C (**102**)
unassigned configuration at C3

tricycloalterfurene D (**103**)
unassigned configuration at C3

tricycloalterfurene E (**104**) R = OH
tricycloalterfurene G (**106**) R = OMe

tricycloalterfurene F (**105**)
17*S*/17*R* (1:0.57) epimeric mixture

Figure 25. Structure of tricycloalterfurenes and proposed structural revisions (in pink) by Fraga.

3.5.3. Marinoterpins

Marinoterpins A–C (**107–109**) (Figure 26) are linear merosesterterpenoids that were recently isolated (2021) by Winter and Fenical from the marine-derived actinomycete bacteria *Streptomyces* sp. AJS-327 and CNQ-253 [96]. Due to their similarity to the aurachin family of compounds, a marinoterpin biosynthetic cluster (*mrt*) was identified. Thus, a biosynthetic route for the 3-geranylfarnesyl-2-methylquinoline core was proposed, although the reactions that lead to the tetrahydrofuran rings as well as the N-oxidation still remain unknown.

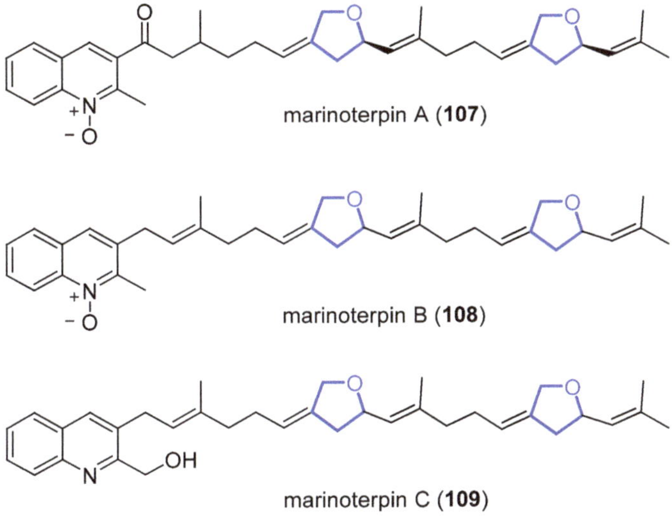

Figure 26. Structure of marinoterpins A–C (**107–109**).

4. Other Tetrahydrofuran Derivatives

4.1. Substituted Tetrahydrofurans

4.1.1. Pachastrissamine (Jaspine B)

Pachastrissamine (**110**) was first isolated by Higa and coworkers from a marine sponge of the genus *Pachastrissa* [97]. A year later, Debitus reported its isolation from another sponge *Jaspis* sp. and, thus, named the compound jaspine B [98]. Other related compounds were also isolated, including jaspine A (**111**) (Figure 27). Pachastrissamine is a sphingolipid—in particular, a derivative from anhydrophytosphingosine. Its biological activity and synthetic endeavors until 2016 were summarized by Martinková in a mini-review [99].

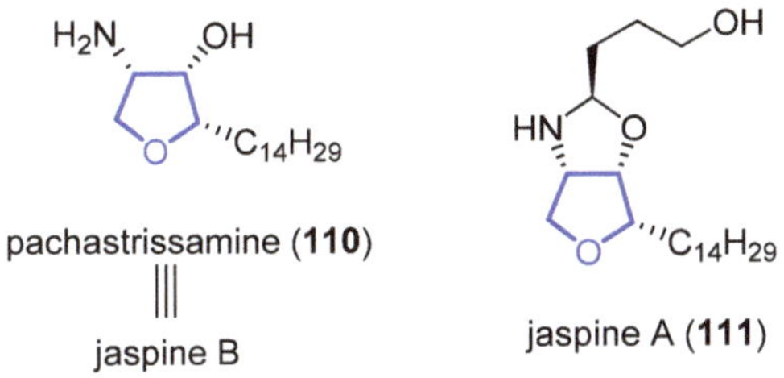

Figure 27. Structures of pachastrissamine (jaspine B, **110**) and jaspine A (**111**).

4.1.2. Myrothecols

In 2020, (−)-1*S*-myrothecol ((−)-**112**), (+)-1*R*-myrothecol ((+)-**112**), and methoxymyrothecol (**113**) (Figure 28) were isolated from deep-sea fungus *Myrothecium sp.* BZO-L062 [100]. Enantiomers (−)-**112** and (+)-**112** were separated by normal-phase chiral

HPLC, and their absolute configurations were established by ECD spectra. Compounds (−)-**112** and (+)-**112** display anti-inflammatory activity, inhibit nitric oxide formation in lipopolysaccharide-treated cells (RAW264.7), and present antioxidant activity in the 2,2-azino-*bis*(3-ethylbenzothiazoline-6-sulfonic acid) and oxygen-radical absorbance capacity assays.

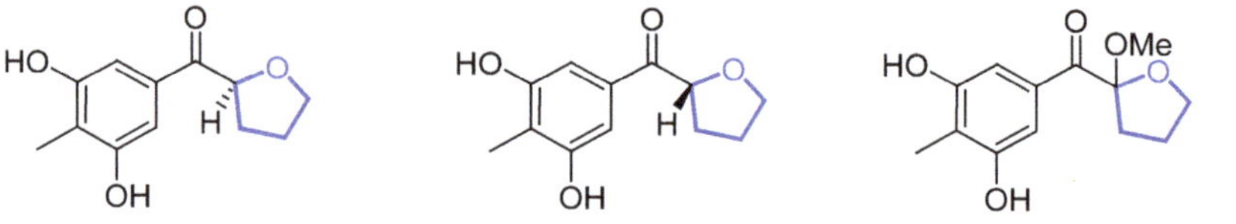

(-)-myrothecol (**-**)-**112**   (+)-myrothecol (**+**)-**112**   methoxy-myrothecol (**113**)

Figure 28. Structure of (−)-1*S*-myrothecol ((−)-**112**), (+)-1*R*-myrothecol ((+)-**112**), and methoxy-myrothecol (**113**).

4.1.3. Astronypyrone, Astronyquinone, and Astronyurea

In 2016, astronypyrone (**114**), astronyquinone (**115**), and astronyurea (**116**) (Figure 29) were isolated from the marine fungus *Astrosphaeriella nypae* BCC 5335 [101]. Compound **115** shows weak antituberculosis activity (with a MIC value of 50 µg/mL) and presents cytotoxicity against African green monkey kidney fibroblast cell lines (IC$_{50}$ = 17.4 µg/mL).

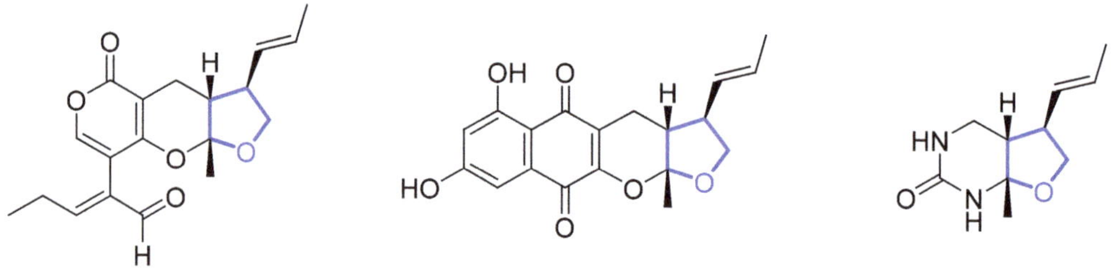

astronypyrone (**114**)   astronyquinone (**115**)   astronyurea (**116**)

Figure 29. Structure of astronypyrone (**114**), astronyquinone (**115**), and astronyurea (**116**).

4.1.4. Sinularones

Sinularones A-I were isolated in 2012 from the marine soft coral *Sinularia* sp. [102]. Their structures were elucidated by IR, MS, CD, 1D, and 2D NMR. Among them, sinularones E (**117**) and F (**118**) contain a tetrahydrofuran moiety (Figure 30).

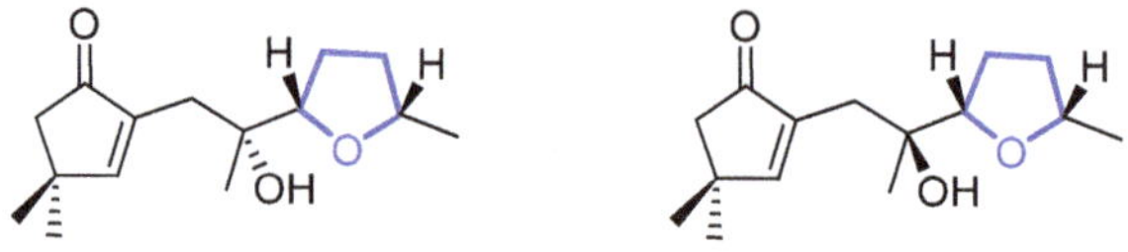

sinularone E (**117**)   sinularone F (**118**)

Figure 30. Structure of sinularones E (**117**) and F (**118**).

Their first total synthesis, based on a hydrogenative metathesis of enynes, was reported in 2020 by Fürstner and coworkers [103]. The required 2,5-*cis*-tetrahydrofuran derivative **119** was readily obtained by hydrogenation (over Rh/Al$_2$O$_3$) of commercial furane **120**. Three further steps were needed to obtain silyl ether **121**, which in the presence of ruthenium catalyst **122** and H$_2$ undergoes a hydrogenative metathesis. Later deprotection with TBAF produces **117** with 65% yield over both steps. Sinularone F (**118**) synthesis utilizes the same strategy (Scheme 13).

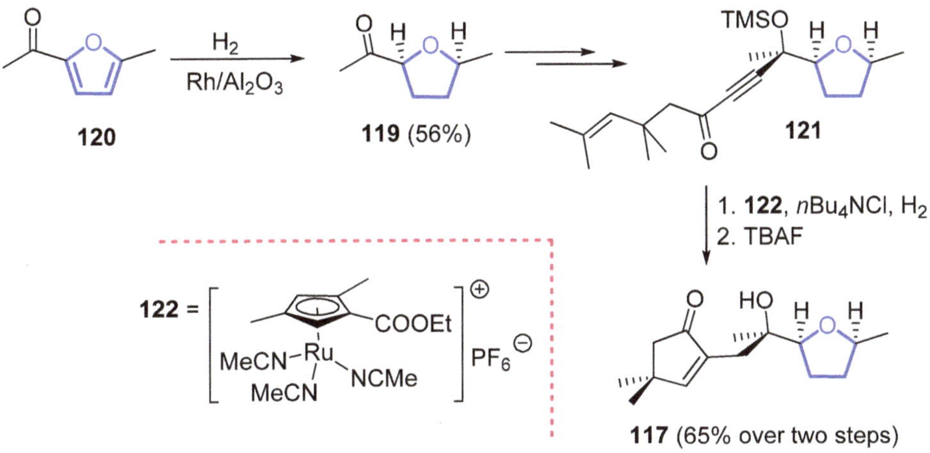

Scheme 13. Synthesis of sinularone E (**117**). A similar strategy was applied to sinularone F (**118**).

4.1.5. (+)-Varitriol

(+)-Varitriol (**(+)-123**) (Figure 31) was isolated in 2002 from a marine-derived strain of the fungus *Emericella variecolor* [104]. Its structure and relative stereochemistry were determined by NMR studies. It displays low cytotoxic activity against leukemia, ovarian, and colon cells, but its response to renal, CNS, and breast cancer cell lines was very promising (of the range of GI_{50} = 1.63–2.44·10^{-7} M). In 2006, Jennings and coworkers achieved the first total synthesis of its enantiomer **(-)-123** and, thus, determined its absolute stereochemistry [105].

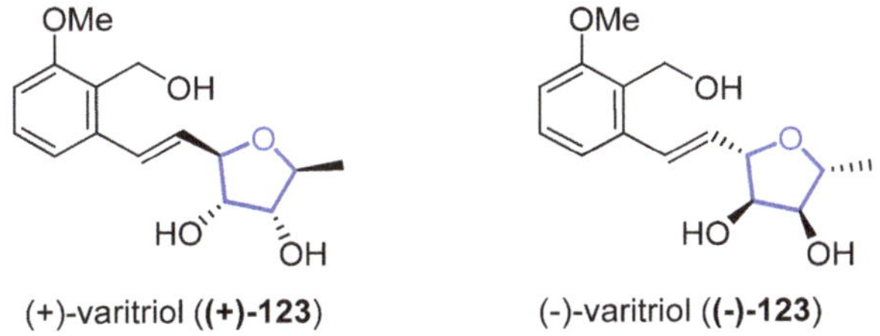

Figure 31. Structure of (+)-varitriol (**(+)-123**) and (−)-varitriol (**(−)-123**).

Its activity towards the mentioned cancer cell lines attracted the attention of synthetic chemists; different synthetic approaches for **(+)-123** appeared in the next few years [106]. Taylor employed a known tetrahydrofuran-2,3,4-triol derivative as the starting material for the synthesis (in three further steps) of the desired **(−)-123** and its 3′-epi-derivative [107]. Srihari also achieved the synthesis of **(−)-123**, **(+)-123**, and its 6′-epi-derivative starting from commercial D-(−)-ribose [108,109]. Krause performed a modular synthesis of **(+)-123** in 10 steps, with an overall yield of 6,4% [110]. The key tetrahydrofuran with the appropriate four stereocenters **124** was prepared in four linear steps from a known enyne. Thus, Sharpless epoxidation and benzylation of (*E*)-hex-2-en-4-yn-1-ol provided propargyl epoxide **125** in 47% yield over two steps. A copper hydride-catalyzed reduction of **125**, followed by a gold-catalyzed cycloisomerization, furnished the key dihydrofuranyl intermediate **126**, with two of the required stereogenic centers. Final Sharpless dihydroxylation of **126** afforded **124** as a satisfactory 78:22 mixture of diastereoisomers. The desired natural product was obtained in a further four steps (Scheme 14).

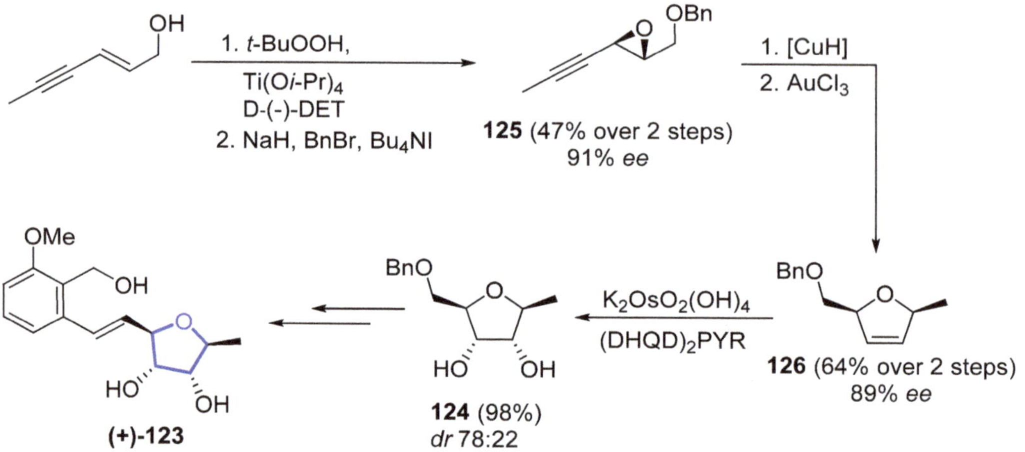

Scheme 14. Modular synthesis of (+)-varitriol ((+)-**123**) by Krause.

A recent example of the total synthesis of **(+)-123** was reported by Cordero-Vargas [111]. In this approach, the tetrahydrofuranyl key intermediate **127**, bearing the four precise sterocenters, was obtained from commercial L-ribono-1,4-lactone in six steps. The key step in this process is the stereocontrolled nucleophilic addition to five-membered oxocarbenium ions directed by the protecting groups. Thus, TBS-protected lactone **128**, obtained in four conventional steps from L-ribono-1,4-lactone, undergoes acetylide addition; a subsequent Lewis acid promoted oxocarbenium ion formation. The following stereoselective hydride attack provides tetrahydrofuran **127** as a single diastereomer in 60% yield. The final synthesis of **(+)-123** is achieved in a further four steps with 31% yield over them (Scheme 15).

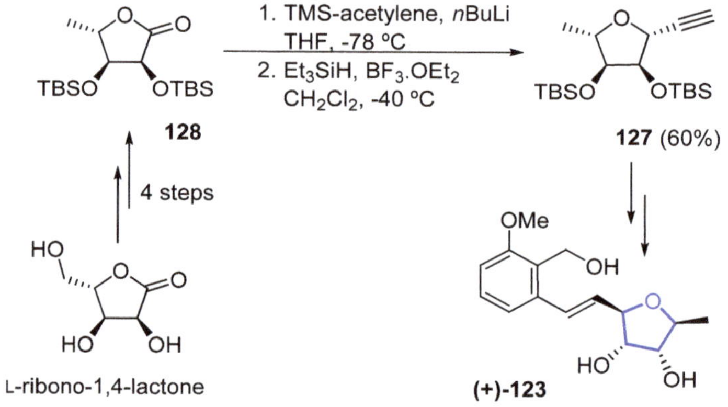

Scheme 15. Protecting group-directed nucleophilic addition for the synthesis of (+)-varitriol (**123**).

Later on, Qin developed a direct cross-coupling between terminal alkynes and glycosyl acetates, which was applied to the formal synthesis of **(+)-123** and analogues [112]. More recently, Wang and coworkers reported another formal synthesis of **(+)-123** [113]. They developed a chromium-catalyzed enantioconvergent allenylation of aldehydes to synthesize α-allenols from racemic propargyl halides. Starting from silylated propargyl bromide **129** and benzyloxyacetaldehyde, allenol **130** can be accessed through the developed procedure. The chromium catalyst was formed in situ by the addition of chromium chloride and the oxazoline ligand **(R,S)-131**. Manganese acted as a reducing agent, and Cp_2ZrCl_2 as a dissociation reagent. Then, removal of the silyl group with tetrabutylammonium fluoride gave advanced intermediate **132** in 82% yield, thus accomplishing the formal synthesis of the desired **(+)-123** (Scheme 16).

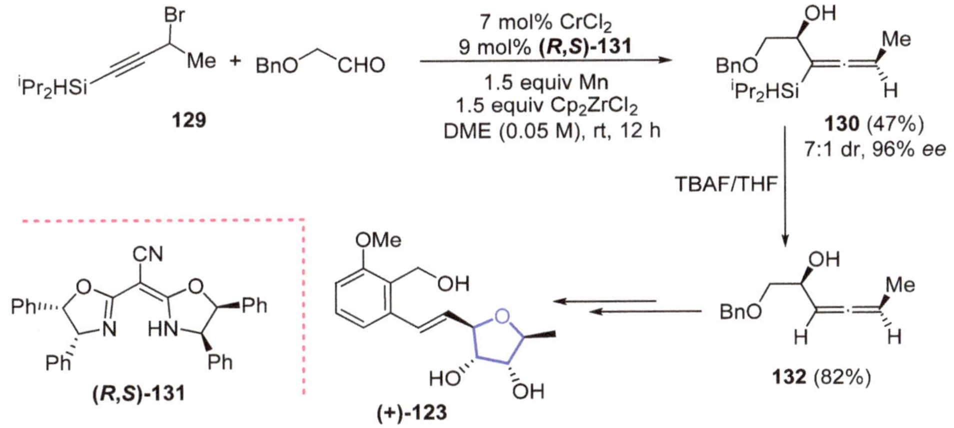

Scheme 16. Application of allenylation of aldehydes to the formal synthesis of (+)-varitriol by Wang.

5. Conclusions

Terpenes and related compounds represent an important family of marine-derived metabolites. The great number of studies focused on their biological activities and total synthesis remark their importance. We have summarized the most active compounds for a variety of bioactivities (see Table 2). *Trans*-oxylipid has shown nematocidal properties against *Haemonchus contortus* (LD_{50} = 1.8 ppm) and *Trichostrongyllus colubriformis* (LD_{50} = 9.9 ppm). These values, comparable to the commercial levamisole and closantel, make this compound an interesting scaffold for the development of antihelmintic substances. Though not related to drug development, we want to remark the biological interest of (+)-PMA. Its potent olfactory response in sea lampreys makes it very valuable for the control and conservation of lamprey populations. Efforts should be made in developing a total synthesis for this compound, as none has been reported to date. Mutafuran D has antifungal activity, showing a moderate value of MIC = 4 mg/mL against *Cryptococcus neoformans var. grubii*. Although not an impressive value, further studies could shed light on the structure–activity relationship of this brominated ene-yne tetrahydrofuran derivative. Furoplocamioid C could serve as a lead for novel biopesticides, as it has shown a potent antifeedant effect against *Leptinotarsa decemlineata*, with an EC_{50} of 19.1 nmol/cm^2, *Myzus Persicae* (EC_{50} of 3.7 nmol/cm^2), and *Ropalosiphum Padi* (EC_{50} of 1.6 nmol/cm^2) but it has low mammalian toxicity and phytotoxic effects. With respect to antibacterial activity, heranopyrrole D has shown very good values against *Staphylococcus aureus* ATCC 25923 (IC_{50} = 1.8 mM), *Staphylococcus epidermidis* ATCC 12228 (IC_{50} = 0.9 mM), and *Bacillus subtilis* ATCC 6633 (IC_{50} = 1.8 mM); thus, the nitropyrrole moiety should be further studied to determine whether it plays an important role in its antibacterial behavior. On the other hand, though (+)-darwinolide shows a more moderate value against *Staphylococcus aureus* (IC_{50} = 33.2 μM), its selectivity towards the biofilm phase and its low toxicity makes it a very good lead for the development of antibiofilm-specific antibiotics.

Regarding antitumoral applications, there are several compounds that have shown very promising activities. Uprolide D acetate has cytotoxic activity against different tumor cell lines: HeLa cells (IC_{50} = 2.5 mM), CCRF-CEM T-cell leukemia (IC_{50} = 7.0 mM), HCT-116 colon cancer (IC_{50} = 7.0 mM), and MCF-7 breast adenocarcinoma (IC_{50} = 0.6 mM). Thyrsenol B has an impressive potential against murine lymphoid neoplasm P-388 cells (IC_{50} = 0.016 mM). Saiyacenol B shows antiproliferative activity against tumor cell lines MM144 human multiple myeloma (IC_{50} = 11.0 mM), HeLa human cervical carcinoma

(IC$_{50}$ = 24.5 mM), CADO-ES1 human Ewing's sarcoma (IC$_{50}$ = 14.0 mM), and possesses a very good value for Jurkat (human T-cell acute leukemia): IC$_{50}$ = 2.7 mM. Furthermore, it presents antifouling activity against *Navicula* cf. *salinicola* (IC$_{50}$ = 17.2 mM) and *Cylindrotheca* sp. (IC$_{50}$ = 17.0 mM). Finally, (+)-varitriol is a very interesting example, as it is quite a simple molecule with powerful properties. It presents submicromolar activities against different cancer cell lines, namely RXF-393 (Renal cancer cell) GI$_{50}$ = 0.16 µM; SNB-75 (CNS cancer cell) GI$_{50}$ = 0.24 µM; and DU-145 (breast cancer cell) GI$_{50}$ = 0.11 µM. Although some efforts have already been made and different total syntheses reported, we believe that further studies should point to the synthesis of analogs and the study of structure–activity relationships in this simple scaffold.

Regarding antiprotozoal activity, saiyacenol B shows a good IC$_{50}$ of 10.3 mM against *Leishmania amazonensis*. Interestingly it was surpassed by its synthetic counterpart, 28-iodo-saiyacenol B, with a value of IC$_{50}$ = 5.4 mM pointing to an interesting effect of this 28-iodo-substitution. Alisiaquinone C presents antimalarial activity in vitro against the chloroquine-resistant strains MC29 CQR (IC$_{50}$ = 0.08 mM) and B1 CQR (IC$_{50}$ = 0.21 mM), and the chloroquine-sensitive strain F32 CQS (IC$_{50}$ = 0.15 mM). Though it presents a high toxicity, similar structures that preserve antimalarial activity and have reduced toxicity values could be developed. A possible lead for anti-inflammatory development is myrothecol: it shows antioxidant activity with an EC$_{50}$ = 1.2 mg/mL (*S* isomer) and EC$_{50}$ = 1.4 mg/mL (*R* isomer), inhibits nitric oxide formation, and displays anti-inflammatory activity. It is also a small molecule and, thus, its synthesis will require lower effort.

In conclusion, the tetrahydrofuran moiety is a common motif found in a variety of such compounds, which has meant a particular emphasis of researchers on the development of new methodologies for the synthesis of such derivatives. In this context, total synthesis is a powerful tool to have access to these natural products. Firstly, it is an invaluable means for the determination of the structure and total configuration of natural compounds since, in some cases, the available NMR methods are insufficient in definitively determining the structures of biologically relevant substances. Secondly, since extracting and purifying compounds from natural sources are difficult and time-consuming processes, total synthesis has emerged as a suitable solution for the production of larger amounts of compounds, thus bringing possibilities for further biological studies, the discovery of novel drug candidates, and the expansion of the medicinal chemistry frontiers.

Table 2. Summary of most active compounds for a range of bioactivities within this review.

Compound	Biological Activity	Cell Line or Organism	Biological Result	Assay	Reference
trans-oxylipid	Nematocidal	*Haemonchus contortus*	LD$_{50}$ = 1.8 ppm	Parasitic nematode larval development assay	[21]
		Trichostrongylus colubriformis	LD$_{50}$ = 9.9 ppm		
(+)-PMA	Pheromone	*Petromyzon marinus*	10^{-11} molL^{-1}	Electro-olfactogram	[26]
Mutafuran D	Antifungal activity	*Cryptococcus neoformans var. grubii*	MIC = 4 µg/mL	Pathogenic fungus assay	[27]
Furoplocamioid C	Antifeedant effects	*Leptinotarsa decemlineata*	EC$_{50}$ = 19.1 nmol/cm^2	Insect bioassay	[32]
		Myzus persicae	EC$_{50}$ = 3.7 nmol/cm^2		
		Ropalosiphum padi	EC$_{50}$ = 1.6 nmol/cm^2		

Table 2. Cont.

Compound	Biological Activity	Cell Line or Organism	Biological Result	Assay	Reference
Heranopyrrole D	Antibacterial activity	*Staphylococcus aureus* ATCC 25923	IC_{50} = 1.8 μM	Antibacterial assay	[36]
		Staphylococcus epidermidis ATCC 12228	IC_{50} = 0.9 μM		
		Bacillus subtilis ATCC 6633	IC_{50} = 1.8 μM		
(+)-Darwinolide	Antibacterial activity	*Staphylococcus aureus*	IC_{50} = 33.2 μM	MRSA biofilm assay	[49]
Uprolide D acetate	Cytotoxic Activity Against Tumor Cell Lines	HeLa cells	IC_{50} = 2.5 μg/mL	Cytotoxicity assay on human cells	[52]
		CCRF-CEM T-cell leukemia	IC_{50} = 7.0 μg/mL		
		HCT 116 colon cancer	IC_{50} = 7.0 μg/mL		
		MCF-7 breast adenocarcinoma	IC_{50} = 0.6 μg/mL		
Thyrsenol B	Cytotoxic Activity Against Tumor Cell Lines	Murine lymphoid neoplasm P-388 cells	IC_{50} = 0.016 μM	Cytotoxicity assays on human cells	[74]
	Inhibitory activity	Protein phosphatase PP2A	Inhibition > 90% ([PP2A] > 10 μM)	Enzymatic assay	[75]
Saiyacenol B	Antiproliferative activity Against Tumor Cell Lines	MM144 (human multiple myeloma) Jurkat (human T-cell acute leukemia)	IC_{50} = 11.0 μM	Cytotoxicity assays on human cells	[78]
		HeLa (human cervical carcinoma)	IC_{50} = 24.5 μM		
		CADO-ES1 (human Ewing's sarcoma)	IC_{50} = 14.0 μM		
		Jurkat (human T-cell acute leukemia)	IC_{50} = 2.7 μM		
	Antifouling activity	*Navicula* cf. *salinicola*	IC_{50} = 17.2 μM	Diatom growth inhibition	
		Cylindrotheca sp.	IC_{50} = 17.0 μM	Inhibition of macroalgal spore germination	
	Anti-protozoal activity	*Leishmania amazonensis*	IC_{50} = 10.3 μM	In vitro susceptibility assay	[80]
28-iodo-saiyacenol B	Anti-protozoal activity	*Leishmania amazonensis*	IC_{50} = 5.4 μM	In vitro susceptibility assay	[80]
Alisiaquinone C	Antimalarial activity (in vitro)	MC29 CQR	IC_{50} = 0.08 μM	[^{3}H]-Hypoxanthine incorporation	[90]
		B1 CQR	IC_{50} = 0.21 μM		
		F32 CQS	IC_{50} = 0.15 μM		
	Antimalarial activity (in vivo)	Rodent malaria	Mortality day 5 = 0 (5 mg/kg/day) Mortality day 5 = 80 (20 mg/kg/day)	four-day suppressive in vivo assay	

Table 2. Cont.

Compound	Biological Activity	Cell Line or Organism	Biological Result	Assay	Reference
(−)-1S-Myrothecol	Antioxidant activity		EC_{50} = 1.2 µg/mL	ABTS assay	[100]
			µM Trolox Equiv/µM = 1.4	ORAC assay	
(+)-1R-Myrothecol	Antioxidant activity		EC_{50} = 1.4 µg/mL	ABTS assay	
			µM Trolox Equiv/µM = 1.2	ORAC assay	
(+)-Varitriol	Cytotoxic activity to cancer cell lines	RXF-393 (Renal cancer cell)	GI_{50} = 0.16 µM	Cytotoxicity assays	[104]
		SNB-75 (CNS cancer cell)	GI_{50} = 0.24 µM	Cytotoxicity assays	
		DU-145 (breast cancer cell)	GI_{50} = 0.11 µM	Cytotoxicity assays	

Author Contributions: Writing—original draft preparation, L.F.-P. and P.G.-A.; writing—reviewing and editing, C.D.-P. and A.B. All authors have read and agreed to the published version of the manuscript.

Funding: This research was funded by the "Junta de Castilla y León", grant number VA294-P18.

Institutional Review Board Statement: Not applicable.

Informed Consent Statement: Not applicable.

Data Availability Statement: Data sharing not applicable.

Acknowledgments: L.F.-P. and P.G.-A. acknowledge predoctoral grants funded by the "Junta de Castilla y León" and the University of Valladolid, respectively.

Conflicts of Interest: The authors declare no conflict of interest.

Abbreviations

Ac: acetate; Aq.: aqueous; BDSB: bromodiethylsulfonium bromopentachloroantimonate; Bn: benzyl; Boc: tert-butyloxy carbonyl; Bu: butyl; Bz: benzoyl; Cat.: catalyst; CD: circular dichroism; Cp: cyclopentadienyl; CSA: camphorsulfonic acid; Cy: cyclohexyl; D-(−)-DET: (−)-diethyl D-tartrate; DDQ: 2,3-Dichloro-5,6-dicyano-1,4-benzoquinone; DFT: density functional theory; $(DHQD)_2PYR$: hydroquinidine-2,5-diphenyl-4,6-pyrimidinediyl diether; DIAD: diisopropyl azodicarboxylate; DME: dimethoxyethane; DMSO: dimethylsulfoxide; *dr*: diastereomeric ratio; ECD: electronic circular dichroism; *ee*: enantiomeric excess; HMDS: hexamethyl disilazide; HPLC: high-performance liquid chromatography; IBX: orto-iodoxybenzoic acid; IR: infrared; M: molar; MS: mass spectrometry; Ms: methanesulfonyl; NMR: nuclear magnetic resonance; PAB: para-aminobenzoate; PG: protecting group; Ph: phenyl; PMA: petromyric acid A; PMB: petromyric acid B or *para*-methoxybenzyl; PNB: *para*-nitrobenzoate; *p*-NBA: *para*-nitrobenzoic acid; Pr: propyl; TBAF: tetrabutylammonium fluoride; TBHP: tert-butyl hydroperoxide; TIPS: triisopropylsilyl; TfOH: trifluoromethanesulfonic acid; TMS: trimethylsilyl.

References

1. Jiménez, C. Marine Natural Products in Medicinal Chemistry. *ACS Med. Chem. Lett.* **2018**, *9*, 959–961. [CrossRef] [PubMed]
2. Carroll, A.R.; Copp, B.R.; Davis, R.A.; Keyzers, R.A.; Prinsep, M.R. Marine Natural Products. *Nat. Prod. Rep.* **2021**, *38*, 362–413. [CrossRef]
3. Carroll, A.R.; Copp, B.R.; Davis, R.A.; Keyzers, R.A.; Prinsep, M.R. Marine Natural Products. *Nat. Prod. Rep.* **2020**, *37*, 175–223. [CrossRef] [PubMed]
4. Carroll, A.R.; Copp, B.R.; Davis, R.A.; Keyzers, R.A.; Prinsep, M.R. Marine Natural Products. *Nat. Prod. Rep.* **2019**, *36*, 122–173. [CrossRef] [PubMed]

5. Fuwa, H. Structure determination, correction, and disproof of marine macrolide natural products by chemical synthesis. *Org. Chem. Front.* **2021**, *8*, 3990–4023. [CrossRef]
6. Caso, A.; da Silva, F.B.; Esposito, G.; Teta, R.; Sala, G.D.; Cavalcanti, L.P.A.N.; Valverde, A.L.; Martins, R.C.C.; Costantino, V. Exploring Chemical Diversity of Phorbas Sponges as a Source of Novel Lead Compounds in Drug Discovery. *Mar. Drugs* **2021**, *19*, 667. [CrossRef]
7. Ebada, S.S.; Lin, W.H.; Proksch, P. Bioactive sesterterpenes and tripterpenes from marine sponges: Ocurrence and pharmacological significance. *Mar. Drugs* **2010**, *8*, 313–346. [CrossRef] [PubMed]
8. Ebel, R. Terpenes from Marine-Derived Fungi. *Mar. Drugs* **2010**, *8*, 2340–2368. [CrossRef] [PubMed]
9. Elissawy, A.M.; El-Shazly, M.; Ebada, S.S.; Singab, A.B.; Proksch, P. Bioactive Terpenes from Marine-Derived Fungi. *Mar. Drugs* **2015**, *13*, 1966–1992. [CrossRef] [PubMed]
10. Jiang, M.; Wu, Z.; Guo, H.; Liu, L.; Chen, S. A Review of Terpenes from Marine-Derived Fungi: 2015–2019. *Mar. Drugs* **2020**, *18*, 321. [CrossRef] [PubMed]
11. Wu, Q.; Sun, J.; Chen, J.; Zhang, H.; Guo, Y.-W.; Wang, H. Terpenoids from Marine Soft Coral of the Genus Lemnalia: Chemistry and Biological Activities. *Mar. Drugs* **2018**, *16*, 320. [CrossRef]
12. Chang, Y.-C.; Sheu, J.-H.; Wu, Y.-C.; Sung, P.-J. Terpenoids from Octocorals of the Genus Pachyclavularia. *Mar. Drugs* **2017**, *15*, 382. [CrossRef]
13. Avila, C. Terpenoids in Marine Heterobranch Molluscs. *Mar. Drugs* **2020**, *18*, 162. [CrossRef] [PubMed]
14. Hegazy, M.E.F.; Mohamed, T.A.; Alhammady, M.A.; Shaheen, A.M.; Reda, E.H.; Elshamy, A.I.; Aziz, M.; Paré, P.W. Molecular Architecture and Biomedical Leads of Terpenes from Red Sea Marine Invertebrates. *Mar. Drugs* **2015**, *13*, 3154–3181. [CrossRef] [PubMed]
15. Nasir, N.M.; Ermanis, K.; Clarke, P.A. Strategies for the construction of tetrahydropyran rings in the synthesis of natural products. *Org. Biomol. Chem.* **2014**, *12*, 3323–3335. [CrossRef] [PubMed]
16. Fuwa, H. Contemporary Strategies for the Synthesis of Tetrahydropyran Derivatives: Application to Total Synthesis of Neopeltolide, a Marine Macrolide Natural Product. *Mar. Drugs* **2016**, *14*, 65. [CrossRef] [PubMed]
17. Barbero, H.; Díez-Poza, C.; Barbero, A. The Oxepane Motif in Marine Drugs. *Mar. Drugs* **2017**, *15*, 361. [CrossRef] [PubMed]
18. Fernandes, R.A.; Pathare, R.S.; Gorve, D.A. Advances in Total Synthesis of Some 2,3,5-Trisubstituted Tetrahydrofuran Natural Products. *Chem. Asian J.* **2020**, *15*, 2815–2837. [CrossRef]
19. Fernandes, R.A.; Gorve, D.A.; Pathare, R.S. Emergence of 2,3,5-trisubstituted tetrahydrofuran natural products and their synthesis. *Org. Biomol. Chem.* **2020**, *18*, 7002–7025. [CrossRef] [PubMed]
20. Fernández-Peña, L.; Díez-Poza, C.; González-Andrés, P.; Barbero, A. The Tetrahydrofuran Motif in Polyketide Marine Drugs. *Mar. Drugs* **2022**, *20*, 120. [CrossRef]
21. Warren, R.G.; Wells, R.J.; Blount, J.F. A novel lipid from the brown alga Notheia anomala. *Aust. J. Chem.* **1980**, *33*, 891–898. [CrossRef]
22. Capon, R.J.; Barrow, R.A.; Rochfort, S.; Jobling, M.; Skene, C.; Lacey, E.; Gill, J.H.; Friedel, T.; Wadsworth, D. Marine nematocides: Tetrahydrofurans from a southern Australian brown alga, Notheia anomala. *Tetrahedron* **1998**, *54*, 2227–2242. [CrossRef]
23. Jang, H.; Shin, I.; Lee, D.; Kim, H.; Kim, D. Stereoselective Substrate-Controlled Asymmetric Syntheses of both 2,5-cis- and 2,5-trans-Tetrahydrofuranoid Oxylipids: Stereodivergent Intramolecular Amide Enolate Alkylation. *Angew. Chem. Int. Ed.* **2016**, *55*, 6497–6501. [CrossRef] [PubMed]
24. Li, K.; Huertas, M.; Brant, C.; Chung-Davidson, Y.-W.; Bussy, U.; Hoye, T.R.; Li, W. (+)- and (−)-Petromyroxols: Antipodal Tetrahydrofurandiols from Larval Sea Lamprey (Petromyzon marinus L.) That Elicit Enantioselective Olfactory Responses. *Org. Lett.* **2015**, *17*, 286–289. [CrossRef]
25. Mullapudi, V.; Ahmad, I.; Senapati, S.; Ramana, C.V. Total Synthesis of (+)-Petromyroxol, (−)-iso-Petromyroxol, and Possible Diastereomers. *ACS Omega* **2020**, *5*, 25334–25348. [CrossRef] [PubMed]
26. Li, K.; Brant, C.O.; Huertas, M.; Hessler, E.J.; Mezei, G.; Scott, A.M.; Hoye, T.R.; Li, W. Fatty-acid derivative acts as a sea lamprey migratory pheromone. *PNAS* **2018**, *115*, 8603. [CrossRef]
27. Morinaka, B.I.; Skepper, C.K.; Molinski, T.F. Ene-yne Tetrahydrofurans from the Sponge Xestospongia muta. Exploiting a Weak CD Effect for Assignment of Configuration. *Org. Lett.* **2007**, *9*, 1975–1978. [CrossRef] [PubMed]
28. Zhou, X.; Lu, Y.; Lin, X.; Yang, B.; Yang, X.; Liu, Y. Brominated aliphatic hydrocarbons and sterols from the sponge Xestospongia testudinaria with their bioactivities. *Chem. Phys. Lipids* **2011**, *164*, 703–706. [CrossRef]
29. Liu, Y.; Ding, L.; Zhang, Z.; Yan, X.; He, S. New antifungal tetrahydrofuran derivatives from a marine sponge-associated fungus Aspergillus sp. LS78. *Fitoterapia* **2020**, *146*, 104677. [CrossRef] [PubMed]
30. Cueto, M.; Darias, J. Uncommon tetrahydrofuran monoterpenes from Antarctic Pantoneura plocamioides. *Tetrahedron* **1996**, *52*, 5899–5906. [CrossRef]
31. Blanc, A.; Toste, F.D. Enantioselective Synthesis of Cyclic Ethers through a Vanadium-Catalyzed Resolution/Oxidative Cyclization. *Angew. Chem. Int. Ed.* **2006**, *45*, 2096–2099. [CrossRef] [PubMed]
32. Darias, J.; Rovirosa, J.; San Martin, A.; Díaz, A.-R.; Dorta, E.; Cueto, M. Furoplocamioids A− C, Novel Polyhalogenated Furanoid Monoterpenes from Plocamium c artilagineum. *J. Nat. Prod.* **2001**, *64*, 1383–1387. [CrossRef]
33. Díaz-Marrero, A.R.; Cueto, M.; Dorta, E.; Rovirosa, J.; San-Martín, A.; Darias, J. New halogenated monoterpenes from the red alga Plocamium cartilagineum. *Tetrahedron* **2002**, *58*, 8539–8542. [CrossRef]

34. Argandoña, V.H.; Rovirosa, J.; San-Martín, A.; Riquelme, A.; Díaz-Marrero, A.R.; Cueto, M.; Darias, J.; Santana, O.; Guadaño, A.; González-Coloma, A. Antifeedant Effects of Marine Halogenated Monoterpenes. *J. Agric. Food. Chem.* **2002**, *50*, 7029–7033. [CrossRef] [PubMed]
35. Raju, R.; Piggott, A.M.; Barrientos Diaz, L.X.; Khalil, Z.; Capon, R.J. Heronapyrroles A−C: Farnesylated 2-Nitropyrroles from an Australian Marine-Derived *Streptomyces* sp. *Org. Lett.* **2010**, *12*, 5158–5161. [CrossRef] [PubMed]
36. Schmidt, J.; Khalil, Z.; Capon, R.J.; Stark, C.B. Heronapyrrole D: A case of co-inspiration of natural product biosynthesis, total synthesis and biodiscovery. *Beilstein J. Org. Chem.* **2014**, *10*, 1228–1232. [CrossRef]
37. Schmidt, J.; Stark, C.B.W. Biomimetic Synthesis and Proposal of Relative and Absolute Stereochemistry of Heronapyrrole C. *Org. Lett.* **2012**, *14*, 4042–4045. [CrossRef]
38. Schmidt, J.; Stark, C.B.W. Synthetic Endeavors toward 2-Nitro-4-Alkylpyrroles in the Context of the Total Synthesis of Heronapyrrole C and Preparation of a Carboxylate Natural Product Analogue. *J. Org. Chem.* **2014**, *79*, 1920–1928. [CrossRef]
39. Ding, X.-B.; Furkert, D.P.; Capon, R.J.; Brimble, M.A. Total Synthesis of Heronapyrrole C. *Org. Lett.* **2014**, *16*, 378–381. [CrossRef]
40. Ding, X.-B.; Brimble, M.A.; Furkert, D.P. Nitropyrrole natural products: Isolation, biosynthesis and total synthesis. *Org. Biomol. Chem.* **2016**, *14*, 5390–5401. [CrossRef]
41. Ding, X.-B.; Furkert, D.P.; Brimble, M.A. 2-Nitropyrrole cross-coupling enables a second generation synthesis of the heronapyrrole antibiotic natural product family. *Chem. Commun.* **2016**, *52*, 12638–12641. [CrossRef]
42. Ding, X.-B.; Brimble, M.A.; Furkert, D.P. Reactivity of 2-Nitropyrrole Systems: Development of Improved Synthetic Approaches to Nitropyrrole Natural Products. *J. Org. Chem.* **2018**, *83*, 12460–12470. [CrossRef]
43. Suzuki, T.; Koizumi, K.; Suzuki, M.; Kurosawa, E. Kumausalle, a new bromoallene from the marine red alga laurencia nipponica yamada. *Chem. Lett.* **1983**, *12*, 1639–1642. [CrossRef]
44. Grese, T.A.; Hutchinson, K.D.; Overman, L.E. General approach to halogenated tetrahydrofuran natural products from red algae of the genus Laurencia. Total synthesis of (.+-.)-kumausallene and (.+-.)-1-epi-kumausallene. *J. Org. Chem.* **1993**, *58*, 2468–2477. [CrossRef]
45. Werness, J.B.; Tang, W. Stereoselective Total Synthesis of (−)-Kumausallene. *Org. Lett.* **2011**, *13*, 3664–3666. [CrossRef]
46. Das, S.; Ramana, C.V. A formal total synthesis of (−)-kumausallene. *Tetrahedron* **2015**, *71*, 8577–8584. [CrossRef]
47. Suzuki, T.; Koizumi, K.; Suzuki, M.; Kurosawa, E. Kumausynes and deacetylkumausynes, four new halogenated C-15 acetylenes from the red alga Laurencia nipponica Yamada. *Chem. Lett.* **1983**, *12*, 1643–1644. [CrossRef]
48. Brown, M.J.; Harrison, T.; Overman, L.E. General approach to halogenated tetrahydrofuran natural products from red algae of the genus Laurencia. Total synthesis of (.+-.)-trans-kumausyne and demonstration of an asymmetric synthesis strategy. *J. Am. Chem. Soc.* **1991**, *113*, 5378–5384. [CrossRef]
49. Von Salm, J.L.; Witowski, C.G.; Fleeman, R.M.; McClintock, J.B.; Amsler, C.D.; Shaw, L.N.; Baker, B.J. Darwinolide, a New Diterpene Scaffold That Inhibits Methicillin-Resistant Staphylococcus aureus Biofilm from the Antarctic Sponge Dendrilla membranosa. *Org. Lett.* **2016**, *18*, 2596–2599. [CrossRef]
50. Shilling, A.J.; Witowski, C.G.; Maschek, J.A.; Azhari, A.; Vesely, B.A.; Kyle, D.E.; Amsler, C.D.; McClintock, J.B.; Baker, B.J. Spongian Diterpenoids Derived from the Antarctic Sponge Dendrilla antarctica Are Potent Inhibitors of the Leishmania Parasite. *J. Nat. Prod.* **2020**, *83*, 1553–1562. [CrossRef]
51. Siemon, T.; Steinhauer, S.; Christmann, M. Synthesis of (+)-Darwinolide, a Biofilm-Penetrating Anti-MRSA Agent. *Angew. Chem. Int. Ed.* **2019**, *58*, 1120–1122. [CrossRef]
52. Rodríguez, A.D.; Piña, I.C.; Soto, J.J.; Rojas, D.R.; Barnes, C.L. Isolation and structures of the uprolides. I. Thirteen new cytotoxic cembranolides from the Caribbean gorgonian Euniceamammosa. *Can. J. Chem.* **1995**, *73*, 643–654. [CrossRef]
53. Rodríguez, A.D.; Soto, J.J.; Piña, I.C. Uprolides D-G, 2. A Rare Family of 4,7-Oxa-bridged Cembranolides from the Caribbean Gorgonian Eunicea mammosa. *J. Nat. Prod.* **1995**, *58*, 1209–1216. [CrossRef]
54. Rodríguez, A.D.; Soto, J.J.; Barnes, C.L. Synthesis of Uprolide D− G Analogues. Revision of Structure of the Marine Cembranolides Uprolide F Diacetate and Uprolide G Acetate. *J. Org. Chem.* **2000**, *65*, 7700–7702. [CrossRef]
55. Zhu, L.; Tong, R. Structural Revision of (+)-Uprolide F Diacetate Confirmed by Asymmetric Total Synthesis. *Org. Lett.* **2015**, *17*, 1966–1969. [CrossRef]
56. Zhu, L.; Liu, Y.; Ma, R.; Tong, R. Total Synthesis and Structural Revision of (+)-Uprolide G Acetate. *Angew. Chem. Int. Ed.* **2015**, *54*, 627–632. [CrossRef]
57. Zhu, L.; Tong, R. Structural Revision of Uprolide G Acetate: Effective Interplay between NMR Data Analysis and Chemical Synthesis. *Synlett* **2015**, *26*, 1643–1648. [CrossRef]
58. Ramana, C.V.; Salian, S.R.; Gurjar, M.K. Central core of uprolides D and E: A survey of some ring closing metathesis approaches. *Tetrahedron Lett.* **2007**, *48*, 1013–1016. [CrossRef]
59. Marshall, J.A.; Griot, C.A.; Chobanian, H.R.; Myers, W.H. Synthesis of a Lactone Diastereomer of the Cembranolide Uprolide D. *Org. Lett.* **2010**, *12*, 4328–4331. [CrossRef]
60. Torres-Mendoza, D.; González, Y.; Gómez-Reyes, J.F.; Guzmán, H.M.; López-Perez, J.L.; Gerwick, W.H.; Fernandez, P.L.; Gutiérrez, M. Uprolides N, O and P from the Panamanian Octocoral Eunicea succinea. *Molecules* **2016**, *21*, 819. [CrossRef]
61. Suzuki, M.; Matsuo, Y.; Takeda, S.; Suzuki, T. Intricatetraol, a halogenated triterpene alcohol from the red alga Laurencia intricata. *Phytochemistry* **1993**, *33*, 651–656. [CrossRef]

62. Morimoto, Y.; Takaishi, M.; Adachi, N.; Okita, T.; Yata, H. Two-directional synthesis and stereochemical assignment toward a C2 symmetric oxasqualenoid (+)-intricatetraol. *Org. Biomol. Chem.* **2006**, *4*, 3220–3222. [CrossRef] [PubMed]
63. Morimoto, Y.; Okita, T.; Takaishi, M.; Tanaka, T. Total Synthesis and Determination of the Absolute Configuration of (+)-Intricatetraol. *Angew. Chem. Int. Ed.* **2007**, *46*, 1132–1135. [CrossRef] [PubMed]
64. Matsuo, Y.; Suzuki, M.; Masuda, M.; Iwai, T.; Morimoto, Y. Squalene-Derived Triterpene Polyethers from the Red Alga Laurencia omaezakiana. *Helv. Chim. Acta* **2008**, *91*, 1261–1266. [CrossRef]
65. Morimoto, Y.; Okita, T.; Kambara, H. Total Synthesis and Determination of the Absolute Configuration of (+)-Omaezakianol. *Angew. Chem. Int. Ed.* **2009**, *48*, 2538–2541. [CrossRef]
66. Xiong, Z.; Busch, R.; Corey, E.J. A Short Total Synthesis of (+)-Omaezakianol via an Epoxide-Initiated Cationic Cascade Reaction. *Org. Lett.* **2010**, *12*, 1512–1514. [CrossRef]
67. Morimoto, Y.; Takeuchi, E.; Kambara, H.; Kodama, T.; Tachi, Y.; Nishikawa, K. Biomimetic Epoxide-Opening Cascades of Oxasqualenoids Triggered by Hydrolysis of the Terminal Epoxide. *Org. Lett.* **2013**, *15*, 2966–2969. [CrossRef]
68. Itokawa, H.; Kishi, E.; Morita, H.; Takeya, K.; Iitaka, Y. A New Squalene-type Triterpene from the Woods of Eurycoma longifolia. *Chem. Lett.* **1991**, *20*, 2221–2222. [CrossRef]
69. Morita, H.; Kishi, E.; Takeya, K.; Itokawa, H.; Iitaka, Y. Squalene derivatives from Eurycoma longifolia. *Phytochemistry* **1993**, *34*, 765–771. [CrossRef]
70. Morimoto, Y.; Iwai, T.; Kinoshita, T. Total synthesis and determination of the absolute configuration of (−)-longilene peroxide. *Tetrahedron Lett.* **2001**, *42*, 6307–6309. [CrossRef]
71. Morimoto, Y.; Iwai, T.; Nishikawa, Y.; Kinoshita, T. Stereospecific and biomimetic synthesis of CS and C2 symmetric 2,5-disubstituted tetrahydrofuran rings as central building blocks of biogenetically intriguing oxasqualenoids. *Tetrahedron Asymmetry* **2002**, *13*, 2641–2647. [CrossRef]
72. Cen-Pacheco, F.; Pérez Manríquez, C.; Luisa Souto, M.; Norte, M.; Fernández, J.J.; Hernández Daranas, A. Marine Longilenes, Oxasqualenoids with Ser-Thr Protein Phosphatase 2A Inhibition Activity. *Mar. Drugs* **2018**, *16*, 131. [CrossRef] [PubMed]
73. Cen-Pacheco, F.; Santiago-Benítez, A.J.; Tsui, K.Y.; Tantillo, D.J.; Fernández, J.J.; Daranas, A.H. Structure and Computational Basis for Backbone Rearrangement in Marine Oxasqualenoids. *J. Org. Chem.* **2021**, *86*, 2437–2446. [CrossRef]
74. Norte, M.; Fernández, J.; Souto, M.L.; Gavín, J.; García-Grávalos, M.D. Thyrsenols A and B, two unusual polyether squalene derivatives. *Tetrahedron* **1997**, *53*, 3173–3178. [CrossRef]
75. Fernández, J.; Souto, M.L.; Norte, M. Evaluation of the cytotoxic activity of polyethers isolated from Laurencia. *Biorg. Med. Chem.* **1998**, *6*, 2237–2243. [CrossRef]
76. Souto, M.A.L.; Manríquez, C.P.; Norte, M.; Leira, F.; Fernández, J.J. The inhibitory effects of squalene-derived triterpenes on protein phosphatase PP2A. *Bioorg. Med. Chem. Lett.* **2003**, *13*, 1261–1264. [CrossRef]
77. Cen-Pacheco, F.; Villa-Pulgarin, J.A.; Mollinedo, F.; Norte, M.; Daranas, A.H.; Fernández, J.J. Cytotoxic oxasqualenoids from the red alga Laurencia viridis. *Eur. J. Med. Chem.* **2011**, *46*, 3302–3308. [CrossRef] [PubMed]
78. Cen-Pacheco, F.; Mollinedo, F.; Villa-Pulgarín, J.A.; Norte, M.; Fernández, J.J.; Hernández Daranas, A. Saiyacenols A and B: The key to solve the controversy about the configuration of aplysiols. *Tetrahedron* **2012**, *68*, 7275–7279. [CrossRef]
79. Cen-Pacheco, F.; Santiago-Benítez, A.J.; García, C.; Álvarez-Méndez, S.J.; Martín-Rodríguez, A.J.; Norte, M.; Martín, V.S.; Gavín, J.A.; Fernández, J.J.; Daranas, A.H. Oxasqualenoids from Laurencia viridis: Combined Spectroscopic–Computational Analysis and Antifouling Potential. *J. Nat. Prod.* **2015**, *78*, 712–721. [CrossRef] [PubMed]
80. Díaz-Marrero, A.R.; López-Arencibia, A.; Bethencout-Estrella, C.J.; Cen-Pacheco, F.; Sifaoui, I.; Hernández Creus, A.; Duque-Ramírez, M.C.; Souto, M.L.; Hernández Daranas, A.; Lorenzo-Morales, J.; et al. Antiprotozoal activities of marine polyether triterpenoids. *Bioorg. Chem.* **2019**, *92*, 103276. [CrossRef] [PubMed]
81. Nishikibe, K.; Nishikawa, K.; Kumagai, M.; Doe, M.; Morimoto, Y. Asymmetric Total Syntheses, Stereostructures, and Cytotoxicities of Marine Bromotriterpenoids Aplysiol B (Laurenmariannol) and Saiyacenol A. *Chem. Asian J.* **2022**, *17*, e202101137. [CrossRef] [PubMed]
82. Suzuki, T.; Suzuki, M.; Furusaki, A.; Matsumoto, T.; Kato, A.; Imanaka, Y.; Kurosawa, E. Teurilene and thyrsiferyl 23-acetate, meso and remarkably cytotoxic compounds from the marine red alga laurencia obtusa (hudson) lamouroux. *Tetrahedron Lett.* **1985**, *26*, 1329–1332. [CrossRef]
83. Sheikh, N.S. Synthetic endeavours towards oxasqualenoid natural products containing 2,5-disubstituted tetrahydrofurans–eurylene and teurilene. *Nat. Prod. Rep.* **2014**, *31*, 1088–1100. [CrossRef] [PubMed]
84. Blunt, J.W.; Hartshorn, M.P.; McLennan, T.J.; Munro, M.H.G.; Robinson, W.T.; Yorke, S.C. Thyrsiferol: A squalene-derived metabolite of laurencia thyrsifera. *Tetrahedron Lett.* **1978**, *19*, 69–72. [CrossRef]
85. Sakemi, S.; Higa, T.; Jefford, C.W.; Bernardinelli, G. Venustatriol. A new, anti-viral, triterpene tetracyclic ether from Laurencia venusta. *Tetrahedron Lett.* **1986**, *27*, 4287–4290. [CrossRef]
86. Little, R.D.; Nishiguchi, G.A. Synthetic Efforts Toward, and Biological Activity of, Thyrsiferol and Structurally-Related Analogues. In *Studies in Natural Products Chemistry*; Attaur, R., Ed.; Elsevier: Amsterdam, The Netherlands, 2008; Volume 35, pp. 3–56.
87. Lorenzo-Morales, J.; Díaz-Marrero, A.R.; Cen-Pacheco, F.; Sifaoui, I.; Reyes-Batlle, M.; Souto, M.L.; Hernández Daranas, A.; Piñero, J.E.; Fernández, J.J. Evaluation of Oxasqualenoids from the Red Alga Laurencia viridis against Acanthamoeba. *Mar. Drugs* **2019**, *17*, 420. [CrossRef] [PubMed]

88. Hirashima, M.; Tsuda, K.; Hamada, T.; Okamura, H.; Furukawa, T.; Akiyama, S.-i.; Tajitsu, Y.; Ikeda, R.; Komatsu, M.; Doe, M.; et al. Cytotoxic Isomalabaricane Derivatives and a Monocyclic Triterpene Glycoside from the Sponge Rhabdastrella globostellata. *J. Nat. Prod.* **2010**, *73*, 1512–1518. [CrossRef] [PubMed]
89. Lai, K.-H.; Huang, Z.-H.; El-Shazly, M.; Peng, B.-R.; Wei, W.-C.; Su, J.-H. Isomalabaricane Triterpenes from the Marine Sponge *Rhabdastrella* sp. *Mar. Drugs* **2021**, *19*, 206. [CrossRef]
90. Desoubzdanne, D.; Marcourt, L.; Raux, R.; Chevalley, S.; Dorin, D.; Doerig, C.; Valentin, A.; Ausseil, F.; Debitus, C. Alisiaquinones and alisiaquinol, dual inhibitors of Plasmodium falciparum enzyme targets from a New Caledonian deep water sponge. *J. Nat. Prod.* **2008**, *71*, 1189–1192. [CrossRef]
91. Shi, Z.-Z.; Miao, F.-P.; Fang, S.-T.; Liu, X.-H.; Yin, X.-L.; Ji, N.-Y. Sesteralterin and Tricycloalterfurenes A-D: Terpenes with Rarely Occurring Frameworks from the Marine-Alga-Epiphytic Fungus Alternaria alternata k21-1. *J. Nat. Prod.* **2017**, *80*, 2524–2529. [CrossRef] [PubMed]
92. Hwang, J.-Y.; Park, S.C.; Byun, W.S.; Oh, D.-C.; Lee, S.K.; Oh, K.-B.; Shin, J. Bioactive Bianthraquinones and Meroterpenoids from a Marine-Derived Stemphylium sp. Fungus. *Mar. Drugs* **2020**, *18*, 436. [CrossRef]
93. Fraga, B.M.; Díaz, C.E. Proposal for structural revision of several monosubstituted tricycloalternarenes. *Phytochemistry* **2022**, *198*, 113141. [CrossRef] [PubMed]
94. Duan, X.; Tan, X.; Gu, L.; Liu, J.; Hao, X.; Tao, L.; Feng, H.; Cao, Y.; Shi, Z.; Duan, Y.; et al. New secondary metabolites with immunosuppressive activity from the phytopathogenic fungus Bipolaris maydis. *Bioorg. Chem.* **2020**, *99*, 103816. [CrossRef] [PubMed]
95. Shi, X.; Wei, W.; Zhang, W.-J.; Hua, C.-P.; Chen, C.-J.; Ge, H.-M.; Tan, R.-X.; Jiao, R.-H. New tricycloalternarenes from fungus *Alternaria* sp. *J. Asian Nat. Prod. Res.* **2015**, *17*, 143–148. [CrossRef] [PubMed]
96. Kim, M.C.; Winter, J.M.; Asolkar, R.N.; Boonlarppradab, C.; Cullum, R.; Fenical, W. Marinoterpins A–C: Rare Linear Merosesterterpenoids from Marine-Derived Actinomycete Bacteria of the Family Streptomycetaceae. *J. Org. Chem.* **2021**, *86*, 11140–11148. [CrossRef]
97. Kuroda, I.; Musman, M.; Ohtani, I.I.; Ichiba, T.; Tanaka, J.; Gravalos, D.G.; Higa, T. Pachastrissamine, a Cytotoxic Anhydrophytosphingosine from a Marine Sponge, *Pachastrissa* sp. *J. Nat. Prod.* **2002**, *65*, 1505–1506. [CrossRef] [PubMed]
98. Ledroit, V.; Debitus, C.; Lavaud, C.; Massiot, G. Jaspines A and B: Two new cytotoxic sphingosine derivatives from the marine sponge *Jaspis* sp. *Tetrahedron Lett.* **2003**, *44*, 225–228. [CrossRef]
99. Martinková, J.; Gonda, J. Marine cytotoxic jaspine B and its stereoisomers: Biological activity and syntheses. *Carbohydr. Res.* **2016**, *423*, 1–42. [CrossRef]
100. Lu, X.; He, J.; Wu, Y.; Du, N.; Li, X.; Ju, J.; Hu, Z.; Umezawa, K.; Wang, L. Isolation and Characterization of New Anti-Inflammatory and Antioxidant Components from Deep Marine-Derived Fungus Myrothecium sp. Bzo-l062. *Mar. Drugs* **2020**, *18*, 597. [CrossRef]
101. Chokpaiboon, S.; Unagul, P.; Kongthong, S.; Danwisetkanjana, K.; Pilantanapak, A.; Suetrong, S.; Bunyapaiboonsri, T. A pyrone, naphthoquinone, and cyclic urea from the marine-derived fungus Astrosphaeriella nypae BCC 5335. *Tetrahedron Lett.* **2016**, *57*, 1171–1173. [CrossRef]
102. Shi, H.; Yu, S.; Liu, D.; Van Ofwegen, L.; Proksch, P.; Lin, W. Sinularones A–I, New Cyclopentenone and Butenolide Derivatives from a Marine Soft Coral *Sinularia* sp. and Their Antifouling Activity. *Mar. Drugs* **2012**, *10*, 1331. [CrossRef] [PubMed]
103. Peil, S.; Bistoni, G.; Goddard, R.; Fürstner, A. Hydrogenative Metathesis of Enynes via Piano-Stool Ruthenium Carbene Complexes Formed by Alkyne gem-Hydrogenation. *J. Am. Chem. Soc.* **2020**, *142*, 18541–18553. [CrossRef] [PubMed]
104. Malmstrøm, J.; Christophersen, C.; Barrero, A.F.; Oltra, J.E.; Justicia, J.; Rosales, A. Bioactive Metabolites from a Marine-Derived Strain of the Fungus Emericella variecolor. *J. Nat. Prod.* **2002**, *65*, 364–367. [CrossRef] [PubMed]
105. Clemens, R.T.; Jennings, M.P. An efficient total synthesis and absolute configuration determination of varitriol. *Chem. Commun.* **2006**, *25*, 2720–2721. [CrossRef]
106. Mahesh, S.M.; Supriya, T.; Prakash, T.P. Recent Developments Towards the Synthesis of Varitriol: An Antitumour Agent from Marine Derived Fungus Emericella Variecolor. *Curr. Org. Synth.* **2014**, *11*, 268–287. [CrossRef]
107. McAllister, G.D.; Robinson, J.E.; Taylor, R.J.K. The synthesis of (−)-varitriol and (−)-3′-epi-varitriol via a Ramberg–Bäcklund route. *Tetrahedron* **2007**, *63*, 12123–12130. [CrossRef]
108. Vamshikrishna, K.; Srihari, P. A conventional approach to the total synthesis of (−)-varitriol. *Tetrahedron: Asymmetry* **2012**, *23*, 1584–1587. [CrossRef]
109. Vamshikrishna, K.; Srihari, P. Total synthesis of (+)-varitriol and (+)-6′-epi-varitriol. *Tetrahedron* **2012**, *68*, 1540–1546. [CrossRef]
110. Sun, T.; Deutsch, C.; Krause, N. Combined coinage metal catalysis in natural product synthesis: Total synthesis of (+)-varitriol and seven analogs. *Org. Biomol. Chem.* **2012**, *10*, 5965–5970. [CrossRef]
111. Sánchez-Eleuterio, A.; García-Santos, W.H.; Díaz-Salazar, H.; Hernández-Rodríguez, M.; Cordero-Vargas, A. Stereocontrolled Nucleophilic Addition to Five-Membered Oxocarbenium Ions Directed by the Protecting Groups. Application to the Total Synthesis of (+)-Varitriol and of Two Diastereoisomers Thereof. *J. Org. Chem.* **2017**, *82*, 8464–8475. [CrossRef] [PubMed]
112. He, H.; Qin, H.-B. ZnBr2-catalyzed direct C-glycosylation of glycosyl acetates with terminal alkynes. *Org. Chem. Front.* **2018**, *5*, 1962–1966. [CrossRef]
113. Zhang, F.-H.; Guo, X.; Zeng, X.; Wang, Z. Catalytic Enantioconvergent Allenylation of Aldehydes with Propargyl Halides. *Angew. Chem. Int. Ed.* **2022**, *61*, e202117114. [CrossRef]

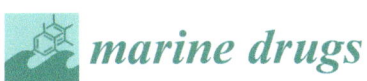

Review

The Tetrahydrofuran Motif in Polyketide Marine Drugs

Laura Fernández-Peña, Carlos Díez-Poza, Paula González-Andrés and Asunción Barbero *

Department of Organic Chemistry, Campus Miguel Delibes, University of Valladolid, 47011 Valladolid, Spain; laura.fernandez.pena@uva.es (L.F.-P.); carlos.diez@uva.es (C.D.-P.); paula.gonzalez.andres@alumnos.uva.es (P.G.-A.)
* Correspondence: asuncion.barbero@uva.es

Abstract: Oxygen heterocycles are units that are abundant in a great number of marine natural products. Among them, marine polyketides containing tetrahydrofuran rings have attracted great attention within the scientific community due to their challenging structures and promising biological activities. An overview of the most important marine tetrahydrofuran polyketides, with a focused discussion on their isolation, structure determination, approaches to their total synthesis, and biological studies is provided.

Keywords: marine natural products; oxygen heterocycles; tetrahydrofuran; total synthesis; biological activity

1. Introduction

The ocean is the biggest ecosystem of our planet. Plenty of organisms live in the ocean, and new species are discovered every year. As well, being the oldest ecosystem, marine organisms have evolved for a longer time than terrestrial living beings, and thus have different and sometimes better mechanisms of defense. These are represented by specific compounds, like toxins found in fish and algae and other bioactive substances found in sponges or tunicates. Usually, the real producers of these compounds are microorganisms such as bacteria, cyanobacteria, or dinoflagellates. The interesting properties of some of these metabolites have attracted the attention of the scientific community. As they are usually scarce and difficult to obtain in large amounts, total synthesis has emerged in the last decades as a necessary tool to tackle this problem. It has helped to clarify the structure of some intriguing compounds, and to obtain higher amounts of them in order to perform proper biological studies. Total synthesis is still a crucial tool, as even with today's advanced NMR techniques, misassignment of the structure of biologically relevant macrolides is a common issue [1].

Polyketides are a diverse class of metabolites, comprising linear as well as macrolide compounds with a range of biological activities. Some of them have promising potential as drug candidates [2]. Common sources of this class of compounds are dinoflagellates of the genus *Amphidinium* [3]. To understand how to access the macrolide core present in these and other structures within natural products, we encourage the reader to review general macrolactonization methods [4].

On the other hand, oxygenated heterocycles are common motifs in marine bioactive compounds, and therefore the development of methods for their synthesis also requires attention. The most common are six-membered oxacycles, tetrahydropyrans, and thus numerous works focus on their synthesis [5,6]. Oxepanes and tetrahydrofurans also appear in a very large number of marine natural products with interesting properties. Oxepane-containing marine compounds were recently reviewed by our group [7]. Total syntheses of marine and non-marine products containing 2,3,5-trisubstituted tetrahydrofurans (such as kumausallene or petromyroxol) have been recently reviewed by Fernandes [8,9].

Continuing our interest for marine heterocyclic compounds, here we provide an overview, from 2013 to October 2021, of tetrahydrofuran-containing marine polyketides.

Citation: Fernández-Peña, L.; Díez-Poza, C.; González-Andrés, P.; Barbero, A. The Tetrahydrofuran Motif in Polyketide Marine Drugs. *Mar. Drugs* 2022, 20, 120. https://doi.org/10.3390/md20020120

Academic Editor: Vassilios Roussis

Received: 2 January 2022
Accepted: 1 February 2022
Published: 3 February 2022

Publisher's Note: MDPI stays neutral with regard to jurisdictional claims in published maps and institutional affiliations.

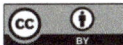

Copyright: © 2022 by the authors. Licensee MDPI, Basel, Switzerland. This article is an open access article distributed under the terms and conditions of the Creative Commons Attribution (CC BY) license (https://creativecommons.org/licenses/by/4.0/).

The compilation of literature on THF-containing macrolides up to 2012 was covered in an excellent review [10]. Macrolides is such a fertile field that some particular families of compounds have already been reviewed, such as haterumalides and biselides [11], or more recently, mandelalides [12]. In recent years, numerous synthetic approaches to the polyketide family continue to emerge, and here we offer an overview of them.

2. Polyketide Marine Drugs Containing Tetrahydrofuran Rings

2.1. Macrolides

Marine invertebrates, such as sponges, algae or dinoflagellate, are a source of a large number of secondary metabolites with relevant biological activities. Within them marine polyketide macrolides have attracted high attention, due to their biological properties and pharmacological potential. Consequently, the development of new synthetic approaches to study their properties has been the goal of many researchers [10,13].

2.1.1. Amphidinolides

Amphidinolides belong to the macrolide family and more than forty members have been isolated from marine dinoflagellates of the genus *Amphidinium* sp. In the last thirty years. Within these structurally rich compounds, only a few contain tetrahydrofuran units embedded in the macrolactone ring. The studies published in the literature about tetrahydrofuran-containing amphidinolides up to 2013 have been already reviewed by Álvarez and coworkers [10].

Amphidinolides C and F

Amphidinolides C (**1**), C2 (**2**), C3 (**3**), and F (**4**) are structurally similar (Figure 1), bearing a complex 25-membered macrolide core, which contains 11 chiral carbons and a functionalized side chain. The nature of this chain drastically affects biological activity. Amphidinolide C, which possesses an (*S*)-hydroxyl group, is active against murine lymphoma L1210 (IC50 = 5.8 ng/mL) and human epidermoid carcinoma KB cell lines (IC50 = 4.6 ng/mL). Strikingly, compounds **2-4** are three orders of magnitude less toxic to the same cell lines.

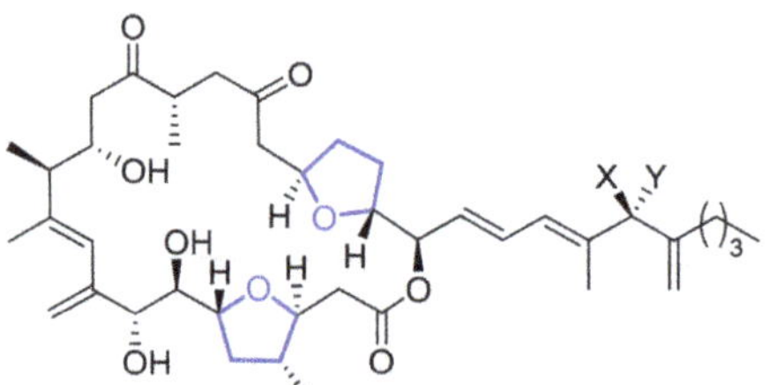

1 Amphidinolide C, X = OH, Y = H
2 Amphidinolide C2, X = OAc, Y = H
3 Amphidinolide C3, X = Y = O

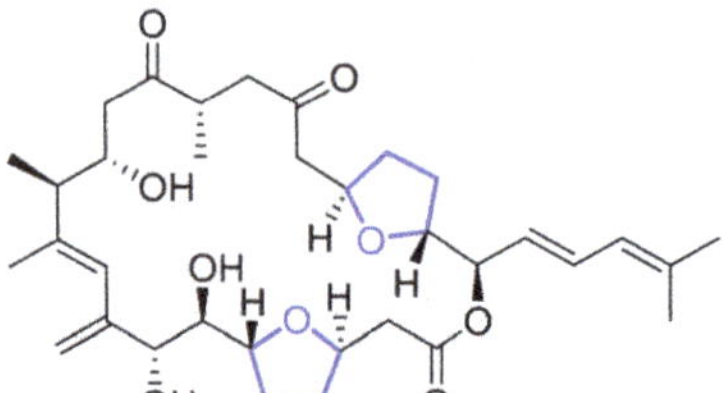

4 Amphidinolide F

Figure 1. Structure of amphidinolides C, C2, C3, and F.

In 2016, a new amphidinolide C4 (**5**) was isolated from octocoral *Stragulum bicolor* (Figure 2). Toxicity was tested against the colon adenocarcinoma cell line HCT-116, finding an IC50 of 10.3 µM. Compound **5** is therefore surprisingly inactive, although it contains a hydroxyl group in the side chain [14].

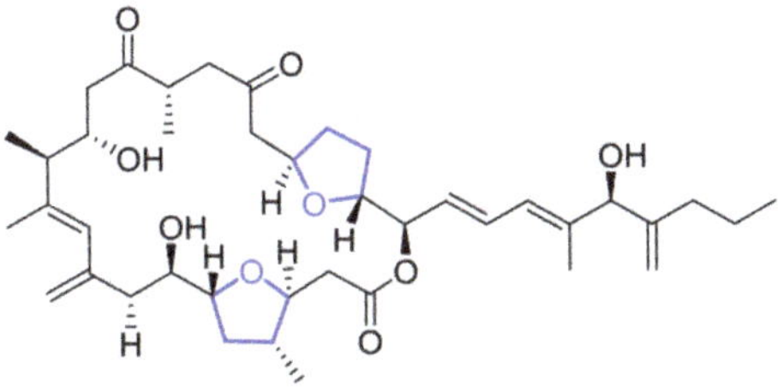

5 Amphidinolide C4

Figure 2. Structure of amphidinolide C4.

The interesting biological properties of these compounds have attracted the attention of different authors who have described either total syntheses [15,16] or synthetic approaches to various molecular fragments [17–19]. For instance, Fürstner and coworkers took advantage of the structural similarity of **1** and **4** to perform an elegant total synthesis of both compounds [15]. In these syntheses, the formation of the trisubstituted tetrahydrofuran unit was performed using a TBAF-mediated oxa-Michael addition, which selectively led to the desired 1,4-*trans* tetrahydrofuran ring **7**. Parallelly, a chemoselective cobalt-catalyzed cyclization of an appropriate bishomoallylic alcohol **8** provided the required *trans*-disubstituted tetrahydrofuran **9** (Scheme 1).

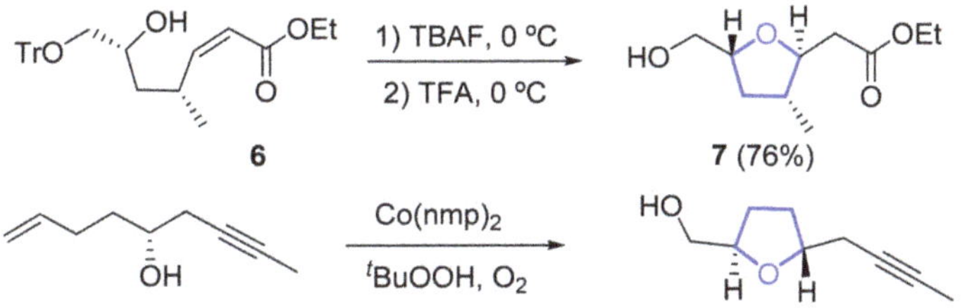

Scheme 1. Synthesis of the THF moiety in amphidinolides C and F by Fürstner.

Amphidinolide E

Amphidinolide E (**10**) presents a 19-membered macrolactone ring, bearing a tetrahydrofuran moiety and eight stereocenters (Figure 3).

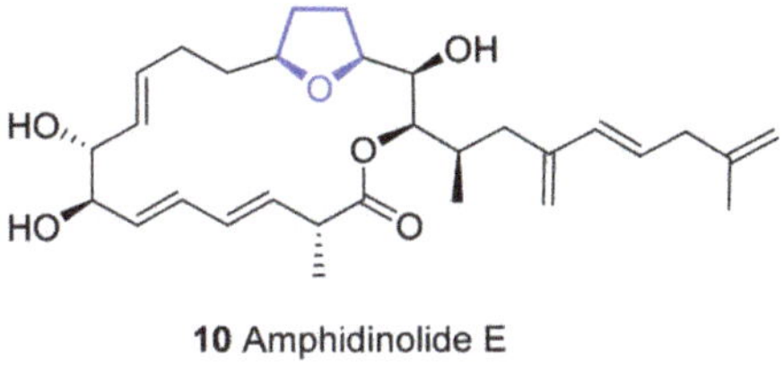

10 Amphidinolide E

Figure 3. Structure of amphidinolide E.

Total syntheses of **10** have already been developed by Lee [20,21] and Roush [22–24]. Recently, Vilarrasa and Costa presented a different approach to its total synthesis. Though no significant improvement was made in terms of yield or number of steps, this work provides interesting insights into Julia-Kocienski olefinations [25]. Thus, epoxidation of alcohol **11** directly afforded tetrahydrofuran **12**, through a tandem epoxidation-cyclization reaction. Subsequent Swern oxidation, followed by Julia-Kocienski reaction with sulfone **13**, provided the northern C10–C21 fragment of amphidinolide E (Scheme 2).

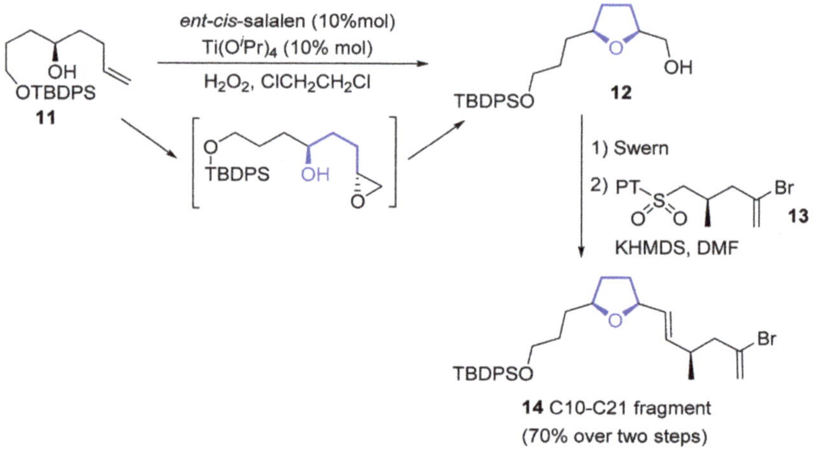

Scheme 2. Synthesis of C10-C21 fragment of amphidinolide E.

Amphidinolide K

Amphidinolide K (**15**) (Figure 4) has also a 19-membered macrolactone, but with a simpler side chain. Regarding its biological properties, amphidinolide K has shown a strong stabilizing effect on actin filaments (F-actin).

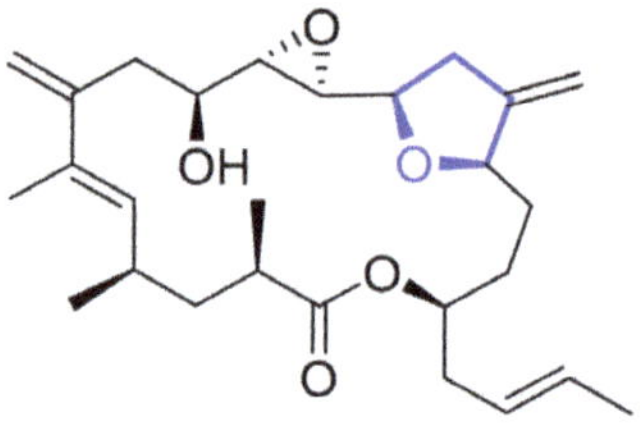

Figure 4. Structure of amphidinolide K.

Vilarrasa proposed a total synthesis of **15** relying on a Hosomi-Sakurai reaction as a key step [26]. The tetrahydrofuran ring **17** was formed by cyclization of alcohol **16**, followed by elimination of the pyridylselenenyl group with Dess-Martin oxidation. Further deprotection of the O-PMB group and extension of the chain, through Swern oxidation and Wittig reaction, led to the C9–C22 fragment **18** (Scheme 3). Subsequent Hosomi-Sakurai reaction with allylsilane **19**, using Yamamoto's chiral (acyloxy)borane (CAB), provided **20** with a good yield.

Amphidinolide N/caribenolide I

Amphidinolide N (**21**) is a 25-membered macrolide which contains a 2,5-*trans*-disubstituted tetrahydrofuran, an allylic epoxide, and 13 stereocenters (Figure 5). Amphidinolide N is the most potent cytotoxic member of this family against murine lymphoma L1210 (IC50 = 0.05 ng/mL) and human epidermoid carcinoma KB cell lines (IC50 = 0.06 ng/mL). However, despite the efforts of different researchers, no total synthesis of this compound has been reported so far. There are different approaches focused on the synthesis of the fragment which contains the tetrahydrofuran ring [27–30], a total synthesis of 7,10-epimer [31,32], and a recently described enantioselective synthesis of des-epoxy-amphidinolide N, which failed in the last epoxidation step towards amphidinolide N [33].

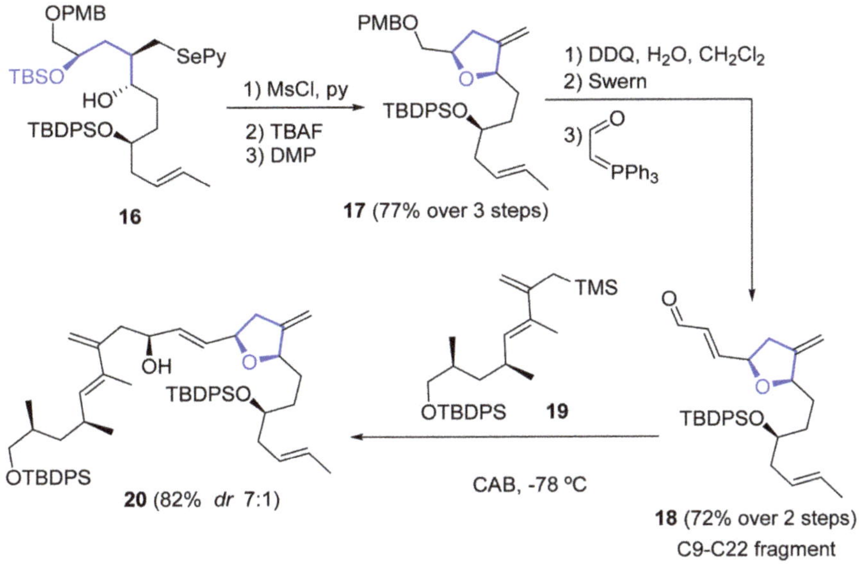

Scheme 3. Synthesis of C9–C22 fragment of amphidinolide K.

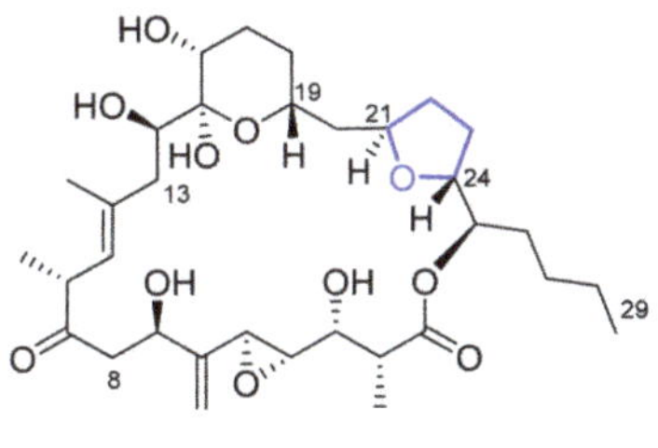

21 Amphidinolide N

Figure 5. Structure of amphidinolide N.

Both Sasaki's [27] and Kuwahara's [29] strategies to build the tetrahydrofuran moiety consisted of an intramolecular cyclization of a diol mesylate obtained by Sharpless asymmetric dihydroxylation (SAD) of mesyl protected alkenol **22** using AD-mix-β. Subsequent cyclization, mediated by base, afforded the desired 2,5-*trans*-disubstituted tetrahydrofuran **23** (Scheme 4).

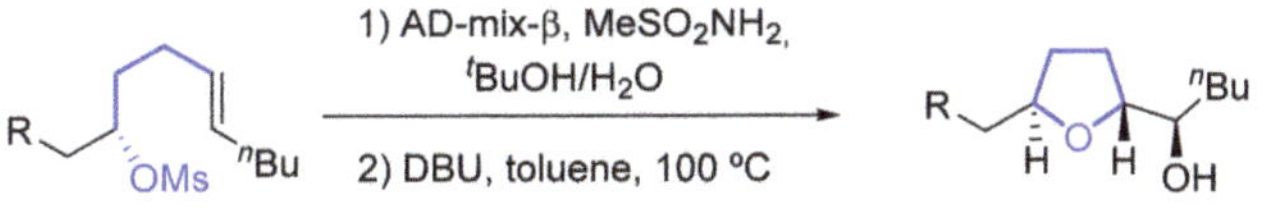

Scheme 4. Synthesis of THF of amphidinolide N by Sasaki and Kuwahara.

Recently, Fuwa proposed the application of cobalt-catalyzed Hartung-Mukaiyama cyclization of γ-hydroxy olefins to obtain the tetrahydrofuran fragment [30]. Mukaiyama cyclization is known to afford 2,5-*trans* substituted tetrahydrofurans with a 2-hydroxy substituent. Hartung's modification allows the access to 2-alkyl-substituted tetrahydrofurans, ideal for the synthesis of tetrahydrofuran-containing fragment **25** of amphidinolide N from alkenol **24** (Scheme 5). It is remarkable that unprotected hydroxy groups and somewhat bulky substituents are well-tolerated.

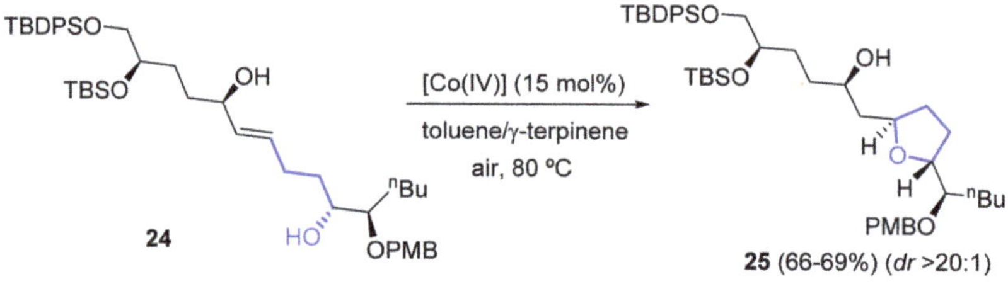

Scheme 5. Synthesis of THF fragment of amphidinolide N by Fuwa.

With close structural similarity, other macrolides have been discovered recently, namely isocaribenolide-I (**26**) and chlorohydrin (**27**) [34]. They were isolated from a free-swimming dinoflagellate Amphidinium species (KCA09053 and KCA09056 strains), together with amphidinolide N. Both have a 26-membered macrolide core, and present high cytotoxicity against human cervix adenocarcinoma HeLa cells (IC50 = 0.02 for isocaribenolide-I and 0.06 nM for chlorohydrin). Isocaribenolide-I presents a characteristic isobutyl side chain, and chlorohydrin is distinguished by a homonymous moiety (Figure 6).

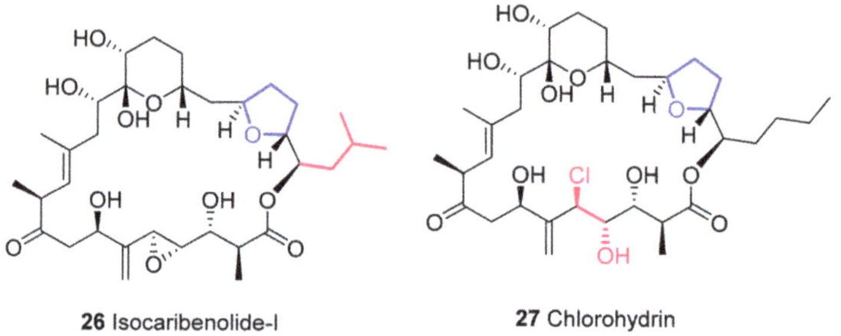

Figure 6. Structure of isocaribenolide I and chlorohydrin.

Amphidinolides T

Amphidinolides T (**28–32**), 19-membered lactones containing a trisubstituted tetrahydrofuran ring and seven or eight stereocenters (Figure 7), were first isolated by Kobayashi [35–37]. They showed cytotoxic activity against murine leukemia L1210 cells in vitro with an IC50 value of 18 µg/mL.

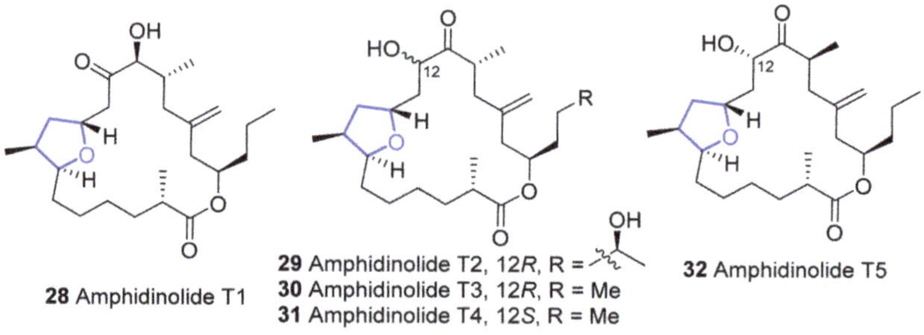

28 Amphidinolide T1
29 Amphidinolide T2, 12R, R =
30 Amphidinolide T3, 12R, R = Me
31 Amphidinolide T4, 12S, R = Me
32 Amphidinolide T5

Figure 7. Structure of amphidinolides T.

In 2013, Clark reported a total synthesis of T1, T2, and T4 from a common intermediate **33** (Scheme 6) [38]. Synthesis of the tetrahydrofuran-containing fragment **35** started from the allyl ether **36** of a commercially available alcohol, which was transformed into the α-diazo ketone **37** by sequential saponification, formation of the corresponding mixed anhydride derivative and reaction with diazomethane. Treatment of **37** with a catalytic amount of (Cu(acac)$_2$) stereoselectively afforded the *trans* dihydrofuranone **38** in high yield. Six further steps led to the desired THF-containing fragment (Scheme 7). The total syntheses of amphidinolide T1, T3, and T4 were completed in 17 steps from a common precursor with 6.9%, 5.9%, and 5.5% overall yield, respectively.

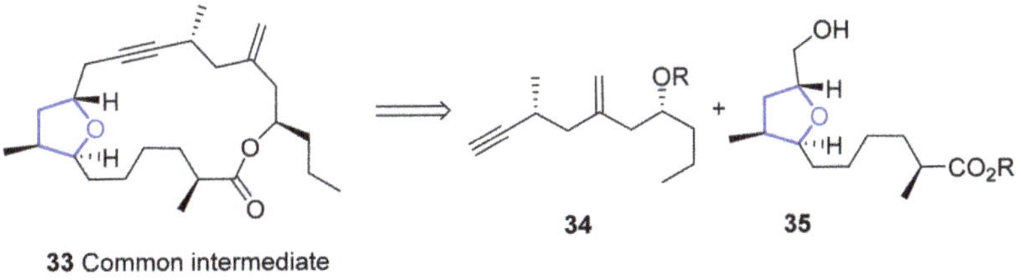

Scheme 6. Retrosynthesis of amphidinolides T from a common intermediate.

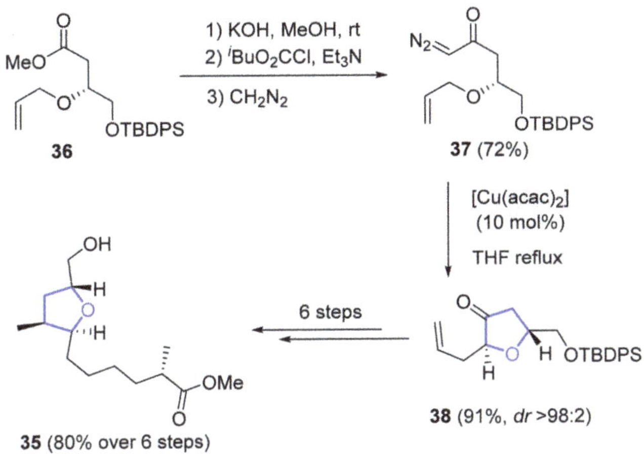

Scheme 7. Synthesis of THF fragment of amphidinolides T.

2.1.2. Haterumalides and Biselides

Haterumalides (**39–44**) (Figure 8) were isolated at the end of the 20th century from the Okinawan ascidian *Lissoclinum* sp. (haterumalide B) [39] and the Okinawan sponge *Iricinia* sp. (haterumalides NA-NE) [40]. Their cytotoxic activity against different targets made them secondary metabolites of great interest. However, no approaches towards their synthesis have been described in recent years [10,11].

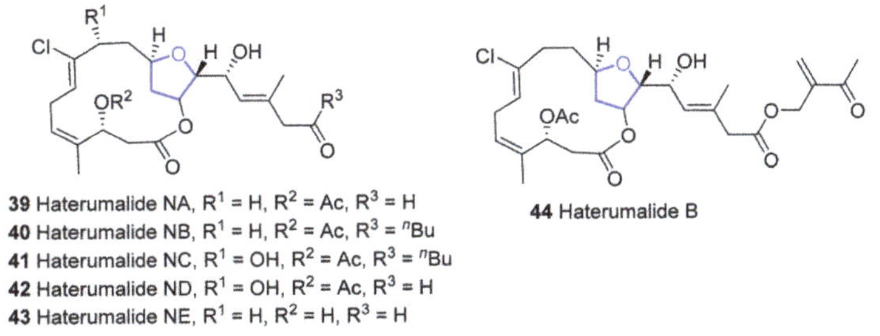

39 Haterumalide NA, R^1 = H, R^2 = Ac, R^3 = H
40 Haterumalide NB, R^1 = H, R^2 = Ac, R^3 = ^{n}Bu
41 Haterumalide NC, R^1 = OH, R^2 = Ac, R^3 = ^{n}Bu
42 Haterumalide ND, R^1 = OH, R^2 = Ac, R^3 = H
43 Haterumalide NE, R^1 = H, R^2 = H, R^3 = H

44 Haterumalide B

Figure 8. Structure of haterumalides.

Biselides (**45–49**) (Figure 9), C-20 oxygenated analogues of haterumalides, are a family of polyketides which were isolated from the Okinawan ascidian *Didemnidae* sp. [41]. Their structure was determined by spectroscopic analysis and their biological activity was tested against tumor cell lines, due to their similarity to haterumalides. Cytotoxic activity of biselides A and C against various human cancer cells are comparable to cisplatin, the known anticancer drug. Notably, and unlike their haterumalide congeners, biselides A and C did not show toxicity against brine shrimp even at 50 µg mL^{-1}, which makes them potential anticancer drug candidates.

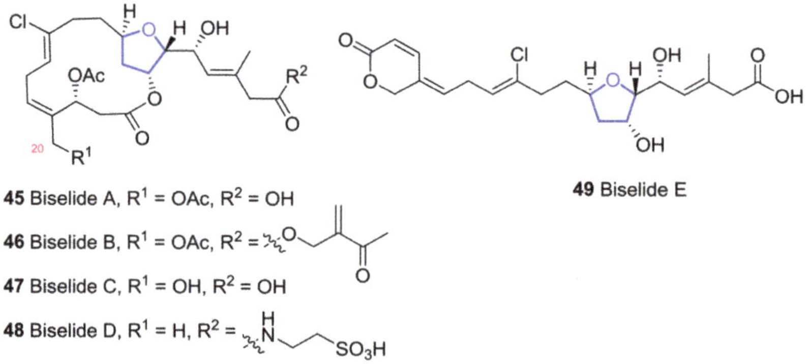

45 Biselide A, R^1 = OAc, R^2 = OH
46 Biselide B, R^1 = OAc, R^2 =
47 Biselide C, R^1 = OH, R^2 = OH
48 Biselide D, R^1 = H, R^2 =
49 Biselide E

Figure 9. Structure of biselides.

In the last years, two total syntheses of biselide A have been published [42,43]. Kigoshi developed synthetic approaches towards both the core carbon fragment [44] and the macrolactone moiety [45]. Relying on these methodologies, Kigoshi and Hayakawa finally accomplished the total synthesis of biselide A [42]. The key step for the construction of the 3-hydroxy tetrahydrofuran unit was accomplished by intramolecular oxy-Michael cyclization of intermediate **50**, which was obtained in four steps from D-mannose. Further 27 steps were required to obtain natural biselide A (Scheme 8).

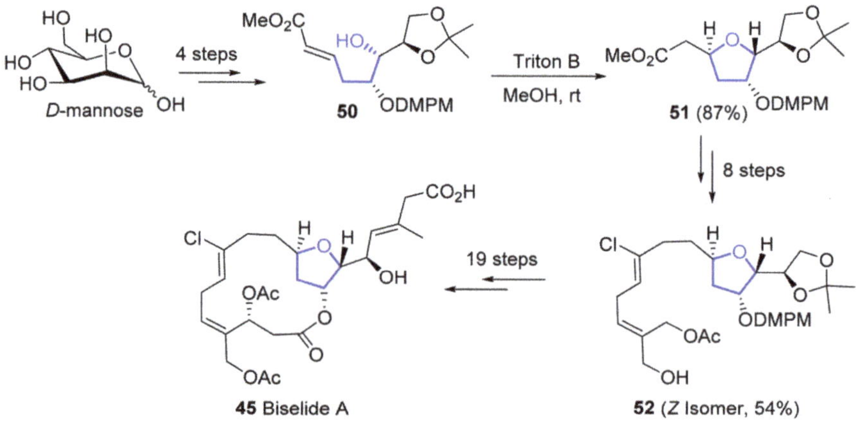

Scheme 8. Synthesis of biselide A by Kigoshi, Hayakawa, and co-workers.

Likewise, Kigoshi has also described the total synthesis of biselide E, from common advanced intermediate **52** [46].

On the other hand, Britton and coworkers have proposed a concise synthesis of biselide A in 20 linear steps from L-serine [43]. In this case the stereoselective formation of the tetrahydrofuran moiety **55** was done by microwave cyclization of chlorodiol intermediate **54** (Scheme 9).

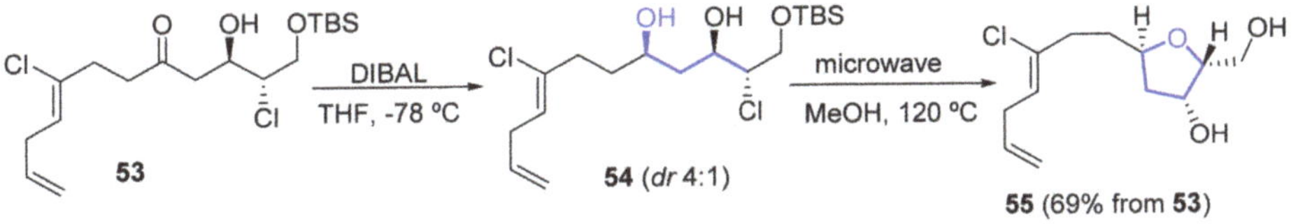

Scheme 9. Synthesis of THF moiety of biselide A in Britton's total synthesis.

The key to building the macrocyclic ring was the use of an intramolecular Reformatsky cyclization from intermediate **56**, which led to a 3.5:1 ratio of epimers of the desired macrolactone. A sequence of oxidation/reduction was used to convert **57** in the desired epimer **58**. Further five steps, including deprotection and installation of the side chain, provided biselide A with ca. 2% overall yield in 20 steps from L-serine (Scheme 10).

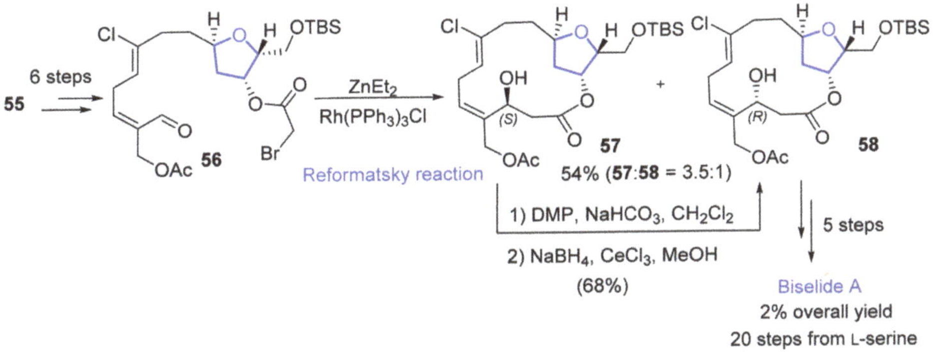

Scheme 10. Reformatsky macrocyclization to biselide A by Britton and coworkers.

2.1.3. Chagosensine

Chagosensine (**59**) (Figure 10), a chloro-substituted macrolide, was isolated from the calcareous sponge *Leucetta chagosensis*. Its structure, consisting of a sixteen-membered macrolide, two 2,5-*trans*-disubstituted tetrahydrofuran rings embedded within, a unique Z,Z-configured chloro-1,3-diene unit, and eleven chiral centers, was assigned by spectroscopic techniques and degradation experiments [47]. Chagosensine structure is similar to the haterumalide and biselide families, but the conjugated chlorodiene unit is only present in this natural product. Nevertheless, Fürstner and co-workers have shown disagreement with the proposed structure and have carried out different synthetic studies in order to demonstrate their arguments [48,49].

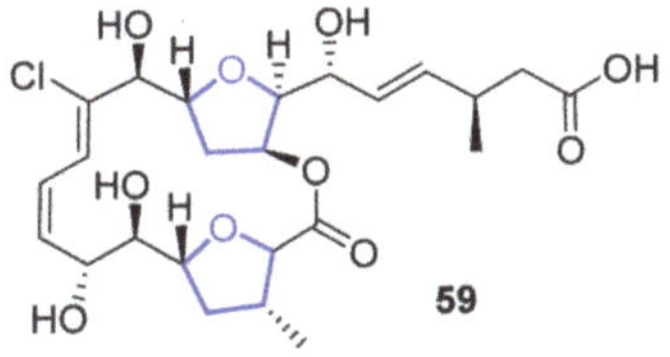

Figure 10. Initially proposed structure of chagosensine.

The synthesis of putative chagosensine proposed by Fürstner relied on Mukaiyama cyclizations using Co(II) catalyst to obtain 2,5-*trans*-tetrahydrofuran derivatives **60** and **61** from the appropriate alkenols **62** and **63** [48]. After further elaboration, optimized Stille coupling of 1,2-bisstannane derivative **64** and vinyl iodide **65** provided the precursor diene **66** in moderate yield. Finally, six additional steps, including a Yamaguchi lactonization, produced the desired macrocycle (Scheme 11). The product proved unstable and had to be transformed into the known methyl ester, though huge deviations in the NMR seemed to indicate that the structure was misassigned. More recently, further efforts were made to access eight different diastereomers in order to find the correct structure [49]. Unfortunately, none of the structures synthesized matched the original spectroscopic data. Thus, the structure of this intriguing marine macrolide remains unresolved.

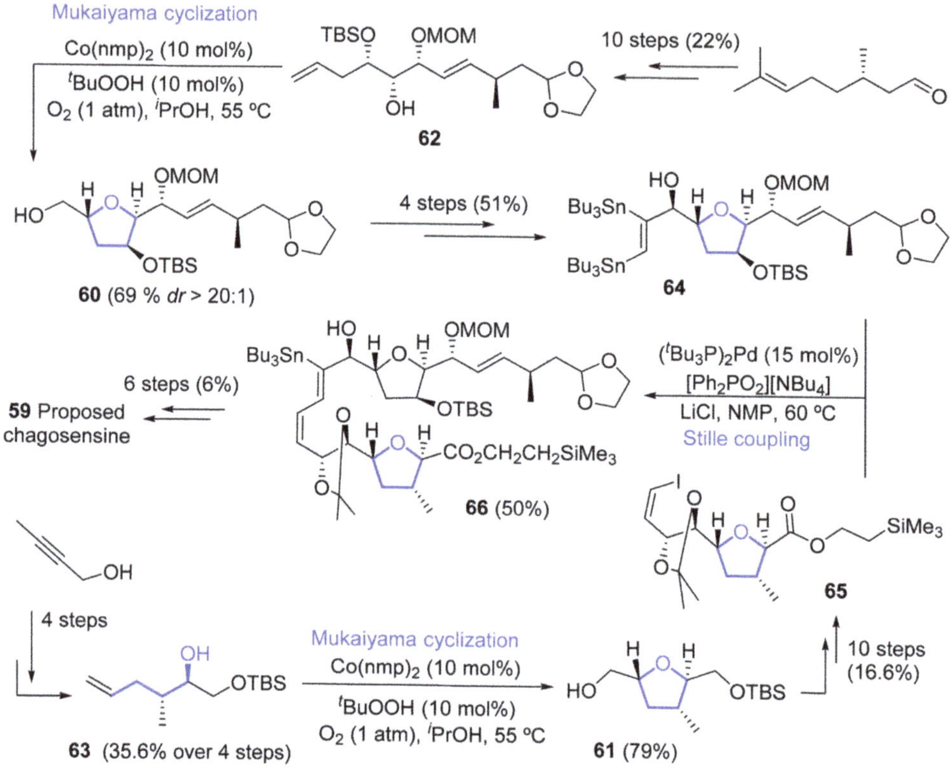

Scheme 11. Synthesis of putative chagosensine.

2.1.4. Formosalides

Formosalides A and B (Figure 11) are 17-membered macrolides isolated from marine dinoflagellate *Prorocentrum* sp. [50]. Their structures and relative stereochemistries were determined by spectroscopic techniques. Cytotoxicty of the formosalides was significantly lower than amphidinolide N or caribenolide I, despite their structural similarity. Formosalides A and B showed in vitro moderate cytotoxic activity against CCRF-CEM human T-cell acute lymphoblastic leukemia cells (LD50 [A] = 0.54 µg/mL and LD50 [B] = 0.43 µg/mL) and DLD-1 human colon adenocarcinoma cells (LD50 [A] > 40 µg/mL and LD50 [B] = 2.73 µg/mL) [50]. The structure and absolute configuration were confirmed by Fürstner and co-workers recently by total synthesis of different stereoisomers [51].

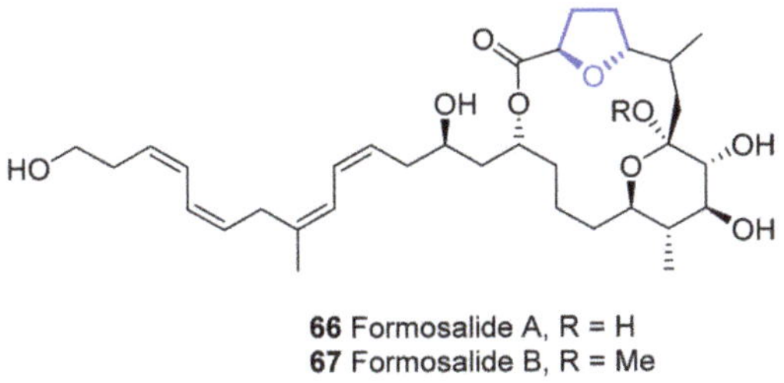

66 Formosalide A, R = H
67 Formosalide B, R = Me

Figure 11. Structure of formosalides A and B.

As said, Fürstner's group has accomplished the synthesis of both macrolides and two other isomers [51]. The required *trans*-disubstituted tetrahydrofuran ring **68** was prepared by stereoselective cobalt-catalyzed oxidative cyclization of bishomoallylic alcohol **69**, with excellent yield and selectivity (Scheme 12).

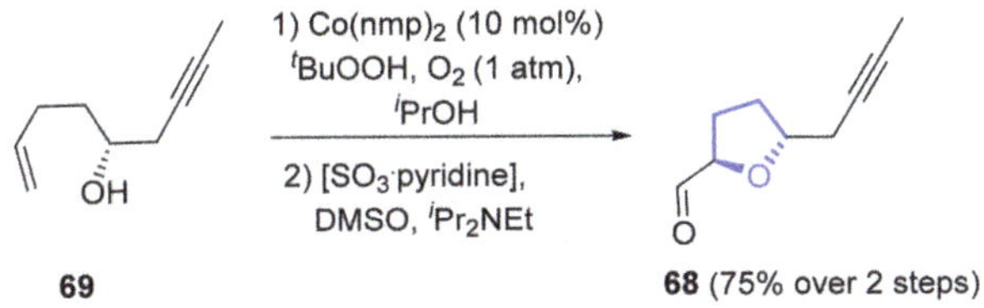

Scheme 12. Synthesis of THF in formosalides.

Following, the coupling of THF-carbaldehyde **68** with fragment **70** by an Evans–Tishchenko reaction led to intermediate **71**, which was subjected to ring closing alkyne metathesis to yield macrocycle **72** with good yield. The final installation of the side chain, achieved by Stille-Migita coupling of vinyliodide **73** with the appropriate vinylstannane derivative, and deprotection of the TBS group led to both formosalides due to unexpected partial hydrolysis of the ketal (Scheme 13).

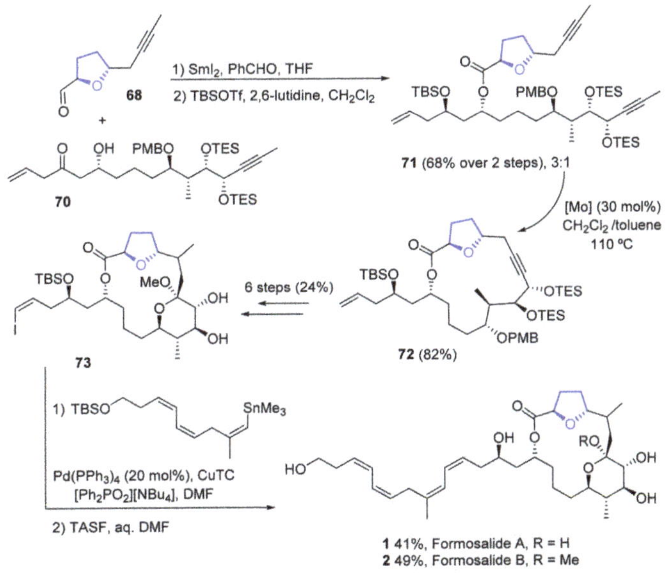

1 41%, Formosalide A, R = H
2 49%, Formosalide B, R = Me

Scheme 13. Synthesis of formosalides by Fürstner.

Mohapatra and co-workers have also reported a stereoselective synthesis of the C1-C16 fragment of formosalide B [52]. A one-pot Sharpless asymmetric dihydroxylation of α,β-unsaturated ester **74**, followed by intramolecular S$_N$2 displacement, produced the desired *trans*-tetrahydrofuran **75** with a high 88% yield and total stereoselectivity (Scheme 14).

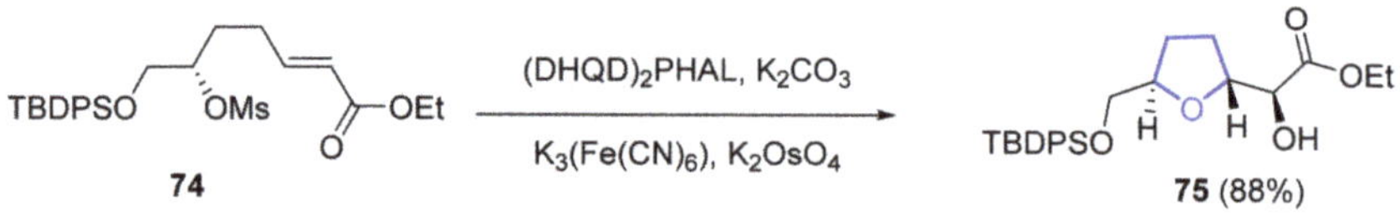

Scheme 14. Synthesis of THF-containing fragment in formosalides by Mohapatra and co-workers.

2.1.5. Halichondrins

Halichondrins (**76–84**) (Figure 12) are a family of polyether macrolides isolated in the 20th century from a marine sponge, *Halichondria okadai* Kadota [53]. According to their structure, they are classified in A–C halichondrins, norhalichondrins, and homohalichondrins (Figure 12). All have been found in natural sources except halichondrin A. Their complex structure is composed of a polyether macrolide with several fused five- and six-membered oxacycles.

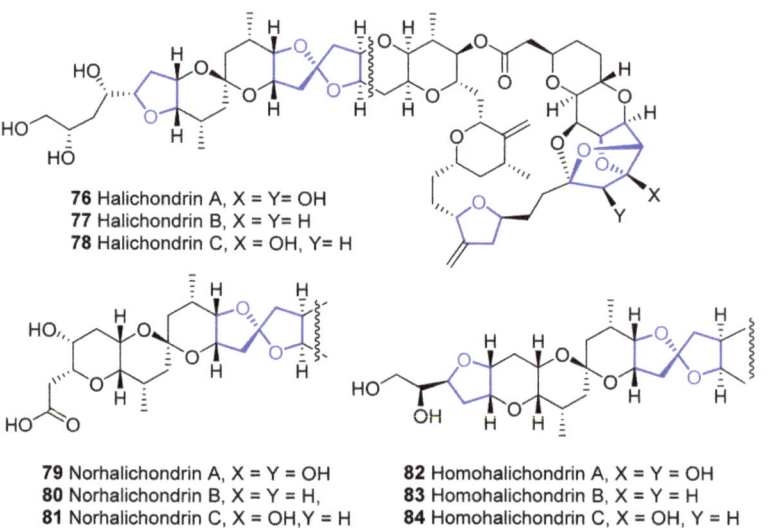

76 Halichondrin A, X = Y = OH
77 Halichondrin B, X = Y = H
78 Halichondrin C, X = OH, Y = H

79 Norhalichondrin A, X = Y = OH
80 Norhalichondrin B, X = Y = H,
81 Norhalichondrin C, X = OH, Y = H

82 Homohalichondrin A, X = Y = OH
83 Homohalichondrin B, X = Y = H
84 Homohalichondrin C, X = OH, Y = H

Figure 12. Structure of halichondrins, norhalichondrins and homohalichondrins.

Great efforts by Kishi's group have been devoted to the synthesis of this family of compounds. To finally reach the total synthesis, Kishi et al. first established the synthesis of different fragments of halichondrins such as: C1–C19, through key Ni/Cr-mediated coupling of polyhalogenated nucleophiles [54,55], C14–C38 fragment, by oxy-Michael cyclization [56,57], and those combined led to the C1–C37 right halves of halichondrins A–C [58]. In 2017, Kishi and co-workers accomplished a general and scalable total synthesis of halichondrins [59]. In this paper, a new Zr/Ni-mediated one-pot ketone synthesis gave the key to couple the right (**85**) and the left (**86**) halves of all types of halichondrins, including homo- and reluctant norhalichondrins (Scheme 15). Then, after fluoride deprotection of the silyl groups, ketone **87** was transformed to the spiroketal **88**. By coupling different halves, halichondrins, norhalichondrins and homohalichondrins were accessed. To exemplify the success of this strategy, an overall yield of 14.3% was obtained for the synthesis of halichondrin B from commercial D-galactal.

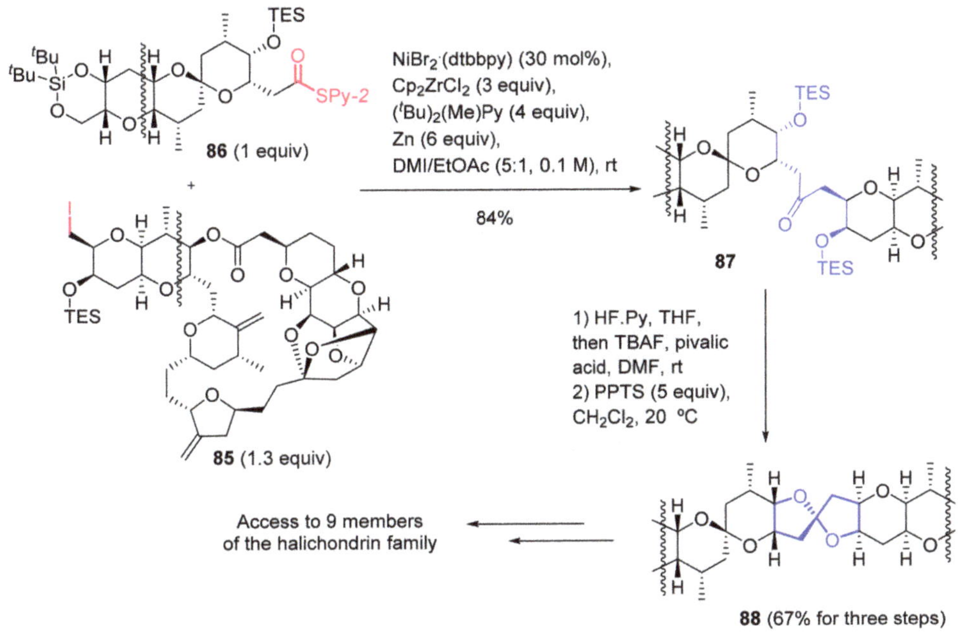

Scheme 15. Key step in the total synthesis of halichondrins by Kishi.

Recently, Nicolaou and coworkers described a reverse approach for the total synthesis of halichondrin B [60]. The strategy consisted of first forming the C-O bonds and then the C-C bonds of the cyclic moieties, which is opposite of the usual methods that first form C-C bonds and then rely on C-O bond-forming cyclizations. As an example, we can see in Scheme 16 the formation of linear ethers **89a** and **89b** by Nicholas etherification of alcohols **90** and **91**. The required diastereoisomer **89b** was subjected to radical cyclization to close the THF ring in **92**. This methodology was applied throughout the total synthesis of halichondrin B, which was synthesized in just 25 linear steps from commercial materials.

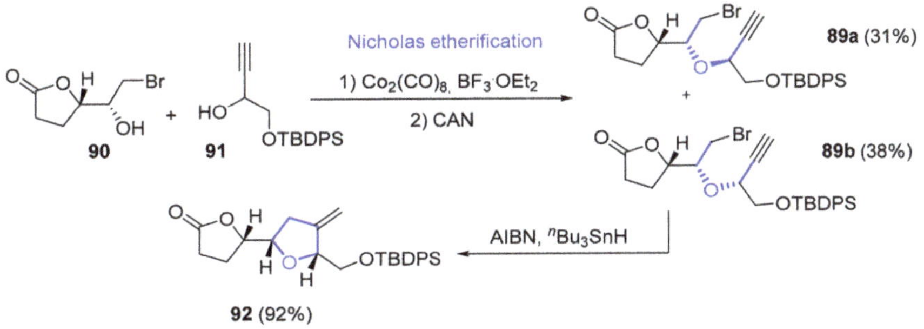

Scheme 16. Reverse approach to halichondrin B by Nicolaou.

Biological studies demonstrated that the right half of this class of natural products showed potent in vitro and in vivo antitumor activity [61], which led to the approval of eribulin mesylate (Figure 13) by the FDA for the treatment of late-stage breast cancer.

This compound is known under the commercial name of Halaven®. The mechanism and pharmacokinetics of eribulin and its use in numerous Phase I, II, and III clinical trials have been described in different reviews [62,63].

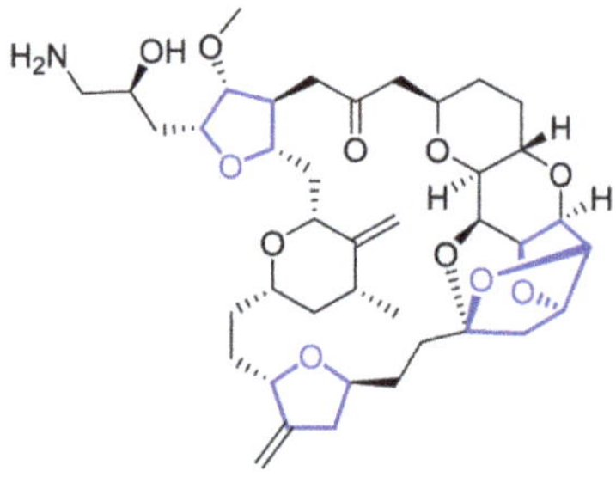

93 Eribulin (synthetic product)

Figure 13. Structure of the anticancer drug eribulin.

2.1.6. Iriomoteolides

Iriomoteolides are a recent class of macrolides isolated from a marine benthic dinoflagellate of the *Amphidinium* species [64]. Among all members of this family, iriomoteolide-2a (**94**) [65], 10a (**95**) [66], and 13a (**96**) [67] present at least a substituted tetrahydrofuran ring (Figure 14). They stand up for their potent biological activity against human cervix adenocarcinoma HeLa cells (IC50 = 0.03 µg/mL, 1.5 µM and 0.5 µg/mL, respectively) and other cell lines, human B lymphocyte DG-75 (IC50 [2a] = 6 ng/mL and IC50 [10a] = 1.2 µM), and murine hepatocellular carcinoma MH134 cells (IC50 [10a] = 3.3 µM).

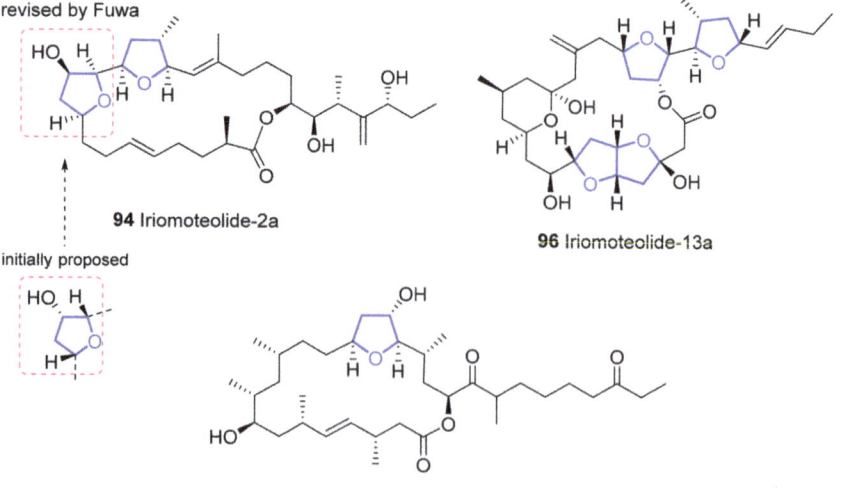

Figure 14. Structure of THF-containing iriomoteolides.

Despite their biological interest, there is no total synthesis reported for the 21-membered macrolide **95**, nor the 22-membered macrolide **96**, probably due to their complexity. On the contrary, the synthesis of **94** was accomplished by Fuwa and co-workers recently and it led to a structural revision [68,69].

Iriomoteolide-2a was the first 23-membered macrolide isolated from nature. Its structure contains two contiguous tetrahydrofuran rings embedded in the macrolide skeleton and a side chain containing three chiral centers. Two key steps made up the synthetic approach devised by Fuwa [68], a Suzuki-Miyaura coupling reaction between a vinyl iodide **97** and an olefin **98**, and a ring closing metathesis with **99** to build the macrolactone (Scheme 17).

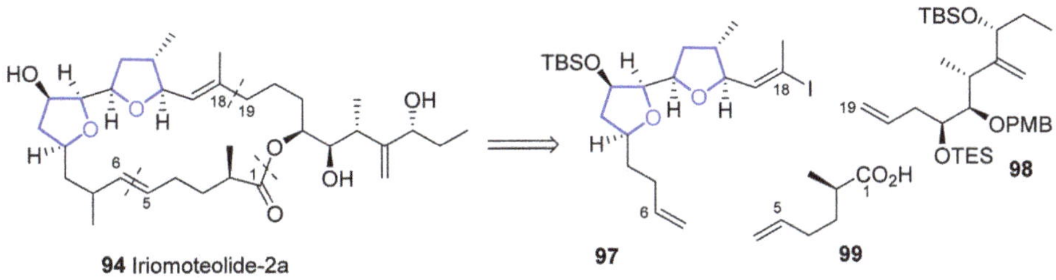

Scheme 17. Retrosynthesis of iriomoteolide-2a.

A convergent strategy allowed the synthesis of the different possible stereoisomers of iriomoteolide-2a. Having discarded the original proposed configuration, the construction of the correct bis-THF fragment was achieved by two sequential cycloetherifications. Thus, Sharpless asymmetric epoxidation of **100** provided diepoxide **101**, which in situ underwent epoxide opening cascade with formation of the desired bis-THF **102**. The relative configuration of this bis-tetrahydrofuran was established by ROE experiments (Scheme 18).

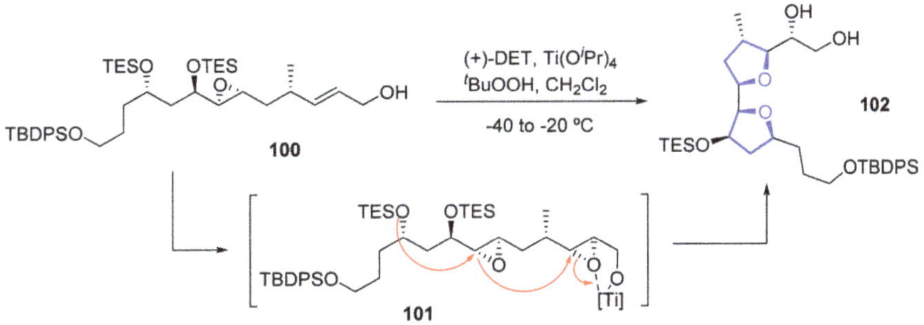

Scheme 18. Synthesis of contiguous THF in iriomoteolide-2a.

In this synthesis macrocyclization was performed at a very late stage. Thus, ring closing methathesis of precursor **103**, with a second-generation Grubbs catalyst (G-II), led to macrocycle **104**, which after final deprotection step afforded the desired iriomoteolide-2a (Scheme 19).

Thanks to this total synthesis it was possible to establish the absolute configuration of iriomoteolide-2a and to re-study the biological activity of synthetic compounds [69]. By comparing the spectral data, the correct stereochemistry of the natural compound could be assigned, which differed from the first proposed assignment [65]. Surprisingly, in contrast to the potent cytotoxic activity reported for the natural product, the synthetic iriomoteolide-2a only showed marginal antiproliferative activity in HeLa cells (IC50 = 60 μM). A plausible explanation for the high cytotoxicity measured in natural iriomoteolide-2a is the presence of traces of a highly potent contaminant in the sample.

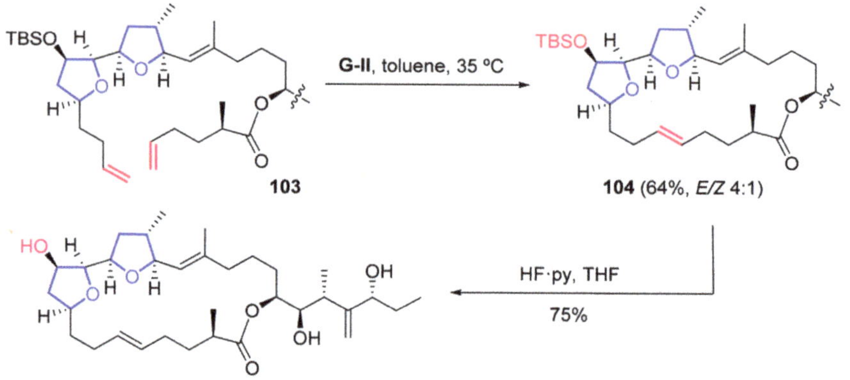

Scheme 19. Engame to iriomoteolide-2a by Fuwa.

2.1.7. Mandelalides

Mandelalides A-D (**105-108**) (Figure 15) are a group of marine macrolides isolated in 2012 from a species of *lissoclinum* ascidian [70]. Their macrocyclic core has two cyclic moieties embedded, a glycosylated 2,6-*cis*-substituted tetrahydropyran and a 2,5-*cis*-substituted tetrahydrofuran. Within them, the natural isolated compounds **105** and **106** yielded nanomolar IC50 values against mouse Neuro2A neuroblastoma cells and human NCI-H460 lung cancer cell lines. Their complex structure was elucidated by 1D and 2D NMR experiments and mass spectrometry, although the stereochemistry of Mandelalide A was definitively established after its total synthesis by Xu and Ye [71].

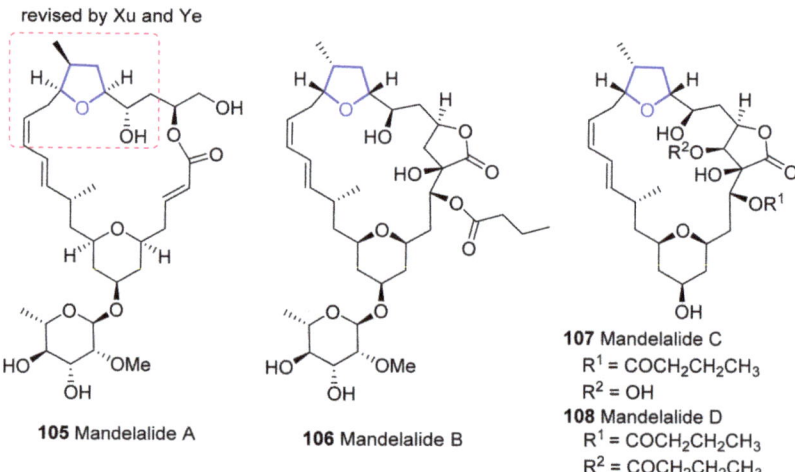

Figure 15. Structure of mandelalides.

Years later, new members of this family were isolated, namely mandelalide E-L [72,73]. This has permitted the study of structure-activity relationship, showing that glycosylation is essential for their biological activity.

Since the discovery of mandelalide A, different researchers have proposed approaches for its total synthesis [12]. The main difference between them lies in the key reaction steps. Tao Ye and co-workers reported the use of Rychnovsky–Bartlett cyclization for the preparation of the tetrahydrofuran moiety and an Horner–Wadsworth–Emmons for the macrocyclization [71]. Amos B. Smith developed an anion relay chemistry (ARC) strategy [74] to synthesize the tetrahydrofuran and tetrahydropyran structural motifs which were joined by Yamaguchi esterification [75]. Intramolecular Heck cyclization [76], Sharpless asymmetric dihydroxylation [77] or Julia olefination [78] were also employed in other total syntheses.

As an example, we want to highlight the convergent total synthesis reported by Altmann [79]. In this synthesis, the highly oxygenated tetrahydrofuran **109** was constructed from compound **110** by acetal cleavage/epoxide opening cascade reaction. Then, substitution of the primary OH with iodine (**111**) and subsequent radical alkynylation with sulfone **112** afforded **113**. After further elaboration, the tetrahydrofuran fragment **114** was accessed (Scheme 20).

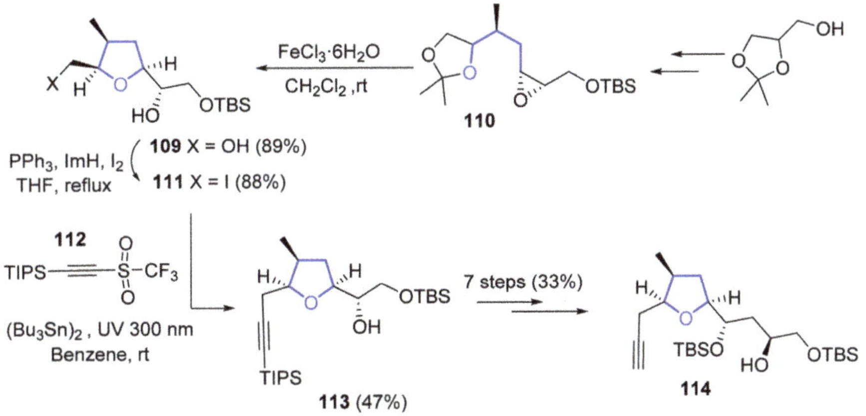

Scheme 20. Synthesis of the trisubstituted THF in mandelalides.

With the needed building blocks in hand, tetrahydropyran **115** and tetrahydrofuran **114** moieties were united via Sonogashira coupling to afford enyne **116**. Then, Shiina macrolactonization was used to access macrolactone **117**, which was transformed to the desired natural product in four additional steps and a 2.15% overall yield (Scheme 21).

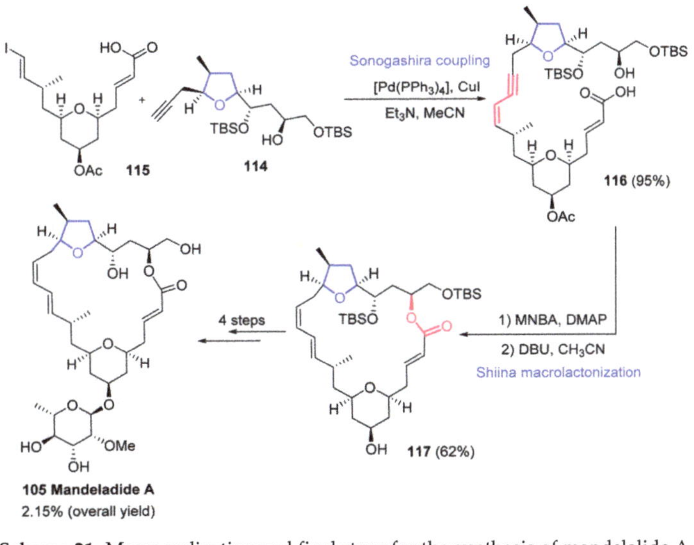

Scheme 21. Macrocyclization and final steps for the synthesis of mandelalide A.

Biological studies of synthetic mandelalide A revealed a potent inhibitory activity of the proliferation of H460 and A549 lung carcinoma cells, but not cytotoxic activity at least within the concentration range studied [70,79]. In general, mandelalides have shown to have highly cell-type dependent bioactive effects.

2.1.8. Mangromicins

Mangromicin A (**118**) and B (**119**) (Figure 16) were the first members of this family isolated from actinomycete *Lechevalieria aerocolonigenes* [80], followed by six new analogues, mangromicins D-I [81]. The mangromicins contain a cyclopentadecaene skeleton with a 5,6-dihydro-4-hidroxy-2-pyrone moiety and a tetrahydrofuran unit. All mangromicins show important biological activities. Special effects have been found in Mangromicin A, which exhibits potent antitrypanosomal activity against Trypanosoma brucei brucei GUTat 3.1 strain (IC50 = 2.4 in vitro essays) and cytotoxicity against MRC-5 cells.

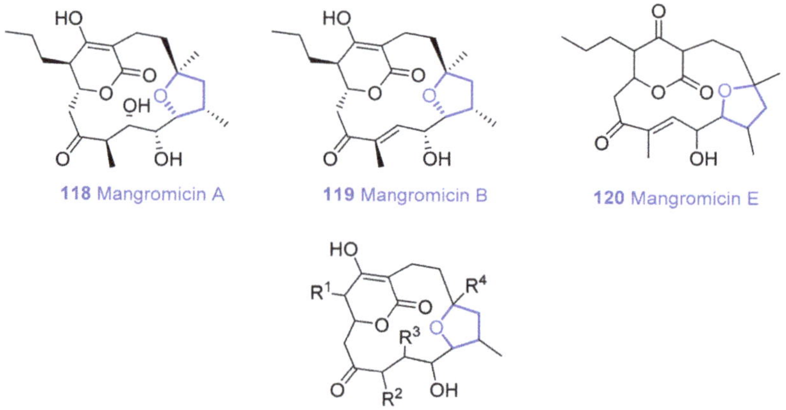

118 Mangromicin A
119 Mangromicin B
120 Mangromicin E

121 Mangromicin D, R^1 = $CH_2CH_2CH_3$, R^2 = CH_2OH, R^3 = H, R^4 = CH_3
122 Mangromicin F, R^1 = C_2H_5, R^2 = CH_2OH, R^3 = H, R^4 = CH_3
123 Mangromicin G, R^1 = $CH_2CH_2CH_3$, R^2 = CH_3, R^3 = H, R^4 = CH_2OH
124 Mangromicin H, R^1 = C_2H_5, R^2 = CH_3, R^3 = H, R^4 = CH_3
125 Mangromicin I, R^1 = C_2H_5, R^2 = $=CH_2$, R^3 = OCH_3, R^4 = CH_3

Figure 16. Structure of mangromicins.

The first and unique enantioselective total synthesis of mangromicin A was reported by Takahashi and coworkers [82]. Deprotection of the OTBS group in compound **126** led to hydroxyketone **127**, in equilibrium with its hemiketal. Then, a Mukaiyama-type vinylogous alkylation was used as key step to synthesize the desired tetrahydrofuran moiety (-)-**128**, bearing a C-2 quaternary carbon with the desired configuration. A further 21 steps, including a crucial Dieckmann cyclization to generate the 4-hydroxydihydropyrone unit, were needed to complete the total synthesis of mangromicin A (Scheme 22) [82].

2.1.9. Nonalides: Cytospolides

Cytospolides (Figure 17), which belong to a nonalide family, are a group of compounds which were isolated in Gomera island (Spain) from an endophytic fungus, *Cytospora* sp., by Zhang and co-workers in 2011 [83]. The different structures and absolute configurations of cytospolides were first elucidated and established by spectroscopic analysis, chemical derivatization, and X-ray diffraction [83]. Almost all members of this family contain a 10-membered lactone. Additionally, cytospolides M (**129**), cytospolide N (**130**), and cytospolide O (**131**) are tetrahydrofuran-containing nonalides. Cytospolide Q (**132**) is the exception, containing a 15-carbon skeleton with two different rings, a tetrahydrofuran and a γ-butyrolactone.

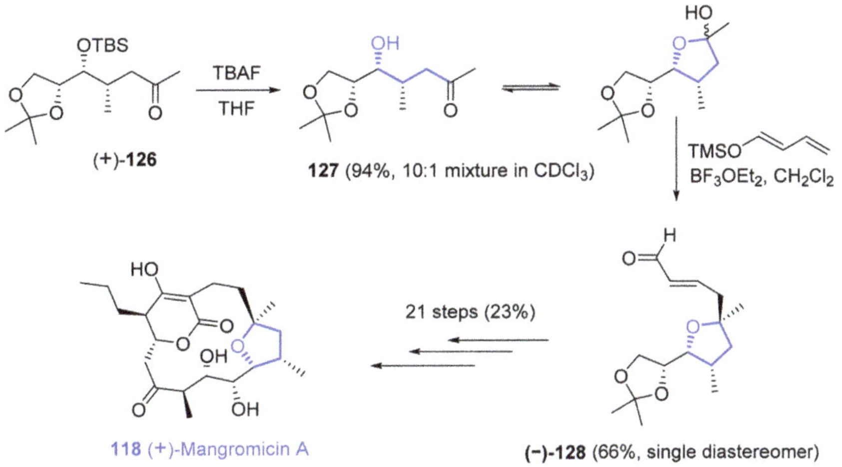

Scheme 22. Synthesis of THF segment of mangromicin A.

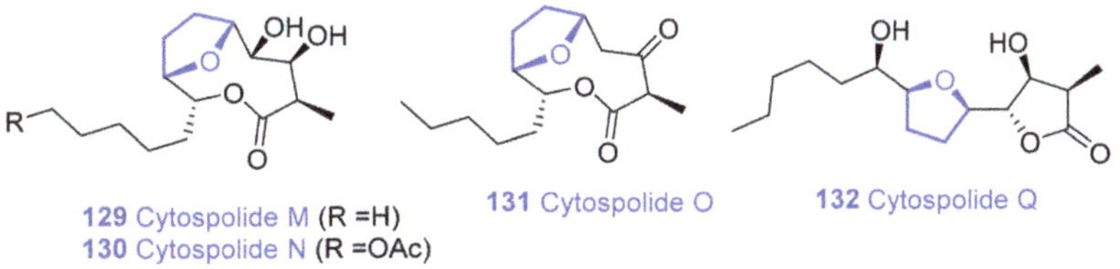

Figure 17. Structure of cytospolides.

Stark et al. have reported the total synthesis of cytospolide D and its conversion into cytospolides M, O, and Q (Scheme 23) [84]. Cytospolide M was obtained in a single step with a 86% yield from cytospolide D, by diastereoselective epoxidation. Subsequent opening of cytospolide M with potassium trimethylsilanolate, followed by spontaneous recyclization during the workup, allowed the preparation of the desired cytospolide Q. On the other hand, cytospolide O was obtained through an oxa-Michael addition from a close precursor of cytospolide D in three steps.

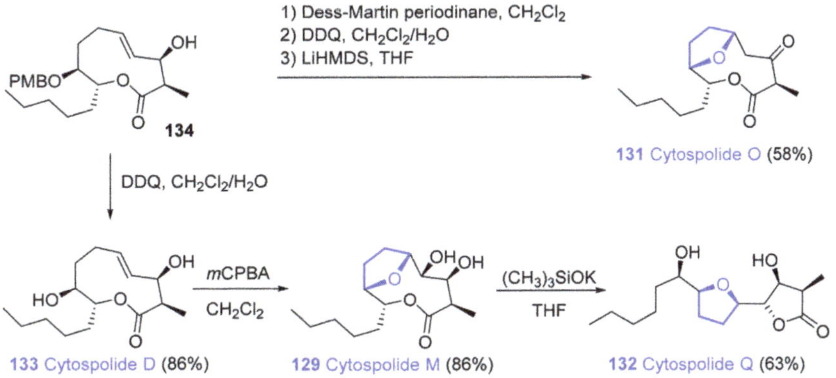

Scheme 23. Synthesis of cytospolides.

In a different approach, a convergent route for the total synthesis of cytospolide Q has been proposed in 10 linear steps, with an overall yield of 2.8%, from known intermediate

135 [85]. A set of cascade reactions are the key to build the tetrahydrofuran ring and the γ-butyrolactone moiety (Scheme 24).

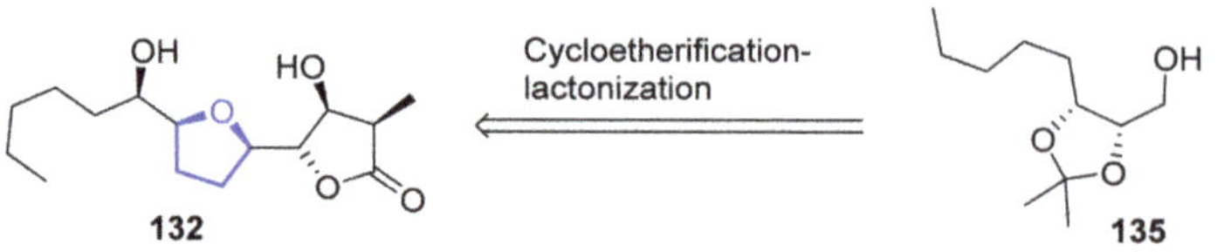

Scheme 24. Retrosynthesis of cytospolide Q.

Nine linear steps from **136** were needed to prepare the required precursor (**137**). A set of convenient cascade reactions, such as acid-catalyzed acetal deprotection, subsequent tetrahydropyranyl formation by epoxide opening with the appropriate hydroxyl group and final γ-lactonization allowed the formation of cytospolide Q in a single step from **137** (Scheme 25).

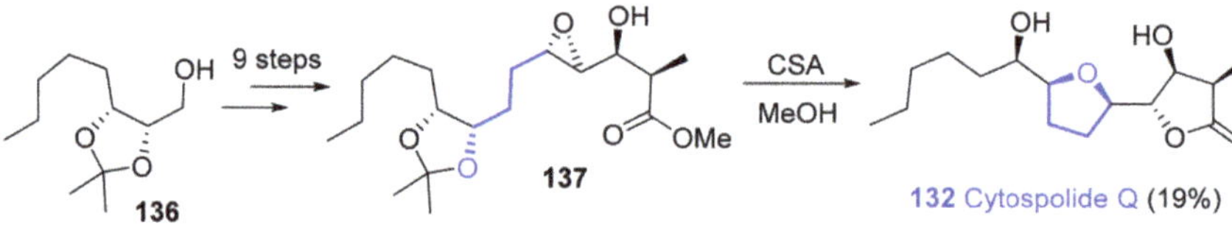

Scheme 25. Total synthesis of cytospolide Q.

The moderate cytotoxic activity against tumor cell lines of some members of the cytospolide family [83] has prompted researchers to synthesize structurally diverse derivatives which may have improved properties [85]. Thus, Stark and Erlich [86] envisioned the synthesis of cytospolide analogues **138** and **139** from a modified cytospolide D intermediate **140** in which an alkynyl side chain was used as a versatile handle for further functionalization (Scheme 26).

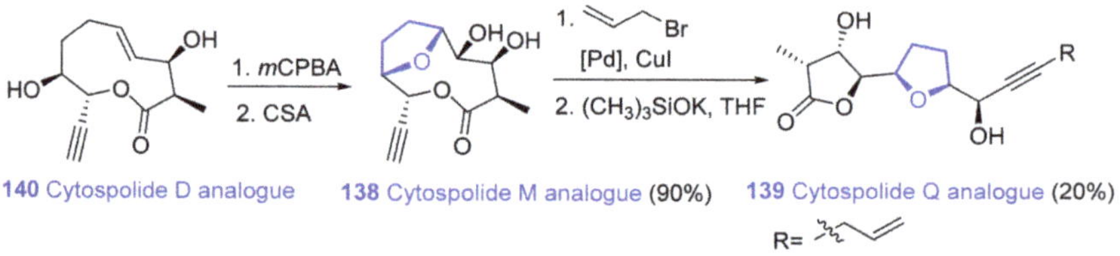

Scheme 26. Synthesis of cytospolide analogues.

2.1.10. Oscillariolide

Murakami and co-workers isolated a new macrolide from a marine blue-green alga *Oscillatoria* sp. in 1991 [87]. Oscillariolide (Figure 18) has a complex structure which was established on the basis of extensive spectral analysis. Interestingly, its determination has been very useful for the discovery of phormidolides.

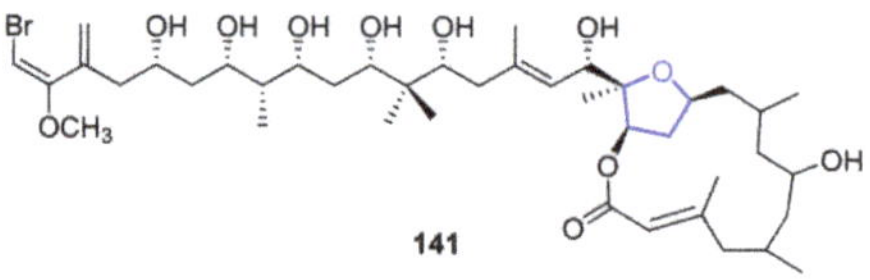

Figure 18. Structure of oscillariolide.

Despite the interesting inhibition activity of oscillariolide towards the cell division of fertilized starfish eggs, no total synthesis of this compound has been reported.

2.1.11. Phormidolides

The first member of this family, Phormidolide A (**142**) (Figure 19), was isolated in 2002 from the marine cyanobacterium *Leptolyngbya* sp. [88]. Although it was an inactive metabolite in cell line essays, phormidolide A showed high toxicity to brine shrimp (LC50 = 1.5 µM). At that moment, a complex structure was proposed on the basis of spectroscopic techniques. Eleven stereocentres, a tetrahydrofuran-embedded macrolactone, a polyol side chain and a terminal bromomethoxydiene motif composed the polyketide. Almost 20 years later, the assignment of eight chiral centers was corrected thanks to the contribution of Gerwick, Paterson, Britton, and Piel and colleagues, who used synthetic methods [89], computational information, and anisotropic NMR studies [90].

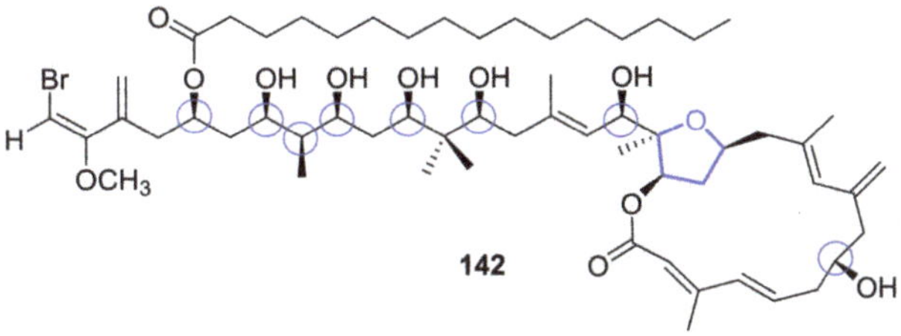

Figure 19. Structure of phormidolide A.

In 2015, the study of an active organic extract of *Petrosiidae* sponge concluded with the discovery of two important novel phormidolides, phormidolide B and phormidolide C (Figure 20) [91]. Their structural similarity to phormidolide A [90] and oscillariolide [87] helped in the establishment of their overall structure by NMR techniques.

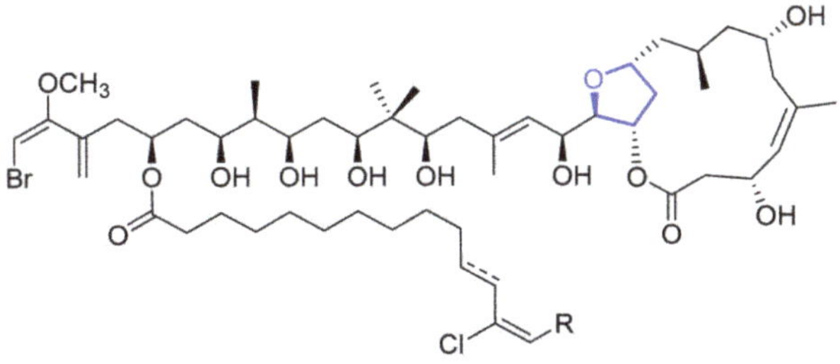

143 Phormidolide B, R = Cl, double bond
144 Phormidolide C, R = Br
145 Phormidolide D, R = Cl

Figure 20. Structure of phormidolides B-D.

These new compounds present cytotoxic activity against three human tumor cell lines, lung (A-549), colon (HT-29), and breast (MDA-MB-231), with an unknown mechanism of action. Their challenging structure has attracted the interest of synthetic chemists who have developed different strategies to access either the macrolide ring [91–93] or the polyhydroxylated chain [94,95].

Phormidolides could be divided into three molecular fragments with two main disconnections: a macrocyclic core, a polyhydroxylated chain containing a tetradecanoic fatty acid, and a propargylic organometallic (Scheme 27). Synthetic approaches to each individual fragment have been described, although no completed synthesis of any of these compounds has been reported so far [93].

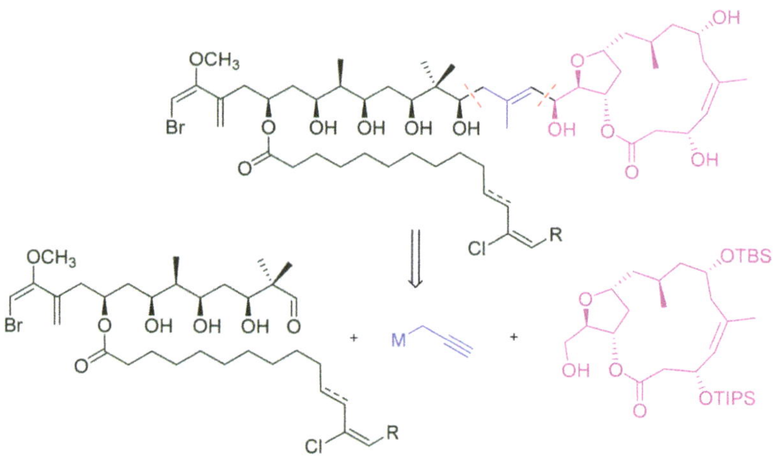

Scheme 27. Retrosynthesis of phormidolides.

Focusing on the tetrahydrofuran-containing macrolactone, Álvarez et al. published an approach to its synthesis starting from commercially available 2-D-deoxyribose [91]. The key steps of this synthesis are the simultaneous formation of a trisubstituted double bond and a new stereocenter through the stereoselective 1,5-*anti*-addition of an allylstannane **146** and ribose-derived aldehyde **147**. Then, **148** was subjected to final Shiina macrolactonization affording the desired **149** (Scheme 28).

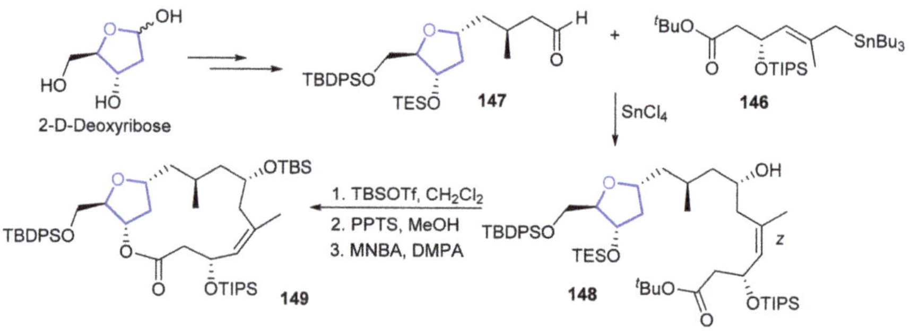

Scheme 28. Retrosynthesis of phormidolide macrocycle.

2.2. Linear Polyketides

Ionostatin

Ionostatin (Figure 21) [96], extracted from an actinomycite of *Streptomycetaceae* family, is the most recently discovered polyether ionophore [97–99]. Its structure and absolute stereochemistry were determined by NMR experiments, X-ray diffraction (calcium salt) and bioinformatic approach. The compound, a close analog to ionomycin (Figure 22) [100], contains 15 chiral centers and two tetrahydrofuran rings.

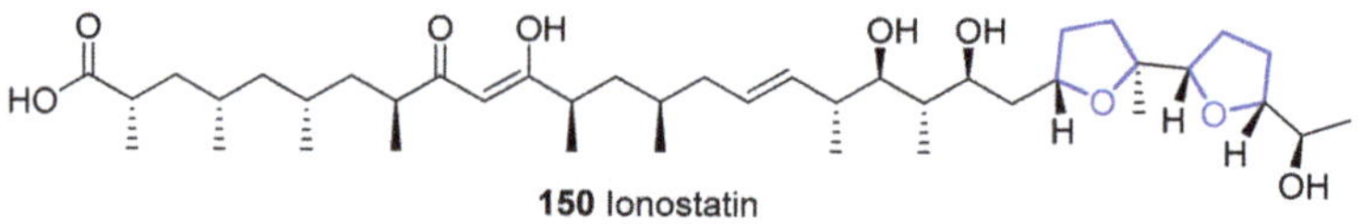

150 Ionostatin

Figure 21. Structure of ionostatin.

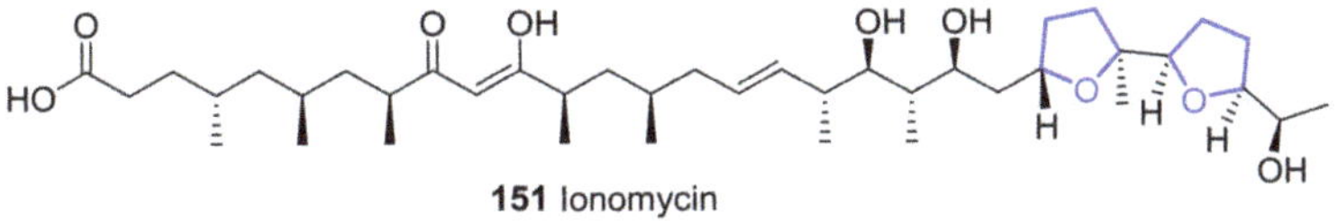

151 Ionomycin

Figure 22. Structure of ionomycin.

Polyether ionophores are chemotherapeutic agents for the treatment of cancer [101]. Initial bioactivity essays of ionostatin revealed inhibition (LD50 = 7.4 µg/mL) against two important cancer cell lines such as U87 glioblastama and SKOV3 ovarian carcinoma.

2.3. Polycyclic Polyketides
Akaeolide

Akaeolide (Figure 23) is another polycyclic polyketide isolated from a culture extract of a marine-derived actinomycete, *Streptomyces* sp., in 2013 [102]. Its 15-membered carbocyclic structure possesses a five-membered cyclic ether and a β-keto-δ-lactone unit. The biological essays of this compound have shown modest cytotoxicity against 3Y1 rat fibroblasts with an IC50 of 8.5 µM [103].

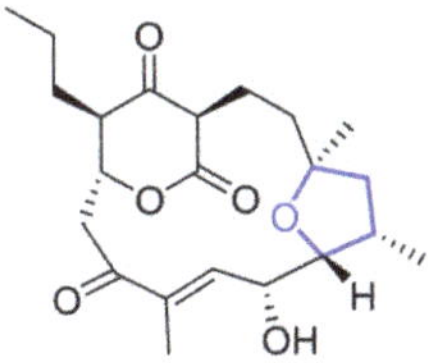

152 Akaeolide

Figure 23. Structure of akaeolide.

2.4. Acetogenin Metabolites

Acetogenins are secondary metabolites derived from polyketides. Acetogenins from marine algae are mostly halogenated and are thought to have a common C15 precursor derived from a C16 fatty acid. The majority of these marine C15 acetogenins are different-sized cyclic ethers with a terminal enyne or bromoallene. Among them, tetrahydrofuran and bis-tetrahydrofuran acetogenins are quite abundant. Acetogenins are known to be chemotaxonomic markers from red algae to the genus *Laurencia*. A general overview of C15 acetogenins from 1965 till 2015 was provided by Falkenberg [104].

In 2016, three new tetrahydrofuran-containing acetogenins with potent and selective antiproliferative activity against human nasopharyngeal carcinoma (NPC) cell lines and their methotrexate-resistant counterparts have been described [105].

In 2019, a synthetic route for the bis-tetrahydrofuran core of acetogenins based on a chemoenzymatic cascade reaction was reported [106]. Catalytic hydrogenation of benzylidene acetal **153** produces the inside-out cyclization to afford bis-tetrahydrofuran-ditosylate **154** in 66% yield. It was also possible to obtain a different stereochemistry on the bis-tetrahydrofuran moiety **156**, through a double Payne rearrangement of epoxide **155** followed by 5-*exo*-tet cycloetherification (Scheme 29).

Obtusallenes

Obtusallenes are C15-halogenated acetogenins that contain a 12-membered ether ring. Obtusallene I was isolated in 1982 from red algae *Laurencia obtusa* and its structure was elucidated by NMR and X-ray crystallographic methods. Since, other obtusallenes have been described: obtusallene II (**157**) and III (**158**) [107], obtusallene IV (**159**) [108], obtusallenes V-VII (**160-162**), and obtusallenes VIII-IX [109]. The structure of **160-162** was corrected in 2008 by Braddock due to unambiguously solved X-ray crystallography and biosynthetic studies [110,111]. Among the obtusallenes, compounds **157-162** contain a tetrahydrofuran motif (Figure 24).

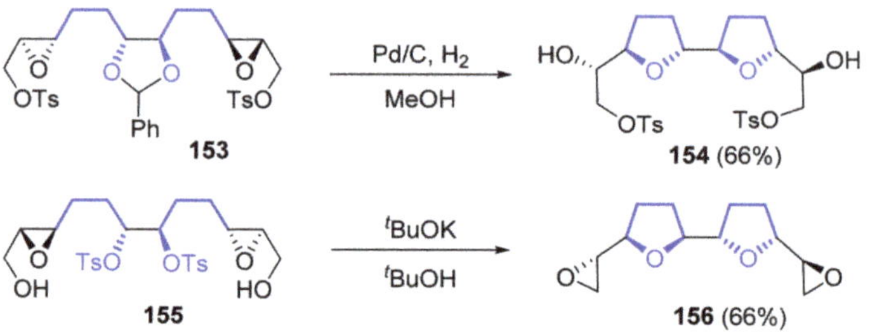

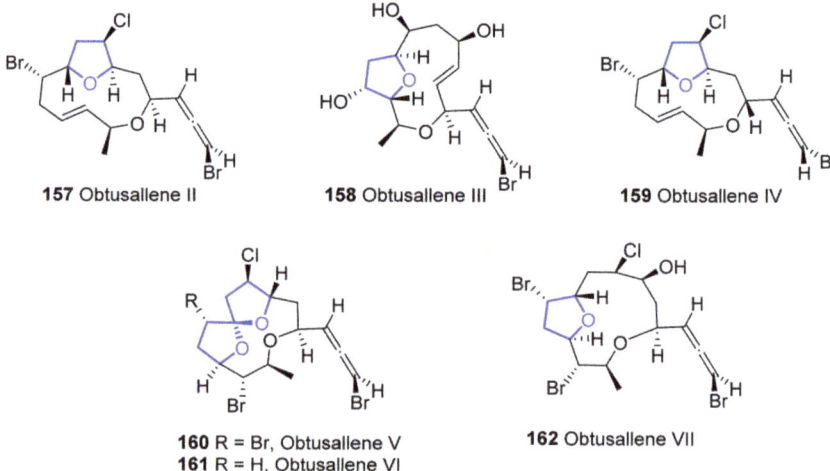

Scheme 29. Synthesis of bis-THF core of acetogenins.

Figure 24. Structures of tetrahydrofuran-containing obtusallenes II–VII.

The first synthesis of tetrahydrofuran rings of compounds **157** and **159** was reported in 2007 [112]. In this synthesis, diene **163** was transformed into tetrahydrofuran **164** with 18% yield and >95% purity in a one-pot reaction (with the sequential addition of *m*-CPBA, TMSCl and PPh₃, TBAF, and then TBCO) (Scheme 30).

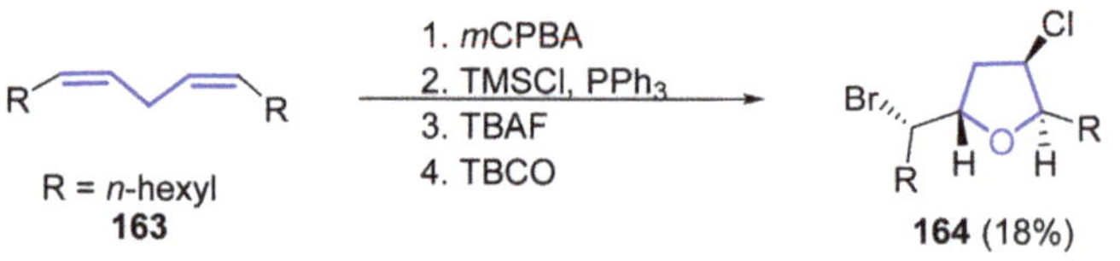

Scheme 30. One pot reaction for THF core of obtusallenes 157 and 159.

Parallelly, a synthesis of the C8–C15 fragment of obtusallene III **158** was described [113]. The Pd-catalyzed cyclization of triol **165** produced 2,5-disubstituted 3-hydroxytetrahydrofuran **166** with an 82% yield. The chemo- and diastereoselective cyclization implies the direct effect of a noncovalent interaction of the counterion carboxylate with the OH groups of the cationic π-allyl-Pd(II) intermediate (Scheme 31).

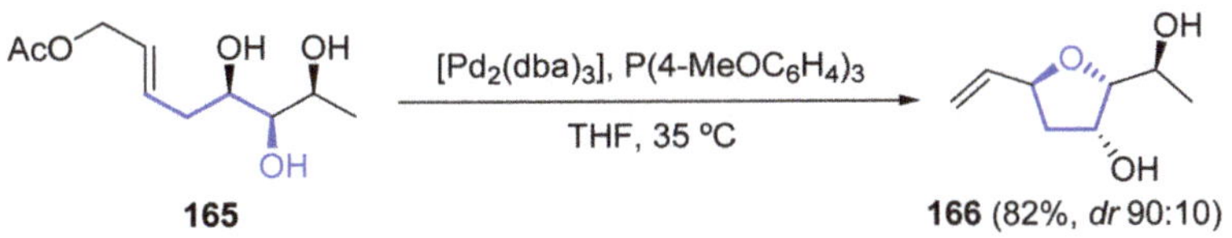

Scheme 31. Synthesis of C8-C15 fragment of obtusallene **158**.

Braddock reported the only known total synthesis of a member of this family to date: obtusallene X (**167**) [114]. The key step of this synthesis is the cyclization of clorhydrine intermediate **168** through a stereoselective bromoetherification process.

Five additional steps from **169** afforded acyclic diene **170**, which, under ring-closing metathesis with a second-generation Hoveyda–Grubbs precatalyst, produces macrocyclic **171**. Six additional steps were needed to obtain **167** with a 7% overall yield from **168** (Scheme 32).

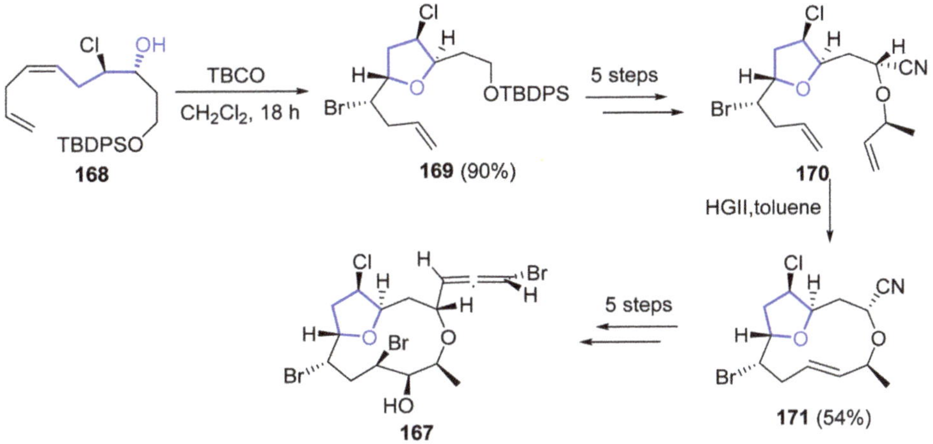

Scheme 32. Synthesis of obtusallene X (**167**).

2.5. Polyhydroxyl

Amphezonol A

The dinoflagelatte *Amphidinium* sp. has been extensively studied in order to discover and isolate new compounds bearing interesting biological properties, such as macrolides, amphidinolides or polyhydroxyl compounds. In 2006, a novel polyhydroxyl metabolite was isolated, amphenozol A (**172**) [115], the structure of which consists of a C60 linear aliphatic chain with two tetrahydropyran rings, one tetrahydrofuran ring, and twenty-one hydroxyl groups (Figure 25). Its structure was established by NMR experiments. Additionally, the biological analysis showed a modest inhibitory activity against DNA polymerase α.

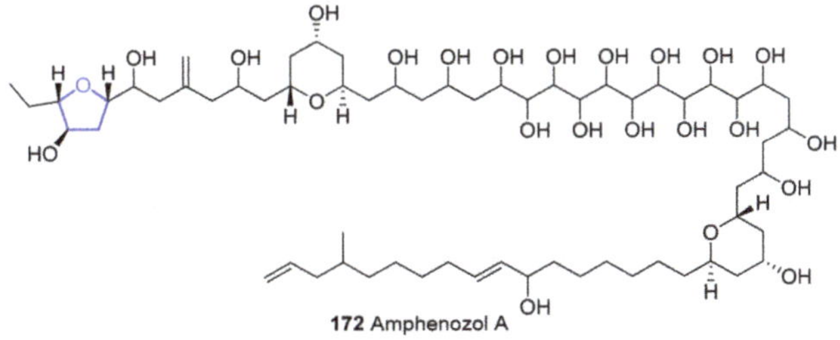

Figure 25. Structure of amphenozol A.

2.6. Bycyclic

2.6.1. Asperpentenone

Recently, J. Wang et al. isolated a novel polyketide, asperpentenone A, from the fungus *Aspergillus* sp. [116]. Its structure, elucidated by nuclear magnetic resonance techniques and X-ray diffraction, contains a cyclopentenone-tetrahydrofuran moiety (Figure 26). So far, no biological activity of asperpentenone A has been described.

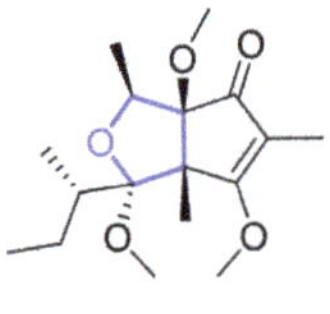

173 Asperpentenone A

Figure 26. Structure of asperpentenone A.

2.6.2. Plakortones

Ten lactone metabolites, known as plakortones (**174–183**), have been isolated from the marine sponge of the genus *Plakortis*. Plakortones belong to a big family of oxygenated polyketide metabolites, the structures of which contain a bicyclic system composed of a tetrahydrofuran fused to a γ-butyrolactone ring (Figure 27). Some of them have been discovered and characterized during the 20th century [117,118], while plakortone L, N, P, and Q were recently isolated [119,120].

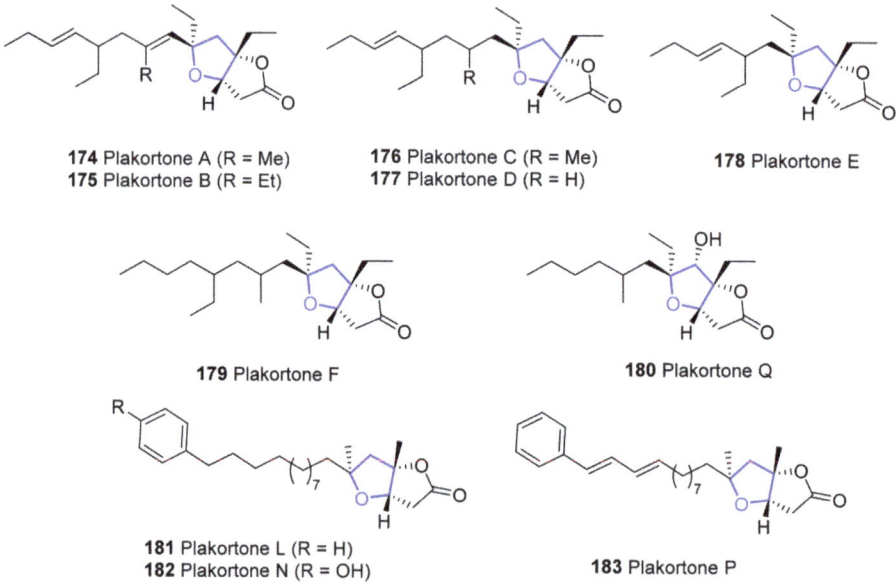

174 Plakortone A (R = Me)
175 Plakortone B (R = Et)

176 Plakortone C (R = Me)
177 Plakortone D (R = H)

178 Plakortone E

179 Plakortone F

180 Plakortone Q

181 Plakortone L (R = H)
182 Plakortone N (R = OH)

183 Plakortone P

Figure 27. Structure of plakortones.

Since their discovery, numerous studies can be found in the literature with different approaches towards the synthesis of these natural products, their epimers [121] or analogues [122]. A palladium-(II)-mediated hydroxycyclization-carbonylation-lactonization cascade [123] was the general methodology applied to obtain the plakortone core in some cases [122,124,125]. There, from diols **184**, the byciclic diastereomers **185** or **186** can be accessed (Scheme 33).

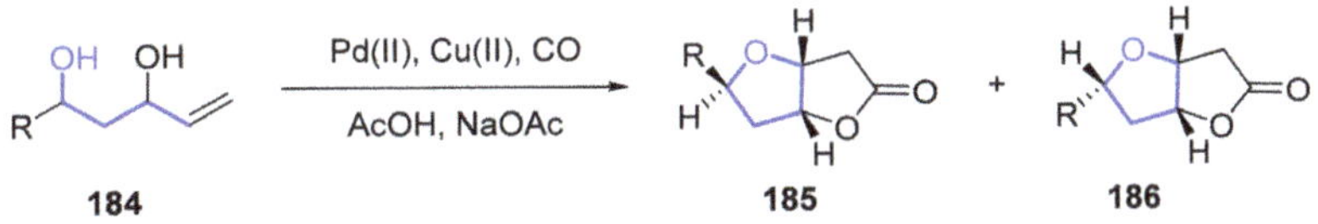

Scheme 33. Synthesis of plakortone core.

The synthesis of the four possible diastereoisomers and comparison with the natural product allowed Wong and co-workers to determine the absolute configuration of the four stereocenters of plakortone B [126]. Thus, retrosynthetic analysis revealed butenolide **187** as the potential precursor of the bicyclic lactone. Formation of butenolide required ten steps from D-mannitol. The bicyclic framework **188** was directly formed with a 90% yield by the reaction of butenolide with 1,5-diazabicyclo[5.4.0]undec-5-ene (DBU), in a domino Michael addition followed by transesterification. Total synthesis of plakortone B was achieved in 22 further steps with a low overall yield (<1%) (Scheme 34).

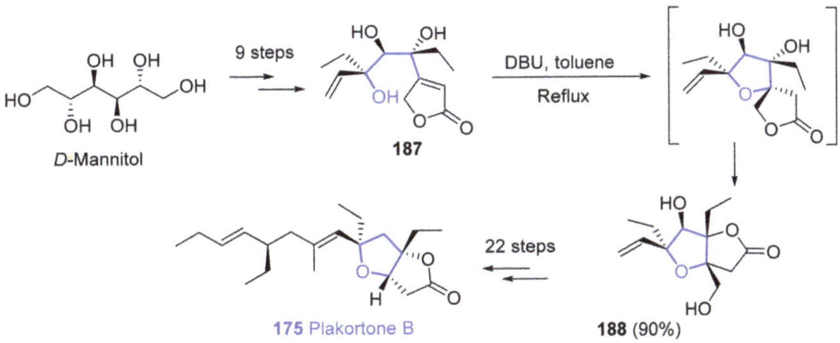

Scheme 34. Total synthesis of plakortone B.

Another biomimetic approach converted plakortide E derivative **189** into plakortone B [127]. Treatment of **189** with zinc in acetic acid broke the peroxy O-O bond and provided diol intermediate **190**. Further intramolecular oxa-Michael addition/lactonization cascade reaction afforded the desired product with high yield (90%) (Scheme 35).

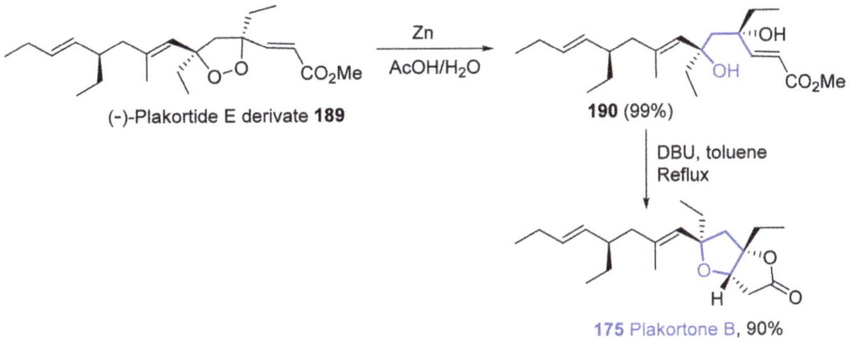

Scheme 35. Synthesis of plakortone B via plakortide E derivative.

In 2014, the total synthesis of plakortone L was also reported [128]. In this case, the strategy to obtain the tetrahydrofuran ring was a [3+2] annulation. Thus, the tetrahydrofuranyl ring **191** was obtained by the reaction of isopropylidene-protected D-arabinose **192** and protected methallyl alcohol **193** in the presence of $BF_3 \cdot OEt_2$. Fourteen further steps were required to accomplish the total synthesis of plakortone L with 6% overall yield (Scheme 36).

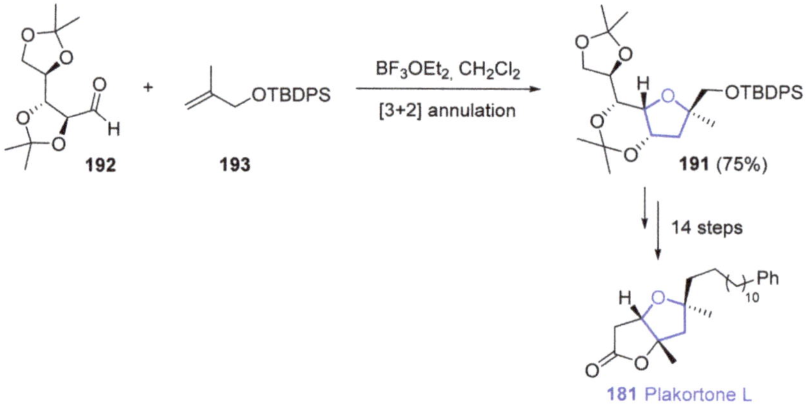

Scheme 36. Synthesis of plakortone L.

In terms of their biological activity, plakortones A-D belong to the class of activators of cardiac sarcoplasmic reticulum Ca^{2+}-pumping ATPase at micromolar concentrations, specially plakortone D [117]. Plakortones B-F exhibit in vitro cytotoxic activity on a murine fibrosarcome cell line [122]. However, plakortone Q, being the only member of the family which contains a hydroxyl group in the ring system, is not active against any of the tested tumor cell lines [129].

3. Conclusions

Polyketides are a class of marine natural products with immense structural and biological diversity. They have interesting biological properties that sometimes make them potential drug candidates, such as in eribulin mesylate. Here, organic synthesis in general, and total synthesis in particular still play an important dual role. First, it is the final way of determining the correct structure of a product. Even though, nowadays, there are cutting-edge NMR techniques available, we still see many cases of structure misassignment in marine bioactive products. Secondly, the scarcity of some marine products makes them unavailable for research, and synthesis provides sufficient amounts for proper biological studies. The tetrahydrofuran motif is common among marine polyketides; thus, the development of new methodologies for the synthesis of tetrahydrofurans is a current need.

Author Contributions: Writing—original draft preparation, L.F.-P. and P.G.-A.; writing—review and editing, C.D.-P. and A.B. All authors have read and agreed to the published version of the manuscript.

Funding: This research was funded by Junta de Castilla y León, grant number VA294-P18.

Acknowledgments: C.D.-P. and L.F.-P. acknowledge predoctoral Grants funded by the European Social Fund and the "Junta de Castilla y León".

Conflicts of Interest: The authors declare no conflict of interest.

Abbreviations

Acac: acetylacetone; AIBN: azobisisobutyronitrile; CAB: (acyloxy)borane; CAN: ceric ammonium nitrate; CSA: camphorsulfonic acid; CuTC: copper(I) thiophene-2-carboxylate; DBU: 1,8-diazabicyclo[5.4.0]undec-7-ene; dba: dibenzylideneacetone; DDQ: 2,3-dichloro-5,6-dicyano-*p*-benzoquinone; (+)-DET: diethyl tartrate; (DHQD)$_2$PHAL: hydroquinidine 1,4-phthalazinediyl diether; DMAP: 4-dimethylaminopyridine; DMI: 1,3-dimethyl-2-imidazolidinone; DMF: dimethylformamide; DMI: 1,3-dimethyl-2-imidazolidinone; DMP: Dess-Martin periodinane; DMPA: dimethylol propionic acid; DMPM: 3,4-dimethoxybenzyl; DMSO: dimethyl sulphoxide; KHMDS: potassium bis(trimethylsilyl)amide; LiHDMS: lithium bis(trimethylsilyl)amide; mCPBA: meta-chloroperoxybenzoic acid; MNBA: 2-methyl-6-nitrobenzoic anhydride; MOM: methoxymethyl; Ms: methanesulfonyl; NMP: *n*-methylpyrrolidone; PMB: *p*-methoxybenzyl; PPTS: pyridinium *p*-toluenesulfonate; PT: 1-phenyltetrazol-5-yl; TASF: tris(dimethylamino)sulfonium difluorotrimethylsilicate; TBAF: tetrabutylammonium fluoride; TBCO: 2,4,4,6-tetrabromo-2,5-cyclohexadienone; TBDPS: *tert*-butyldiphenylsilyl; TES: triethylsilyl; TFA: trifluoroacetic acid; TIPS: triisopropylsilyl; TMS: trimethylsilyl; Tr: triphenyl methyl; Ts: tosyl.

References

1. Fuwa, H. Structure determination, correction, and disproof of marine macrolide natural products by chemical synthesis. *Org. Chem. Front.* **2021**, *8*, 3990–4023. [CrossRef]
2. Lorente, A.; Makowski, K.; Albericio, F.; Álvarez, M. Bioactive Marine Polyketides as Potential and Promising Drugs. *Ann. Mar. Biol. Res.* **2014**, *1*, 1003.
3. Kobayashi, J.; Kubota, T. Bioactive Macrolides and Polyketides from Marine Dinoflagellates of the Genus *Amphidinium*. *J. Nat. Prod.* **2007**, *70*, 451–460. [CrossRef] [PubMed]
4. Parenty, A.; Moreau, A.X.; Campagne, J.-M. Macrolactonizations in the Total Synthesis of Natural Products. *Chem. Rev.* **2006**, *106*, 911–939. [CrossRef] [PubMed]
5. Nasir, N.M.; Ermanis, K.; Clarke, P.A. Strategies for the construction of tetrahydropyran rings in the synthesis of natural products. *Org. Biomol. Chem.* **2014**, *12*, 3323–3335. [CrossRef] [PubMed]
6. Fuwa, H. Contemporary Strategies for the Synthesis of Tetrahydropyran Derivatives: Application to Total Synthesis of Neopeltolide, a Marine Macrolide Natural Product. *Mar. Drugs* **2016**, *14*, 65. [CrossRef] [PubMed]
7. Barbero, H.; Díez-Poza, C.; Barbero, A. The Oxepane Motif in Marine Drugs. *Mar. Drugs* **2017**, *15*, 361. [CrossRef]
8. Fernandes, R.A.; Pathare, R.S.; Gorve, D.A. Advances in Total Synthesis of Some 2,3,5-Trisubstituted Tetrahydrofuran Natural Products. *Chem. Asian J.* **2020**, *15*, 2815–2837. [CrossRef]
9. Fernandes, R.A.; Gorve, D.A.; Pathare, R.S. Emergence of 2,3,5-trisubstituted tetrahydrofuran natural products and their synthesis. *Org. Biomol. Chem.* **2020**, *18*, 7002–7025. [CrossRef]
10. Lorente, A.; Lamariano-Merketegi, J.; Albericio, F.; Álvarez, M. Tetrahydrofuran-Containing Macrolides: A Fascinating Gift from the Deep Sea. *Chem. Rev.* **2013**, *113*, 4567–4610. [CrossRef]
11. Kigoshi, H.; Hayakawa, I. Marine cytotoxic macrolides haterumalides and biselides, and related natural products. *Chem. Rec.* **2007**, *7*, 254–264. [CrossRef] [PubMed]
12. Shabir, G.; Saeed, A. A Comparative Study of Synthetic Approaches Towards Total Synthesis of Mandelalide A, An Anti-Lung Cancer Metabolite from Lissoclinum Ascidian. *Curr. Org. Chem.* **2018**, *22*, 101–127. [CrossRef]
13. Zhang, H.; Zou, J.; Yan, X.; Chen, J.; Cao, X.; Wu, J.; Liu, Y.; Wang, T. Marine-Derived Macrolides 1990–2020: An Overview of Chemical and Biological Diversity. *Mar. Drugs* **2021**, *19*, 180. [CrossRef] [PubMed]
14. Nuzzo, G.; Gomes, B.A.; Luongo, E.; Torres, M.C.M.; Santos, E.A.; Cutignano, A.; Pessoa, O.D.L.; Costa-Lotufo, L.V.; Fontana, A. Dinoflagellate-Related Amphidinolides from the Brazilian Octocoral Stragulum bicolor. *J. Nat. Prod.* **2016**, *79*, 1881–1885. [CrossRef] [PubMed]
15. Valot, G.; Mailhol, D.; Regens, C.S.; O'Malley, D.P.; Godineau, E.; Takikawa, H.; Philipps, P.; Fürstner, A. Concise Total Syntheses of Amphidinolides C and F. *Chem. A Eur. J.* **2015**, *21*, 2398–2408. [CrossRef]
16. Ferrié, L.; Fenneteau, J.; Figadère, B. Total Synthesis of the Marine Macrolide Amphidinolide F. *Org. Lett.* **2018**, *20*, 3192–3196. [CrossRef] [PubMed]
17. Akwaboah, D.C.; Wu, D.; Forsyth, C.J. Stereoselective Synthesis of the C1–C9 and C11–C25 Fragments of Amphidinolides C, C2, C3, and F. *Org. Lett.* **2017**, *19*, 1180–1183. [CrossRef]
18. Su, Y.-X.; Dai, W.-M. Synthesis of the C18–C26 tetrahydrofuran-containing fragment of amphidinolide C congeners via tandem asymmetric dihydroxylation and S$_N$2 cyclization. *Tetrahedron* **2018**, *74*, 1546–1554. [CrossRef]
19. Namirembe, S.; Yan, L.; Morken, J.P. Studies toward the Synthesis of Amphidinolide C1: Stereoselective Construction of the C(1)–C(15) Segment. *Org. Lett.* **2020**, *22*, 9174–9177. [CrossRef]
20. Kim, C.H.; An, H.J.; Shin, W.K.; Yu, W.; Woo, S.K.; Jung, S.K.; Lee, E. Total Synthesis of (−)-Amphidinolide E. *Angew. Chem. Int. Ed.* **2006**, *45*, 8019–8021. [CrossRef]
21. Kim, C.H.; An, H.J.; Shin, W.K.; Yu, W.; Woo, S.K.; Jung, S.K.; Lee, E. Stereoselective Synthesis of (−)-Amphidinolide E. *Chem. Asian J.* **2008**, *3*, 1523–1534. [CrossRef]
22. Va, P.; Roush, W.R. Total Synthesis of Amphidinolide E. *J. Am. Chem. Soc.* **2006**, *128*, 15960–15961. [CrossRef] [PubMed]
23. Va, P.; Roush, W.R. Synthesis of 2-epi-Amphidinolide E: An Unexpected and Highly Selective C(2) Inversion during an Esterification Reaction. *Org. Lett.* **2007**, *9*, 307–310. [CrossRef] [PubMed]
24. Va, P.; Roush, W.R. Total synthesis of amphidinolide E and amphidinolide E stereoisomers. *Tetrahedron* **2007**, *63*, 5768–5796. [CrossRef] [PubMed]

25. Bosch, L.; Mola, L.; Petit, E.; Saladrigas, M.; Esteban, J.; Costa, A.M.; Vilarrasa, J. Formal Total Synthesis of Amphidinolide E. *J. Org. Chem.* **2017**, *82*, 11021–11034. [CrossRef] [PubMed]
26. Sanchez, D.; Andreou, T.; Costa, A.M.; Meyer, K.G.; Williams, D.R.; Barasoain, I.; Díaz, J.F.; Lucena-Agell, D.; Vilarrasa, J.; Sánchez-Pérez, D. Total Synthesis of Amphidinolide K, a Macrolide That Stabilizes F-Actin. *J. Org. Chem.* **2015**, *80*, 8511–8519. [CrossRef]
27. Sasaki, M.; Kawashima, Y.; Fuwa, H. Studies toward the Total Synthesis of Amphidinolide N: Stereocontrolled Synthesis of the C13–C29 Segment. *Heterocycles* **2015**, *90*, 579. [CrossRef]
28. Kawashima, Y.; Toyoshima, A.; Fuwa, H.; Sasaki, M. Toward the Total Synthesis of Amphidinolide N: Synthesis of the C8–C29 Fragment. *Org. Lett.* **2016**, *18*, 2232–2235. [CrossRef]
29. Fujishima, Y.; Ogura, Y.; Towada, R.; Enomoto, M.; Kuwahara, S. Stereoselective synthesis of the C17–C29 fragment of amphidinolide N. *Tetrahedron Lett.* **2016**, *57*, 5240–5242. [CrossRef]
30. Ohta, M.; Kato, S.; Sugai, T.; Fuwa, H. Cobalt-Catalyzed Hartung–Mukaiyama Cyclization of γ-Hydroxy Olefins: Stereocontrolled Synthesis of the Tetrahydrofuran Moiety of Amphidinolide N. *J. Org. Chem.* **2021**, *86*, 5584–5615. [CrossRef] [PubMed]
31. Ochiai, K.; Kuppusamy, S.; Yasui, Y.; Okano, T.; Matsumoto, Y.; Gupta, N.R.; Takahashi, Y.; Kubota, T.; Kobayashi, J.; Hayashi, Y. Total Synthesis of the 7,10-Epimer of the Proposed Structure of Amphidinolide N, Part I: Synthesis of the C1-C13 Subunit. *Chem. A Eur. J.* **2016**, *22*, 3282–3286. [CrossRef]
32. Ochiai, K.; Kuppusamy, S.; Yasui, Y.; Harada, K.; Gupta, N.R.; Takahashi, Y.; Kubota, T.; Kobayashi, J.; Hayashi, Y. Total Synthesis of the 7,10-Epimer of the Proposed Structure of Amphidinolide N, Part II: Synthesis of C17-C29 Subunit and Completion of the Synthesis. *Chem. A Eur. J.* **2016**, *22*, 3287–3291. [CrossRef] [PubMed]
33. Trost, B.M.; Bai, W.-J.; Stivala, C.E.; Hohn, C.; Poock, C.; Heinrich, M.; Xu, S.; Rey, J. Enantioselective Synthesis of des-Epoxy-Amphidinolide N. *J. Am. Chem. Soc.* **2018**, *140*, 17316–17326. [CrossRef]
34. Tsuda, M.; Akakabe, M.; Minamida, M.; Kumagai, K.; Tsuda, M.; Konishi, Y.; Tominaga, A.; Fukushi, E.; Kawabata, J. Structure and Stereochemistry of Amphidinolide N Congeners from Marine Dinoflagellate *Amphidinium* Species. *Chem. Pharm. Bull.* **2021**, *69*, 141–149. [CrossRef] [PubMed]
35. Tsuda, M.; Endo, T.; Kobayashi, J. Amphidinolide T, Novel 19-Membered Macrolide from Marine Dinoflagellate *Amphidinium* sp. *J. Org. Chem.* **2000**, *65*, 1349–1352. [CrossRef]
36. Kobayashi, J.; Kubota, T.; Endo, A.T.; Tsuda, M. Amphidinolides T2, T3, and T4, New 19-Membered Macrolides from the Dinoflagellate *Amphidinium* sp. and the Biosynthesis of Amphidinolide T1. *J. Org. Chem.* **2001**, *66*, 134–142. [CrossRef]
37. Kubota, T.; Endo, T.; Tsuda, M., Shiro, M.; Kobayashi, J. Amphidinolide T5, a new 19-membered macrolide from a dinoflagellate and X-ray structure of amphidinolide T1. *Tetrahedron* **2001**, *57*, 6175–6179. [CrossRef]
38. Clark, J.S.; Romiti, F. Total Syntheses of Amphidinolides T1, T3, and T4. *Angew. Chem.* **2013**, *125*, 10256–10259. [CrossRef]
39. Ueda, K.; Hu, Y. Haterumalide B: A new cytotoxic macrolide from an Okinawan ascidian *Lissoclinum* sp. *Tetrahedron Lett.* **1999**, *40*, 6305–6308. [CrossRef]
40. Takada, N.; Sato, H.; Suenaga, K.; Arimoto, H.; Yamada, K.; Ueda, K.; Uemura, D. Isolation and structures of haterumalides NA, NB, NC, ND, and NE, novel macrolides from an Okinawan Sponge *Ircinia* sp. *Tetrahedron Lett.* **1999**, *40*, 6309–6312. [CrossRef]
41. Teruya, T.; Suenaga, K.; Maruyama, S.; Kurotaki, M.; Kigoshi, H. Biselides A–E: Novel polyketides from the Okinawan ascidian *Didemnidae* sp. *Tetrahedron* **2005**, *61*, 6561–6567. [CrossRef]
42. Hayakawa, I.; Kigoshi, H.; Okamura, M.; Suzuki, K.; Shimanuki, M.; Kimura, K.; Yamada, T.; Ohyoshi, T. Total Synthesis of Biselide A, A Cytotoxic Macrolide of Marine Origin. *Synthesis* **2017**, *49*, 2958–2970. [CrossRef]
43. Challa, V.R.; Kwon, D.; Taron, M.; Fan, H.; Kang, B.; Wilson, D.; Haeckl, F.P.J.; Keerthisinghe, S.; Linington, R.G.; Britton, R. Total synthesis of biselide A. *Chem. Sci.* **2021**, *12*, 5534–5543. [CrossRef] [PubMed]
44. Satoh, Y.; Kawamura, D.; Yamaura, M.; Ikeda, Y.; Ochiai, Y.; Hayakawa, I.; Kigoshi, H. Synthetic studies toward biselides. Part 1: Synthesis of the core carbon framework of biselides A, B, and E using Stille coupling. *Tetrahedron Lett.* **2012**, *53*, 1390–1392. [CrossRef]
45. Satoh, Y.; Yamada, T.; Onozaki, Y.; Kawamura, D.; Hayakawa, I.; Kigoshi, H. Synthetic studies toward biselides. Part 2: Synthesis of the macrolactone part of biselides A and B using allylic oxidation. *Tetrahedron Lett.* **2012**, *53*, 1393–1396. [CrossRef]
46. Hayakawa, I.; Suzuki, K.; Okamura, M.; Funakubo, S.; Onozaki, Y.; Kawamura, D.; Ohyoshi, T.; Kigoshi, H. Total Synthesis of Biselide E, a Marine Polyketide. *Org. Lett.* **2017**, *19*, 5713–5716. [CrossRef]
47. Řezanka, T.; Hanuš, L.; Dembitsky, V.M. Chagosensine, a New Chlorinated Macrolide from the Red Sea Sponge *Leucetta chagosensis*. *Eur. J. Org. Chem.* **2003**, *2003*, 4073–4079. [CrossRef]
48. Heinrich, M.; Murphy, J.J.; Ilg, M.K.; Letort, A.; Flasz, J.; Philipps, P.; Fürstner, A. Total Synthesis of Putative Chagosensine. *Angew. Chem. Int. Ed.* **2018**, *57*, 13575–13581. [CrossRef]
49. Heinrich, M.; Murphy, J.J.; Ilg, M.K.; Letort, A.; Flasz, J.T.; Philipps, P.; Fürstner, A. Chagosensine: A Riddle Wrapped in a Mystery Inside an Enigma. *J. Am. Chem. Soc.* **2020**, *142*, 6409–6422. [CrossRef]
50. Lu, C.-K.; Chen, Y.-M.; Wang, S.-H.; Wu, Y.-Y.; Cheng, Y.-M. Formosalides A and B, cytotoxic 17-membered ring macrolides from a marine dinoflagellate *Prorocentrum* sp. *Tetrahedron Lett.* **2009**, *50*, 1825–1827. [CrossRef]
51. Schulthoff, S.; Hamilton, J.Y.; Heinrich, M.; Kwon, Y.; Wirtz, C.; Fürstner, A. The Formosalides: Structure Determination by Total Synthesis. *Angew. Chem. Int. Ed.* **2021**, *60*, 446–454. [CrossRef] [PubMed]

52. Gajula, S.; Reddy, A.V.V.; Reddy, D.P.; Yadav, J.S.; Mohapatra, D.K. Stereoselective Synthesis of the C1–C16 Fragment of the Purported Structure of Formosalide B. *ACS Omega* **2020**, *5*, 10217–10224. [CrossRef]
53. Hirata, Y.; Uemura, D. Halichondrins-antitumor polyether macrolides from a marine sponge. *Pure Appl. Chem.* **1986**, *58*, 701–710. [CrossRef]
54. Li, J.; Yan, W.; Kishi, Y. Unified Synthesis of C1–C19 Building Blocks of Halichondrins via Selective Activation/Coupling of Polyhalogenated Nucleophiles in (Ni)/Cr-Mediated Reactions. *J. Am. Chem. Soc.* **2015**, *137*, 6226–6231. [CrossRef]
55. Yan, W.; Li, Z.; Kishi, Y. Selective Activation/Coupling of Polyhalogenated Nucleophiles in Ni/Cr-Mediated Reactions: Synthesis of C1–C19 Building Block of Halichondrin Bs. *J. Am. Chem. Soc.* **2015**, *137*, 6219–6225. [CrossRef] [PubMed]
56. Kim, D.-S.; Dong, C.-G.; Kim, J.T.; Guo, H.; Huang, J.; Tiseni, P.S.; Kishi, Y. New Syntheses of E7389 C14−C35 and Halichondrin C14−C38 Building Blocks: Double-Inversion Approach. *J. Am. Chem. Soc.* **2009**, *131*, 15636–15641. [CrossRef]
57. Dong, C.-G.; Henderson, J.A.; Kaburagi, Y.; Sasaki, T.; Kim, D.-S.; Kim, J.T.; Urabe, D.; Guo, H.; Kishi, Y. New Syntheses of E7389 C14−C35 and Halichondrin C14−C38 Building Blocks: Reductive Cyclization and Oxy-Michael Cyclization Approaches. *J. Am. Chem. Soc.* **2009**, *131*, 15642–15646. [CrossRef]
58. Yahata, K.; Ye, N.; Iso, K.; Naini, S.R.; Yamashita, S.; Ai, Y.; Kishi, Y. Unified Synthesis of Right Halves of Halichondrins A–C. *J. Org. Chem.* **2017**, *82*, 8792–8807. [CrossRef]
59. Yahata, K.; Ye, N.; Ai, Y.; Iso, K.; Kishi, Y. Unified, Efficient, and Scalable Synthesis of Halichondrins: Zirconium/Nickel-Mediated One-Pot Ketone Synthesis as the Final Coupling Reaction. *Angew. Chem.* **2017**, *129*, 10936–10940. [CrossRef]
60. Nicolaou, K.C.; Pan, S.; Shelke, Y.; Das, D.; Ye, Q.; Lu, Y.; Sau, S.; Bao, R.; Rigol, S. A Reverse Approach to the Total Synthesis of Halichondrin B. *J. Am. Chem. Soc.* **2021**, *143*, 9267–9275. [CrossRef]
61. Towle, M.J.; Salvato, K.A.; Budrow, J.; Wels, B.F.; Kuznetsov, G.; Aalfs, K.K.; Welsh, S.; Zheng, W.; Seletsky, B.M.; Palme, M.H.; et al. In vitro and in vivo anticancer activities of synthetic macrocyclic ketone analogues of halichondrin B. *Cancer Res.* **2001**, *61*.
62. Cigler, T.; Vahdat, L.T. Eribulin mesylate for the treatment of breast cancer. *Expert Opin. Pharmacother.* **2010**, *11*, 1587–1593. [CrossRef] [PubMed]
63. Swami, U.; Shah, U.; Goel, S. Eribulin in Cancer Treatment. *Mar. Drugs* **2015**, *13*, 5016–5058. [CrossRef]
64. Tsuda, M.; Oguchi, K.; Iwamoto, R.; Okamoto, Y.; Kobayashi, J.; Fukushi, E.; Kawabata, J.; Ozawa, T.; Masuda, A.; Kitaya, A.Y.; et al. Iriomoteolide-1a, a Potent Cytotoxic 20-Membered Macrolide from a Benthic Dinoflagellate *Amphidinium* Species. *J. Org. Chem.* **2007**, *72*, 4469–4474. [CrossRef] [PubMed]
65. Kumagai, K.; Tsuda, M.; Masuda, A.; Fukushi, E.; Kawabata, J. Iriomoteolide-2a, a Cytotoxic 23-Membered Macrolide from Marine Benthic Dinoflagellate *Amphidinium* Species. *Heterocycles* **2015**, *91*, 265. [CrossRef]
66. Akakabe, M.; Kumagai, K.; Tsuda, M.; Konishi, Y.; Tominaga, A.; Kaneno, D.; Fukushi, E.; Kawabata, J.; Masuda, A.; Tsuda, M. Iriomoteolides-10a and 12a, Cytotoxic Macrolides from Marine Dinoflagellate *Amphidinium* Species. *Chem. Pharm. Bull.* **2016**, *64*, 1019–1023. [CrossRef]
67. Akakabe, M.; Kumagai, K.; Tsuda, M.; Konishi, Y.; Tominaga, A.; Tsuda, M.; Fukushi, E.; Kawabata, J. Iriomoteolide-13a, a cytotoxic 22-membered macrolide from a marine dinoflagellate *Amphidinium* species. *Tetrahedron* **2014**, *70*, 2962–2965. [CrossRef]
68. Sakamoto, K.; Hakamata, A.; Tsuda, M.; Fuwa, H. Total Synthesis and Stereochemical Revision of Iriomoteolide-2a. *Angew. Chem. Int. Ed.* **2018**, *57*, 3801–3805. [CrossRef] [PubMed]
69. Sakamoto, K.; Hakamata, A.; Iwasaki, A.; Suenaga, K.; Tsuda, M.; Fuwa, H. Total Synthesis, Stereochemical Revision, and Biological Assessment of Iriomoteolide-2a. *Chem. A Eur. J.* **2019**, *25*, 8528–8542. [CrossRef]
70. Sikorska, J.; Hau, A.M.; Anklin, C.; Parker-Nance, S.; Davies-Coleman, M.; Ishmael, J.E.; McPhail, K.L. Mandelalides A–D, Cytotoxic Macrolides from a New *Lissoclinum* Species of South African Tunicate. *J. Org. Chem.* **2012**, *77*, 6066–6075. [CrossRef]
71. Lei, H.; Yan, J.; Yu, J.; Liu, Y.; Wang, Z.; Xu, Z.; Ye, T. Total Synthesis and Stereochemical Reassignment of Mandelalide A. *Angew. Chem.* **2014**, *126*, 6651–6655. [CrossRef]
72. Nazari, M.; Serrill, J.D.; Sikorska, J.; Ye, T.; Ishmael, J.E.; McPhail, K.L. Discovery of Mandelalide E and Determinants of Cytotoxicity for the Mandelalide Series. *Org. Lett.* **2016**, *18*, 1374–1377. [CrossRef]
73. Nazari, M.; Serrill, J.D.; Wan, X.; Nguyen, M.H.; Anklin, C.; Gallegos, D.A.; Smith, A.B.; Ishmael, J.E.; McPhail, K.L. New Mandelalides Expand a Macrolide Series of Mitochondrial Inhibitors. *J. Med. Chem.* **2017**, *60*, 7850–7862. [CrossRef] [PubMed]
74. Nguyen, M.H.; Imanishi, M.; Kurogi, T.; Smith, A.B., III. Total Synthesis of (−)-Mandelalide A Exploiting Anion Relay Chemistry (ARC): Identification of a Type II ARC/CuCN Cross-Coupling Protocol. *J. Am. Chem. Soc.* **2016**, *138*, 3675–3678. [CrossRef]
75. Nguyen, M.H.; Imanishi, M.; Kurogi, T.; Wan, X.; Ishmael, J.E.; McPhail, K.L.; Smith, A.B., III. Synthetic Access to the Mandelalide Family of Macrolides: Development of an Anion Relay Chemistry Strategy. *J. Org. Chem.* **2018**, *83*, 4287–4306. [CrossRef] [PubMed]
76. Reddy, K.M.; Yamini, V.; Singarapu, K.K.; Ghosh, S. Synthesis of Proposed Aglycone of Mandelalide A. *Org. Lett.* **2014**, *16*, 2658–2660. [CrossRef] [PubMed]
77. Yamini, V.; Reddy, K.M.; Krishna, A.S.; Lakshmi, J.K.; Ghosh, S. Formal total synthesis of mandelalide A. *J. Chem. Sci.* **2019**, *131*, 25. [CrossRef]
78. AnkiReddy, P.; AnkiReddy, S.; Sabitha, G. Synthetic Studies toward the Revised Aglycone of Mandelalide A. *ChemistrySelect* **2017**, *2*, 1032–1036. [CrossRef]
79. Brütsch, T.M.; Bucher, P.; Altmann, K.-H. Total Synthesis and Biological Assessment of Mandelalide A. *Chem. A Eur. J.* **2016**, *22*, 1292–1300. [CrossRef]

80. Nakashima, T.; Iwatsuki, M.; Ochiai, J.; Kamiya, Y.; Nagai, K.; Matsumoto, A.; Ishiyama, A.; Otoguro, K.; Shiomi, K.; Takahashi, Y.; et al. Mangromicins A and B: Structure and antitrypanosomal activity of two new cyclopentadecane compounds from *Lechevalieria aerocolonigenes* K10-0216. *J. Antibiot.* **2013**, *67*, 253–260. [CrossRef]
81. Nakashima, T.; Kamiya, Y.; Iwatsuki, M.; Takahashi, Y.; Omura, S. Mangromicins, six new anti-oxidative agents isolated from a culture broth of the actinomycete, *Lechevalieria aerocolonigenes* K10-0216. *J. Antibiot.* **2014**, *67*, 533–539. [CrossRef] [PubMed]
82. Takada, H.; Yamada, T.; Hirose, T.; Ishihara, T.; Nakashima, T.; Takahashi, Y.K.; Omura, S.; Sunazuka, T. Total Synthesis and Determination of the Absolute Configuration of Naturally Occurring Mangromicin A, with Potent Antitrypanosomal Activity. *Org. Lett.* **2017**, *19*, 230–233. [CrossRef] [PubMed]
83. Lu, S.; Sun, P.; Li, T.; Kurtán, T.; Mándi, A.; Antus, S.; Krohn, K.; Draeger, S.; Schulz, B.; Yi, Y.; et al. Bioactive Nonanolide Derivatives Isolated from the Endophytic Fungus *Cytospora* sp. *J. Org. Chem.* **2011**, *76*, 9699–9710. [CrossRef]
84. Ehrlich, G.; Stark, C.B.W. Total Synthesis of Cytospolide D and Its Biomimetic Conversion to Cytospolides M, O, and Q. *Org. Lett.* **2016**, *18*, 4802–4805. [CrossRef]
85. Chatterjee, S.; Mandal, G.H.; Goswami, R.K. Total Synthesis of Cytospolide Q. *ACS Omega* **2018**, *3*, 7350–7357. [CrossRef]
86. Ehrlich, G.; Stark, C.B.W. Synthesis of Cytospolide Analogues and Late-State Diversification Thereof. *J. Org. Chem.* **2019**, *84*, 3132–3147. [CrossRef] [PubMed]
87. Murakami, M.; Matsuda, H.; Makabe, K.; Yamaguchi, K. Oscillariolide, a novel macrolide from a blue-green alga *Oscillatoria* sp. *Tetrahedron Lett.* **1991**, *32*, 2391–2394. [CrossRef]
88. Williamson, R.T.; Boulanger, A.; Vulpanovici, A.; Roberts, M.A.; Gerwick, W.H. Structure and Absolute Stereochemistry of Phormidolide, a New Toxic Metabolite from the Marine Cyanobacterium *Phormidium* sp. *J. Org. Chem.* **2002**, *67*, 7927–7936. [CrossRef]
89. Lam, N.Y.S.; Muir, G.; Challa, V.R.; Britton, R.; Paterson, I. A counterintuitive stereochemical outcome from a chelation-controlled vinylmetal aldehyde addition leads to the configurational reassignment of phormidolide A. *Chem. Commun.* **2019**, *55*, 9717–9720. [CrossRef]
90. Ndukwe, I.E.; Wang, X.; Lam, N.Y.S.; Ermanis, K.; Alexander, K.L.; Bertin, M.J.; Martin, G.E.; Muir, G.; Paterson, I.; Britton, R.; et al. Synergism of anisotropic and computational NMR methods reveals the likely configuration of phormidolide A. *Chem. Commun.* **2020**, *56*, 7565–7568. [CrossRef]
91. Lorente, A.; Gil, A.; Fernández, R.; Cuevas, C.; Albericio, F.; Álvarez, M. Phormidolides B and C, Cytotoxic Agents from the Sea: Enantioselective Synthesis of the Macrocyclic Core. *Chem. Eur. J.* **2015**, *21*, 150–156. [CrossRef] [PubMed]
92. Gil, A.; Lorente, A.; Albericio, F.; Alvarez, M. Stereoselective Allylstannane Addition for a Convergent Synthesis of a Complex Molecule. *Org. Lett.* **2015**, *17*, 6246–6249. [CrossRef] [PubMed]
93. Gil, A.; Giarrusso, M.; Lamariano-Merketegi, J.; Lorente, A.; Albericio, F.; Álvarez, M. Toward the Synthesis of Phormidolides. *ACS Omega* **2018**, *3*, 2351–2362. [CrossRef] [PubMed]
94. Gil, A.; Lamariano-Merketegi, J.; Lorente, A.; Albericio, F.; Álvarez, M. Enantioselective Synthesis of the Polyhydroxylated Chain of Oscillariolide and Phormidolides A–C. *Org. Lett.* **2016**, *18*, 4485–4487. [CrossRef] [PubMed]
95. Gil, A.; Lamariano-Merketegi, J.; Lorente, A.; Albericio, F.; Álvarez, M. Synthesis of (E)-4-Bromo-3-methoxybut-3-en-2-one, the Key Fragment in the Polyhydroxylated Chain Common to Oscillariolide and Phormidolides A-C. *Chem. A Eur. J.* **2016**, *22*, 7033–7035. [CrossRef] [PubMed]
96. Kim, M.C.; Winter, J.M.; Cullum, R.; Li, Z.; Fenical, W. Complementary Genomic, Bioinformatics, and Chemical Approaches Facilitate the Absolute Structure Assignment of Ionostatin, a Linear Polyketide from a Rare Marine-Derived Actinomycete. *ACS Chem. Biol.* **2020**, *15*, 2507–2515. [CrossRef]
97. Liu, H.; Lin, S.; Jacobsen, K.M.; Poulsen, T.B. Chemical Syntheses and Chemical Biology of Carboxyl Polyether Ionophores: Recent Highlights. *Angew. Chem. Int. Ed.* **2019**, *58*, 13630–13642. [CrossRef]
98. Kevin, D.A., II; Meujo, D.A.F.; Hamann, M.T. Polyether ionophores: Broad-spectrum and promising biologically active molecules for the control of drug-resistant bacteria and parasites. *Expert Opin. Drug Discov.* **2009**, *4*, 109–146. [CrossRef]
99. Rutkowski, J.; Brzezinski, B. Structures and Properties of Naturally Occurring Polyether Antibiotics. *BioMed Res. Int.* **2013**, *2013*, 162513. [CrossRef]
100. Toeplitz, B.K.; Cohen, A.I.; Funke, P.T.; Parker, W.L.; Gougoutas, J.Z. Structure of ionomycin-A novel diacidic polyether antibiotic having high affinity for calcium ions. *J. Am. Chem. Soc.* **1979**, *101*, 3344–3353. [CrossRef]
101. Huczyński, A. Polyether ionophores—Promising bioactive molecules for cancer therapy. *Bioorganic Med. Chem. Lett.* **2012**, *22*, 7002–7010. [CrossRef] [PubMed]
102. Igarashi, Y.; Zhou, T.; Sato, S.; Matsumoto, T.; Yu, L.; Oku, N. Akaeolide, a Carbocyclic Polyketide from Marine-Derived Streptomyces. *Org. Lett.* **2013**, *15*, 5678–5681. [CrossRef] [PubMed]
103. Zhou, T.; Komaki, H.; Ichikawa, N.; Hosoyama, A.; Sato, S.; Igarashi, Y. Biosynthesis of Akaeolide and Lorneic Acids and Annotation of Type I Polyketide Synthase Gene Clusters in the Genome of *Streptomyces* sp. NPS554. *Mar. Drugs* **2015**, *13*, 581–596. [CrossRef] [PubMed]
104. Blunt, J.W.; Hartshorn, M.P.; McLennan, T.J.; Munro, M.H.G.; Robinson, W.T.; Yorke, S.C. Thyrsiferol: A squalene-derived metabolite of *Laurencia thyrsifera*. *Tetrahedron Lett.* **1978**, *19*, 69–72. [CrossRef]

105. Juang, S.-H.; Chiang, C.-Y.; Liang, F.-P.; Chan, H.-H.; Yang, J.-S.; Wang, S.-H.; Lin, Y.-C.; Kuo, P.-C.; Shen, M.-R.; Thang, T.D.; et al. Mechanistic Study of Tetrahydrofuran- acetogenins In Triggering Endoplasmic Reticulum Stress Response-apotoposis in Human Nasopharyngeal Carcinoma. *Sci. Rep.* **2016**, *6*, 39251. [CrossRef]
106. van Lint, M.J.; Hall, M.; Faber, K.; van Spanning, R.J.M.; Ruijter, E.; Orru, R.V.A. Stereoselective Chemoenzymatic Cascade Synthesis of the bis-THF Core of Acetogenins. *Eur. J. Org. Chem.* **2019**, *2019*, 1092–1101. [CrossRef]
107. Öztunç, A.; Imre, S.; Lotter, H.; Wagner, H. Two C15 bromoallenes from the red alga *Laurencia obtusa*. *Phytochemistry* **1991**, *30*, 255–257. [CrossRef]
108. Guella, G.; Chiasera, G.; Mancini, I.; Öztunç, A.; Pietra, F. Twelve-Membered O-Bridged Cyclic Ethers of Red Seaweeds in the Genus *Laurencia* Exist in Solution as Slowly Interconverting Conformers. *Chem. A Eur. J.* **1997**, *3*, 1223–1231. [CrossRef]
109. Guella, G.; Mancini, I.; Öztunç, A.; Pietra, F. Conformational Bias in Macrocyclic Ethers and Observation of High Solvolytic Reactivity at a Masked Furfuryl (=2-Furylmethyl) C-Atom. *Helv. Chim. Acta* **2000**, *83*, 336–348. [CrossRef]
110. Braddock, D.C.; Rzepa, H.S. Structural Reassignment of Obtusallenes V, VI, and VII by GIAO-Based Density Functional Prediction. *J. Nat. Prod.* **2008**, *71*, 728–730. [CrossRef]
111. Braddock, D.C.; Millan, D.S.; Pérez-Fuertes, Y.; Pouwer, R.H.; Sheppard, R.N.; Solanki, S.; White, A.J.P. Bromonium Ion Induced Transannular Oxonium Ion Formation−Fragmentation in Model Obtusallene Systems and Structural Reassignment of Obtusallenes V−VII. *J. Org. Chem.* **2009**, *74*, 1835–1841. [CrossRef] [PubMed]
112. Braddock, D.C.; Bhuva, R.; Millan, D.S.; Pérez-Fuertes, Y.; Roberts, C.A.; Sheppard, R.N.; Solanki, S.; Stokes, E.S.E.; White, A.J.P. A Biosynthetically-Inspired Synthesis of the Tetrahydrofuran Core of Obtusallenes II and IV. *Org. Lett.* **2007**, *9*, 445–448. [CrossRef]
113. Arthuis, M.; Beaud, R.; Gandon, V.; Roulland, E. Counteranion-Directed Catalysis in the Tsuji-Trost Reaction: Stereocontrolled Access to 2,5-Disubstituted 3-Hydroxy-Tetrahydrofurans. *Angew. Chem. Int. Ed.* **2012**, *51*, 10510–10514. [CrossRef]
114. Clarke, J.; Bonney, K.J.; Yaqoob, M.; Solanki, S.; Rzepa, H.S.; White, A.J.P.; Millan, D.S.; Braddock, D.C. Epimeric Face-Selective Oxidations and Diastereodivergent Transannular Oxonium Ion Formation Fragmentations: Computational Modeling and Total Syntheses of 12-Epoxyobtusallene IV, 12-Epoxyobtusallene II, Obtusallene X, Marilzabicycloallene C, and Marilzabicycloallene D. *J. Org. Chem.* **2016**, *81*, 9539–9552. [CrossRef]
115. Kubota, T.; Sakuma, Y.; Shimbo, K.; Tsuda, M.; Nakano, M.; Uozumi, Y.; Kobayashi, J. Amphezonol A, a novel polyhydroxyl metabolite from marine dinoflagellate *Amphidinium* sp. *Tetrahedron Lett.* **2006**, *47*, 4369–4371. [CrossRef]
116. Chen, W.; Liu, H.; Long, J.; Tao, H.; Lin, X.; Liao, S.; Yang, B.; Zhou, X.; Liu, Y.; Wang, J. Asperpentenone A, A novel polyketide isolated from the deep-sea derived fungus *Aspergillus* sp. SCSIO 41024. *Phytochem. Lett.* **2020**, *35*, 99–102. [CrossRef]
117. Patil, A.D.; Freyer, A.J.; Bean, M.F.; Carte, B.K.; Westley, J.W.; Johnson, R.K.; Lahouratate, P. The plakortones, novel bicyclic lactones from the sponge *Plakortis halichondrioides*: Activators of cardiac SR-Ca^{2+}-pumping ATPase. *Tetrahedron* **1996**, *52*, 377–394. [CrossRef]
118. Cafieri, F.; Fattorusso, E.; Taglialatela-Scafati, O.; di Rosa, M.; Ianaro, A. Metabolites from the sponge *plakortis simplex*. II.: Isolation of four bioactive lactone compounds and of a novel related amino acid. *Tetrahedron* **1999**, *55*, 13831–13840. [CrossRef]
119. Chianese, G.; Yu, H.-B.; Yang, F.; Sirignano, C.; Luciano, P.; Han, B.-N.; Khan, S.; Lin, H.-W.; Taglialatela-Scafati, O. PPAR Modulating Polyketides from a Chinese *Plakortis simplex* and Clues on the Origin of Their Chemodiversity. *J. Org. Chem.* **2016**, *81*, 5135–5143. [CrossRef]
120. Yong, K.W.L.; de Voss, J.J.; Hooper, J.N.A.; Garson, M.J. Configurational Assignment of Cyclic Peroxy Metabolites Provides an Insight into Their Biosynthesis: Isolation of Plakortolides, *seco*-Plakortolides, and Plakortones from the Australian Marine Sponge *Plakinastrella clathrata*. *J. Nat. Prod.* **2011**, *74*, 194–207. [CrossRef]
121. Akiyama, M.; Isoda, Y.; Nishimoto, M.; Narazaki, M.; Oka, H.; Kuboki, A.; Ohira, S. Total synthesis and absolute stereochemistry of plakortone E. *Tetrahedron Lett.* **2006**, *47*, 2287–2290. [CrossRef]
122. Semmelhack, M.F.; Hooley, R.J.; Kraml, C.M. Synthesis of Plakortone B and Analogs. *Org. Lett.* **2006**, *8*, 5203–5206. [CrossRef] [PubMed]
123. Paddon-Jones, G.C.; Hungerford, N.L.; Hayes, P.; Kitching, W. Efficient Palladium(II)-Mediated Construction of Functionalized Plakortone Cores. *Org. Lett.* **1999**, *1*, 1905–1907. [CrossRef]
124. Hayes, P.Y.; Kitching, W. Total Synthesis and Absolute Stereochemistry of Plakortone D. *J. Am. Chem. Soc.* **2002**, *124*, 9718–9719. [CrossRef]
125. Hayes, P.Y.; Kitching, W. Synthesis in the Plakortone Series: Plakortone E. *Heterocycles* **2004**, *35*, 173–177. [CrossRef]
126. Xie, X.-G.; Wu, X.-W.; Lee, H.-K.; Peng, X.-S.; Wong, H.N.C. Total Synthesis of Plakortone B. *Chem. A Eur. J.* **2010**, *16*, 6933–6941. [CrossRef] [PubMed]
127. Sun, X.-Y.; Tian, X.-Y.; Li, Z.-W.; Peng, X.-S.; Wong, H.N.C. Total Synthesis of Plakortide E and Biomimetic Synthesis of Plakortone B. *Chem. A Eur. J.* **2011**, *17*, 5874–5880. [CrossRef] [PubMed]
128. Sugimura, H.; Sato, S.; Tokudome, K.; Yamada, T. Stereoselective Formation of Tetrahydrofuran Rings via [3 + 2] Annulation: Total Synthesis of Plakortone L. *Org. Lett.* **2014**, *16*, 3384–3387. [CrossRef]
129. Li, J.; Li, C.; Riccio, R.; Lauro, G.; Bifulco, G.; Li, T.-J.; Tang, H.; Zhuang, C.-L.; Ma, H.; Sun, P.; et al. Chemistry and Selective Tumor Cell Growth Inhibitory Activity of Polyketides from the South China Sea Sponge *Plakortis* sp. *Mar. Drugs* **2017**, *15*, 129. [CrossRef]

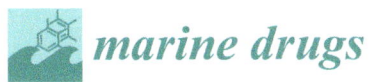

Article

Bacillimidazoles A–F, Imidazolium-Containing Compounds Isolated from a Marine *Bacillus*

Jia-Xuan Yan [1,†,‡], Qihao Wu [1,‡,§], Eric J. N. Helfrich [2,∥], Marc G. Chevrette [3,¶], Doug R. Braun [1], Heino Heyman [4,**], Gene E. Ananiev [5], Scott R. Rajski [1], Cameron R. Currie [3], Jon Clardy [2] and Tim S. Bugni [1,5,*]

- [1] Pharmaceutical Sciences Division, University of Wisconsin-Madison, 777 Highland Ave, Madison WI 53705, USA; jiaxuan.yan@merck.com (J.-X.Y.); qihao.wu@yale.edu (Q.W.); drbraun1@wisc.edu (D.R.B.); scott.rajski@wisc.edu (S.R.R.)
- [2] Harvard Medical School, Harvard University, 240 Longwood Ave, Boston, MA 02115, USA; eric.helfrich@bio.uni-frankfurt.de (E.J.N.H.); jon_clardy@hms.harvard.edu (J.C.)
- [3] Department of Bacteriology, University of Wisconsin-Madison, 1550 Linden Ave, Madison, WI 53706, USA; chevrette@wisc.edu (M.G.C.); currie@bact.wisc.edu (C.R.C.)
- [4] Bruker Daltonics, Bruker Scientific LLC., 40 Manning Rd, Billerica, MA 01821, USA; heino@metabolon.com
- [5] The Small Molecule Screening Facility (SMSF), University of Wisconsin-Madison, 600 Highland Ave, Madison, WI 53792, USA; geananiev@wisc.edu
- * Correspondence: tim.bugni@wisc.edu
- † Current addresses: Merck & Co. LLC., 126 E. Lincoln Ave, Rahway, NJ 07065, USA.
- ‡ These authors contributed equally to this work.
- § Current addresses: Departments of Chemistry & Microbial Pathogenesis, Institute of Biomolecular Design & Discovery, Yale University, West Haven, CT 06516, USA.
- ∥ Current address: LOEWE Centre for Translational Biodiversity Genomics, Institute of Molecular Bio-Science, Goethe University Frankfurt, 60487 Frankfurt am Main, Germany.
- ¶ Current address: Department of Plant Pathology, Wisconsin Institute for Discovery, University of Wisconsin-Madison, 425 G Henry Mall, Madison, WI 53706, USA.
- ** Current address: Metabolon Inc., 617 Davis Drive. Suite 100, Morrisville, NC 27560, USA.

Abstract: Chemical investigations of a marine sponge-associated *Bacillus* revealed six new imidazolium-containing compounds, bacillimidazoles A–F (**1–6**). Previous reports of related imidazolium-containing natural products are rare. Initially unveiled by timsTOF (trapped ion mobility spectrometry) MS data, extensive HRMS and 1D and 2D NMR analyses enabled the structural elucidation of **1–6**. In addition, a plausible biosynthetic pathway to bacillimidazoles is proposed based on isotopic labeling experiments and invokes the highly reactive glycolytic adduct 2,3-butanedione. Combined, the results of structure elucidation efforts, isotopic labeling studies and bioinformatics suggest that **1–6** result from a fascinating intersection of primary and secondary metabolic pathways in *Bacillus* sp. WMMC1349. Antimicrobial assays revealed that, of **1–6**, only compound **six** displayed discernible antibacterial activity, despite the close structural similarities shared by all six natural products.

Keywords: marine-derived *Bacillus*; antibacterial; biosynthetic gene cluster; isotopic enrichment; heterocycles; imidazolium

1. Introduction

Heterocyclic scaffolds are commonly encountered in natural products isolated from both terrestrial and marine organisms [1–4]. Their vast structural diversity, drug-like features, and biological properties have inspired both intensive efforts to discover new heterocyclic compounds, as well as imaginative total syntheses [4]. Nitrogen-containing heterocycles, such as pyrroles, imidazoles, oxazoles, pyridines, and quinolones, exhibit a diverse array of biological activities; these include, but are by no means limited to, antibacterial [5], antifungal [6], and anticancer [7] activities.

Marine-derived imidazole alkaloids have been one of the most fruitful families of bioactive compounds giving rise to many pharmaceutical leads [8]. Historically, marine-derived imidazole alkaloids have been most often isolated from sponges; imidazole alkaloids [9] featuring bromopyrrole-imidazoles [10], indole-containing imidazoles [11], and 2-aminoimidazoles are among the species most often identified from marine sponges [12]. Furthermore, in recent years, marine microorganisms have come to be viewed as sustainable and productive sources of new bioactive imidazole-containing natural products [9]. However, reports of positively charged imidazolium natural products remain relatively rare. Most reports of imidazolium-containing compounds feature 1,3-dimethyl-5-methylthiol [13–15] or 2-aminoimidazolium containing structures (guanidinium-like) [10,11]. A wide array of applications in ionic liquids [16], important biological activities [17], and their amenability to further structural modifications have made imidazolium salts an attractive target of contemporary research [18]. Therefore, discovering new imidazolium-based species and gaining further insight into their biosynthetic origins has become an interesting, yet challenging, task for natural product scientists.

2. Results & Discussion

As part of our ongoing efforts to discover new natural products from marine invertebrate-associated bacteria [19], we developed a streamlined discovery platform that includes strain prioritization by metabolomics [20] and an LC/MS fractionation platform to generate screening libraries [21]. Strain WMMC1349, a marine *Bacillus* sp. cultivated from the sponge *Cinachyrella apion*, drew our attention since one of its fractions displayed activity against methicillin-resistant *Staphylococcus aureus* (MRSA). Further purification of the active fraction by HPLC resulted in enrichment of an active subfraction. Interestingly, subsequent analytical HPLC revealed this fraction to be a represented by a broad peak (Figure S1) despite the clear presence of a mixture of compounds as revealed by ^{1}H NMR (Figure S1). Fortunately, Bruker timsTOF (trapped ion mobility spectrometry) MS data for this subfraction indicated a series of new molecules with m/z values of 305.2, 319.2, 344.4, 358.2, 383.2, and 397.2, respectively (Figure 1). Exhaustive attempts to separate each different m/z species (see Figures S1–S55), as initially visualized by timsTOF MS, ultimately afforded HPLC conditions amenable to clean separation and isolation of each discreet compound. The six new imidazolium-containing compounds, now differentiated from each other, were termed bacillimidazoles A–F (**1–6**, Figure 2), and all were assessed for in vitro activity against MRSA, *B. subtilis*, and *E. coli*; only compound **6** was found to be active (MRSA). Isotopic labelling of these metabolites using isotopically enriched culture media, and bioinformatic analysis were conducted to decipher the means by which the bacillimidazoles are biosynthesized.

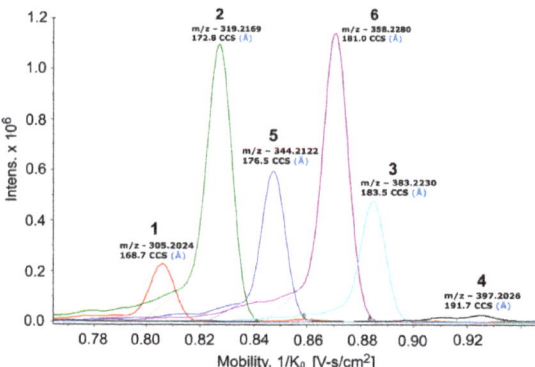

Figure 1. Bruker timsTOF MS spectrum of the bioactive wells against MRSA. Peak/compound assignments are shown above each relevant signal.

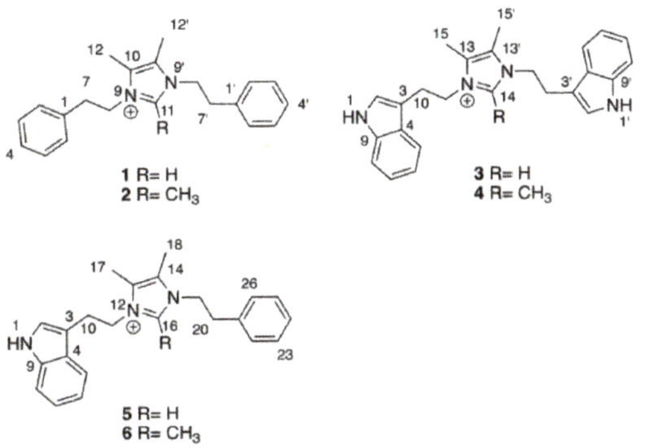

Figure 2. Structures of bacillimidazoles A–F (**1**–**6**) with central imidazolium numberings indicated for each subgroup.

The molecular formulae of bacillimidazoles A (**1**) and B (**2**) were determined to be $C_{21}H_{25}N_2^+$ (m/z = 305.2029, M$^+$, calcd 305.2012, Figure S37) and $C_{22}H_{27}N_2^+$ (m/z = 319.2171, M$^+$, calcd 319.2169, Figure S38), respectively, based on HRESIMS data. In the ^{13}C NMR spectra of **1** and **2** in Table 1, only 11 and 12 carbon signals were observed, respectively, suggesting symmetric scaffolds for both **1** and **2**. Furthermore, comparisons of ^{1}H and ^{13}C NMR data revealed a high degree of similarity between compound **1** and lepidiline A, an imidazolium-containing alkaloid isolated from the South American plants *Lepidium meyenii* Walp [22]. These similarities suggested the presence of a 4,5-dimethyl imidazolium cyclic structure and two phenyl-ring containing substituents in compound **1**. More highly refined datasets revealed that H$_2$-7 (δ_H 3.06) and H$_2$-8 (δ_H 4.35) showed COSY correlations (Figure 3) to each other. The HMBC correlations (Figure 3) were also observed from H$_2$-7 to C-2 (δ_C 130.0) and from H$_2$-8 (δ_H 4.35) to C-10 (δ_C 128.5), C-11 (δ_C 135.5), suggesting that –CH$_2$CH$_2$– groups linked the central imidazolium ring to two terminal phenyl rings, one on either side of the imidazolium. Therefore, the structure of **1** was assigned as a 1,3-difunctionalized imidazolium-containing structure. The NMR dataset of **2** was compared to that obtained for **1** and the only observable difference was an additional methyl group (δ_H, 2.01, H$_3$-13; δ_C 9.7, CH$_3$) substitution on C-11 (δ_C 144.0), which was determined by careful interpretation of the well resolved HMBC correlation from H$_3$-13 to C-11 (Figure 3).

Table 1. Summary of ^{1}H and ^{13}C NMR data for **1**–**4** (600 MHz for ^{1}H (500 MHz for **4**), 125 MHz for ^{13}C, CD$_3$OD).

Position	1		2		3		4	
	δ_C, Type	δ_H, (J in Hz)	δ_C, Type	δ_H, (J in Hz)	δ_C, Type	δ_H, (J in Hz)	δ_C, Type	δ_H, (J in Hz)
1, 1'	137.8, qC		138.2, qC					
2, 2'	130.0, CH	7.12, dd (8.0, 1.8)	130.2, CH	7.11, dd (8.0, 1.8)	124.4, CH	6.96, s	124.5, CH	6.98, s
3, 3'	130.0, CH	7.34, t (7.4)	130.1, CH	7.34, t (7.8)	110.5, qC		110.8, qC	
4, 4'	128.4, CH	7.30, t (7.4)	128.6, CH	7.32, t (7.8)	128.3, qC		128.4, qC	
5, 5'	130.0, CH	7.34, t (7.4)	130.1, CH	7.34, t (7.8)	118.4, CH	7.32, d (7.6)	118.2, CH	7.24, d (8.0)
6, 6'	130.0, CH	7.12, dd (8.0, 1.8)	130.2, CH	7.11, dd (8.0, 1.8)	120.1, CH	7.03, t (7.6)	120.2, CH	7.03, t (8.0)
7, 7'	37.1, CH$_2$	3.06, t (6.6)	36.3, CH$_2$	3.02, t (6.8)	122.8, CH	7.15, t (7.6)	122.9, CH	7.14, t (8.0)
8, 8'	49.3, CH$_2$	4.35, t (6.6)	47.9, CH$_2$	4.31, t (6.8)	112.6, CH	7.39, d (7.8)	112.7, CH	7.39, d (8.0)
9, 9'					138.1, qC		138.0, qC	
10, 10'	128.5, qC		127.1, qC		26.8, CH$_2$	3.07, t (6.8)	26.0, CH$_2$	3.03, t (6.0)
11, 11'	135.5 CH	8.51, s	144.0, qC		48.7, CH$_2$	4.25, t (6.8)	47.5, CH$_2$	4.19, t (6.0)
12, 12'	7.9, CH$_3$	2.08, s	8.2, CH$_3$	2.08, s				
13, 13'			9.7, CH$_3$	2.01, s	128.2, qC		127.0, qC	
14					135.4, CH	8.12, s	144.0, qC	
15, 15'					7.9, CH$_3$	2.09, s	8.3, CH$_3$	2.18, s
16							9.3, CH$_3$	1.64, s

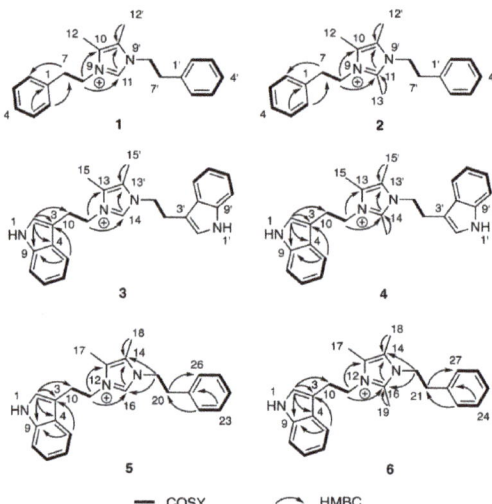

Figure 3. ¹H–¹H COSY and key HMBC correlations of compounds **1–6**.

The molecular formulae of bacillimidazole C (**3**) and bacillimidazole D (**4**) were identified as $C_{25}H_{27}N_4^+$ (m/z = 383.2228, M⁺, calcd 383.2230) and $C_{26}H_{29}N_4^+$ (m/z = 397.2385, M⁺, calcd 397.2387), respectively, by analyzing their HRMS data (Figures S39 and S40). Analysis of their ¹³C NMR data also suggested symmetrical structures for both **3** and **4**. In particular, detailed 1D NMR data analyses of **3** and **4** suggested that the central portion of each molecule bore a common imidazolium functionality. Overall, five sets of unassigned aromatic protons (H-2, δ_H 6.96; H-5, δ_H 7.32; H-6, δ_H 7.03; H-7, δ_H 7.15; H-8, δ_H 7.39) and eight unassigned aromatic carbons (C-2, δ_C 124.4; C-3, δ_C 110.5; C-4, δ_C 128.3; C-5, δ_C 118.4; C-6, δ_C 120.1; C-7, δ_C 122.8; C-8, δ_C 112.6; C-9, δ_C 138.1) were characteristic of the 3-indoyl structural motifs in **3**; the validity of this idea was verified by the observation of HMBC correlations from H-2 to C-3/C-4/C-9 and from H-5 to C-3/C-9 (Figure 3). Similar to **1** and **2**, the connection between –CH₂CH₂– groups and the aromatic building blocks in **3**, as well as the central imidazolium ring, was deduced by HMBC correlations from H-3 to C-10 and from H₂-11 to C-13/C-14 (Figure 3), respectively, establishing the full structural assignment of bacillimidazole C (**3**). Finally, in a fashion similar to that applied to **3**, the structure of **4**, with its additional imidazolium-linked methyl group, was elucidated.

Approaches employed to solve the structures of **1–4** also were applied to determine the structures of **5** and **6** in Table 2. Analysis of HRMS data for bacillimidazole E (**5**) and bacillimidazole F (**6**) made clear their molecular formulae as $C_{23}H_{26}N_3^+$ (m/z = 344.2134, M⁺, calcd 344.2121) and $C_{24}H_{28}N_3^+$ (m/z = 358.2283, M⁺, calcd 358.2278), respectively. In addition, review of their ¹³C NMR data suggested asymmetrical structures for both **5** and **6** since 23 ¹³C NMR signals were observed in **5** (24 signals for **6**). Additionally, comparisons of NMR data for **5** to those of **1** and **3** suggested the presence of an imidazolium ring, a phenyl ring, and a 3-indole ring in **5**. Furthermore, H-2 (δ_H 7.03), assigned to the indole ring, showed an HMBC correlation to C-10 (δ_H 26.5); and H-22 (δ_H 7.04), assigned to the phenyl ring, showed an HMBC correlation to C-20 (δ_C 36.7) (Figure 3). COSY correlations were observed between H₂-10 (δ_H 3.23) and H₂-11 (δ_H 4.36), H₂-19 (δ_H 4.18) and H₂-20 (δ_H 2.84). H₂-11 and H₂-19 both showed HMBC correlations to C-16 (δ_C 135.4), which was assigned to the imidazolium ring (Figure 3). Therefore, **5** was believed to contain an indole ring, an imidazolium ring, and a phenyl moiety (Figure 2). In addition, two –CH₂CH₂– groups were found to intervene the three different cyclic structural motifs. In applying the established correlation data, we thus elucidated structure **5** as shown in Figure 2. The structure of **6** was determined in a fashion similar to that employed for **5**, and was ultimately identified as an analog of **5** bearing a methyl group on the central imidazolium ring.

Table 2. Summary of ^{1}H and ^{13}C NMR data for 5 and 6 (600 MHz for ^{1}H. (500 MHz for 6), 125 MHz for ^{13}C, CD$_3$OD).

Position	5		6	
	δ_C, Type	δ_H, (J in Hz)	δ_C, Type	δ_H, (J in Hz)
1				
2	124.6, CH	7.03, s	124.6, CH	7.02, s
3	110.4, qC		110.8, qC	
4	128.4, qC		128.5, qC	
5	112.7, CH	7.40, dd (8.2, 1.0)	112.7, CH	7.37, d (7.8)
6	120.2, CH	7.04, dt (7.6, 1.2)	120.3, CH	7.00, t (7.8)
7	122.9, CH	7.15, dt (8.0, 1.0)	123.9, CH	7.12, t (7.8)
8	118.4, CH	7.34, dd (8.0, 1.0)	118.2, CH	7.23, d (7.8)
9	138.1, qC		138.1, qC	
10	26.5, CH$_2$	3.23, t (6.6)	26.0, CH$_2$	3.17, t (6.2)
11	48.9, CH$_2$	4.38, t (6.6)	47.7, CH$_2$	4.30, t (6.2)
12				
13	128.3, qC		127.1, qC	
14	128.3, qC		127.0, qC	
15				
16	135.4, CH	8.27, s	144.0, qC	
17	8.0, CH$_3$	2.12, s	8.3, CH$_3$	2.15, s
18	7.9, CH$_3$	2.04, s	8.2, CH$_3$	2.07, s
19	48.7, CH$_2$	4.18, t (7.2)	9.4, CH$_3$	1.77, s
20	36.7, CH$_2$	2.84, t (7.2)	47.6, CH$_2$	4.11, t (6.8)
21	137.8, qC		36.3, CH$_2$	2.77, t (6.8)
22	130.0, CH	7.04, d (7.2)	138.0, qC	
23	129.9, CH	7.29, m	130.1, CH	7.03, dd (7.3, 1.6)
24	128.3, CH	7.28, m	130.0, CH	7.30, m
25	129.9, CH	7.29, m	128.5, CH	7.26, m
26	130.0, CH	7.04, d (7.2)	130.0, CH	7.30, m
27			130.1, CH	7.03, dd (7.3, 1.6)

Following their structural elucidation, bacillimidazoles A–F (1–6) were tested for antibacterial activity against MRSA, *B. subtilis*, and *E. coli* (Table S1). All compounds failed to show any significant activity against *B. subtilis* and *E. coli*, although bacillimidazole F (6) did display weak activity against MRSA with an MIC of 38.3 µM.

To better understand the biosynthetic mechanisms involved in generating the uncommon imidazolium structures found in the bacillimidazoles, isotopic enrichment studies were carried out. In particular, we employed ^{13}C enriched culture media to glean vital insight into how the bacillimidazoles are constructed. By substituting two carbon sources, starch and D-glucose, with ^{13}C$_6$-D-glucose, we found that the four carbons composing the vicinal dimethyl olefin of bacillimidazoles C (3) and E (5) (Figures S43–S48) underwent substantial ^{13}C enrichment relative to all other carbons (Figure 4a). On the basis of these findings, we theorized that all carbons of the basic framework originate from amino acids whereas the dimethyl olefin elements of the bacillimidazoles are derived from glucose, presumably via a glycolytic process (Figure 4b). This logic is, of course, buoyed by the resemblance of the bacillimidazole sidechains to those found in phenylalanine and tryptophan. On the basis of these findings, we investigated the possibility of a biosynthetic pathway, as shown in Figure 4. It is well known that glucose is readily converted to 2,3-butadione along the canonical glycolytic pathway to acetolactate and subsequent processing of acetolactate to the essential 2,3-butadione, which can spontaneously react with either tryptamine or phenethylamine, both of which are common bacterial metabolites formed from the aromatic amino acids tryptophan and phenylalanine. These three components—two amines and a dione—provide most of the atoms of the imidazole moiety tethered through both nitrogens to various side chains. This diimine could undergo further spontaneous reactions with either one or two carbon carboxylic acids, or derivatives, and appropriate redox agents (or enzymes) to form the central imidazolium ring. Acetyl-CoA, or an equivalent, would produce the methylated compounds and formate, or a derivative, would produce the unmethylated bacillimidazoles. There is an alternative possibility in which the relevant amino acids condense with the butadione moiety prior to decarboxylation, and that the decarboxylation(s) of such intermediates might expedite imidazolium ring formation. While it is not possible at this stage to propose a detailed stepwise biosynthesis for the bacillimidazoles, an overall path with both enzymatic and spontaneous steps is likely, and the ^{13}C-glucose feeding studies clearly indicate the importance of glucose processing en route to imidazole assembly. That the production of bacillimidazoles by WMMC1349 is driven by secondary metabolism biosynthetic machineries and is not relegated only to primary metabolic events and/or extract workup conditions, is supported by the fact that, of six *bacilli* strains evaluated, only two (including WMMC1349) proved to be bacillimidazole producers (Figures S4–S6, S49–S54 and Table S2).

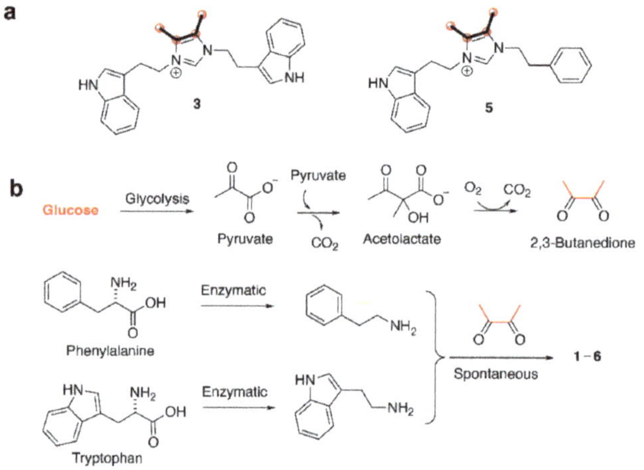

Figure 4. Biosynthesis of bacillimidazoles. (**a**) Isotopic labeling of bacillimidazoles C (**3**) and E (**5**). Carbons highlighted with bold bonds and red spheres showed high levels of ^{13}C incorporation. (**b**) Proposed biosynthetic pathway to compounds **1–6** calls for enzymatic production of tryptamine, phenethylamine and 2,3-butanedione (from glucose); all subsequent steps may proceed spontaneously.

Based on the biosynthetic insights gained from labelling experiments, we set out to identify the gene cluster responsible for the biosynthesis of **1–6**. We sequenced and assembled the genome of the producer, *Bacillus* sp. WMMC1349 [23]. The genome sequence was analyzed with state-of-the-art biosynthetic pipelines, yet no likely biosynthetic pathway for the biosynthesis of **1–6** was identified. We therefore mined the genome for the presence of the genes involved in acetoin biosynthesis, of which 2,3-butanedione, the proposed building block of **1–6**, is a precursor. We identified all of the genes responsible for acetoin biosynthesis in the genome of *Bacillus* sp. WMMC1349. Acetoin is biosynthesized from two molecules of pyruvate that are condensed to generate acetolactate. Acetolactate can either be enzymatically transformed into acetoin by a decarboxylase or can undergo spontaneous decarboxylation to yield the building block of **1–6**, 2,3-butanedione. A diacetyl reductase subsequently converts 2,3-butanedione into acetoin. Whole genome alignments of different *Bacillus* spp. revealed that the region upstream of the acetoin biosynthetic genes differs significantly from other *Bacillus* spp., including the model strain *B. subtilis* 168 (insertion of a large low-density coding region in *Bacillus* sp. WMMC1349), while the downstream region is homologous in all analyzed genomes. To our surprise, we were not able to identify a copy of the gene family encoding butanediol-dehydrogenases which was present in all other analyzed *Bacillus* spp. The absence of genes involved in acetoin catabolism would be expected to increase the concentration of the precursor 2,3-butanedione. Genome mining

(Section 4.5 below) of the bacillimidazole producer revealed the presence of a gene encoding an aromatic-L-amino acid decarboxylase, which is the proposed second enzyme essential for **1–6** biosynthesis en route to building blocks tryptamine and phenethylamine, respectively. No homologs of the aromatic-L-amino acid decarboxylase gene were identified in any other *Bacillus* genome analyzed, including the model strain *Bacillus subtilis* 168, indicating that the gene is facultative for the genus *Bacillus*. Relative to the biosynthetic machineries of most bacterial secondary metabolites, genes involved in acetoin biosynthesis and the aromatic-L-amino acid decarboxylase gene are not clustered. This observation suggests that the bacillimidazoles may form spontaneously from high-abundance primary metabolites with congruent reactivities. The biosynthesis of the bacillimidazoles is yet another example of the growing number of natural products that are produced partly by genetically coded instructions and partly by spontaneous reactivity—the joining of reactive intermediates, or products, from different pathways [24–26]. The initial formation of the bis-imines represents, for example, the unsurprising coupling of highly reactive primary amines with a very reactive alpha-diketone.

3. Conclusions

The isolation and structural elucidation of bacillimidazoles A–F, six imidazolium-containing heterocycles from marine *Bacillus* sp. WMMC1349 represent the discovery of a new class of marine-derived heterocyclic natural products. Isotopic labeling of **1–6** using ^{13}C enriched culture media, biomimetic synthetic approaches and bioinformatic analyses were performed in order to gain insights into the biosynthetic assembly of these interesting compounds. To the best of our knowledge, there are only a few reports of natural products containing 1,3-difunctionalized imidazolium moieties, and this is the first report of naturally occurring imidazolium-containing heterocycles. We contend, based on these findings, that the discovery of **1–6** contributes to our advancing knowledge of significantly underexplored biosynthetic pathways, specifically those that intersect primary and secondary metabolic pathways. We anticipate that the lessons learned here will help to expedite efforts to more fully understand and exploit the full biosynthetic potential of *Bacillus* spp.

4. Materials and Methods

4.1. General Experimental Procedures

UV spectra were recorded on an Aminco/OLIS UV-Vis spectrophotometer. IR spectra were measured with a Bruker Equinox 55/S FT-IR spectrophotometer. NMR spectra were obtained in CD$_3$OD (δ_H 3.34 ppm, δ_C 49.0 ppm) with a Bruker Avance 600 III MHz (Billerica, MA, USA) spectrometer equipped with a ^{1}H{^{13}C/^{15}N/^{31}P} cryoprobe, a Bruker Avance III 500 MHz (Billerica, MA, USA) spectrometer equipped with a ^{13}C/^{15}N{^{1}H} cryoprobe, and a Bruker Avance III HD 400 MHz (Billerica, MA, USA) spectrometer. HRMS data were acquired with a Bruker MaXis™ 4G ESI-QTOF (Billerica, MA, USA) mass spectrometer. RP HPLC was performed using a Shimadzu Prominence HPLC system and a Phenomenex Gemini C18 column (250 × 30 mm). UHPLC-HRMS was acquired using a Bruker MaXis™ 4G ESI-QTOF (Billerica, MA, USA) mass spectrometer coupled with a Waters Acquity UPLC system operated by Bruker Hystar software and a C18 column (Phenomenex Kinetex 2.6 μm, 2.1 mm × 100 mm). Bruker timsTOF Pro instrument (Billerica, MA, USA) was used for the trapped ion mobility MS analysis using direct infusion with 0.003 mL/min of flow rate and ESI+ ionization source. Nebulizer gas 0.4 bar, dry gas 3.5 L/min, source temperature 220 °C, ESI voltage 4200V (+). MS spectra were collected using the following parameters: tims ramp time = 350 ms, PASEF on, scan range (m/z, 20–1000; $1/k_0$, 0.70–1.00 V·s/cm^2.

4.2. Biological Material

Sponge specimens were collected on 27 May 2015 near the west shore of Ramrod Key (24°39′38.1″ N, 81°25′25.0″ W) in Florida. A voucher specimen is housed at the University of Wisconsin–Madison. For cultivation, a sample of sponge (1 cm^3) was ground in 500 µL sterile seawater, and dilutions were made using 500 µL sterile seawater. Subsequently, 400 µL of diluted sponge sample was added to 200 µL of sterile artificial seawater and 100 µL was plated using a sterile L-shaped spreader. Diluted samples were plated on Gauze 1 media supplemented with artificial seawater. Each medium was supplemented with 50 µg/mL cycloheximide, 25 µg/mL nystatin, and 25 µg/mL nalidixic acid. Plates were incubated at 28 °C and colonies were isolated over the course of two months.

4.3. Fermentation, Extraction and Isolation

Two 10 mL seed cultures (25 × 150 mm tubes) in medium DSC (20 g soluble starch, 10 g glucose, 5 g peptone, 5 g yeast extract per liter of artificial seawater) were inoculated with strain WMMC-1349 and shaken (200 RPM, 28 °C) for seven days. Two-liter flasks (1 × 500 mL) containing ASW-A (20 g soluble starch, 10 g D-glucose, 5 g peptone, 5 g yeast extract, 5 g CaCO$_3$ per liter of artificial seawater. For ^{13}C enriched ASW-A media, 10 g D-glucose (U-^{13}C$_6$, 99%) was used instead of soluble starch and D-glucose) were inoculated with 20 mL seed culture and were incubated (200 RPM, 28 °C) for seven days. Four-liter flasks (10 × 1 L) containing medium ASW-A with Diaion HP20 (7% by weight) were inoculated with 50 mL from the 500 mL culture and shaken (200 RPM, 28 °C) for seven days. For producing artificial sea water, solutions I (415.2 g NaCl, 69.54 g Na$_2$SO$_4$, 11.74 g KCl, 3.40 g NaHCO$_3$, 1.7 g KBr, 0.45 g H$_3$BO$_3$, 0.054 g NaF) and II (187.9 g MgCl$_2$·6H$_2$O, 22.72 g CaCl$_2$·2H$_2$O, 0.428 g SrCl$_2$·6H$_2$O) were made up separately using distilled water and combined to give a total volume of 20 L.

Filtered HP20 and cells were washed with H$_2$O and extracted with acetone. The acetone extract was subjected to liquid-liquid partitioning using 30% aqueous MeOH and CHCl$_3$ (1:1). The CHCl$_3$-soluble partition (3.12 g) was fractionated by Sephadex LH20 column chromatography (column size 500 × 40 mm, CHCl$_3$:MeOH = 1:1, 20 mL for each fraction). Fractions containing **1–6** (1.1 g) were subjected to RP HPLC (20%/80% to 100%/0% MeOH/H$_2$O (with 0.1% acetic acid), 23.5 min, 20 mL/min) using a Phenomenex Gemini C18 column (250 × 30 mm). The fraction collected between 16–18 min was further fractionated by RP HPLC (22%/78% to 51%/49% MeCN/H$_2$O (with 0.05% trifluoroacetic acid), 29.5 min, 20 mL/min) using a Phenomenex Gemini C18 column (250 × 30 mm), yielding **1** (50.2 mg, t_R 28.2 min), **2** (35.8 mg, t_R 27.6 min), **3** (2.2 mg, t_R 27.3 min), **4** (3.1 mg, t_R 28.9 min), **5** (40.5 mg, t_R 28.6 min), **6** (32.3 mg, t_R 29.3 min).

Bacillimidazole A (**1**): light yellow solid, UV-Vis (MeOH): λ_{max} (log ε) 211 nm (3.83), 259 nm (2.65), 279 nm (2.55), 291 nm (2.55); IR (ATR): υ_{max} 3385, 3144, 3033, 2935, 2873, 2834, 1781, 1679, 1563, 1498, 1456, 1399, 1357, 1199, 1129, 1083, 1029, 831, 801, 751, 720, 702 cm^{-1}; HRMS M$^+$ m/z = 305.2029 (calcd. for C$_{21}$H$_{25}$N$_2^+$ 305.2012). ^{1}H NMR (600 MHz, MeOD) δ_H 8.51 (s, 1H), 7.34 (t, J = 7.2 Hz, 4H), 7.31 (d, J = 7.2 Hz, 2H), 7.12 (d, J = 7.0 Hz, 4H), 4.35 (t, J = 7.0 Hz, 4H), 3.06 (t, J = 6.9 Hz, 4H), 2.08 (s, 6H). ^{13}C NMR (126 MHz, MeOD) δ_C 137.83, 135.53, 130.02, 129.97, 128.45, 128.44, 49.28, 37.07, 7.94.

Bacillimidazole B (**2**): light yellow solid, UV-Vis (MeOH): λ_{max} (log ε) 217 nm (3.85), 274 nm (3.02), 282 nm (3.04), 290 (2.97); IR (ATR): υ_{max} 3383, 3065, 3034, 2934, 2870, 1681, 1564, 1525, 1497, 1440, 1400, 1355, 1200, 1128, 1030, 934, 840, 801, 749, 722, 703 cm^{-1}; HRMS M$^+$ m/z = 319.2171 (calcd. for C$_{22}$H$_{27}$N$_2^+$ 319.2169). ^{1}H NMR (600 MHz, MeOD) δ_H 7.36–7.33 (m, 6H), 7.11 (d, J = 6.4 Hz, 4H), 4.31 (t, J = 6.7 Hz, 4H), 3.02 (t, J = 6.7 Hz, 4H), 2.08 (s, 6H), 2.01 (s, 3H). ^{13}C NMR (126 MHz, MeOD) δ_C 144.04, 138.15, 130.22, 130.08, 128.56, 127.14, 47.87, 36.33, 9.67, 8.21.

Bacillimidazole C (**3**): light yellow solid, UV-Vis (MeOH): λ_{max} (log ε) 223 nm (4.25), 274 nm (3.67), 282 nm (3.69), 290 nm (3.61); IR (ATR): υ_{max} 3357, 2946, 2835, 1679, 1564, 1449, 1432, 1341, 1203, 1185, 1137, 1024, 838, 802, 746, 722 cm^{-1}; HRMS M$^+$ m/z = 383.2228 (calcd. for C$_{25}$H$_{27}$N$_4^+$ 383.2230). ^{1}H NMR (600 MHz, MeOD) δ_H 8.12 (s, 1H), 7.39 (d, J = 8.1 Hz, 2H), 7.32 (d, J = 7.9 Hz, 2H), 7.15 (t, J = 7.4 Hz, 2H), 7.03 (t, J = 7.4 Hz, 2H), 6.96 (s, 2H), 4.25 (t, J = 6.7 Hz, 4H), 3.07 (t, J = 6.7 Hz, 4H), 2.09 (s, 9H). ^{13}C NMR (126 MHz, MeOD) δ_C 138.05, 135.37, 128.30, 128.19, 124.42, 122.83, 120.13, 118.43, 112.64, 110.49, 26.81, 7.94.

Bacillimidazole D (**4**): light yellow solid, UV-Vis (MeOH): λ_{max} (log ε) 224 nm (3.98), 281 nm (3.44), 290 nm (3.38); IR (ATR): υ_{max} 3360, 3292, 2925, 2854, 1729, 1648, 1561, 1456, 1411, 1342, 1256, 1235, 1181, 1105, 1073, 1025, 926, 744 cm^{-1}; HRMS M$^+$ m/z = 397.2385 (calcd. for $C_{26}H_{29}N_4^+$ 397.2387). ^{1}H NMR (500 MHz, MeOD) δ_H 7.39 (d, J = 8.0 Hz, 1H), 7.24 (d, J = 7.9 Hz, 1H), 7.14 (t, J = 7.5 Hz, 1H), 7.03 (t, J = 7.5 Hz, 1H), 6.98 (s, 1H), 4.19 (t, J = 5.9 Hz, 2H), 3.03 (t, J = 5.7 Hz, 2H), 2.18 (s, 3H), 1.64 (s, 1H). ^{13}C NMR (126 MHz, MeOD) δ_C 143.95, 138.00, 128.40, 126.96, 124.50, 122.88, 120.21, 118.23, 112.67, 110.76, 47.50, 25.97, 9.30, 8.29.

Bacillimidazole E (**5**): light yellow solid, UV-Vis (MeOH): λ_{max} (log ε) 221 nm (3.87), 274 nm (3.17), 282 nm (3.18), 290 (3.11); IR (ATR): υ_{max} 3376, 2991, 2950, 2836, 1677, 1564, 1497, 1456, 1398, 1356, 1341, 1201, 1134, 1078, 1025, 934, 834, 801, 747, 721, 703 cm^{-1}; HRMS M$^+$ m/z = 344.2134 (calcd. for $C_{23}H_{26}N_3^+$ 344.2121). ^{1}H NMR (600 MHz, MeOD) δ_H 8.27 (s, 1H), 7.40 (d, J = 8.2 Hz, 1H), 7.34 (d, J = 7.9 Hz, 1H), 7.32–7.26 (m, 3H), 7.15 (t, J = 7.4 Hz, 1H), 7.07–7.02 (m, 4H), 4.38 (t, J = 6.5 Hz, 2H), 4.18 (t, J = 7.2 Hz, 2H), 3.23 (t, J = 6.5 Hz, 2H), 2.84 (t, J = 7.2 Hz, 2H), 2.12 (s, 3H), 2.04 (s, 3H). ^{13}C NMR (126 MHz, MeOD) δ_C 138.08, 137.82, 135.44, 129.95, 129.87, 128.38, 128.34, 128.29, 128.27, 124.55, 122.85, 120.17, 118.37, 112.68, 110.42, 37.03, 26.76, 7.97, 7.89.

Bacillimidazole F (**6**): light yellow solid, UV-Vis (MeOH): λ_{max} (log ε) 225 nm (3.96), 274 nm (3.55), 282 nm (3.56), 290 nm (3.5^1); IR (ATR): υ_{max} 3356, 3275, 3062, 3001, 2971, 2928, 2830, 1647, 1562, 1497, 1454, 1401, 1353, 1234, 1203, 1179, 1108, 1077, 1028, 924, 745, 703 cm^{-1}; HRMS M$^+$ m/z = 358.2283 (calcd. for $C_{24}H_{28}N_3^+$ 358.2278). ^{1}H NMR (500 MHz, MeOD) δ_H 7.37 (d, J = 8.0 Hz, 1H), 7.28 (m, 3H), 7.23 (d, J = 7.9 Hz, 1H), 7.11 (t, J = 7.5 Hz, 1H), 7.06 – 6.97 (m, 3H), 4.31 (t, J = 5.5 Hz, 2H), 4.11 (t, J = 6.6 Hz, 2H), 3.17 (t, J = 5.5 Hz, 2H), 2.76 (t, J = 6.6 Hz, 2H), 2.15 (s, 2H), 2.07 (s, 3H), 1.77 (s, 3H). ^{13}C NMR (126 MHz, MeOD) δ_C 143.99, 138.09, 138.03, 130.07, 130.02, 128.47, 128.45, 127.06, 127.00, 124.64, 122.91, 120.28, 118.18, 112.72, 110.76, 47.74, 47.59, 36.27, 26.00, 9.43, 8.32, 8.18.

4.4. Antibacterial Testing

Bacillimidazoles A–F (**1**–**6**) were tested for antibacterial activity against *E. coli* (ATCC #25922), *B. subtilis* strain NRS-231, and Methicillin-resistant *Staphylococcus aureus* (MRSA) (ATCC #33591), and MICs were determined using a dilution antimicrobial susceptibility test for aerobic bacteria. Compounds **1**–**6** were dissolved in DMSO and serially diluted to 10 concentrations (0.25–128 µg/mL) in 96-well plates. Vancomycin was used as a positive control against *B. subtilis* and MRSA, and exhibited MIC values of 0.25 µg/mL. Gentamicin was used as a positive control against *E. coli*, and exhibited an MIC of 4 µg/mL. Bacillimidazoles, vancomycin, and gentamicin were tested in triplicate. On each plate, there were six untreated media controls. The plates were incubated at 37 °C for 18 h. The MICs were determined as the lowest concentration that inhibited visible growth of bacteria.

4.5. Sequencing and Identification of Candidate Bacillimidazole Biosynthetic Genes

16S rDNA sequencing was conducted as previously described [27]. WMMC1349 was identified as a *Bacillus* sp. The 16S sequence for WMMC1349 was deposited in GenBank (accession number MK892477). PacBio sequencing data were converted from BAM to FASTQ format using bedtools [28], and this fastq file was then corrected, trimmed, and assembled using Canu v1.8 [29], with an estimated genome size of 4.5 megabases (Mb). The resulting assembly was 4.677Mb over 10 contigs. It has an N50 of 4.03Mb and an L50 of 1.

Genome sequence (accession number JABJUQ000000000) was subjected to antiSMASH 5.0 analysis [30]. Results were analyzed by BLAST analysis. Acetoin and amino acid biosynthetic genes (KEGG) were identified in the bacillimidazole producer and selected model *Bacillus* spp. By BLAST analysis using Geneious 11.1.3 [31], and verified using additional online platforms such as Phyre2 [32]. Genomes of the producer of **1**–**6** and selected model *Bacillus* spp. were aligned using the MAUVE algorithm [33]. Promoter regions were identified using the BPROM algorithm [34].

Supplementary Materials: The following are available online at https://www.mdpi.com/article/10.3390/md20010043/s1. Detailed experimental discussions of isotopic enrichment studies and validation of bacillimidazoles as genuine natural products as well as Tables S1 & S2 summarizing all antibacterial data (Table S1), and bacillimidazole productivity of six *Bacilli* strains (Table S2). Also: Figure S1. Analytical HPLC analysis and ^{1}H NMR analysis of active subfractions. Figure S2. LC-MS analysis (EIC *m/z* 383) of 3. Figure S3. LC-MS analysis (EIC *m/z* 397) of 4. Figure S4. LC-MS analysis of chemical reaction of tryptamine (10.0 mg/mL) and 2,3 butanedione (0.5 equivalent) in MeOH solution without HP-20 resin for 2 h. Figure S5. LC-MS analysis of chemical reaction of tryptamine (10.0 mg/mL) and 2,3 butanedione (0.5 equivalent) in MeOH solution with HP-20 resin for 2 h. Figure S6. LC-MS analysis of chemical reaction of tryptamine (10.0 mg/mL) and 2,3 butanedione (0.5 equivalent) in CHCl$_3$:MeOH = 1:1 solution for 24 h. Figure S7. ^{1}H NMR Spectrum of Bacillimidazole A (1, 600 MHz, CD$_3$OD). Figure S8. ^{13}C NMR Spectrum of Bacillimidazole A (1, 125 MHz, CD$_3$OD). Figure S9. gCOSY Spectrum of Bacillimidazole A (1, 600 MHz, CD$_3$OD). Figure S10. gHSQC Spectrum of Bacillimidazole A (1, 600 MHz, CD$_3$OD). Figure S11. gHMBC Spectrum of Bacillimidazole A (1, 600 MHz, CD$_3$OD). Figure S12. ^{1}H NMR Spectrum of Bacillimidazole B (2, 600 MHz, CD$_3$OD). Figure S13. ^{13}C NMR Spectrum of Bacillimidazole B (2, 125 MHz, CD$_3$OD). Figure S14. gCOSY Spectrum of Bacillimidazole B (2, 600 MHz, CD$_3$OD). Figure S15. gHSQC Spectrum of Bacillimidazole B (2, 600 MHz, CD$_3$OD). Figure S16. gHMBC Spectrum of Bacillimidazole B (2, 600 MHz, CD$_3$OD). Figure S17. ^{1}H NMR Spectrum of Bacillimidazole C (3, 600 MHz, CD$_3$OD). Figure S18. ^{13}C NMR Spectrum of Bacillimidazole C (3, 125 MHz, CD$_3$OD). Figure S19. gCOSY Spectrum of Bacillimidazole C (3, 600 MHz, CD$_3$OD). Figure S20. gHSQC Spectrum of Bacillimidazole C (3, 600 MHz, CD$_3$OD). Figure S21. gHMBC Spectrum of Bacillimidazole C (3, 600 MHz, CD$_3$OD). Figure S22. ^{1}H NMR Spectrum of Bacillimidazole D (4, 500 MHz, CD$_3$OD). Figure S23. ^{13}C NMR Spectrum of Bacillimidazole D (4, 125 MHz, CD$_3$OD). Figure S24. gCOSY Spectrum of Bacillimidazole D (4, 500 MHz, CD$_3$OD). Figure S25. gHSQC Spectrum of Bacillimidazole D (4, 500 MHz, CD$_3$OD). Figure S26. gHMBC Spectrum of Bacillimidazole D (4, 500 MHz, CD$_3$OD). Figure S27. ^{1}H NMR Spectrum of Bacillimidazole E (5, 600 MHz, CD$_3$OD). Figure S28. ^{13}C NMR Spectrum of Bacillimidazole E (5, 125 MHz, CD$_3$OD). Figure S29. gCOSY Spectrum of Bacillimidazole E (5, 600 MHz, CD$_3$OD). Figure S30. gHSQC Spectrum of Bacillimidazole E (5, 600 MHz, CD$_3$OD). Figure S31. gHMBC Spectrum of Bacillimidazole E (5, 600 MHz, CD$_3$OD). Figure S32. ^{1}H NMR Spectrum of Bacillimidazole F (6, 500 MHz, CD$_3$OD). Figure S33. ^{13}C NMR Spectrum of Bacillimidazole F (6, 125 MHz, CD$_3$OD). Figure S34. gCOSY Spectrum of Bacillimidazole F (6, 500 MHz, CD$_3$OD). Figure S35. gHSQC Spectrum of Bacillimidazole F (6, 500 MHz, CD$_3$OD). Figure S36. gHMBC Spectrum of Bacillimidazole F (6, 500 MHz, CD$_3$OD). Figure S37. Positive Ion HRESIMS of Bacillimidazole A (1). Figure S38. Positive Ion HRESIMS of Bacillimidazole B (2). Figure S39. Positive Ion HRESIMS of Bacillimidazole C (3). Figure S40. Positive Ion HRESIMS of Bacillimidazole D (4). Figure S41. Positive Ion HRESIMS of Bacillimidazole E (5). Figure S42. Positive Ion HRESIMS of Bacillimidazole F (6). Figure S43. ^{1}H NMR Spectrum of ^{13}C Labeled Bacillimidazole C (3, 500 MHz, CD$_3$OD). Figure S44. ^{13}C NMR Spectrum of ^{13}C Labeled Bacillimidazole C (3, 125 MHz, CD$_3$OD). Figure S45. ^{1}H NMR Spectrum of ^{13}C Labeled Bacillimidazole E (5, 500 MHz, CD$_3$OD). Figure S46. ^{13}C NMR Spectrum of ^{13}C Labeled Bacillimidazole E (5, 125 MHz, CD$_3$OD). Figure S47. Positive Ion HRESIMS of ^{13}C Enriched Bacillimidazole C (3). Figure S48. Positive Ion HRESIMS of ^{13}C Enriched Bacillimidazole E (5). Figure S49. LC-MS analysis of strain *Bacillus* sp. WMMC325. Figure S50. LC-MS analysis of strain *Bacillus* sp. WMMC331. Figure S51. LC-MS analysis of strain *Bacillus* sp. WMMC1349. Figure S52. LC-MS analysis of strain *Bacillus* sp. WMMC1350. Figure S53. LC-MS analysis of strain *Bacillus* sp. WMMC1351. Figure S54. LC-MS analysis of strain *Bacillus* sp. WMMC1352. Figure S55. Culture broth of six different marine *Bacillus* strains. Figure S56. Pictures for sponge hosts of six different marine *Bacillus* strains.

Author Contributions: Conceptualization, C.R.C., J.C. and T.S.B.; methodology, J.-X.Y., Q.W., J.C. and T.S.B.; formal analysis, J.-X.Y., Q.W., E.J.N.H., M.G.C., H.H.; investigation, J.-X.Y., Q.W., E.J.N.H., M.G.C., D.R.B., G.E.A.; resources, H.H. and T.S.B.; writing—original draft preparation, J.-X.Y., Q.W., E.J.N.H. and S.R.R.; writing—review and editing, Q.W., S.R.R., J.C., M.G.C. and T.S.B.; supervision, C.R.C., J.C. and T.S.B.; project administration, C.R.C., J.C. and T.S.B.; funding acquisition, C.R.C., J.C. and T.S.B. All authors have read and agreed to the published version of the manuscript.

Funding: This work was funded by NIH Grants U19AI109673, U19AI142720, and R01AT009874 in addition to the University of Wisconsin-Madison School of Pharmacy and the Graduate School at the University of Wisconsin. E.J.N.H. gratefully acknowledges funding by the Swiss National Science Foundation (Postdoctoral Mobility Fellowship). We would like to thank the Analytical Instrumentation Center at the School of Pharmacy, University of Wisconsin-Madison for the facilities to acquire spectroscopic data. This study made use of the National Magnetic Resonance Facility at Madison, which is supported by NIH grant P41GM103399 (NIGMS). Additional equipment was purchased with funds from the University of Wisconsin, the NIH (RR02781, RR08438), the NSF (DMB-8415048, OIA-9977486, BIR-9214394), and the USDA.

Conflicts of Interest: The authors declare no conflict of interest.

References

1. Lewis, J.R. Amaryllidaceae, Sceletium, imidazole, oxazole, thiazole, peptide and miscellaneous alkaloids. *Nat. Prod. Rep.* **2001**, *18*, 95–128. [CrossRef] [PubMed]
2. Jin, Z.; Li, Z.; Huang, R. Muscarine, imidazole, oxazole, thiazole, Amaryllidaceae and Sceletium alkaloids. *Nat. Prod. Rep.* **2002**, *19*, 454–476. [CrossRef] [PubMed]
3. Blunt, J.W.; Copp, B.R.; Keyzers, R.A.; Munro, M.H.G.; Prinsep, M.R. Marine Natural Products. *Nat. Prod. Rep.* **2017**, *34*, 235–294. [CrossRef] [PubMed]
4. Jin, Z. Muscarine, imidazole, oxazole and thiazole alkaloids. *Nat. Prod. Rep.* **2016**, *33*, 1268–1317. [CrossRef] [PubMed]
5. Ziar, N.; Montalvão, S.; Hodnik, Z.; Nawrot, D.A.; Žula, A.; Ilaš, J.; Kikelj, D.; Tammela, P.; Mašič, L.P. Antimicrobial activity of the marine alkaloids clathrodin and oroidin, and their synthetic analogues. *Mar. Drugs* **2014**, *12*, 940–963.
6. Hassan, W.; Edrada, R.; Ebel, R.; Wray, V.; Berg, A.; van Soest, R.; Wiryowidagdo, S.; Proksch, P. New imidazole alkaloids from the Indonesian sponge *Leucetta chagosensis*. *J. Nat. Prod.* **2004**, *67*, 817–822. [CrossRef] [PubMed]
7. Dyson, L.; Wright, A.D.; Young, K.A.; Sakoff, J.A.; McCluskey, A. Synthesis and anticancer activity of focused compound libraries form the natural product lead, oroidin. *Bioorg. Med. Chem.* **2014**, *22*, 1690–1699. [CrossRef]
8. Jin, Z. Muscarine, imidazole, oxazole and thiazole alkaloids. *Nat. Prod. Rep.* **2013**, *30*, 869–915. [CrossRef]
9. Jin, Z. Muscarine, imidazole, oxazole and thiazole alkaloids. *Nat. Prod. Rep.* **2011**, *28*, 1143–1191. [CrossRef] [PubMed]
10. Tanaka, N.; Kusama, T.; Takahashi-Nakaguchi, A.; Gonoi, T.; Fromont, J.; Kobayashi, J. Nagelamides X-Z, dimeric bromopyrrole alkaloids from a marine sponge *Agelas* sp. *Org. Lett.* **2013**, *15*, 3262–3265. [CrossRef]
11. Zhang, F.; Wang, B.; Prasad, P.; Capon, R.J.; Jia, Y. Asymmetric total synthesis of (+)-dragmacidin D reveals unexpected stereocomplexity. *Org. Lett.* **2015**, *17*, 1529–1532. [CrossRef]
12. Gong, K.-K.; Tang, X.-L.; Liu, Y.-S.; Li, P.-L.; Li, G.-Q. Imidazole alkaloids form the South China Sea Sponge *Pericharax heteroraphis* and their cytotoxi and antiviral activities. *Molecules* **2016**, *21*, 150. [CrossRef]
13. Bourguet-Kondracki, M.L.; Martin, M.T.; Guyot, M. A New—Carboline Alkaloid Isolated from the Marine Sponge *Hyrtios erecta*. *Tetrahedron Lett.* **1996**, *37*, 3457–3460. [CrossRef]
14. Pedpradab, S.; Edrada, R.; Ebel, R.; Wray, V.; Proksch, P. New beta-carboline alkaloids form the Andaman Sea sponge *Dragmacidon* sp. *J. Nat. Prod.* **2004**, *67*, 2113–2116. [CrossRef] [PubMed]
15. Carroll, A.R.; Avery, V.M. Leptoclinidamines A-C, indole alkaloids from the Australian ascidian *Leptoclinides durus*. *J. Nat. Prod.* **2009**, *72*, 696–699. [CrossRef] [PubMed]
16. Malhotra, S.V.; Kumar, V.A. A profile of the in vitro anti-tumor activity of imidazolium-based ionic liquids. *Bioorg. Med. Chem. Lett.* **2010**, *20*, 581–585. [CrossRef] [PubMed]
17. Liu, L.-P.; Zong, M.-H.; Linhardt, R.J.; Lou, W.-Y.; Li, N.; Huang, C.; Wu, H. Mechanistic insights into the effect of imidazolium ionic liquid on liquid production by *Geotrichum fermentas*. *Biotechnol. Biofuels* **2016**, *9*, 266. [CrossRef] [PubMed]
18. Wright, B.D.; Deblock, M.C.; Wagers, P.O.; Duah, E.; Robishaw, N.K.; Shelton, K.L.; Southerland, M.R.; DeBord, M.A.; Kersten, K.M.; McDonald, L.J.; et al. Anti-tumor activity of lipophilic imidazolium salts on select NSCLC cell lines. *J. Med. Chem. Res.* **2015**, *24*, 2838–2861. [CrossRef] [PubMed]
19. Wyche, T.P.; Piotrowski, J.S.; Hou, Y.; Braun, D.; Deshpande, R.; Mcllwain, S.; Ong, I.M.; Myers, C.L.; Guzei, I.A.; Westler, W.M.; et al. Forazoline A: Marine-derived polyketide with antifungal in vivo activity. *Angew. Chem. Int. Ed.* **2014**, *53*, 11583–11586. [CrossRef] [PubMed]
20. Hou, Y.; Braun, D.R.; Michel, C.R.; Klassen, J.L.; Adnani, N.; Wyche, T.P.; Bugni, T.S. Microbial strain prioritization using metabolomics tools for the discovery of natural products. *Anal. Chem.* **2012**, *84*, 4277–4283. [CrossRef] [PubMed]
21. Zhang, F.; Barns, K.; Hoffmann, F.M.; Braun, D.R.; Andes, D.R.; Bugni, T.S. Thalassosamide, a Siderophore Discovered from the Marine-Derived Bacterium *Thalassospira profundimaris*. *J. Nat. Prod.* **2017**, *80*, 2551–2555. [CrossRef]
22. Cui, B.; Zheng, B.L.; He, K.; Zheng, Q.Y. Imidazole alkaloids from *Lepidium meyenii*. *J. Nat. Prod.* **2003**, *66*, 1101–1103. [CrossRef]
23. Wu, Q.; Throckmorton, K.; Maity, M.; Chevrette, M.G.; Braun, D.R.; Rajski, S.R.; Currie, C.R.; Thomas, M.G.; Bugni, T.S. Bacillibactins E and F from a Marine Sponge-Associated *Bacillus* sp. *J. Nat. Prod.* **2021**, *84*, 136–141. [CrossRef] [PubMed]

24. Hu, Y.; Potts, M.B.; Colosimo, D.; Herrera-Herrera, M.L.; Legako, A.G.; Yousufuddin, M.; White, M.A.; MacMillan, J.B. Discoipyrroles A–D: Isolation, structure determination, and synthesis of potent migration inhibitors from *Bacillus hunanensis*. *J. Am. Chem. Soc.* **2013**, *135*, 13387–13392. [CrossRef]
25. Mevers, E.; Saurí, J.; Helfrich, E.J.N.; Henke, M.; Barns, K.J.; Bugni, T.S.; Andes, D.; Currie, C.R.; Clardy, J. Pyronitrins A–D: Chimeric Natural Products Produced by *Pseudomonas protegens*. *J. Am. Chem. Soc* **2019**, *141*, 17098–17101. [CrossRef] [PubMed]
26. Wu, Q.; Li, S.W.; Xu, H.; Wang, H.; Hu, P.; Zhang, H.; Luo, C.; Chen, K.X.; Nay, B.; Guo, Y.W.; et al. Complex Polypropionates from a South China Sea Photosynthetic Mollusk: Isolation and Biomimetic Synthesis Highlighting Novel Rearrangements. *Angew. Chem. Int. Ed.* **2020**, *59*, 12105–12112. [CrossRef]
27. Wyche, T.P.; Hou, Y.; Braun, D.; Cohen, H.C.; Xiong, M.; Bugni, T.S. First natural analogs of the cytotoxic thiodepsipeptide thiocoraline A from a marine *Verrucosispora* sp. *J. Org. Chem.* **2011**, *76*, 6542–6547. [CrossRef] [PubMed]
28. Quinlan, A.R.; Hall, I.M. BEDTools: A flexible suite of utilities for comparing genomic features. *Bioinformatics* **2010**, *26*, 841–842. [CrossRef]
29. Koren, S.; Walenz, B.P.; Berlin, K.; Miller, J.R.; Bergman, N.H.; Phillippy, A.M. Canu: Scalable and accurate long-read assembly via adaptive *k*-mer weighting and repeat separation. *Genome Res.* **2017**, *27*, 722–736. [CrossRef]
30. Blin, K.; Shaw, S.; Steinke, K.; Villebro, R.; Ziemert, N.; Lee, S.Y.; Medema, M.H.; Weber, T. antiSMASH 5.0: Updates to the secondary metabolite genome mining pipeline. *Nucleic. Acids. Res.* **2019**, *47*, 81–87. [CrossRef]
31. For related approach see: Kerkhof, L.J.; Dillon, K.P.; Häggblom, M.M.; McGuinnes, L.R. Profiling bacterial communities by MinION sequencing of ribosomal operons. *Microbiome* **2017**, *5*, 116.
32. Kelley, L.A.; Mezulis, S.; Yates, C.M.; Wass, M.N.; Sternberg, M.J. The Phyre2 web portal for protein modeling, prediction and analysis. *Nat. Protoc.* **2015**, *10*, 845–858. [CrossRef]
33. Darling, A.E.; Mau, B.; Perna, N.T. progressiveMauve: Multiple genome alignment with gene gain, loss and rearrangement. *PLoS ONE* **2010**, *5*, e11147. [CrossRef] [PubMed]
34. Cassiano, M.H.A.; Silva-Rocha, R. Benchmarking Bacterial Promoter Prediction Tools: Potentialities and Limitations. *mSystems* **2020**, *5*, e00438-20. [CrossRef] [PubMed]

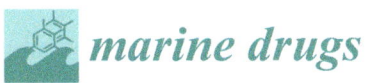

Review

Advances in Phenazines over the Past Decade: Review of Their Pharmacological Activities, Mechanisms of Action, Biosynthetic Pathways and Synthetic Strategies

Junjie Yan [1,†], Weiwei Liu [2,†], Jiatong Cai [1], Yiming Wang [1], Dahong Li [1,*], Huiming Hua [1,*] and Hao Cao [1,3,*]

1. Key Laboratory of Structure-Based Drug Design & Discovery, Ministry of Education, School of Traditional Chinese Materia Medica, Shenyang Pharmaceutical University, Shenyang 110016, China; yanjunjue0705@sina.cn (J.Y.); caijiatong1@sina.cn (J.C.); w1292720822@sina.cn (Y.W.)
2. Wuya College of Innovation, Shenyang Pharmaceutical University, Shenyang 110016, China; 104040219@syphu.edu.cn
3. School of Life Science and Biopharmaceutics, Shenyang Pharmaceutical University, Shenyang 110016, China
* Correspondence: lidahong@syphu.edu.cn (D.L.); huahuiming@syphu.edu.cn (H.H.); caohao@syphu.edu.cn (H.C.)
† These authors contributed equally to this work.

Abstract: Phenazines are a large group of nitrogen-containing heterocycles, providing diverse chemical structures and various biological activities. Natural phenazines are mainly isolated from marine and terrestrial microorganisms. So far, more than 100 different natural compounds and over 6000 synthetic derivatives have been found and investigated. Many phenazines show great pharmacological activity in various fields, such as antimicrobial, antiparasitic, neuroprotective, insecticidal, anti-inflammatory and anticancer activity. Researchers continued to investigate these compounds and hope to develop them as medicines. Cimmino et al. published a significant review about anticancer activity of phenazines, containing articles from 2000 to 2011. Here, we mainly summarize articles from 2012 to 2021. According to sources of compounds, phenazines were categorized into natural phenazines and synthetic phenazine derivatives in this review. Their pharmacological activities, mechanisms of action, biosynthetic pathways and synthetic strategies were summarized. These may provide guidance for the investigation on phenazines in the future.

Keywords: phenazine; pharmacological activity; mechanism of action; biosynthetic pathway; synthetic strategy

1. Introduction

Natural products are considered to be especially valuable resources for drug discovery. With the rapid development of technologies for isolation, purification and detection, great interest has been shown in the underexplored natural products. Natural phenazines are mainly discovered from microorganisms of marine and terrestrial. More than 100 natural phenazine derivatives and over 6000 synthetic phenazine derivatives have been investigated so far [1–4]. Phenazine derivatives are a large group of planar nitrogen-containing heterocyclic compounds and the most important core structure is a pyrazine ring (1,4-diazabenzene) with two annulated benzenes [5–7]. Phenazine derivatives differ in their chemical and physical properties based on the type and position of present functional groups. Their oxidation–reduction (redox) and fluorescent properties have attracted increasing attention. Some of them are significant dyes applied in medical and biological industry, while others are developed as efficient fluorescent probes to study the change of biochemical profile in vivo [8,9]. Natural phenazines are produced directly from various microorganisms, including *Pseudomonas* spp., *Streptomyces* spp., *Actinomycete* spp. in terrestrial and marine environments. They, like most other important secondary metabolites, possessed various biological activities and have been extensively studied for a long period of time [10,11]. Phenazines and their derivatives exhibit a broad range of biological activities, such as antimicrobial, antiparasitic, neuroprotective, insecticidal, anti-inflammatory, anticancer activity and so on [12–15]. Phenazine derivatives could be used as prodrugs due to biological activities, for which pharmacologists and chemists have committed themselves to make them into patent medicines. For example, clofazimine (Figure 1) is successfully applied in clinic as widely used antileprosy and antitubercular drug due to antimicrobial activity and immunosuppressive properties [16]. XR11576, XR5944, NC-182 and NC-190 (Figure 1) belong to fused aryl phenazine derivatives, also they show significant anticancer activity and are under clinical studies [7]. Phenazine derivatives display antibacterial activity mainly against methicillin-resistant due to redox properties [17]. According to reports in recent years, phenazine derivatives possessed antiproliferative activities against various cancer cell lines [18–21]. Additionally, phenazine derivatives were candidates to be developed as inhibitors of disease-related targets and reported to show activity of inhibition to multiple enzymes [22–25]. Although phenazine derivatives possessed a broad activity spectrum, the in-depth study was hindered due to the limited resource. Many research groups devoted themselves to carrying out the synthetic work to investigate biological activities of synthetic phenazine derivatives.

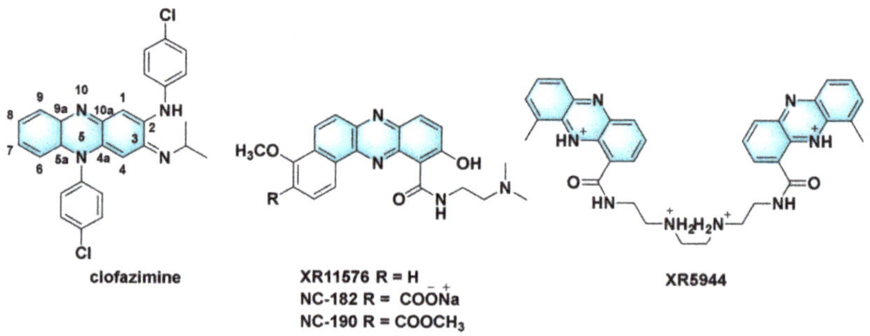

Figure 1. The chemical structures of clofazimine, XR11576, NC-182, NC-190 and XR5944.

Laursen et al. reviewed natural and synthetic phenazine derivatives with regard to biological activities in 2004 [6]. Phenazines and their derivatives had been associated with anticancer activity since 1959. On the basis of significant anticancer activity of phenazines and their derivatives, Cimmino et al. excellently reviewed natural and synthetic phenazines and derivatives about their anticancer activity and mechanisms of action in 2012, covering articles from 2000 to 2011 [26]. In recent years, researchers found various novel structures of natural phenazine derivatives and investigations of pharmacological activity were involved in many aspects. In this review, phenazines isolated from microorganisms, synthetic phenazine derivatives, their pharmacological activities and mechanisms of action were summarized, covering the articles from 2012 to 2021.

2. Natural Phenazine Derivatives

In the past decades, according to the published articles, many researchers investigated known phenazines deeply and further evaluated their potent biological activity. Other researchers tried to find novel phenazines from natural sources. Natural phenazines can be categorized according to the types of functional groups and their linking positions on the phenazine core.

2.1. Biological Activity of Known Phenazines

Compound **1** (phenazine-1-carboxylic acid, Figure 2) is also called tubermycin B due to its antibiotic activity against *Mycobacterium tuberculosis*. It is widely distributed in various microorganisms as a precursor of many natural phenazine derivatives. Gorantla et al. firstly reported its antifungal activity against major human pathogen, *Trichophyton rubrum*, which could be responsible for causing athlete's foot, jock itch, ringworm and fingernail fungus infections. The minimum inhibitory concentration (MIC) was 4 mg/mL [27]. Varsha et al. first isolated it from *Lactococcus* BSN307 and investigated its anticancer activity against HeLa cell line (IC_{50} = 20 µg/mL) and MCF-7 cells (IC_{50} = 24 µg/mL). It showed inhibitory activity towards leucine and proline aminopeptidases; thus, it would be used as a potential metalloenzyme inhibitor [28].

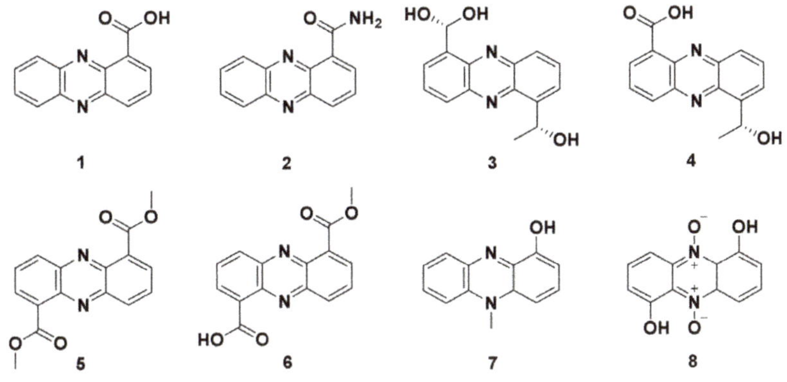

Figure 2. The chemical structures of classical phenazines 1–8.

Compound **2** (Figure 2) is also a significant phenazine-type metabolite produced by various microorganisms. Cardozo et al. investigated its antibacterial activity against MRSA (Methicillin-resistant *Staphylococcus aureus*) strains and found its synergic effect when combined with silver nanoparticles produced by *Fusarium oxysporum* [29]. Thanabalasingam et al. first isolated it from the leaves of a medicinal plant *Coccinia grandis* [30]. Tupe et al. tested its activity against human pathogen *Candida albicans* (MIC = 32–64 µg/mL), demonstrating its mechanism of antibacterial and antifungal activities via reactive oxygen species (ROS)-mediated apoptotic death; **2** could lead to production of intracellular ROS. ROS caused hyperpolarization of mitochondrial membrane, following externalizing phosphatidylserine, chromatin condensation and DNA fragmentation, thus, inducing apoptosis and, finally, cell death [31]. Kennedy et al. and Ali et al. further investigated anticancer mechanism of **2**. The anticancer activity mechanism was also connected with ROS. p53, Bax and cytochrome C (Cyto-C) were overexpressed while caspase-3 was activated and oncogenic, anti-apoptotic proteins such as poly ADP-ribose polymerase (PARP) and B-cell lymphoma-2 (Bcl-2) family proteins (Bcl-2, Bcl-w and Bcl-xL) were inhibited (Figure 3) [32,33].

Pyocyanin (**7**, Figure 2) is a redox-active phenazine. It is a major virulent factor produced by *Pseudomonas aeruginosa*, which exerts damage effects on mammalian cells. Chai et al. explored pathogenesis of **7** on macrophages. Biological data showed it could promote IL-8 secretion and mRNA expression in a concentration-dependent manner. Signal pathways of the protein kinase C (PKC) and nuclear factor-κ-gene binding (NF-κB) were involved in phorbol 12-myristate 13-acetate (PMA)-differentiated U937 cells infected by **7** [34]. Forbes et al. aimed to investigate the pyocyanin role of redox-sensitive mitogen-activated protein kinase (MAPK) by inducing toxicity in A549 cell line. The results showed that pyocyanin-induced cytotoxicity was different from c-Jun N-terminal Kinase (JNK) and p38MAPK signaling pathways. Acute ROS production and subsequent oxidative stress strengthened its toxicity [35]. 1,6-Dihydroxyphenazine 5,10-dioxide (**8**, Figure 2) is also called iodinin. It was discovered to show anti-bacterial activity and weak activity against a mouse tumor model. Sletta et al. firstly isolated it from *Streptosporangium* sp. DSM 45942 from the fjord sediment; **8** showed great antibacterial and antifungal activities against *Candida glabrata* and *Enterococcus faecium*, MIC ranging from 0.35–0.71 µg/mL.

Compared with normal rat kidney (NRK) fibroblasts, **8** showed higher selectivity towards leukemia cell line. It was a promising compound to be developed as an anticancer drug, especially those targeting leukemia [36]. Myhren et al. further investigated its anticancer potential against acute myeloid leukemia (AML) and acute promyelocytic leukemia (APL) cells. The results demonstrated its anticancer potency against two selective cancer cell lines and weak toxicity to normal cells. Molecular modeling results suggested that it could intercalate between bases in the DNA, leading to DNA-strand break. The apoptosis progress was associated with Fms-like tyrosine kinase (FLT3) internal tandem duplications, mutated/deficient p53 and activation of caspase-3 [37].

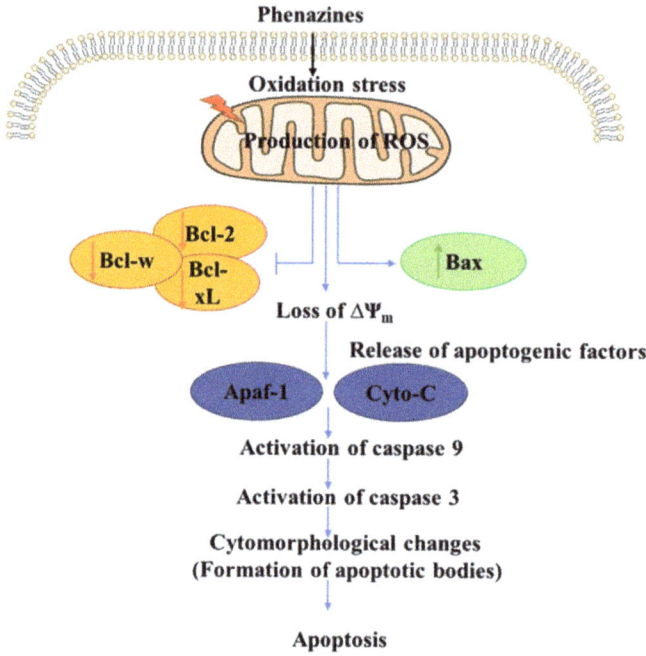

Figure 3. The anticancer mechanisms of action of reported phenazines which induced apoptosis associated via mitochondria mediated apoptotic pathways.

Lee et al. isolated compounds **1**, **3** and **4** (saphenic acid, Figure 2) from a deep-sea sediment-derived yeast-like fungus *Cystobasidium larynigs* IV17-028. These compounds could decrease the production of NO, thus showing inhibitory activity against lipopolysaccharide (LPS)-induced murine macrophage RAW 264.7 cells with EC_{50} values of 17.06 mg/mL (76.1 µM), 14.67 mg/mL (54.7 µM) and 6.15 mg/mL (22.9 µM), respectively [38].

Hifnawy et al. isolated compounds **1**, **5** (phenazine-1,6-dicarboxylate) and **6** (phencomycin) from actinomycetes, *Micromonospora* sp. UR56 and *Actinokineospora* sp. EG49. These compounds demonstrated high to moderate antibacterial and antibiofilm activities against four bacterial strains (*Staphylococcus aureus*, *Bacillus subtilis*, *Escherichia coli* and *Pseudomonas aeruginosa*), with modest cytotoxicity against four cell lines (WI38, HCT116, HepG-2 and MCF-7). They took *Staphylococcus* DNA gyrase-B and pyruvate kinase as targets. Subsequently, in vitro data showed that **1**, **5** and **6** (Figure 2) exerted their bacterial inhibitory activities through inhibiting *Staphylococcus* DNA gyrase-B and pyruvate kinase [39].

2.2. Natural Phenazines

2.2.1. Terpenoid Phenazines

Terpenoid phenazines contain common structural feature of isoprenylated C or N side chains and most of them show moderate or weak antibacterial activity. Kondratyuk et al. isolated marine phenazines **9** and **10** (Figure 4) from *Streptomyces* sp. strain CNS284: **9** demonstrated inhibitory activity of NF-κB and cyclooxygenase-2 (COX-2); **10** showed potent (sub-μM) inhibition activity of prostaglandin E2 (PGE2) production. However, these activities monitored did not have a strong correlation with each other. The mechanism of action was not apparent and needed to be further investigated [40]. Ohlendorf et al. isolated geranylphenazinediol (**11**, Figure 4) from a marine sediment *Streptomyces* sp. strain LB173 [41]: **11** bears geranylation at C-4 side. It showed weak antibacterial activity and great inhibitory activity toward human acetylcholinesterase (IC_{50} = 2.62 ± 0.35 μM). Phenaziterpenes A (**12**) and B (**13**, Figure 4) are structurally related to geranylphenazinediol, bearing *O*-geranylation. Song et al. isolated them from *Streptomyces lusitanus* SCSIO LR32. However, compounds **12** and **13** did not show antibacterial activity and cytotoxicity against tumor cell lines [42].

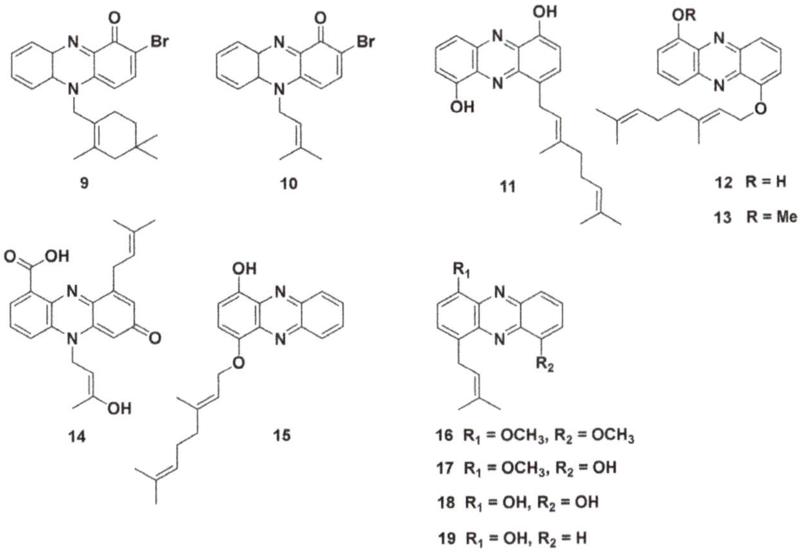

Figure 4. The chemical structures of compounds **9–19**.

Wu et al. isolated N-prenylated endophenazine **14** (Figure 4) from *Kitasatospora* sp. MBT66. **14** inhibited *B. subtilis* better than positive control drugs Ampicillin and Streptomycin [43]. Han et al. isolated several natural phenazines **15–19** (Figure 4) isolated from *Streptomyces* sp. NA04227; **15–19** showed moderate inhibitory activity against human acetylcholinesterase and moderate antibacterial activity against *Micrococcus luteus* (MIC = 4 μmol/L) [44].

2.2.2. Glycosylated Phenazines

A few natural glycosylated phenazines have so far been found and reported. The activity of glycosylated phenazines was not remarkable and needed to be further investigated. Rusman et al. firstly isolated deglycosylated phenazines (compounds **20–25**, Figure 5) from *Streptomyces* sp. Strain DL-93. None of the compounds exhibited any inhibitory activity against tested bacteria and fungi. However, **21**, **22** and **25** showed weak cytotoxicity against HCT-116 cancer cell line with EC_{50} values of 18 μM, 52 μM and 45 μM, respectively. In vitro biological assay data demonstrated that the weak cytotoxic activity was not associated with DNA intercalations and topoisomerase inhibition. The mechanisms of action were uncertain and needed to be further investigated [45].

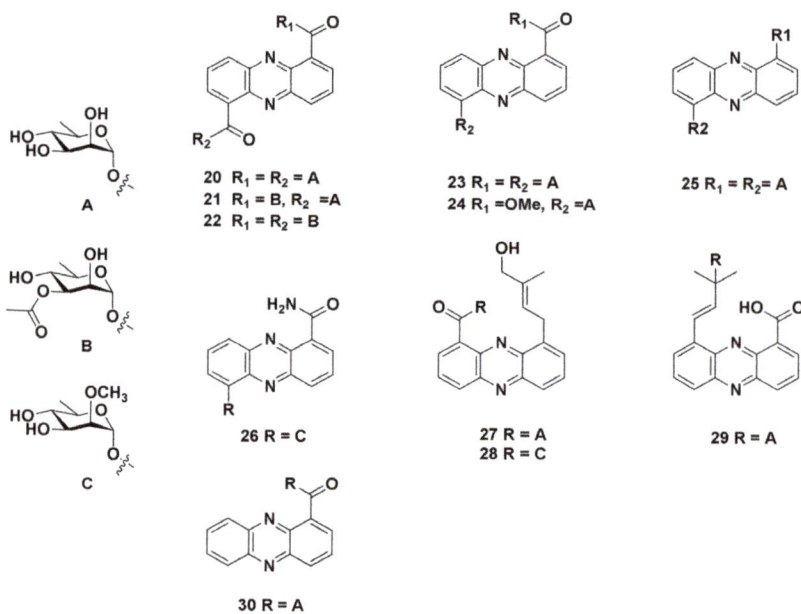

Figure 5. The chemical structures of compounds 20–30.

Wu et al. also isolated glycosylated endophenazines (compounds 26–30, Figure 5) from *Kitasatospora* sp. MBT66; 26 and 28 contain sugar moiety and the sugar is methylated at 2′-O position. These two compounds are rare in nature and firstly reported; 26–30 all showed antibacterial activity to some extent against Gram-positive *B. subtilis*. In addition, 26–28 and 30 also showed antimicrobial activity against Gram-negative *E. coli*. Interestingly, they found that glycosylated 27 and 28, compared with their corresponding aglycone, displayed enhanced activities against Gram-negative *E. coli* [43].

2.2.3. Divergent Fused Phenazines

This class of phenazines contains more than one phenazine-derived moiety. There are a few divergent fused phenazines in nature that have been reported so far. Li et al. isolated diastaphenazine (31, Figure 6) from an endophytic *Streptomyces diastaticus* subsp. *ardesiacus*: 31 was a cytotoxic dimeric phenazine, showing antibacterial activity against *S. aureus* (MIC = 64 μg/mL). However, 31 was inactive against *E. coli* and *C. albicans* even at 128 μg/mL. Compared with positive control (adriamycin), 31 showed weak cytotoxicity against HCT116, BGC-823, HepG2, HeLa and H460 cell lines with IC_{50} values of 14.9 μM, 28.8 μM, 65.2 μM and 82.5 μM, respectively [46].

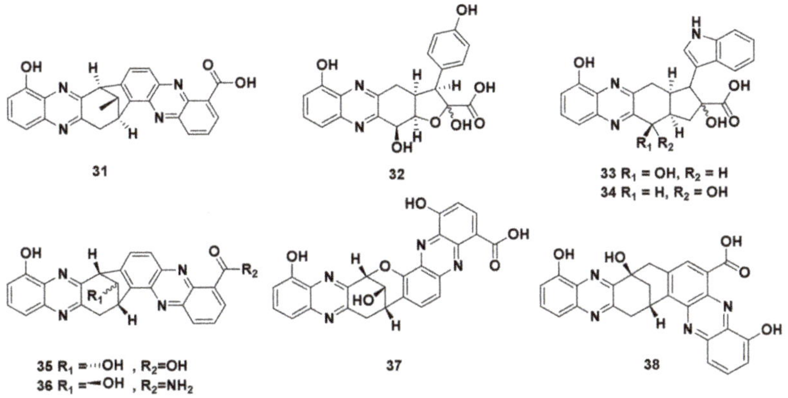

Figure 6. The chemical structures of compounds 31–38.

Baraphenazines A−C (32–34, Figure 6) are fused 5-hydroxyquinoxaline/alpha-keto acid amino acid compounds. Baraphenazines D and E (35 and 36, Figure 6) are special diastaphenazine-type compounds. In addition, baraphenazines F and G (37 and 38, Figure 6) are phenazinolin-type compounds. Wang et al. isolated them from *Streptomyces* sp. PU-10A and investigated their anticancer activity. Only 36 displayed appreciable activity against A549 and PC3 cell lines with IC$_{50}$ values of 2.4 µM and 4.7 µM, respectively. Structure-activity relationship (SAR) indicated that the group of amide on 36 was important to the anticancer activity. On the contrary, the group of free acid on 32−35, 37 and 38 was not benefit to the antiproliferative activity. These bioactivity data could explain a general toxicity-based mechanism of action [47].

2.2.4. Biological Activity of New Phenazines

Kennedy et al. isolated 5-methyl phenazine-1-carboxylic acid (39, Figure 7) from a rhizosphere soil bacterium. It showed selective cytotoxicity against A549 and MDA MB-231 cell lines in a dose-dependent manner, with IC$_{50}$ values of 488.7 nM and 458.6 nM, respectively. It exhibited antiproliferative activity by inhibiting cell viability, DNA synthesis and induced G1 cell cycle arrest and apoptosis in cancer cell lines. It was mediated by mitochondrial apoptotic pathway via activation of caspase-3 and down regulation of Bcl-2 expression [32].

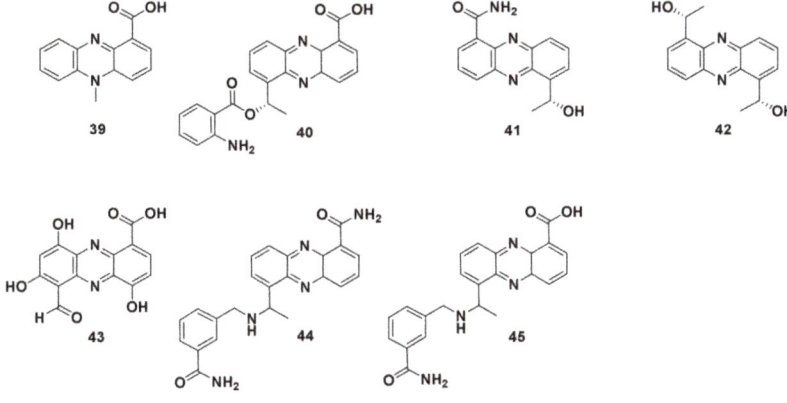

Figure 7. The chemical structures of compounds 39–45.

Lee et al. isolated compounds **40–42** (Figure 7) from yeast-like fungus *Cystobasidium larynigs* IV17-028. These compounds, except for compound **41**, could also inhibit the production of NO, thereby showing inhibitory activity against lipopolysaccharide (LPS)-induced murine macrophage RAW 264.7 cells with EC$_{50}$ values of 18.10 mg/mL (46.8 μM) and 6.15 mg/mL (22.9 μM), respectively [38]. Deng et al. isolated bioactive compound **43** (Figure 7) from *Streptomyces lomondensis* S015, which inhibited *Pythium ultimum*, *Rhizoctonia solani*, *Septoria steviae* and *Fusarium oxysporum* f. sp. *Niveum*, with MIC values of 16 μg/mL, 32 μg/mL, 16 μg/mL and 16 μg/mL, respectively. These biological data showed the potency of **43** as a promising hit for the further development as a biopesticide [48]. Cha et al. isolated compounds **44** and **45** (Figure 7) from *Streptomyces* sp. UT1123. These two compounds had a unique methylamine linker rather than common methyl ether. Additionally, **44** and **45** showed neuronal protective activity on HT-22 mouse hippocampal neuronal cells even in a low concentration [14].

3. The Progresses of Biosynthetic Pathways of Phenazines

McDonald et al. found that 2-amino-2-deoxyisochorismic acid could be completely converted into **1**. These compounds were mainly extracted from *Pseudomonas* spp. *PhzB*, *phzD*, *phzE*, *phzF*, *phzG* and so on, which belong to the *phz* gene family and they were proved to play important roles in phenazine synthesis [49]. Chorismic acid (**56**) was not only a common precursor for many primary and secondary metabolism but also the first substrate in biosynthetic pathway towards natural phenazines. Many important phenazines could be produced from microorganisms by this biosynthetic pathway. Combining with previous reports of Xu et al. and Blankenfeldt et al., the classical biosynthetic pathway towards strain-specific phenazines starting from chorismic acid is shown in Figure 8 [5,50].

Normally, the biosynthetic pathway in *Pseudomonas* mainly focused on simple modification of phenazine cores. Shi et al. reported a different biosynthetic pathway of various complex phenazines from the entomopathogenic bacterium *Xenorhabdus szentirmaii*. By modifying the core structure of phenazine, such as electron-rich aromatic rings, reduced form nitrogen(s) and carboxylic acid, a variety of natural phenazine derivatives can be generated. The synthesis of compound **59** is controlled by the typical *phz* operon in *X. szentirmaii* similar to classical biosynthetic pathway. Further modification of **59** was diversified by the enzymes from two discrete biosynthetic gene clusters. This progress of biosynthetic pathway was involved in multiple enzymatic and non-enzymatic reactions (Figure 9) [51].

Guo et al. developed a biosynthetic pathway to synthesize phenazine N-oxides in *Pseudomonas chlororaphis* HT66 (Figure 10). They used three enzymes, a monooxygenase (*phzS*), a monooxygenase (*phzO*) and the N-monooxygenase (*naphzNO1*). Additionally, *naphzNO1* only catalyzed the conversion of **80**, but failed to convert into **81** in vitro. This study also provided a promising method for the synthesis of aromatic N-oxides by *naphzNO1* [52].

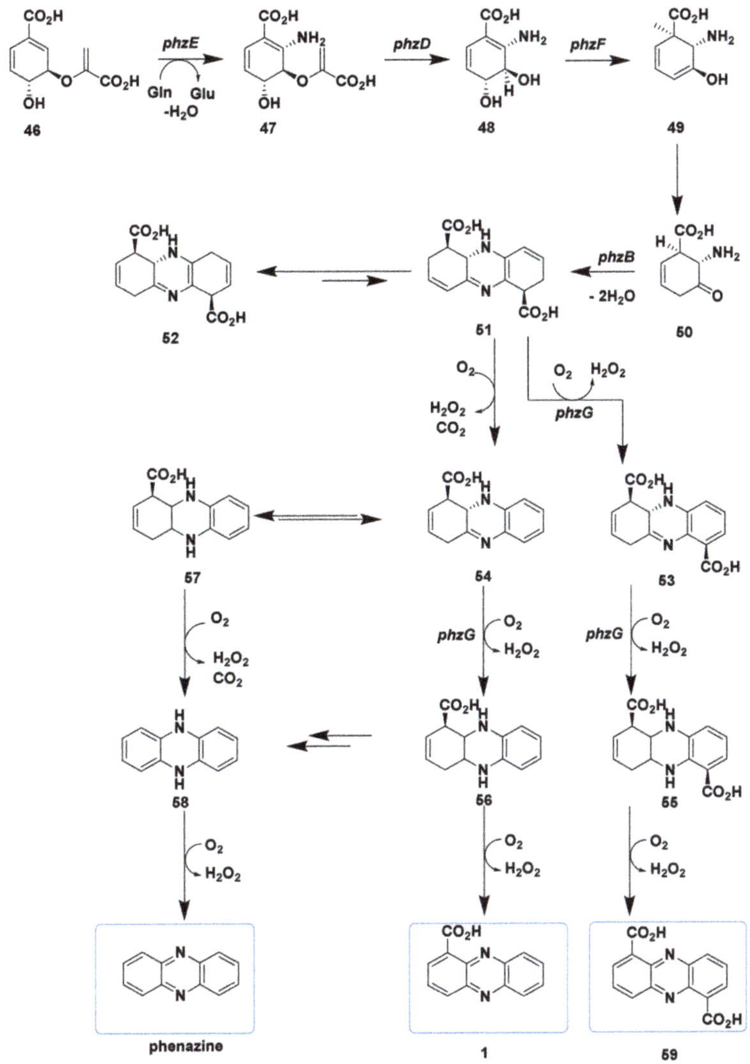

Figure 8. Classical biosynthetic pathway towards strain-specific phenazines starting from chorismic acid.

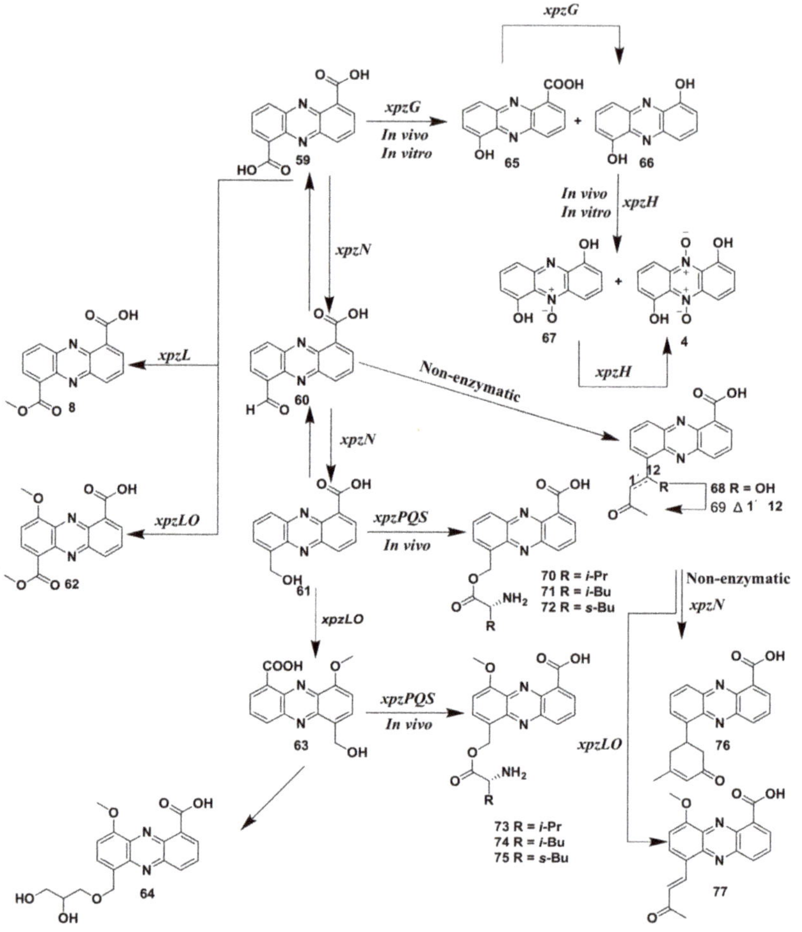

Figure 9. Complex phenazines **4, 8** and **59–77** and their biosynthetic pathway in *X. szentirmaii*.

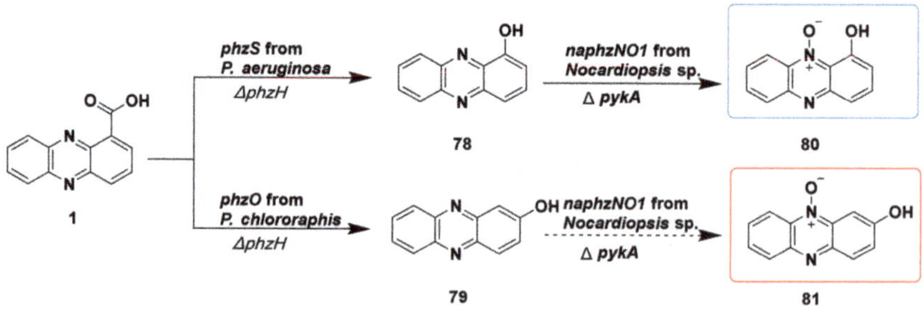

Figure 10. The designed biosynthetic pathway for phenazine N-oxides **80** and **81**.

4. Synthetic Phenazine Derivatives

Although natural phenazines possess a variety of biological activities, most of which show moderate or weak activity, thus lacking the possibility to be used as drugs. Structural modification and total synthesis are used to achieve some phenazine derivatives which show notable activity. Normally, the researchers focus on enhancing one special biological activity. Here, synthetic phenazine derivatives will be classified into the following categories in detail, with the perspective of biological activities and functional groups connected to phenazine core.

4.1. Antimicrobial Activity

4.1.1. Halogenated Phenazine Derivatives

According to related reports, bacterium would stop growth in MIC of 2–4 µg/mL and die in MIC of 2 µg/mL [48]. Halogenated phenazines derivatives are tested as antibacterial agents which could target multiple persistent bacterial phenotypes effectively and show negligible toxicity against mammalian cells. Antibacterial effect of halogenated phenazine derivatives could be attributed to membrane disruption, interference with redox cascades or electron-flow and the production of ROS [13,53]. Halogenated phenazine derivatives needed to be further developed by chemists due to the great antibacterial activity.

Conda-Sheridan et al. synthesized a series of phenazines derivatives inspired by some natural halogenated phenazines. They found N-(methylsulfonyl) amide group in the position of C-4 and halogenated group in the position of C-6 would remarkably improve the activity against MRSA. Compounds **82** and **83** (Figure 11) showed stronger antibacterial activity in these synthetic halogenated phenazines compared to positive drug vancomycin (MIC = 2 µg/mL). The mechanism of action of the most active compound was also investigated, but various tested biological data indicated that **83** did not have correlations with major reported antibacterial mechanisms. The in vitro IC_{50} values of **80** and **81** (Figure 11) against HaCaT cells (immortal keratinocytes) were 118 mM (**82**) and 193 mM (**83**), respectively; **83** seemed to be a promising molecule for the development of MRSA drugs. Additionally, the application of computational methods such as quantitative structure–activity relationship (QSAR) and the prediction of LogP would promote the development of antibacterial drugs [54].

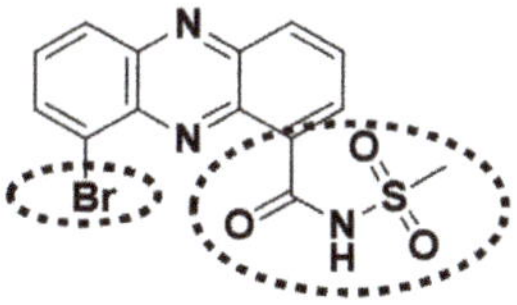

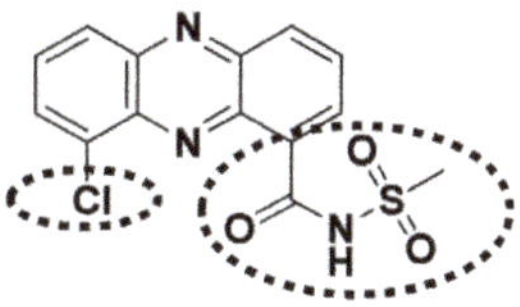

Figure 11. The chemical structures of compounds **82** and **83**.

Garrison et al. synthesized a series of phenazines derivatives modified in the positions of C-2, C-4, C-7 and C-8. Compound **84** (Figure 12) proved to be the most potent biofilm-eradicating agent (≥99.9% persister cell killing) against Methicillin-resistant *Staphylococcus aureus* (minimal biofilm eradication concentration (MBEC) < 10 µM), Methicillin-resistant *Staphylococcus epidermidis* (MBEC = 2.35 µM) and vancomycin-resistant *Enterococcus* (MBEC = 0.20 µM) biofilms, while compound **85** (Figure 12) demonstrated antibacterial activity against *M. tuberculosis* (MIC = 3.13 µM) [55]. Yang et al. explored a series of halogenated phenazines derivatives modified in the positions of C-4, C-6 and C-8. They discovered that 6-substituted halogenated phenazines derivatives could enhance biofilm eradication and antibacterial activities against Methicillin-resistant *Staphylococcus aureus*, Methicillin-resistant *Staphylococcus epidermidis* and vancomycin-resistant *Enterococcus*. In addition, Yang et al. synthesized a polyethylene glycol (PEG)-carbonate phenazine derivative **86** (Figure 12). Its water solubility was improved and demonstrated 30- to 100-fold enhancement of antibacterial activities against Methicillin-resistant *Staphylococcus aureus* strains, likely through a prodrug mechanism [53].

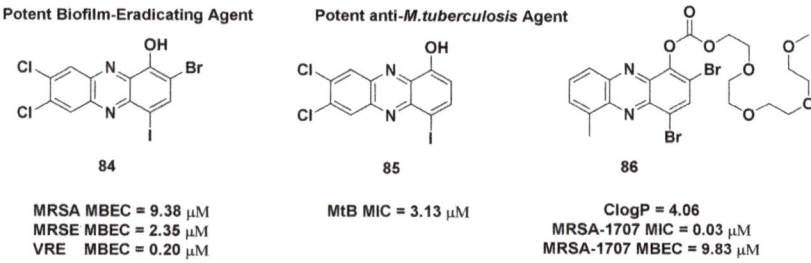

Figure 12. The chemical structures of compounds **84–86** and related activity data.

Borrero et al. synthesized several halogenated phenazine derivatives which were inspired by natural halogenated phenazine **87** (Figure 13); **87** was selected as a lead antibiotic which displayed great inhibitory activity against *S. aureus* (MIC= 1.56 µM). For example, the activity of **88** increased two folds by systematic structural diversification and the SAR was discussed as shown in Figure 13 [56].

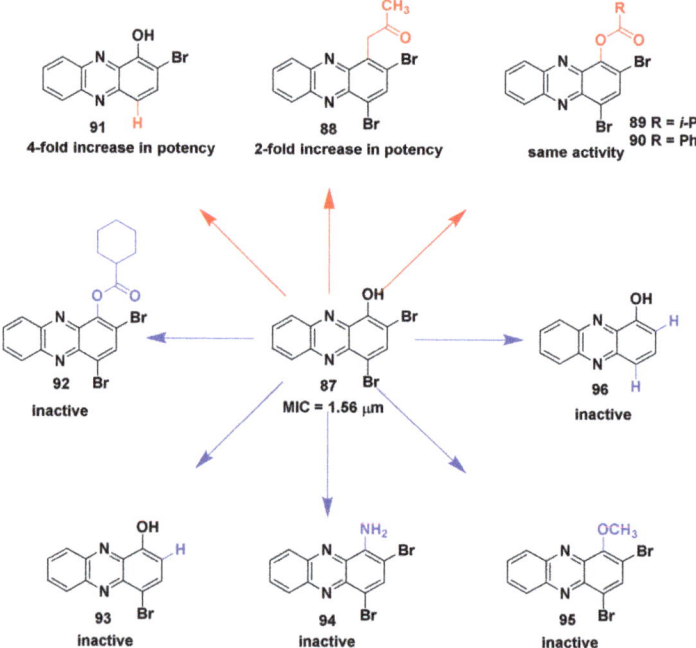

Figure 13. The chemical structures of compounds **87–96** and their inhibitory activity against *S. aureus*.

4.1.2. Derivatives of Clofazimine

Although clofazimine (Figure 14) is an antibiotic against multidrug-resistant *M. tuberculosis*, the clinical utility of this agent is limited by its poor physical and chemical properties and the possibility of skin discoloration. TBI-1004 and B4100, modified at different positions (Figure 14), showed stronger anti-*M. tuberculosis* activity than clofazimine. Zhang et al. designed and synthesized a series of riminophenazine derivatives which contained a pyridyl group at the C-3 position of the phenazine core, inspired by previous investigations about the developments of TBI-1004 and B4100. Among these derivatives, compound **97** (Figure 14) demonstrated similar activity against *M. tuberculosis*. Additionally, reduced the possibility of skin discoloration in an experimental mouse infection model as compared to clofazimine. In addition, physicochemical properties and pharmacokinetic profiles of **97** were improved [57].

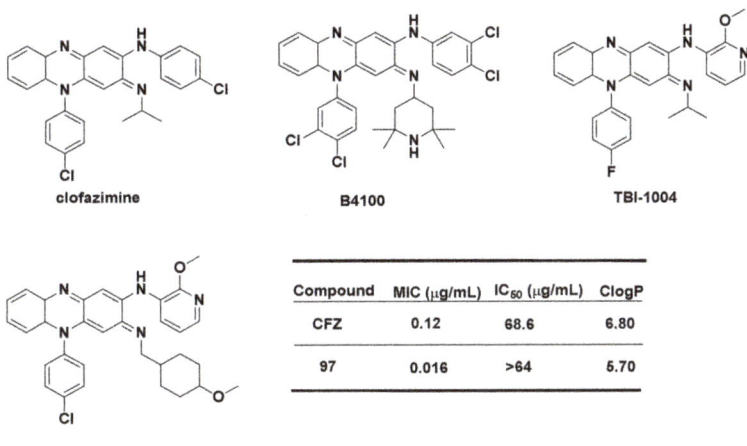

Figure 14. The chemical structures of clofazimine, B4100, TBI-1004, **97** and the data of related biochemical properties (MIC, IC_{50} and ClogP).

Tonelli et al. also synthesized a series of riminophenazine derivatives which contained quinolizidinylalkyl and pyrrolizidinylethyl moieties. These riminophenazine derivatives were tested against *M. tuberculosis* strains H37Rv and H37Ra, six clinical isolates of *M. avium* and *M. tuberculosis* and three mammalian cell lines (HMEC-1, MT-4 and Vero 76). The best compounds **98–101** (Figure 15) showed great inhibition against all strains of *M. tuberculosis* (MIC = 0.82–0.86 µM), **98** showed great inhibition against *M. avium* (MIC = 3.3 µM). The MIC values for clofazimine were 1.06 µM against *M. tuberculosis* and 4.23 µM against *M. avium*, respectively; **98** demonstrated a selectivity index (SI = 5.23) against the human cell line MT-4 comparable with clofazimine (SI = 6.4). Toxicity of **98** against mammalian Vero 76 cell line was quite low (SI = 79) [58].

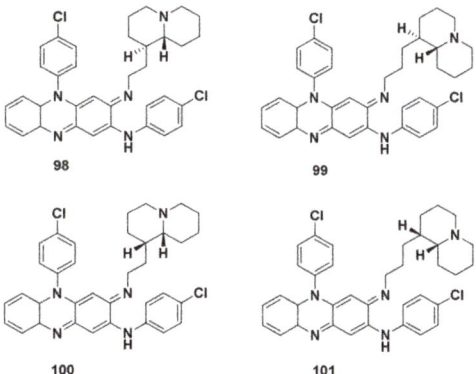

Figure 15. The chemical structures of compounds **98–101**.

4.1.3. Derivatives of Phenazine-1-carboxylic acid

Exemplified by compounds **1** and **2**, simple natural phenazines possess great fungicidal activities. Many groups continued to investigate their derivatives, hoping to discovery new eco-friendly agrochemicals. Niu et al. designed and synthesized derivatives of phenazine-1-carboxylic acid (**1**) linking with different amino-acid esters. Compounds **102–109** (Figure 16) showed greater activity than **1** (EC$_{50}$ = 66 μg/mL) with EC$_{50}$ values between 5.35 to 8.85 μg/mL. Particularly, **107** (EC$_{50}$ = 6.47 μg/mL) and **108** (EC$_{50}$ = 5.35 μg/mL) showed the best fungicidal activities against *Rhizoctonia solani* Kuhn and none of them had phloem mobility [59].

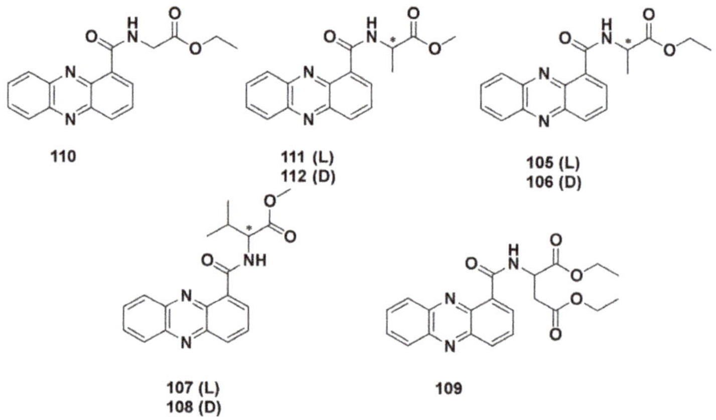

Figure 16. The chemical structures of compounds **102–109**.

Taking compound **2** as the lead compound, Zhu et al. designed and synthesized a series of phenazine-1-carboxylic acid (**1**) diamide derivatives. The fungicidal activities were tested by using the inhibitory ratio under 0.2 mmol/L (%) against six phytopathogenic fungi *Rhizoctonia solani*, *Fusarium graminearum*, *Alternaria solani*, *Fusarium oxysporum*, *Sclerotinia sclerotiorum* and *Pyricularia oryzac*. Although all derivatives had fungicidal activities to some degree, the inhibitory activities of most derivatives were lower than control (compound **1**). Compounds **121–124** (Scheme 1) demonstrated inhibitory rates more than 50% against *R. solani* and *A. solani*. Particularly, **121** showed the most potent fungicidal activity against *R. solani*, with the inhibitory rate of 72.7%. Compound **121** demonstrated the strongest fungicidal activity against *P. oryzae* with the inhibitory rate of 82.0% [60].

Han et al. designed and synthesized a series of phenazine-1-carboxylic (compound **1**) piperazine derivatives. Most phenazine-1-carboxylic piperazine derivatives showed fungicidal activities in vitro. Particularly, compound **125** (Figure 17) showed inhibitory activity against all tested pathogenic fungi (*R. solani*, *A. solani*, *F. oxysporum*, *F. graminearum* and *P. oryzac*) with EC$_{50}$ values of 24.6 μM, 42.9 μM, 73.7 μM, 73.8 μM and 34.2 μM, respectively [61]. Lu et al. designed and synthesized the derivatives based on the skeleton of **1**, which contained a series of 1,3,4-oxadiazol-2-yl thioether derivatives. The results of biological assay demonstrated that target compounds possessed moderate to good fungicidal activities against *R. solani*, *S. sclerotioru* and *P. oryzac Cavgra*. Compounds **126** and **127** showed more than 90% inhibitory rate against *S. sclerotioru*. The EC$_{50}$ values of **126** and **127** were 11.16 μM and 30.47 μM, respectively. In addition, the EC$_{50}$ value of **127** against *S. sclerotioru* was 10.49 mM, similar as that of compound **1** [62].

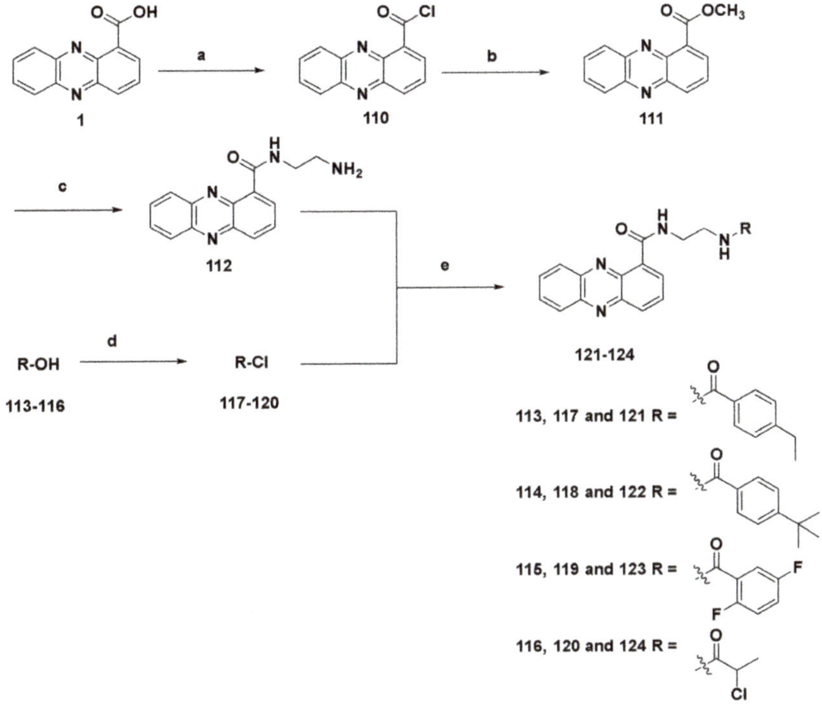

Scheme 1. Synthesis of compounds **121–124**. Reagents and conditions: (**a**) Oxalyl, CH$_2$Cl$_2$, DMF, reflux, 8 h; (**b**) MeOH, rt, 1 h; (**c**) EDA, MeOH, rt, 0 °C to reflux, 2 h; (**d**) SOCl$_2$, reflux, 6 h; (**e**) Intermediates **117–120**, 0 °C, 1 h.

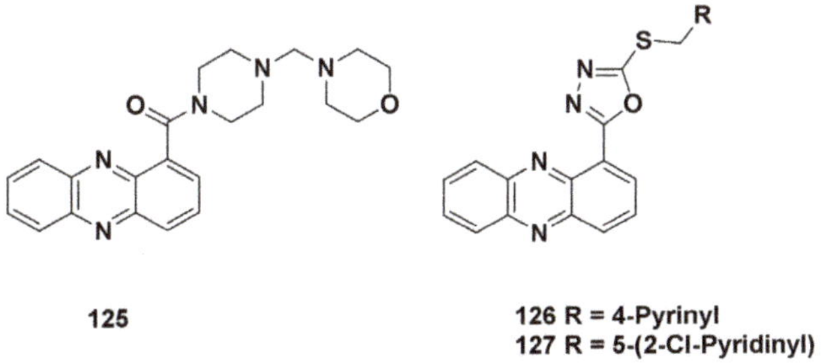

Figure 17. The chemical structures of compounds **125–127**.

Li et al. also designed and synthesized the derivatives of compound **1** containing substituted groups of triazole. Most 3-benzyl mercapto-1,2,4-triazol derivatives demonstrated fungicidal activity against one or multiple plant pathogens in vitro and in vivo. Compounds **137–140** (Scheme 2) displayed better inhibitory activity against rice blast (*P. oryzae*) than **1**. These results provided valuable references for further studies [63].

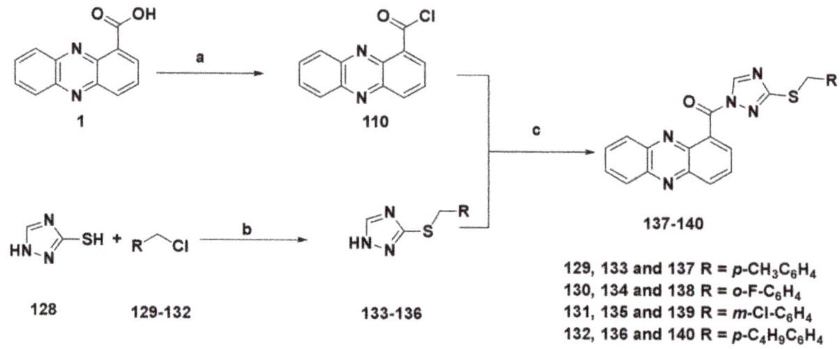

Scheme 2. Synthesis of compounds **137–140**. Reagents and conditions: (**a**) Oxalyl chloride, CH$_2$Cl$_2$, DMF, reflux, 8 h; (**b**) NaOH (4%), EtOH, reflux, 20 min; (**c**) pyridine, C$_4$H$_8$O$_2$, 0 °C, 2 h.

4.1.4. Water-Soluble Triazole Phenazine Derivatives

Hayden et al. evaluated water-soluble triazole phenazine derivatives, which were synthesized previously. Compounds **141–143** (Figure 18) showed high antimicrobial activity at tested concentrations without cytotoxicity against human epithelial cells and tested biological data suggested that **141–143** could interrupt metabolic electron-transfer cascades thereby exhibiting cytotoxicity against *E. coli*, rather than production of ROS [64].

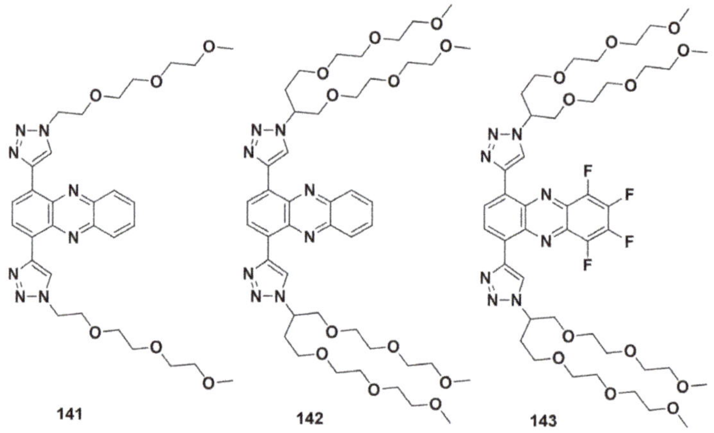

Figure 18. The chemical structures of compounds **141–143**.

4.2. Insecticidal Activity

Podophyllotoxin is a natural product used as the lead compound for the preparation of insecticidal agents. It contains A, B, C, D and E rings. Zhi et al. designed and synthesized a series of podophyllotoxin-based phenazine derivatives modified in the C, D and E rings. In addition, the insecticidal activity of target compounds was investigated which showed insecticidal activity against *Mythimna separata* Walker in vivo. Compounds **148** and **149** (Scheme 3) were phenazine derivatives of 4-acyloxypodophyllotoxin modified in the E ring. They demonstrated stronger insecticidal activity than toosendanin [65]. Then, they designed and synthesized a series of oxime derivatives of podophyllotoxin-based phenazines modified in the C, D and E rings. Compounds **153–157** (Scheme 4) exhibited equal or higher insecticidal activity than toosendanin. The combination of podophyllotoxin and phenazine was proved to enhance insecticidal activity [66].

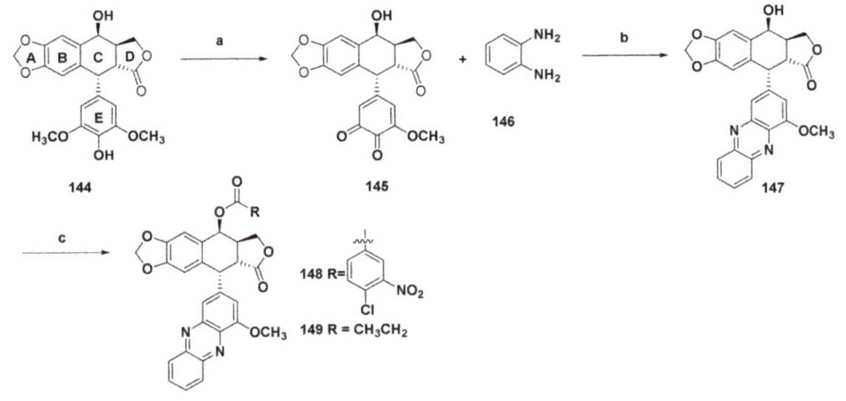

Scheme 3. Synthesis of compounds **148** and **149**. Reagents and conditions: (**a**) NaIO$_4$, HOAc, rt, 17 h; (**b**) CH$_3$Cl, rt, 0.5 h; (**c**) RCOOH, DIC, DMAP, DCM, rt, 0.5–7 h.

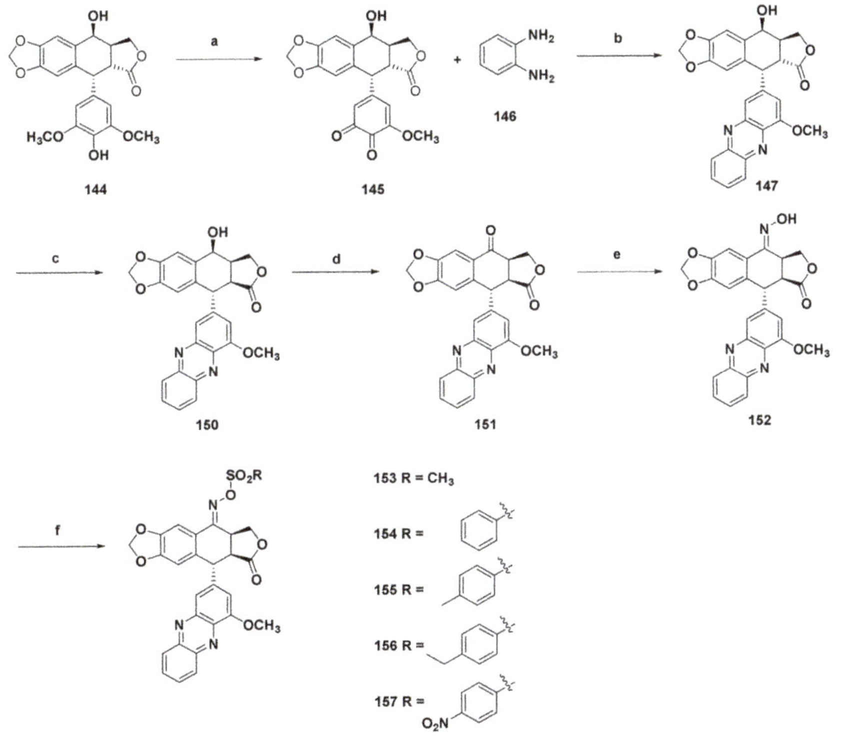

Scheme 4. Synthesis of compounds **153–157**. Reagents and conditions: (**a**) NaIO$_4$, HOAc, rt, 17 h; (**b**) CH$_3$Cl, rt, 0.5 h; (**c**) 10% aq. NaOAc/EtOH, reflux, 15 h; (**d**) CrO$_3$, pyridine, CH$_2$Cl$_2$; (**e**) NH$_4$Cl, pyridine, EtOH, reflux, 54 h; (**f**) RSO$_2$Cl, NaH, THF, rt, overnight.

4.3. Antiparasitic Activity

Chagas' disease, caused by *Trypanosoma cruzi*, is a widely spread endemic disease in American. Alvarez and Minini et al. selected phenazine **158** (Figure 19) from their own chemistry library and investigated its in-depth insight mechanism of inhibition; **158** could bind to a widespread enzyme, triosephosphate isomerase (TIM) from *T. cruzi*. It showed great inhibitory activity against TIM and could be further developed as inhibitors of TIM; **158** showed highly selective inhibition against *T. cruzi* enzyme (TcTIM) and weak inhibition against *T. brucei* (TbTIM), without affecting TIM from *H. sapiens* (HsTIM) and *Leishmania* sp. (LmTIM) [67,68].

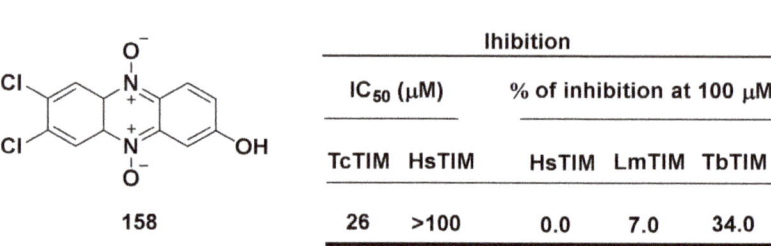

Figure 19. The chemical structure of compound **158** and its inhibition assay data against Tc, Hs, Lm and TbTIMs.

4.4. Anticancer Activity

4.4.1. Phenazine 5,10-dioxide Derivatives

Phenazine-5,10-dioxide derivatives **159–166** are listed in Table 1. Hernández et al. investigated chemosensitizer effect of compounds **159** and **161** to cisplatin. They showed a significant increase of the antiproliferative activity compared with the control group treated with cisplatin alone, demonstrating sensitization to cisplatin therapy. In addition, **159** combined with cisplatin induced cell cycle arrest on bladder cancer cells, resensitizing the invasive and cisplatin resistant 253 J cell line. It also showed great inhibition activity against histone deacetylase (HDAC) and sensitized chemotherapeutic drugs to better access to DNA, which would cause DNA damage, leading to cell death [69].

Table 1. The chemical structures of phenazine-5,10-dioxide derivatives **159–166** and survival rate (%) in normoxia and hypoxia.

Structure/Name	SF [a,b,c]	
	Norm	Hypox
159 R = NH$_2$, Z 160 R = OH, Z	(**159**): 100 ± 10 (**160**): 100 ± 7	(**159**): 45 ± 4 (**160**): 75 ± 2
161	Nd.	Nd.
162 R = NO$_2$, 163 R = Cl, 164 R = SCH$_3$	(**162**): 89 ± 10 (**163**): 100 ± 6 (**164**): 100 ± 6	(**162**): 58 ± 4 (**163**): 44 ± 5 (**164**): 55 ± 3

Table 1. Cont.

Structure/Name	SF [a,b,c]	
	Norm	Hypox
165	(165): 57 ± 7	(165): 66 ± 6
166	(166): 100 ± 8	(166): 73 ± 4

[a] SF norm = survival fraction in normoxia at 20 mM on V79 cells. [b] SF hypox = survival fraction in hypoxia at 20 mM on V79 cells. [c] Values are means of two different experiments. The assays were done by duplicate and using at least three repetitions. Nd = not determined.

Phenazine 5,10-dioxide derivatives have also been reported in development as bioreductive agents. This class of compounds all contain a bioreductive moiety, the N-oxide group and a planar heterocycle moiety, phenazine [70,71]. After the hypoxic selective bioreductive process, the phenazine moiety can interact with DNA causing cytotoxicity in the solid tumour cells [72]. Gonda et al. attempted to find selective hypoxic cytotoxins with additional ability to inhibit DNA topoisomerase II. Inhibitive values in normoxia and hypoxia condition of these compounds were shown in Table 1: **162–164** displayed some degree of selectivity; **165** showed non-selectivity towards both conditions, normoxia and hypoxia. Meanwhile, **159** and **163** showed the best selectivity; **164** exhibited inhibition of topoisomerase II in hypoxia; **166** showed no inhibition of topoisomerase II in hypoxia and normoxia. The DNA interaction abilities of phenazine 5,10-dioxide derivatives were related to cytotoxicity in normoxia or hypoxia. SAR implicated that the arylethenyl moieties were generally responsible for normoxic cytotoxicity. On the contrary, the group of sulfonamido did not produce selective cytotoxicity whether in normoxia or hypoxia [73].

4.4.2. Benzo[a]phenazine Derivatives

According to related reports, benzo[a]phenazine derivatives show significant activity of antiproliferation against HL-60 cell line. Topoisomerases, including topoisomerase I and II, have been proved to be effective anticancer targets in drug discovery due to highly over-expression in cancer cells [74,75].

Benzo[a]phenazine derivatives **167–174** are listed in Table 2. Zhuo et al. designed series of benzo[a]phenazine derivatives, which alkylated the phenolic hydroxyl group on ring B, introducing different substituted groups on ring D by condensation and followed up with amination. This class of compounds showed good antiproliferative activity. Compound **167** demonstrated good Topo I–DNA cleavage complex stabilizing ability in vivo. Compound **168** showed inhibition of ATPase. Compared with **167**, **168** and **169** were introduced a methoxy group, their inhibitory activity was significantly improved and there was a good correlation between the inhibitory activity and cytotoxic activity. Caspase-3/7 activation assay showed that this class of compounds could induce an apoptotic response in HL-60 cell line [76].

Table 2. The chemical structures of benzo[a]phenazine derivatives **167–174**, IC$_{50}$ values of in vitro growth inhibitory, relative activity of Topo I-DNA cleavage and Topo II ATPase inhibition.

Structure/Name	In Vitro Growth Inhibitory ^{a} IC$_{50}$ Values	Relative Activity	
		Topo I Cleavage ^{b}	Topo II ATPase Inhibition ^{c}
167 R$_1$ = R$_2$ = H **168** R$_1$ = H, R$_2$ = OCH$_3$ **169** R$_1$ = OCH$_3$, R$_2$ = H	(**167**): IC$_{50}$ = 3.99 μM (HeLa), 3.65 μM (A549), 5.01 μM (MCF-7), 1.40 μM (HL-60). (**168**): IC$_{50}$ = 4.36 μM (HeLa), 5.45 μM (A549), 2.83 μM (MCF-7), 2.36 μM (HL-60). (**169**): IC$_{50}$ = 2.26 μM (HeLa), 2.24 μM (A549), 2.27 μM (MCF-7), 1.04 μM (HL-60).	(**167**): +++ (**168**): − (**169**): −	(**167**): ++ (**168**): +++ (**169**): ++
170 n = 1 **171** n = 2 **172** n = 3	(**170**): IC$_{50}$ = 0.31 μM (HL-60), 24.56 μM (K562), 9.91 μM (Hela), 22.31 μM (A549). (**171**): IC$_{50}$ = 0.21 μM (HL-60), 5.93 μM (K562), 8.41 μM (Hela), 13.51 μM (A549). (**172**): IC$_{50}$ = 0.38 μM (HL-60), 4.73 μM (K562), 21.44 μM (Hela), 16.28 μM (A549).	(**170**): Nd. (**171**): Nd. (**172**): ++	(**170**): Nd. (**171**): Nd. (**172**): ++++
173 R$_1$ = R$_2$ = H, R$_3$ = OCH$_3$ **174** R$_1$ = H, R$_2$ = R$_3$ = OCH$_3$	(**173**): IC$_{50}$ = 0.22 μM (HL-60), 7.13 μM (K562), 29.95 μM (Hela), 32.96 μM (A549). (**174**): IC$_{50}$ = 0.09 μM (HL-60), 8.73 μM (K562), 18.23 μM (Hela), 26.45 μM (A549).	(**173**): Nd. (**174**): Nd.	(**173**): ++++ (**174**): ++++

^{a} IC$_{50}$ = concentration required for 50% of the antiproliferative effect for a given cell population grown for 2 days in presence of the compound of interest.; ^{b} The relative Topo I cleavage complex stabilizing potencies of the compounds are presented as follows: −, no detectable activity; +, weak activity; ++, weaker activity than that of CPT; +++, activity similar to that of CPT.; ^{c} The relative Topo II ATPase inhibitory potencies of the compounds are presented as follows: −, no detectable activity; +, weak activity; ++, weaker activity than that of 1,4-naphthoquinone; +++, activity similar to that of 1,4-naphthoquinone, higher activity than that of 1,4-naphthoquinone; ++++.; Nd = not determined.

Yao et al. synthesized a series of 7-alkylamino substituted benzo[a]phenazine derivatives. Most of these compounds showed better inhibitory activity in HL-60 cell line than the other tested cell lines. The structure–activity relationship studies revealed that the substitution of amino groups on terminal of side chain at N-7 position could improve the Topo I/II inhibitory activity and cytotoxicity: **170–172** with the dimethylamino terminal showed good Topo I and Topo II inhibitory activity; **170** could stabilize the Topo I-DNA cleavage complexes in vivo; **173** with methoxy group at position C-9 exhibited good Topo I and Topo II inhibitory activity at 25 mM concentration; **173** showed inhibition of ATPase [22].

4.4.3. Pyran[2,3-c]phenazine Derivatives

Phenazine derivatives and pyran derivatives are important heterocyclic compounds which possess good biological activity. The heterocyclic pyran structure usually is a functional framework which appears in amounts of important drugs and natural products. Molecular hybridization strategy shows great prospect in the present drug discovery to reduce the side effects and the occurrence of drug-resistance [77]. The aromatic interlayer coupling structure of phenazine, as well as the structural characteristics of fluted or specific enzyme binders, leads to selective high-affinity binders that target DNA and DNA-enzyme complexes [78]. According to recent articles, pyran[2,3-c] phenazine derivatives mainly showed cytotoxicity against HepG2 cell line. In addition, the mechanism inducing apoptosis against cancer cells about this class of compounds is shown in Figure 3.

Lu et al. designed and synthesized a series of pyran[3,2-*a*] phenazine derivatives. Most pyran[3,2-*a*] phenazine derivatives demonstrated cytotoxicity against HCT116, MCF-7, HepG2 and A549 cancer cell lines in vitro. Especially, compounds **181–183** (Scheme 5) were found to show potent growth inhibitory activity against HepG2 cell line (IC_{50} of 2–6 µM). In addition, they also used experimental mouse models to test in vivo activity of these phenazine derivatives. Among these phenazine derivatives, **181** was selected to do tumor xenografts experiment to test the effect of inhibition. H22 cells was injected into ICR mice, inhibitions were 7.78% (5 mg/kg), 68.89% (10 mg/kg) and 77.78% (20 mg/kg), respectively. Further mechanism studies implicated **181** acted as topoisomerases I and II dual inhibitor, cell cycle arrester and apoptosis inducer against HepG2 cell line [23].

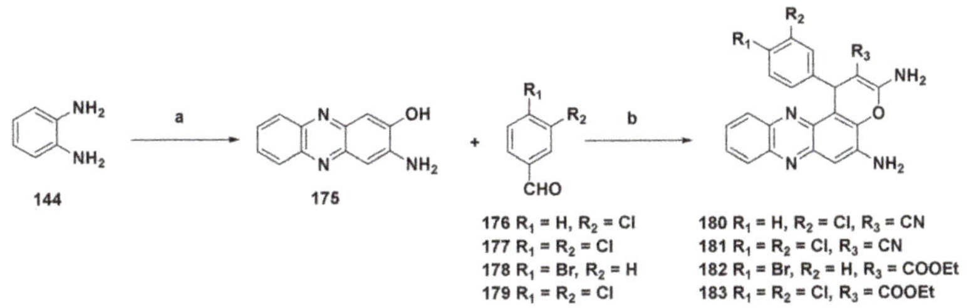

Scheme 5. Synthesis of compounds **180–183**. Reagents and conditions: (**a**) Conc. HCl, $FeCl_3$, rt, overnight; (**b**) malononitrile or ethyl 2-cyanoacetate, DABCO, EtOH, reflux, 0.5–2.5 h.

Additionally, Liao et al. firstly found **181** as thioredoxin reductase I (TrxR1) inhibitor against HepG2 cell line. TrxR1 is a novel anticancer target different from topoisomerases I and II. Molecular docking was carried out to study the inhibitory possibility of compound **181** against TrxR1. Soon afterwards, they investigated the crucial downstream protein TrxR1 to confirm antiproliferation function of **181** against the HepG2 cell line. It supplied valuable information for further development of the TrxR1 inhibitors [24].

Lu et al. also designed phenazine derivatives containing phenazine, pyran, indole and 1,2,3-triazole pharmacophores. Among these derivatives, **187** (Scheme 6) demonstrated the best antiproliferative activity against A549 cancer cell line (IC_{50} of 5.4 µM) and no cytotoxicity against L02 and HUVEC non-cancer cell lines [18].

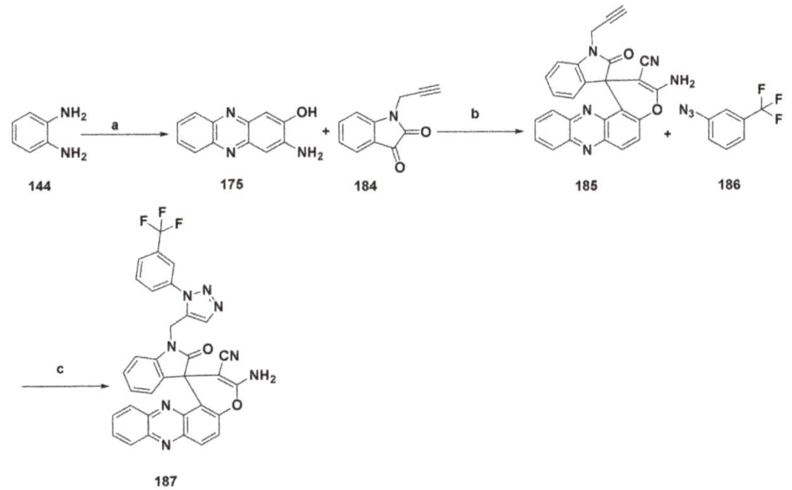

Scheme 6. Synthesis of compound **187**. Reagents and conditions: (**a**) Conc. HCl, $FeCl_3$, rt, overnight; (**b**) malononitrile, DABCO, EtOH; (**c**) sodium ascorbate, $CuSO_4$, THF/H_2O.

4.4.4. Benzo[a]pyran[2,3-c]phenazine Derivatives

This class of phenazine derivatives, which contain phenazine, pyran and benzo core, possess great anticancer activity but rarely reported. Inspired by **XR11576** (Figure 1), benzophenazine derivative has been proved to be a great antitumor compound which could be further modified. Gao et al. synthesized a series of benzo[a]pyran[2,3-c] phenazine derivatives and evaluated their biological activities. Some of them (compounds **188–191**) are listed in Figure 20. Among these compounds, **189** and **191** possessed a p-dimethylamino substituted group in benzo ring and the apparent differences between their structures possessed cyan group and ethyl acetate group, respectively, in 3-position of γ-pyran ring. Compared to the positive control drug (hydroxycamptothecin), **189** showed better inhibition activity against tested cancer cell line HepG2. However, **191** demonstrated no inhibitory activity against all selective cell lines. These experimental data proved that cyan group played an important role in antiproliferative activity: **189** and **190**, possessing a p-dimethylamino group and p-hydroxyl group, respectively, demonstrated some cytotoxic activity to HCT116 cell line, IC$_{50}$ of 0.22 µM and 15.32 µM, respectively; **189** showed cytotoxic activity against HepG2 cell line with IC$_{50}$ of 6.71 µM; **188–191** showed weak or no activity against MCF-7 and A549 cell lines. SAR studies showed that cyan group and p-dimethylamino group played a significant role in antiproliferative activity and resulted in the decrease of cytotoxic activity [79].

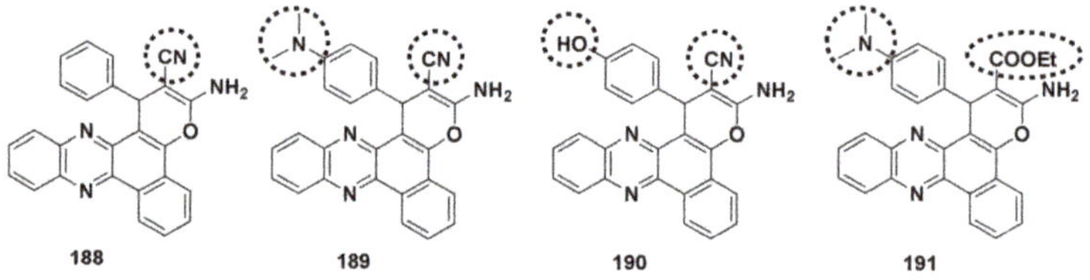

Figure 20. The chemical structures of compounds **188–191**.

4.4.5. Benzo[a]chromeno[2,3-c] phenazine Derivatives

Chromenes are also an important class of heterocyclic compounds which exhibit attractive pharmacological properties, such as antitumor, anti-vascular, antioxidant, antimicrobial, sex pheromone, tumor necrosis factor-α (TNF-α) inhibitor, cancer therapy and central neuroprotective activities [80]. Chromenes and phenazine derivatives both have attracted attention, but benzo[a]chromeno[2,3-c] phenazine derivatives have rarely been investigated [81].

Reddy et al. synthesized a series of phenazine-chromene hybrid molecules by protocol of one pot multi-component reaction. Compounds **192–194** (Figure 21) showed excellent in vitro antioxidant activity which was benefit to the treatment of cancer and prevention of cardiovascular diseases. Compared with anticancer drugs etoposide and camptothecin, **192–194** showed similar antiproliferative activity against selective cancer cell lines with IC$_{50}$ values of 3.28 µM, 4.31 µM and 4.01 µM against HeLa cell line and 2.24 µM, 3.81 µM and 3.12 µM against SK-BR-3 cell line, respectively. These compounds did not show significant toxicity against normal human breast cells (HBL 100) at lower concentrations [19].

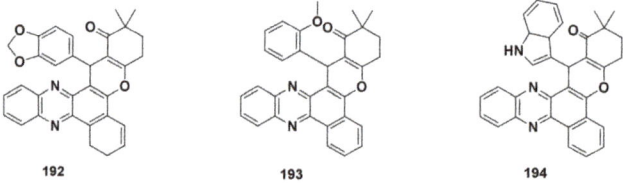

Figure 21. The chemical structures of compounds **192–194**.

4.4.6. Derivatives Derived from 2-Phenazinamine

Inspired by previous reports, Gao et al. isolated a natural derivative derived from 2-phenazinamine, showing high cytotoxicity against selective cancer cell lines. A series of 2-phenazinamine derivatives, including compounds **195–202** (Figure 22), were synthesized. The antiproliferative activity results showed that IC_{50} values of **195** and **197** against HepG2 cell line were 16.46 µM and 15.21 µM, respectively. IC_{50} values of **195** and **198** against K562 cell line were 33.43 µM and 49.20 µM, respectively. In addition, IC_{50} value of **196** against MCF-7 cell line was 11.63 µM. Notably, these active compounds showed no cytotoxicity on the epithelial cells from the 293T non-cancer cells. Moreover, mechanism of **195** was similar to control drug (cisplatin), inhibiting cancer proliferation by inducing apoptosis [82].

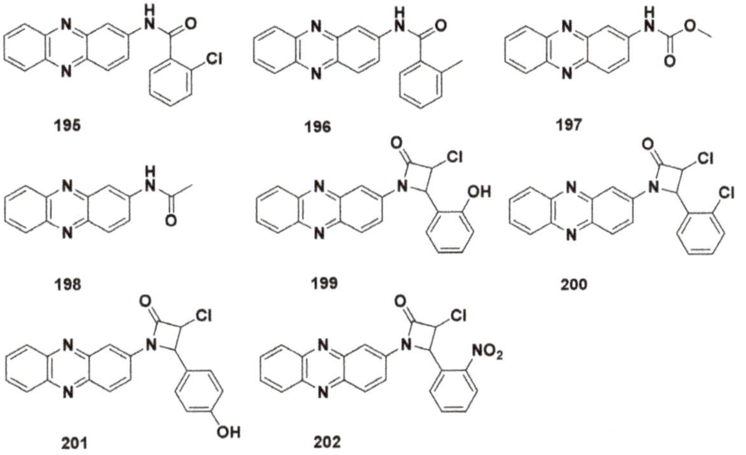

Figure 22. The chemical structures of compounds **195–202**.

According to the report of Gao et al., Kale et al. selected some 2-phenazinamines derivatives and further utilized computational methods to investigate their protein targets. The experimental data of **199–202** showed great binding energy against BCR-ABL tyrosine kinase by Autodock 4.2. Scores of **199–202** were −7.6 kcal/mol, −8.8 kcal/mol, −7.2 kcal/mol and −7.1 kcal/mol, respectively. In addition, the score of imatinib was −8.7 kcal/mol. All the computational data showed 2-phenazinamine derivatives would be inhibitors against BCR-ABL tyrosine kinase and needed to be further investigated [25].

4.4.7. Derivatives Derived from 2,3-Diaminophenazine

Protein kinases (PKs) are essential in many cellular processes, which catalyze phosphorylation of different cellular substrates. Then, phosphorylation in turn regulates various cellular functions. Normally, their activity is strictly regulated. Under pathological conditions, PKs can be deregulated, leading to changes in the phosphorylation, resulting in uncontrolled cell division, inhibiting apoptosis and other abnormalities. Various cancers are known to be caused or accompanied by deregulation of the phosphorylation. Screening new potent, selective and less toxic compounds to inhibit PKs has been proved to be a promising cancer treatment strategy [83].

Mahran et al. prepared some phenazine derivatives, such as compound **203** and its analogues (Figure 23). Among these derivatives, compounds **203–207** displayed antiproliferative activity with IC_{50} values of 8.8 µM, 7.7 µM, 8.4 µM, 6.8 µM and 8.8 µM against A549 cell line and 6.0 µM, 4.4 µM, 5.2 µM, 16 µM and 6.8 µM against HCT116 cell line, respectively. These compounds also showed inhibitory activity of human tyrosine kinases. The experimental results of inhibiting human tyrosine kinase were consistent with cell cytotoxicity activity [20].

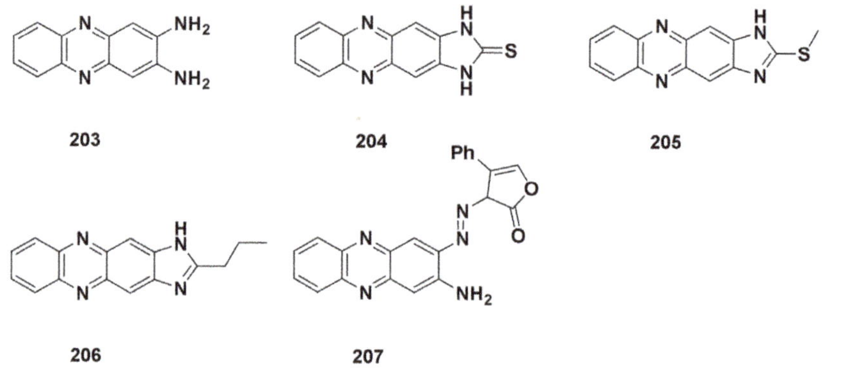

Figure 23. The chemical structures of compounds **203–207**.

4.4.8. 2,3-Dialkoxyphenazine Derivatives

Endo et al. reported the only antitumor activity of 2,3-disubstituted phenazines against sarcoma and carcinoma tumors in 1965 [84]. The presence of long fatty chains could provide a good effect to cross the lipid barrier [85]. Moris et al. synthesized 2,3-dialkoxyphenazine derivatives using an easy, efficient and straightforward condensation method. These compounds **208–211** (Figure 24) were firstly reported to show activity on MiaPaca pancreatic cell lines with IC_{50} of 0.06 µM, 21 µM, 75 µM and 7 µM, respectively. Interestingly, **208** and **209** interacted with DNA through hydrogen bonds remarkably, showing significant anticancer activity. Compared to Gemzar®, **208** and **211** were the most effective ones against pancreatic MiaPaca cell resistant lines. The experimental results showed that the carboxyl substituents on position 7 did not interact with each other through hydrogen bonds. Although possessing planar structures, these derivatives did not have similar mechanism of action as Gemcitabine. In vivo study on mice, **211** was as efficient as Gemzar® at a ten times lower concentration (1 mg/kg vs. 10 mg/kg) [21].

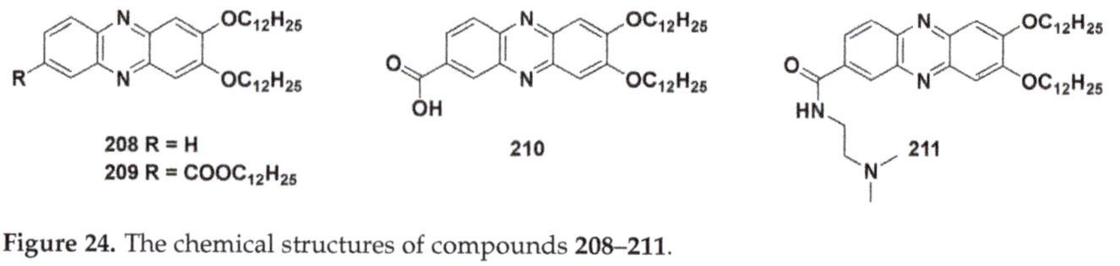

Figure 24. The chemical structures of compounds **208–211**.

5. Conclusions

In this review, we introduced natural phenazines and synthetic phenazine derivatives, which were reported from 2012 to 2021. The biosynthetic pathways of natural phenazines, sources of microorganism and operon genes were illustrated in detail. Additionally, their pharmacological activities, mechanisms of action and structure–activity relationships were also summarized. In future studies, first of all, it is still necessary to find novel structures from natural sources for the screening of lead compounds. Secondly, it is very important to design and synthesize new compounds based on existing SAR through structural modification. The successfully applied drug clofazimine and XR11576, XR5944, NC-182 and NC-190 in clinical studies are good references. The structure modification at C-2, C-3, C-4 and N-6 sites and ring fused derivatives have a good prospect. In addition, target-based drug design can reduce the randomness. Finally, more extensive activity screening will enable more efficient use of compound resources.

Author Contributions: J.Y., investigation, visualization, writing—original draft, writing—review and editing; W.L., investigation, visualization, writing—review and editing; J.C., investigation, visualization, writing—original draft, writing—review and editing; Y.W., investigation, visualization, writing—original draft, writing—review and editing; D.L., funding acquisition, project administration, supervision, writing—original draft, writing—review and editing; H.H., project administration, supervision, writing—original draft, writing—review and editing; H.C., funding acquisition, project administration, supervision, writing—original draft, writing—review and editing. All authors have read and agreed to the published version of the manuscript.

Funding: This paper was financially supported by the Career Development Support Plan for Young and Middle-aged Teachers in Shenyang Pharmaceutical University.

Conflicts of Interest: The authors declare no conflict of interest.

References

1. Guttenberger, N.; Blankenfeldt, W.; Breinbauer, R. Recent developments in the isolation, biological function, biosynthesis, and synthesis of phenazine natural products. *Bioorg. Med. Chem.* **2017**, *25*, 6149–6166. [CrossRef] [PubMed]
2. Valliappan, K.; Sun, W.; Li, Z. Marine actinobacteria associated with marine organisms and their potentials in producing pharmaceutical natural products. *Appl. Microbiol. Biotechnol.* **2014**, *98*, 7365–7377. [CrossRef]
3. Yang, P.; Yang, Q.; Qian, X.; Cui, J. Novel synthetic Aisoquinolino[5,4-*ab*] phenazines: Inhibition toward topoisomerase I, antitumor and DNA photo-cleaving activities. *Bioorg. Med. Chem.* **2005**, *13*, 5909–5914. [CrossRef] [PubMed]
4. Peng, H.; Zhang, P.; Bilal, M.; Wang, W.; Hu, H.; Zhang, X. Enhanced biosynthesis of phenazine-1-carboxamide by engineered *Pseudomonas* chlororaphis HT66. *Microb. Cell Fact.* **2018**, *17*, 117–129. [CrossRef] [PubMed]
5. Blankenfeldt, W.; Parsons, J.F. The structural biology of phenazine biosynthesis. *Curr. Opin. Struct. Biol.* **2014**, *29*, 26–33. [CrossRef]
6. Laursen, J.B.; Nielsen, J. Phenazine natural products: Biosynthesis, synthetic analogues, and biological activity. *Chem. Rev.* **2004**, *104*, 1663–1685. [CrossRef] [PubMed]
7. Hari Narayana Moorthy, N.S.; Pratheepa, V.; Maria, J.R.; Vitor, V.; Pedro, A.F. Fused aryl-phenazines: Scaffold for the development of bioactive molecules. *Curr. Drug Targets.* **2014**, *15*, 681–688. [CrossRef] [PubMed]
8. Gu, P.; Zhao, Y.; Zhang, J.; Wang, C.; Sun, X.; He, J.; Xu, Q.; Lu, J.; Zhang, Q. Synthesis, physical properties, and light-emitting diode performance of phenazine-based derivatives with three, five, and nine fused six-membered rings. *J. Org. Chem.* **2015**, *806*, 3030–3035. [CrossRef]
9. Raymond, Z.; Laure, B.; Pascal, R.; Gilles, U. Isocyanate-, isothiocyanate-, urea-, and thiourea-substituted boron dipyrromethene dyes as fluorescent probes. *J. Org. Chem.* **2006**, *718*, 3093–3102.
10. Tagele, S.B.; Lee, H.G.; Kim, S.W.; Lee, Y.S. Phenazine and 1-undecene producing *Pseudomonas chlororaphis subsp*. aurantiaca strain KNU17Pc1 for growth promotion and disease suppression in Korean maize cultivars. *J. Microbiol. Biotechnol.* **2018**, *29*, 66–78. [CrossRef]
11. Abdel-Mageed, W.M.; Milne, B.F.; Wagner, M.; Schumacher, M.; Sandor, P.; Pathom-aree, W.; Goodfellow, M.; Bull, A.T.; Horikoshi, K.; Ebel, R. Dermacozines, a new phenazine family from deep-sea dermacocci isolated from a Mariana Trench sediment. *Org. Biomol. Chem.* **2010**, *8*, 2352–2362. [CrossRef]
12. Lavaggi, M.L.; Aguirre, G.A.; Boiani, L.; Orelli, L.; García, B.; Cerecetto, H.; González, M. Pyrimido[1,2-*a*] quinoxaline 6-oxide and phenazine 5,10-dioxide derivatives and related compounds as growth inhibitors of *Trypanosoma cruzi*. *Eur. J. Med. Chem.* **2008**, *43*, 1737–1741. [CrossRef]
13. Krishnaiah, M.; Almeida, N.R.; Udumula, V.; Song, Z.; Chhonker, Y.S.; Abdelmoaty, M.M.; Nascimento, V.A.; Murry, D.J.; Conda-Sheridan, M. Synthesis, biological evaluation, and metabolic stability of phenazine derivatives as antibacterial agents. *Eur. J. Med. Chem.* **2018**, *143*, 936–947. [CrossRef] [PubMed]
14. Cha, J.W.; Lee, S.I.; Kim, M.C.; Thida, M.; Lee, J.W.; Park, J.; Kwon, H.C. Pontemazines A and B, phenazine derivatives containing a methylamine linkage from *Streptomyces* sp. UT1123 and their protective effect to HT-22 neuronal cells. *Bioorg. Med. Chem. Lett.* **2015**, *25*, 5083–5086. [CrossRef]
15. Pachón, O.G.; Azqueta, A.; Lavaggi, M.L.; Cerain, A.L.; Creppy, E.; Collins, A.; Cerecetto, H.; González, M.; Centelles, J.J.; Cascante, M. Antitumoral effect of phenazine N_5, N_{10}-dioxide derivatives on Caco-2 Cells. *Chem. Res. Toxicol.* **2008**, *21*, 1578–1585. [CrossRef] [PubMed]
16. Makgatho, E.M.; Mbajiorgu, E.F. In vitro investigation of clofazimine analogues for antiplasmodial, cytotoxic and pro-oxidative activities. *Afr. Health Sci.* **2017**, *17*, 191–198. [CrossRef] [PubMed]
17. Pierson, S.L.; Pierson, E.A. Metabolism and function of phenazines in bacteria: Impacts on the behavior of bacteria in the environment and biotechnological processes. *Appl. Microbiol. Biotechnol.* **2010**, *86*, 1659. [CrossRef]
18. Lu, Y.; Wang, L.; Wang, X.; Xi, T.; Liao, J.; Wang, Z.; Jiang, F. Design, combinatorial synthesis and biological evaluations of novel 3-amino-1'-((1-aryl-1H-1,2,3-triazol-5-yl) methyl)-2'-oxospiro[benzo[*a*] pyrano[2,3-*c*]phenazine-1,3'-indoline]-2-carbonitrile antitumor hybrid molecules. *Eur. J. Med. Chem.* **2017**, *135*, 125–141. [CrossRef] [PubMed]

19. Reddy, M.V.; Valasani, K.R.; Lim, K.T.; Jeong, Y.T. Tetramethylguanidiniumchlorosulfonate ionic liquid (TMG IL): An efficient reusable catalyst for the synthesis of tetrahydro-1H-benzo[a]chromeno[2,3-c] phenazin-1-ones under solvent-free conditions and evaluation for their in vitro bioassay activity. *New J. Chem.* **2015**, *39*, 9931–9941. [CrossRef]
20. Mahran, A.M.; Ragab, S.S.; Hashem, A.I.; Ali, M.M.; Nada, A.A. Synthesis and antiproliferative activity of novel polynuclear heterocyclic compounds derived from 2,3-diaminophenazine. *Eur. J. Med. Chem.* **2015**, *90*, 568–576. [CrossRef]
21. Moris, M.A.; Andrieu, C.; Rocchi, P.; Seillan, C.; Acunzo, J.; Brunel, F.; Garzino, F.; Siri, O.; Camplo, M. 2,3-Dialkoxyphenazines as anticancer agents. *Tetrahedron Lett.* **2015**, *56*, 2695–2698. [CrossRef]
22. Yao, B.; Mai, Y.; Chen, S.; Xie, H.; Yao, P.; Ou, T.; Tan, J.; Wang, H.; Li, D.; Huang, S. Design, synthesis and biological evaluation of novel 7-alkylamino substituted benzo[a]phenazin derivatives as dual topoisomerase I/II inhibitors. *Eur. J. Med. Chem.* **2015**, *92*, 540–553. [CrossRef]
23. Lu, Y.; Yan, Y.; Wang, L.; Wang, X.; Gao, J.; Xi, T.; Wang, Z.; Jiang, F. Design, facile synthesis and biological evaluations of novel pyrano[3,2-a]phenazine hybrid molecules as antitumor agents. *Eur. J. Med. Chem.* **2016**, *127*, 928–943. [CrossRef] [PubMed]
24. Liao, J.; Wang, L.; Wu, Z.; Wang, Z.; Chen, J.; Zhong, Y.; Jiang, F.; Lu, Y. Identification of phenazine analogue as a novel scaffold for thioredoxin reductase I inhibitors against Hep G2 cancer cell lines. *J. Enzym. Inhib. Med. Chem.* **2019**, *34*, 1158–1163. [CrossRef]
25. Kaleza, M.; Sonwane, G.; Choudhari, Y. Searching for potential novel BCR-ABL tyrosine kinase inhibitors through G-QSAR and docking studies of some novel 2-phenazinamine derivatives. *Curr. Comput.-Aid. Drug.* **2020**, *16*, 501–510.
26. Cimmino, A.; Evidente, A.; Mathieu, V.; Andolfi, A.; Lefranc, F.; Kornienko, A.; Kiss, R. Phenazines and cancer. *Nat. Prod. Rep.* **2012**, *29*, 487–501. [CrossRef] [PubMed]
27. Gorantla, J.N.; Nishanth Kumar, S.; Nisha, G.V.; Sumandu, A.S.; Dileep, C.; Sudaresan, A.; Sree Kumar, M.M.; Lankalapalli, R.S.; Dileep Kumar, B.S. Purification and characterization of antifungal phenazines from a fluorescent *Pseudomonas* strain FPO4 against medically important fungi. *J. Mycol. Med.* **2014**, *24*, 185–192. [CrossRef] [PubMed]
28. Varsha, K.K.; Nishant, G.; Sneha, S.; Shilpa, G.; Devendra, L.; Priya, S.; Nampoothiri, K. Antifungal, anticancer and aminopeptidase inhibitory potential of a phenazine compound produced by *Lactococcus* BSN307. *Indian J. Microbiol.* **2016**, *56*, 411–416. [CrossRef]
29. Cardozo, V.F.; Oliveira, A.G.; Nishio, E.K.; Perugini, M.R.; Andrade, C.G.; Silveira, W.; Durán, N.; Andrade, G.; Kobayashi, R.K.; Nakazato, G. Antibacterial activity of extracellular compounds produced by a *Pseudomonas* strain against methicillin-resistant *Staphylococcus aureus* (MRSA) strains. *Ann. Clin. Microbiol. Antimicrob.* **2013**, *12*, 12–20. [CrossRef] [PubMed]
30. Thanabalasingama, D.; Kumara, N.S.; Jayasinghea, L.; Fujimotoa, Y. Endophytic fungus *Nigrospora oryzae* from a medicinal plant *Coccinia grandis*, a high yielding new source of phenazine-1-carboxamide. *Nat. Prod. Commun.* **2015**, *10*, 1659–1660. [CrossRef]
31. Tupe, S.G.; Kulkarni, R.R.; Shirazi, F.; Sant, D.G.; Joshi, S.P.; Deshpande, M.V. Possible mechanism of antifungal phenazine-1-carboxamide from *Pseudomonas* sp. against dimorphic fungi *Benjaminiella poitrasii* and human pathogen *Candida albicans*. *J. Appl. Microbiol.* **2015**, *118*, 39–48. [CrossRef] [PubMed]
32. Kennedy, R.K.; Veena, V.; Naik, P.R.; Lakshmi, P.; Krishna, R.; Sudharani, S.; Sakthivel, N. Phenazine-1-carboxamide (PCN) from *Pseudomonas* sp. strain PUP6 selectively induced apoptosis in lung (A549) and breast (MDA MB-231) cancer cells by inhibition of antiapoptotic Bcl-2 family proteins. *Apoptosis* **2015**, *20*, 858–868. [CrossRef]
33. Ali, H.M.; El-Shikhl, H.; Salem, M.Z.M.; Muzaheed, M. Isolation of bioactive phenazine-1-carboxamide from the soil bacterium *Pantoea agglomerans* and study of its anticancer potency on different cancer cell lines. *J. AOAC Int.* **2016**, *99*, 1233–1239. [CrossRef] [PubMed]
34. Chai, W.; Zhang, J.; Zhu, Z.; Liu, W.; Pan, D.; Li, Y.; Chen, B. Pyocyanin from *Pseudomonas* induces IL-8 production through the PKC and NF-κB pathways in U937 cells. *Mol. Med. Rep.* **2013**, *8*, 1404–1410. [CrossRef] [PubMed]
35. Forbes, A.; Davey, A.K.; Perkins, A.V.; Grant, G.D.; McFarland, A.J.; McDermott, C.M.; Anoopkumar-Dukie, S. ERK1/2 activation modulates pyocyanin-induced toxicity in A549 respiratory epithelial cells. *Chem. Biol. Interact.* **2014**, *208*, 58–63. [CrossRef] [PubMed]
36. Sletta, H.; Degnes, K.F.; Herfindal, L.; Klinkenberg, G.; Fjærvik, E.; Zahlsen, K.; Brunsvik, A.; Nygaard, G.; Aachmann, F.L.; Ellingsen, T.E.; et al. Anti-microbial and cytotoxic 1,6-dihydroxyphenazine-5,10-dioxide (iodinin) produced by *Streptosporangium* sp. DSM 45942 isolated from the fjord sediment. *Appl. Microbiol. Biotechnol.* **2014**, *98*, 603–610. [CrossRef] [PubMed]
37. Myhren, L.E.; Nygaard, G.; Gausdal, G.; Sletta, H.; Teigen, K.; Degnes, K.F.; Zahlsen, K.; Brunsvik, A.; Bruserud, Ø.; Ove Døskeland, S.; et al. Iodinin (1,6-dihydroxyphenazine 5,10-dioxide) from *Streptosporangium* sp. induces apoptosis selectively in myeloid leukemia cell lines and patient cells. *Mar. Drugs* **2013**, *11*, 332–349. [CrossRef] [PubMed]
38. Lee, H.S.; Kang, J.; Choi, B.K.; Lee, H.S.; Lee, Y.J.; Lee, J.; Shin, H.J. Phenazine derivatives with anti-inflammatory activity from the deep-sea sediment-derived yeast-like fungus *Cystobasidium laryngis* IV17-028. *Mar. Drugs* **2019**, *17*, 482. [CrossRef]
39. Hifnawy, M.S.; Hassan, H.M.; Mohammed, R.; Fouda, M.M.; Sayed, A.M.; Hamed, A.A.; Abouzid, S.F.; Rateb, M.E.; Alhadrami, H.A.; Abdelmohsen, U.R. Induction of antibacterial metabolites by co-cultivation of two red-sea-sponge-associated *Actinomycetes Micromonospora* sp. UR56 and *Actinokinespora* sp. EG49. *Mar. Drugs* **2020**, *18*, 243. [CrossRef]
40. Kondratyuk, T.P.; Park, E.J.; Yu, R.; van Breemen, R.B.; Asolkar, R.N.; Murphy, B.T.; Fenical, W.; Pezzuto, J.M. Novel marine phenazines as potential cancer chemopreventive and anti-inflammatory agents. *Mar. Drugs* **2012**, *10*, 451–464. [CrossRef] [PubMed]
41. Ohlendorf, B.; Schulz, D.; Erhard, A.; Nagel, K.; Imhoff, J.F. Geranylphenazinediol, an acetylcholinesterase inhibitor produced by a *Streptomyces* Species. *J. Nat. Prod.* **2012**, *75*, 1400–1404. [CrossRef]

42. Song, Y.; Huang, H.; Chen, Y.; Ding, J.; Zhang, Y.; Sun, A.; Zhang, W.; Ju, J. Cytotoxic and antibacterial marfuraquinocins from the deep south China sea-derived *Streptomyces* niveus SCSIO 3406. *J. Nat. Prod.* **2013**, *76*, 2263–2268. [CrossRef] [PubMed]
43. Wu, C.; van Wezel, G.P.; Choi, Y.H. Identification of novel endophenaside antibiotics produced by *Kitasatospora* sp. MBT66. *J. Antibiot.* **2015**, *68*, 445–452. [CrossRef] [PubMed]
44. Han, H.; Guo, Z.; Zhang, B.; Zhang, M.; Shi, J.; Li, W.; Jiao, R.; Tan, R.; Ge, H. Bioactive phenazines from an earwig-associated *Streptomyces* sp. *Chin. J. Nat. Med.* **2019**, *17*, 475–480. [CrossRef]
45. Rusman, Y.; Oppegard, L.M.; Hiasa, H.; Gelbmann, C.; Salomon, C.E. Solphenazines A−F, glycosylated phenazines from *Streptomyces* sp. Strain DL-93. *J. Nat. Prod.* **2013**, *76*, 91–96. [CrossRef]
46. Li, Y.; Han, L.; Rong, H.; Li, L.; Zhao, L.; Wu, L.; Xu, L.; Jiang, Y.; Huang, X. Diastaphenazine, a new dimeric phenazine from an endophytic *Streptomyces* diastaticus subsp. Ardesiacus. *J. Antibiot.* **2015**, *68*, 210–212. [CrossRef]
47. Wang, X.; Abbas, M.; Zhang, Y.; Elshahawi, S.I.; Ponomareva, L.V.; Cui, Z.; Van Lanen, S.G.; Sajid, I.; Voss, S.R.; Shaaban, K.A.; et al. Baraphenazines A−G, divergent fused phenazine-based metabolites from a himalayan *Streptomyces*. *J. Nat. Prod.* **2019**, *82*, 1686–1693. [CrossRef]
48. Deng, R.; Zhang, Z.; Li, H.; Wang, W.; Hu, H.; Zhang, X. Identification of a novel bioactive phenazine derivative and regulation of phoP on its production in *Streptomyces* lomondensis S015. *J. Agric. Food Chem.* **2021**, *69*, 974–981. [CrossRef] [PubMed]
49. McDonald, M.; Mavrodi, D.V.; Thomashow, L.S.; Floss, H.G. Phenazine biosynthesis in *Pseudomonas* fluorescens: Branchpoint from the primary shikimate biosynthetic pathway and role of phenazine-1,6-dicarboxylic acid. *J. Am. Chem. Soc.* **2001**, *123*, 9459–9460. [CrossRef] [PubMed]
50. Xu, N.; Ahuja, E.G.; Janning, P.; Mavrodi, D.V.; Thomashow, L.S.; Blankenfeldt, W. Trapped intermediates in crystals of the FMN-dependent oxidase phzG provide insight into the final steps of phenazine biosynthesis. *Acta Crystallogr. Sect. D* **2013**, *69*, 1403–1413. [CrossRef]
51. Shi, Y.; Brachmann, A.O.; Westphalen, M.A.; Neubacher, N.; Tobias, N.J.; Bode, H.B. Dual phenazine gene clusters enable diversification during biosynthesis. *Nat. Chem. Biol.* **2019**, *15*, 331–339. [CrossRef] [PubMed]
52. Guo, S.; Liu, R.; Wang, W.; Hu, H.; Li, Z.; Zhang, X. Designing an artificial pathway for the biosynthesis of a novel phenazine N-Oxide in *Pseudomonas* chlororaphis HT66. *ACS Synth. Biol.* **2020**, *9*, 883–892. [CrossRef] [PubMed]
53. Yang, H.; Abouelhassan, Y.; Burch, G.M.; Kallifidas, D.; Huang, G.; Yousaf, H.; Jin, S.; Luesch, H.; Huigens, R.W. A highly potent class of halogenated phenazine antibacterial and biofilm-eradicating agents accessed through a modular Wohl-Aue synthesis. *Sci. Rep.* **2017**, *7*, 2003–2019. [CrossRef] [PubMed]
54. Conda-Sheridan, M.; Udumula, V.; Endres, J.L.; Harper, C.N.; Jaramillo, L.; Zhong, H.A.; Bayles, K.W. Simple synthesis of endophenazine G and other phenazines and their evaluation as anti-methicillin-resistant *Staphylococcus aureus* agent. *Eur. J. Med. Chem.* **2017**, *125*, 710–721. [CrossRef] [PubMed]
55. Garrison, A.T.; Abouelhassan, Y.; Kallifidas, D.; Tan, H.; Kim, Y.S.; Jin, S.; Luesch, H. An efficient buchwald-hartwig/reductive cyclization for the scaffold diversification of halogenated phenazines: Potent antibacterial targeting, biofilm eradication, and prodrug exploration. *J. Med. Chem.* **2018**, *61*, 3962–3983. [CrossRef] [PubMed]
56. Borrero, N.V.; Bai, F.; Perez, C.; Duong, B.Q.; Rocca, J.R.; Jin, S.; Huigens, R.W. Phenazine antibiotic inspired discovery of potent bromophenazine antibacterial agents against *Staphylococcus aureus* and *Staphylococcus epidermidis*. *Org. Biomol. Chem.* **2014**, *12*, 881–886. [CrossRef]
57. Zhang, D.; Lu, Y.; Liu, K.; Liu, B.; Wang, J.; Zhang, G.; Zhang, H.; Liu, Y.; Wang, B.; Zheng, M.; et al. Identification of less lipophilic riminophenazine derivatives for the treatment of drug-resistant tuberculosis. *J. Med. Chem.* **2012**, *55*, 8409–8417. [CrossRef]
58. Tonelli, M.; Novelli, F.; Tasso, B.; Sparatore, A.; Boido, V.; Sparatore, F.; Cannas, S.; Molicotti, P.; Zanetti, S.; Parapini, S.; et al. Antitubercular activity of quinolizidinyl/pyrrolizidinylalkyliminophenazines. *Bioorgan. Med. Chem.* **2014**, *22*, 6837–6845. [CrossRef]
59. Niu, J.; Chen, J.; Xu, Z.; Zhu, X.; Wu, Q.; Li, J. Synthesis and bioactivities of amino acid ester conjugates of phenazine-1-carboxylic acid. *Bioorg. Med. Lett.* **2016**, *26*, 5384–5386. [CrossRef]
60. Zhu, X.; Zhang, M.; Yu, L.; Xu, Z.; Yang, D.; Du, X.; Wu, Q.; Li, J. Synthesis and bioactivities of diamide derivatives containing a phenazine-1-carboxamide scaffold. *Nat. Prod. Res.* **2019**, *33*, 2453–2460. [CrossRef]
61. Han, F.; Yan, R.; Zhang, M.; Xiang, Z.; Wu, Q.; Li, J. Synthesis and bioactivities of phenazine-1-carboxylic piperazine derivatives. *Nat. Prod. Res.* **2020**, *34*, 1282–1287. [CrossRef]
62. Lu, X.; Zhu, X.; Zhang, M.; Wu, Q.; Zhou, X.; Li, J. Synthesis and fungicidal activity of 1,3,4-oxadiazol-2-ylthioether derivatives containing a phenazine-1-carboxylic acid scaffold. *Nat. Prod. Res.* **2019**, *33*, 2145–2150.
63. Li, X.; Zhang, W.; Zhao, C.; Wu, Q.; Li, J.; Xu, Z. Synthesis and fungicidal activity of phenazine-1-carboxylic triazole derivatives. *J. Asian Nat. Prod. Res.* **2021**, *23*, 452–465. [CrossRef] [PubMed]
64. Hayden, S.C.; Bryant, J.J.; Mackey, M.A.; Höfer, K.; Lindner, B.D.; Nguyen, V.P.; Jäschke, A.; Bunz, U.H.F. Antimicrobial activity of water-soluble triazole phenazine clickamers against *E. coli*. *Chem. Eur. J.* **2014**, *20*, 719–723. [CrossRef]
65. Zhi, X.; Yang, C.; Zhang, R.; Hu, Y.; Ke, Y.; Xu, H. Natural products-based insecticidal agents 13. Semisynthesis and insecticidal activity of novel phenazine derivatives of 4 beta-acyloxypodophyllotoxin modified in the E-ring against Mythimna separata Walker in vivo. *Ind. Crops Prod.* **2013**, *42*, 520–526. [CrossRef]
66. Zhi, X.; Yang, C.; Yu, X.; Xu, H. Synthesis and insecticidal activity of new oxime derivatives of podophyllotoxin-based phenazines against Mythimna separata Walker. *Bioorg. Med. Chem. Lett.* **2014**, *24*, 5679–5682. [CrossRef]

67. Alvarez, G.; Martinez, J.; Aguirre-Lopez, B.; Cabrera, N.; Perez-Diaz, L.; Tuena de Gomez-Puyou, M.; Gomez-Puyou, A.; Perez-Montfort, R.; Garat, B.; Merlino, A.; et al. New chemotypes as *Trypanosoma cruzi* triosephosphate isomerase inhibitors: A deeper insight into the mechanism of inhibition. *J. Enzyme Inhib. Med. Chem.* **2014**, *29*, 1–7. [CrossRef]
68. Minini, L.; Álvarez, G.; González, M.; Cerecetto, H.; Merlino, A. Molecular docking and molecular dynamics simulation studies of Trypanosoma cruzi triosephosphate isomerase inhibitors. Insights into the inhibition mechanism and selectivity. *J. Mol. Graph. Model.* **2015**, *58*, 40–49. [CrossRef] [PubMed]
69. Hernández, P.; Alem, D.; Nieves, M.; Cerecetto, H.; González, M.; Martínez-López, W.; Lavaggi, M.L. Chemosensitizer effect of cisplatin-treated bladder cancer cells by phenazine-5,10-dioxides. *Environ. Toxicol. Pharmacol.* **2019**, *69*, 9–15. [CrossRef]
70. Viktorsson, E.Ö.; Grøthe, B.M.; Aesoy, R.; Sabir, M.; Snellingen, S.; Prandina, A.; Høgmoen Åstrand, O.A.; Bonge-Hansen, T.; Døskeland, S.O.; Herfindal, L.; et al. Total synthesis and antileukemic evaluations of the phenazine 5,10-dioxide natural products iodinin, myxin and their derivatives. *Bioorg. Med. Chem.* **2017**, *25*, 2285–2293. [CrossRef]
71. Chowdhury, G.; Sarkar, U.; Pullen, S. DNA strand cleavage by the phenazine di-N-oxide natural product myxin under both aerobic and anaerobic conditions. *Chem. Res. Toxicol.* **2012**, *25*, 197–206. [CrossRef]
72. Lavaggi, M.L.; Cabrera, M.; Celano, L.; Thomson, L.; Cerecetto, H.; González, M. Biotransformation of phenazine 5,10-dioxides under hypoxic conditions as an example of activation of anticancer prodrug: An interdisciplinary experiment for biochemistry or organic chemistry. *J. Chem. Educ.* **2013**, *90*, 1388–1391. [CrossRef]
73. Gonda, M.; Nieves, M.; Nunes, E.; López De Ceráin, A.; Monge, A.; Lavaggi, M.L.; González, M.; Cerecetto, H.; Phenazine, N. N′-dioxide scaffold as selective hypoxic cytotoxin pharmacophore. Structural modifications looking for further DNA topoisomerase II-inhibition activity. *Med. Chem. Commun.* **2013**, *4*, 595–607. [CrossRef]
74. Vos, S.M.; Tretter, E.M.; Schmidt, B.H.; Berger, J.M. All tangled up: How cells direct, manage and exploit topoisomerase function. *Nat. Rev. Mol. Cell Biol.* **2011**, *12*, 827–841. [CrossRef] [PubMed]
75. Nitiss, J.L. Targeting DNA topoisomerase II in cancer chemotherapy. *Nat. Rev. Cancer* **2009**, *9*, 338–350. [CrossRef] [PubMed]
76. Zhuo, S.; Li, C.; Hu, M.; Chen, S.; Yao, P.; Huang, S.; Ou, T.; Tan, J.; An, L.; Li, D. Synthesis and biological evaluation of benzo[a]phenazine derivatives as a dual inhibitor of topoisomerase I and II. *Org. Biomol. Chem.* **2013**, *11*, 3989–4005. [CrossRef] [PubMed]
77. Nepali, K.; Sharma, S.; Sharma, M.; Bedi, P.M.; Dhar, K.L. Rational approaches, design strategies, structure activity relationship and mechanistic insights for anticancer hybrids. *Eur. J. Med. Chem.* **2014**, *77*, 422–487. [CrossRef]
78. Gamage, S.A.; Spicer, J.A.; Rewcastle, G.W.; Milton, J.; Sohal, S.; Dangerfield, W.; Mistry, P.; Vicker, N.; Charlton, P.A.; Denny, W.A. Structure-activity relationships for pyrido-, imidazo-, pyrazolo-, pyrazino-, and pyrrolophenazinecarboxamides as topoisomerase-targeted anticancer agents. *J. Med. Chem.* **2002**, *45*, 740–743. [CrossRef] [PubMed]
79. Gao, J.; Chen, M.; Tong, X.; Zhu, H.; Yan, H.; Liu, D.; Li, W.; Qi, S.; Xiao, D.; Wang, Y.; et al. Synthesis, antitumor activity, and structure-activity relationship of some benzo[a]pyrano[2,3-c] phenazine derivatives. *Comb. Chem. High Throughput Screen.* **2015**, *18*, 960–974. [CrossRef]
80. Whelan, P.; Dietrich, L.E.P.; Newman, D.K. Rethinking 'secondary' metabolism: Physiological roles for phenazine antibiotics. *Nat. Chem. Biol.* **2006**, *2*, 71–78. [CrossRef] [PubMed]
81. Gao, X.; Lu, Y.; Fang, L.; Fang, X.; Xing, Y.; Gou, S.; Xi, T. Synthesis and anticancer activity of some novel 2-phenazinamine Derivatives. *Eur. J. Med. Chem.* **2013**, *69*, 1–9. [CrossRef] [PubMed]
82. Khafagy, M.M.; El-Wahab, A.; Eid, F.A.; El-Agrody, A.M. Synthesis of halogen derivatives of benzo[h]chromene and benzo[a]anthracene with promising antimicrobial activities. *Farmaco* **2002**, *57*, 715–772. [CrossRef]
83. Shchemelinin, I.; Sefc, L.; Nečas, E. Protein kinases, their function and implication in cancer and other diseases. *Folia Biol.* **2006**, *52*, 81–100.
84. Endo, H.; Tada, M.; Katagiri, K. Biological characteristics of phenazine derivatives. IX. Effect on the fungal plant pathogen, *Piricularia oryzae*. *Sci. Rept. Res. Inst. Tohoku Univ. Ser. C* **1965**, *12*, 53.
85. Dai, J.; Punchihewa, C.; Mistry, P.; Ooi, A.T.; Yang, D. Novel DNA bis-intercalation by MLN944, a potent clinical bisphenazine anticancer drug. *J. Biol. Chem.* **2004**, *279*, 46096–46103. [CrossRef] [PubMed]

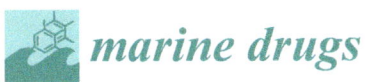

Review

Marine Pyrrole Alkaloids

Kevin Seipp [†], Leander Geske [†] and Till Opatz *

Department of Chemistry, Organic Chemistry Section, Johannes Gutenberg University, Duesbergweg 10–14, 55128 Mainz, Germany; kseipp@uni-mainz.de (K.S.); legeske@uni-mainz.de (L.G.)
* Correspondence: opatz@uni-mainz.de; Tel.: +49-(0)6131-39-24443
† Both authors contributed equally to this work.

Abstract: Nitrogen heterocycles are essential parts of the chemical machinery of life and often reveal intriguing structures. They are not only widespread in terrestrial habitats but can also frequently be found as natural products in the marine environment. This review highlights the important class of marine pyrrole alkaloids, well-known for their diverse biological activities. A broad overview of the marine pyrrole alkaloids with a focus on their isolation, biological activities, chemical synthesis, and derivatization covering the decade from 2010 to 2020 is provided. With relevant structural subclasses categorized, this review shall provide a clear and timely synopsis of this area.

Keywords: pyrroles; alkaloids; marine natural products; nitrogen heterocycles; bromopyrroles; pyrrole-imidazole alkaloids; pyrrole-aminoimidazole alkaloids

1. Introduction

The oceans cover more than 70% of the earth's surface and comprise around 95% of the volume of the biosphere. This impressive size of the marine habitat and its biological diversity known to date lead to the assumption of an enormous, yet still largely unexplored world, carrying an unused potential for research areas such as pharmacology, medicine, crop protection, or food technology. Furthermore, the uniqueness of marine life is reflected by the fact that only a small fraction of the 30,000 marine natural products (MNPs) known at present can also be found in terrestrial sources [1]. Additionally, the isolation and investigation of MNPs is a rapidly expanding field of research at the interface of biology and chemistry [2–10]. Looking back to 2009, when only 20,000 MNPs were known, an impressive increase of 50% has been achieved in the past 11 years, which highlights the importance of the marine habitat in this context [11].

Among the marine alkaloids, which are largely composed of nitrogen-containing heterocycles, the pyrroles form a large group of intriguing natural products which occur in marine organisms ranging from microbes over algae and sponges to animals. Their structural diversity including terpenoid-, polyketide-, carbohydrate-, lipid-, and peptide-frameworks [7,12] accompanied by attractive biological properties, has spurred a considerable interest of chemists [6,13–19].

This review focuses on marine pyrrole alkaloids containing at least one pyrrole moiety, which were discovered during the decade of 2010 to 2020. The number of newly discovered pyrrole MNPs surged in this decade and many structural revisions resulted in a deeper knowledge of their biogenetic origin and structural relations.

In addition to the reported structures and their biological sources, known biological activities and, where applicable, the first total syntheses of these compounds will be shown. Furthermore, this review is subdivided by structural subclasses based on the substitution pattern of the pyrrole core. As a delineation, only MNPs with intact pyrrole functionality are described, whereas indole alkaloids [20], the saturated heterocycles pyrroline and pyrrolidine [21], as well as other fused systems (e.g., carbazoles) and pyrrole derivatives lacking a genuine pyrrole core [22–25], will not be covered. Several other specific overviews

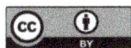

focusing on subclasses such as bromopyrroles [26,27] and pyrrole-imidazole alkaloids (PIA) [13,14,28] or with the focus on the isolation source [14,25,27], have been published. In contrast, we intend to provide the reader with an impression of the multiple facets of pyrrole alkaloids in the marine environment.

The five-membered planar 6π heteroaromatic pyrrole core with its high electron density is a reactive and privileged structural motif found in many biomolecules. It can provide stacking interactions, coordinate metal ions, or form hydrogen bonds when devoid of a substituent in the 1-position. Probably, the most well-known pyrrole derivatives in nature possess a tetrapyrrole skeleton, which can, e.g., be found in heme, chlorophyll, and several other porphyrinoid cofactors [29,30]. However, pyrroles possessing much simpler architectures have also attracted considerable interest, e.g., as promising lead structures in medicinal chemistry [15]. The biggest-selling drug of all time, the blood cholesterol lowering HMG-CoA reductase inhibitor atorvastatin (Lipitor®), is a pyrrole derivative. Not surprisingly, many pyrrole MNPs have also been associated with various pharmacological activities, such as cytotoxic [31,32], anti-bacterial [33,34], anti-fungal [35], and anti-cancer properties [6,36,37].

2. Non-Halogenated Marine Pyrrole Alkaloids

The alkaloids presented in this chapter are identified by a non-halogenated pyrrole core. Despite their structural diversity, the biosynthetic origin of these alkaloids can be traced back to a small number of possible biosynthetic pathways. According to the stunning logic of nature, only a few building blocks such as the amino acids glycine, serine, tryptophan, and proline are necessary to construct their pyrrole units.

A well-known pathway involves δ-aminolevulinic acid (ALA) as a key intermediate, which is produced from glycine and succinyl-CoA. An enzyme-catalyzed Knorr-type condensation–cyclization reaction of two molecules of δ-aminolevulinate yields porphobilinogen as a central intermediate, from which the trialkyl-substituted pyrroles are derived. Porphobilinogen is prone to self-condensation under acidic conditions and can further react to polypyrrolic systems, most notably the tetrapyrroles. Another major biosynthetic pathway is the dehydrogenation of proline to the common pyrrole-2-carboxylate unit. The activation of proline is suggested to involve a peptidyl carrier protein (PCP) forming a thioester linkage. In the next step, a controlled four-electron oxidation process with a flavoprotein desaturase occurs. These two C–N desaturation steps of the prolyl-S-PCP and subsequent tautomerization lead to the desired pyrrolyl-2-carboxyl-S-PCP product. Starting from this activated intermediate, a broad spectrum of reactions such as enzymatic transfer to nucleophiles or enzymatic halogenations can occur to create the world of marine pyrrole alkaloids [25,30,38,39].

2.1. Simple Pyrroles

The pyrrole derivative 1-(4-benzyl-1H-pyrrol-3-yl)ethanone (**1**) was found in a co-culture of the marine-derived fungi *Aspergillus sclerotiorum* and *Penicillium citrinum* in 2017 (Figure 1). The acylated pyrrole **1** shows only medium toxicity against brine shrimp (LC$_{50}$ values of 46.2 μM) and oppositely increases the growth of *Staphylococcus aureus* at 100 μg/mL [40].

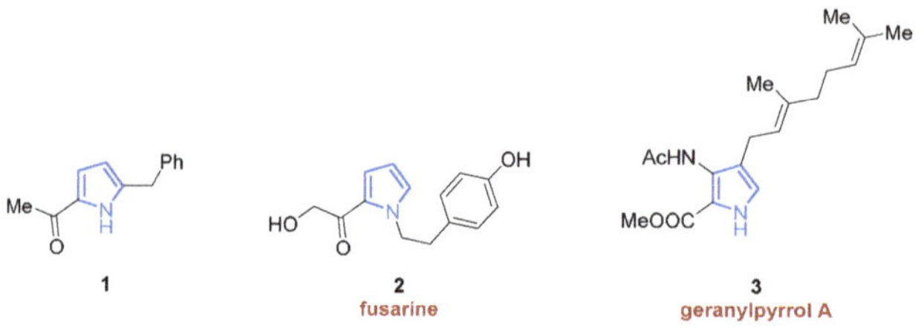

Figure 1. Simple pyrrole alkaloids **1**–**3** isolated from different marine organisms.

Investigation of an endophytic strain of *Fusarium incarnatum* yielded another acylated pyrrole, fusarine (**2**), isolated from the marine mangrove fruit *Aegiceras corniculatum* in 2012 (Figure 1). Alkaloid **2** is expected to be formed biosynthetically via a Paal–Knorr cyclization of a primary amine and a 1,3-dicarbonyl, but showed neither antiproliferative nor cytotoxic potential against HUVEC, K-562, and HeLa human cell lines [41].

Another simple pyrrole is represented by geranylpyrrol A (**3**), which is counted among the small class of pyrrolomonoterpenoids and derives from pyrrolostatin (Figure 1). It was isolated from a mutant strain of *Streptomyces* sp. CHQ-64 in 2017 but did not display any toxicity against eight tested human cancer cell lines [42].

The pyrroloterpenoid glaciapyrrol A (**10b**) was already isolated along with its congeners glaciapyrrols B and C in 2005. Despite extensive investigations, the relative configuration of C-11 and the overall absolute configuration could not be determined at this time [43]. Through the first total synthesis of its four diastereomers by Dickschat in 2011, the relative configuration of the three stereocenters could be unequivocally established [44]. The authors devised an enantioselective synthesis starting from geraniol (**4**) using a Sharpless epoxidation to furnish alcohol **5**. Protection of the alcohol functionality and subsequent Sharpless dihydroxylation followed by intramolecular cyclization served as the key step and stereoselectively generated compound **6**. After several steps including a protection/deprotection sequence followed by oxidation and Horner–Wadsworth–Emmons (HWE) reaction using phosphonate **7**, ester **8** was obtained in 64% over four steps. Saponification, the addition of pyrrolyl Grignard **9**, and final TBS-deprotection finally produced *ent*-(−)-glaciapyrrol A (**10a**) showing the opposite optical rotation as the original publication from 2005. The authors, therefore, identified the natural product as (+)-glaciapyrrol A (**10b**) (Scheme 1) [44].

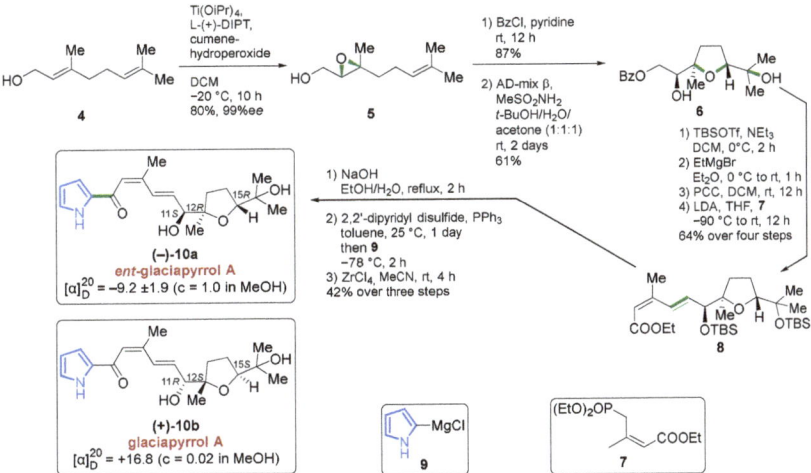

Scheme 1. Enantioselective approach towards the total synthesis of pyrrolosesquiterpenoid **10b** by a Sharpless epoxidation/dihydroxylation sequence, leading to the unnatural *ent*-(−)-glaciapyrrol A (**10a**).

The bromotyrosine-derived pyrrole alkaloid pseudocerolide A (**11**), was isolated from a marine sponge (*Pseudoceratina* sp.) from the South China Sea in 2020 and its proposed structure could be confirmed by X-ray crystallography (Figure 2). Unfortunately, compound **11** exhibited no activities against methicillin-resistant *Staphylococcus aureus*, *Escherichia coli*, or *Candida albicans* [45].

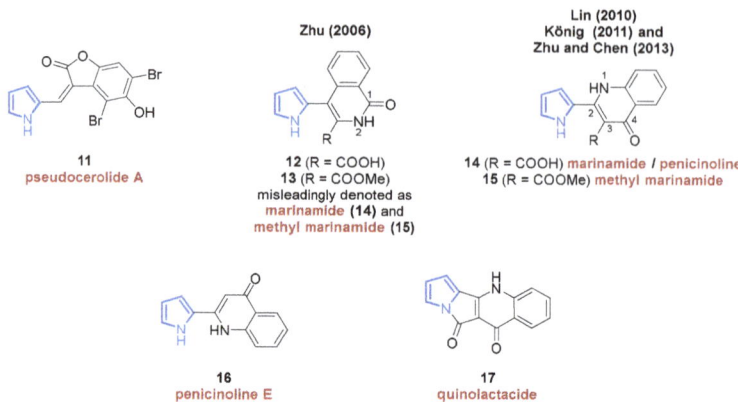

Figure 2. Pseudocerolide A (**11**) and quinolinone alkaloids **12–17** isolated from marine origin.

The unusual pyrrolyl 1-isoquinolone alkaloids **12** and **13** were discovered from a habitat in the South China Sea within a co-culture of two mangrove endophytic fungi (strain No. 1924 and 3893) in 2006 [46]. It took until 2011, when König and co-workers isolated methyl marinamide (**15**) from the marine sponge (*Ircinia variabilis*) and reported a revised structure of **15**, in which the previously assumed 1-isoquinolone of **13** was reassigned as a 4-quinolinone unit on the basis of X-ray crystallography. Unfortunately, **15** showed only weak or no effects in the biological evaluation on cannabinoid receptors [47]. In accordance with the findings of König, Zhu and Chen, chemically modified the previously isolated compound **14** in 2013, which also led to the revision of the structure **12** to **14** for marinamide in the same fashion, further confirming the revision of marinamide by König and co-workers [48]. However, one year before the report of König, the Lin laboratory isolated the same compound **14**, but referred to it as penicinoline (Figure 2) [49]. Both compounds **14** and **15** display promising in vitro cytotoxicity towards 95-D and HepG2 cell lines (IC_{50} values of 0.57 µg/mL and 6.5 µg/mL, respectively) as well as insecticidal activity against *Aphis gossypii* (100% mortality at 1000 ppm) [48,49].

The related congener penicinoline E (**16**) was isolated from an endophytic fungus *Penicillium* sp. ghq208 in 2012 alongside quinolactacide (**17**), which was isolated from a marine source for the first time [50,51]. In biological assays, moderate cytotoxicity against HepG2 was exclusively attributed to 4-quinolinones **14** and **15** (IC_{50} values of 11.3 µg/mL and 13.2 µg/mL, respectively), indicating the importance of the free carboxy function at C3 (Figure 2) [51].

Based on the auspicious pharmacological activities of penicinoline E (**16**), marinamide (**14**), and methyl marinamide (**15**), the Nagarajan group established their total synthesis in 2017 for further biological testing [52]. They achieved a two- to three-step approach, characterized by a Suzuki–Miyaura coupling and subsequent dearomatization as key steps from their starting materials **18**, **19**, and **20**. They were also able to unambiguously confirm the structure of penicinoline E (**16**) by X-ray crystallography (Scheme 2) [52].

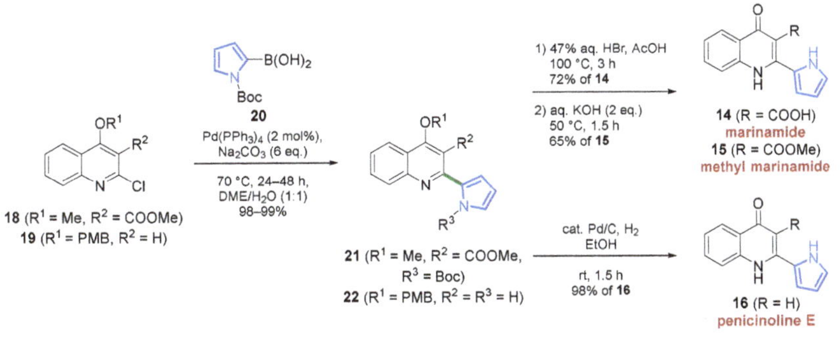

Scheme 2. A high-yield sequence towards pyrrolyl 4-quinolinones **14**, **15**, and **16** starting from 2-chloroquinoline precursors **18** and **19** by Nagarajan et al.

Furthermore, the antimalarial properties against the 3D7 strain of *Plasmodium falciparum* were evaluated and the decarboxylated derivative **16**, as well as the methyl ester **15**, showed significant activity (IC_{50} value of 1.56 µM for both). These results have been confirmed by binding mode studies of the synthesized ligands **14**, **15**, and **16** to the CYTB protein of *Plasmodium falciparum* [52].

Another pharmacologically interesting compound class is the indanomycins, which possess a variety of biological activities such as antibacterial [53], insecticidal [54], and antiprotozoal [55] properties. In 2011, the group of Kelly and co-workers published a study on the biosynthesis of indanomyincs, including an intramolecular Diels–Alder cyclization of a tetraene as the key step [56]. Two years later, researchers isolated three new representatives of these pyrrole ethers from the culture broth of a marine *Streptomyces anibioticus* strain PTZ0016 which possess in vitro activity against *Staphylococccus aureus* (MIC values between 4.0 and 8.0 µg/mL). Based on their previous derivatives and on the α- or β-orientation of the pyran ring, they were named 16-deethylindanomycins. The relative and absolute configurations of iso-16-deethylindanomycin (**23**), iso-16-deethylindanomycin methyl ester (**24**), and 16-deethylindanomycin methyl ester (**25**) were established by extensive NMR and CD spectroscopy (Figure 3) [57].

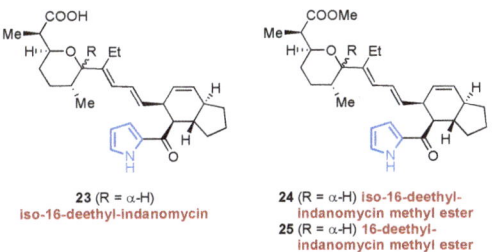

Figure 3. Three new members **23**–**25** of the indanomycin-group, discovered in 2013.

Another important source of bioactive MNPs is represented by the genus *Agelas* (family Agelasidae), which provides a wide diversity of glycolipids [58,59], diterpene alkaloids [60–62], and pyrrole alkaloids [63–66]. To date, more than 130 pyrrole alkaloids have been isolated from over 20 *Agelas* species, all of which share a unique bromo- or debromopyrrole-2-carboxamide moiety alongside several linear side chains, anellated ring systems, or dimeric structural units [67].

In 2017, Li et al. reported the isolation of the nakamurines A–C (**26**–**28**) from the South China Sea sponge *Agelas nakamurai*. They only differ in the side chain of the carboxamide unit, however, no activity could be observed for any of the compounds in cytotoxicity tests and antiviral assays. In antimicrobial assays, only nakamurine B (**27**) showed weak inhibitory effects against *Candida albicans* (MIC = 60 µg/mL, Figure 4) [67].

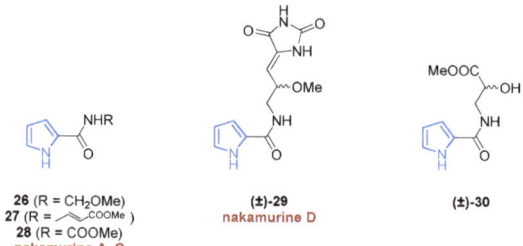

Figure 4. Isolation of five pyrrole-2-carboxamides (**26–30**) from the sea sponge *Agelas nakamurai*.

A few weeks later, the same group published the extraction of two non-brominated pyrroles, **29** and **30**, from the same sponge *Agelas nakamurai* [68]. For structure elucidation, the racemic pairs were resolved by chiral HPLC with the absolute stereochemistries determined by quantum chemical calculations and measurements of molar rotations. The carboxamide **30** was listed in *SciFinder Scholar* with no associated reference at that time, but the analytical data were reported for the first time. In cytotoxicity and antimicrobial tests, no activity could be observed for any of the enantiomers of nakamurine D (**29**) or for compound **30** (Figure 4) [68].

In 2017, Li and co-workers were able to isolate a new class of racemic pyrroles, the nemoechines A–C (**31**, **32**, and **124**), from the species *Agelas* aff. *nemoechinata* (Figure 5) [69]. Nemoechine A (**31**) differs from the two related congeners **32** and **124** by its unusual bicyclic cyclopentane-fused imidazole skeleton, whereas nemoechine B (**124**) features a fused pyrrole core and is therefore specified in Section 2.4. Nemoechine C (**32**), with its butyric acid ester side chain, shows structural similarity to pyrrole **30** and differs only by an additional methylene group. Unfortunately, nemoechine A (**31**) and C (**32**) did not show any promising activities which complies with the inactivity of the structurally related pyrroles **29** and **30** [69].

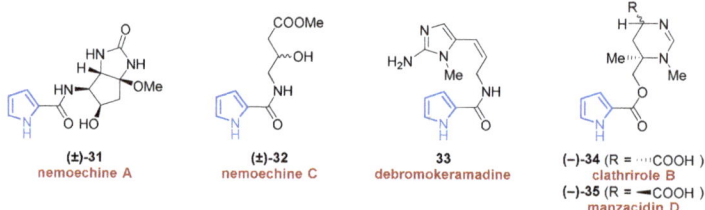

Figure 5. Isolation of nemoechine A (**31**) and C (**32**), debromokeramadine (**33**), and clathrirole B (**34**).

The isolation of pyrrole-2-aminoimidazole (P-2-AI) debromokeramadine (**33**) from the marine sponge *Agelas* cf. *mauritiana* was reported alongside the first total syntheses of **33** and keramadine (**41**) in 2015. Interestingly, **33** and the previously isolated derivative keramadine (**41**), feature a (*Z*)-configuration at the C=C double bond, which is in contrast to the well-known natural key-precursor oroidin featuring an (*E*)-configured double bond (Figure 5) [70,71].

Clathrirole B (**34**), extracted from the marine sponge *Clathria prolifera*, represents another P-2-AI alkaloid. The carboxylic acid ester **34** is a C-11 epimer of manzacidin D (**35**), which was isolated from the marine sponge *Astrosclera willeyana* back in 1997 (Figure 5) [72]. Interestingly, compound **34** completely lacks antifungal activity against *Saccharomyces cerevisiae*, whereas diastereomer **35** and derivatives thereof proved to be potent antifungals against this yeast [35]. Thus, the authors concluded that the absolute configurations at both C-9 and C-11 may have a massive influence on the antifungal activity of this compound class [73].

The authors applied a one-pot approach with a regioselective oxidative addition in which partially brominated *N*-acylpyrrole-1,2-dihydropyridines **36** and **37** were reacted with guanidine **38** in a double nucleophilic substitution to generate the aminoimidazoline moiety. Finally, the cyclic aminal structure is ring-opened by TFA, resulting in the MNPs **33** and **41** (Scheme 3) [71].

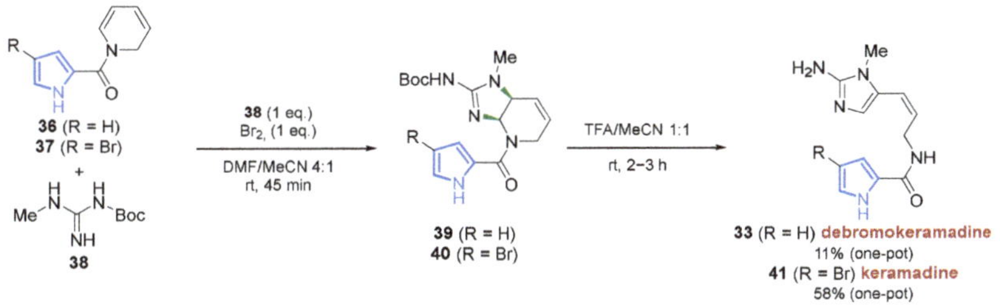

Scheme 3. Synthesis of keramadines **33** and **41**, including a regioselective oxidative addition followed by acid mediated bond cleavage of the aminal.

In the previously reported isolation of MNPs from *Agelas* aff. *nemoechinata* and *nakamurai*, the class of nakamurines and nemoechines were presented [68,69]. It should be mentioned that the group of Li isolated several structurally related pyrrole alkaloids from marine sources and identified them as known compounds that had been synthesized but not isolated from natural sources before. Therefore, carboxamides **42–47**, isolated from marine sources for the first time, are grouped together in Figure 6. The *N*-acylglycine methyl ester **42** identified in both sponges is related to nakamurine C (**28**) but carries an additional methylene group [68,69]. The synthetically known pyrrole **43** bearing two more methylene groups in the side chain, was isolated from *Agelas nakamurai* [68,74,75].

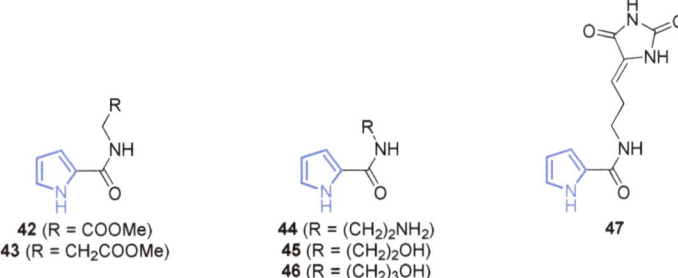

Figure 6. Synthetically known pyrrole-2-carboxamides **42–47**, isolated for the first time from marine origin.

Some reduction products of the methyl esters and an amine derivative are represented by compounds **44–46**, of which **45** occurs in both sponges, whereas **44** and **46** were exclusively isolated from the *Nemoechinata* sp. [68,69,76,77]. The carboxamide **47** is a debromo analog of mukanadin B and is present in *Agelas nakamurai* [68,78,79]. Compounds **42–47** described show neither cytotoxicity nor antimicrobial activity.

The Arctic hydrozoan *Thuiaria breitfussi* (family Sertulariidae) produces a class of indole-oxazole-pyrrole MNPs named breitfussins. Biosynthetically, the breitfussins may share a similar biogenesis as the phorbazoles (cf. Figure 33), arising from the dipeptides Pro-Trp or Pro-Tyr. In the first isolation and analysis of breitfussin A (**48**) in 2012, high-resolution mass spectrometry indicated a ratio of non-hydrogen atoms to hydrogen of 2:1 which makes the structural elucidation by spectroscopic methods challenging [80]. The authors, however, could identify a brominated 4-methoxyindole moiety, a 2-substituted pyrrole core as well as an unresolved C$_3$NO fragment suggestive of an oxazole core, which finally prevented the unambiguous determination of the entire structure. By applying a combined approach of atomic force microscopy (AFM), computer-aided structure elucidation (CASE) and calculation of ^{13}C-NMR shifts through density functional theory (DFT), the structure of breitfussin A (**48**) could be unequivocally determined (Figure 7) [80]. A recently published article describes the isolation of further non-halogenated congeners, namely breitfussins C (**49**), D (**50**), and F (**51**), of which structures **49** and **50** could also be confirmed by total syntheses (Figure 7) [81].

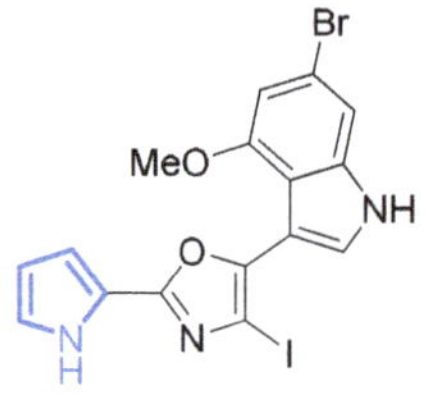

48
breitfussin A

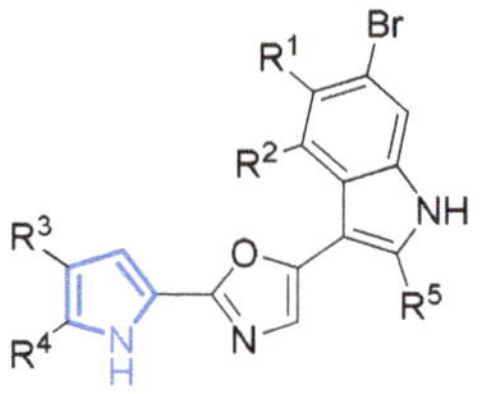

49 (R^1 = OMe, R^2 = R^3 = R^4 = R^5 = H)
50 (R^1 = R^3 = R^4 = R^5 = H, R^2 = OMe)
51 (R^1 = R^3 = R^4 = H, R^2 = OMe, R^5 = I)
breitfussins C, D and F

Figure 7. Molecular structures of breitfussins **48–51** isolated from the marine hydrozoan *Thuiaria breitfussi*.

Given the promising cytotoxic activities of the breitfussins C (**49**) and D (**50**) against several cancer cell lines with IC$_{50}$ values below 10 μM, extensive research on the breitfussin scaffold in search for selective kinase inhibitors has been performed [81]. Due to their promising bioactivity but extremely challenging heteroaromatic core in terms of structure elucidation, the breitfussins are attractive starting points for ongoing synthetic work [82].

The first total synthesis and hence the structure validation of breitfussin A (**48**) was published by the Bayer group in 2015 [83]. They used an approach involving two Suzuki couplings in which the oxazole and pyrrole moieties were installed sequentially. First, indole **52** was converted with oxazole **54** into coupling product **55**, followed by double lithiation of the oxazole core. Coupling with *N*-Boc-2-pyrrole boronic acid (**20**) furnished pyrrole **57**, which, after removal of all protection groups, resulted in the formation of breitfussin A (**48**) [83]. Alongside the isolation of additional breitfussins in 2019, the Bayer laboratory employed the same approach as in their previous publication for the synthesis of breitfussin C (**49**) and D (**50**). Here, only the penultimate step varied by acid-mediated Boc-deprotection, since deiodination of the oxazole core was required (Scheme 4) [81].

Bisindole pyrroles represent a class of MNPs having similar biological activities. The lynamicins F (**59**) and G (**60**) were isolated from a marine-derived *Streptomyces* sp. SCSIO 03032 [84], extending the lynamicin family, of which lynamicins A–E have been isolated back in 2008 (Figure 8) [85]. Unfortunately, no antimicrobial or cytotoxic activities were observed for **59** and **60** against several indicator strains or cancer cell lines. In 2017, the first total synthesis of the antimicrobial lynamicin D (**72**) was achieved, thereby enabling the implementation of further biological assays (Scheme 5). It turned out that lynamicin D (**72**) influenced the splicing of pre-mRNAs by upregulating the level of the key kinase SRPK1, which is involved in both constitutive and alternative splicing [86].

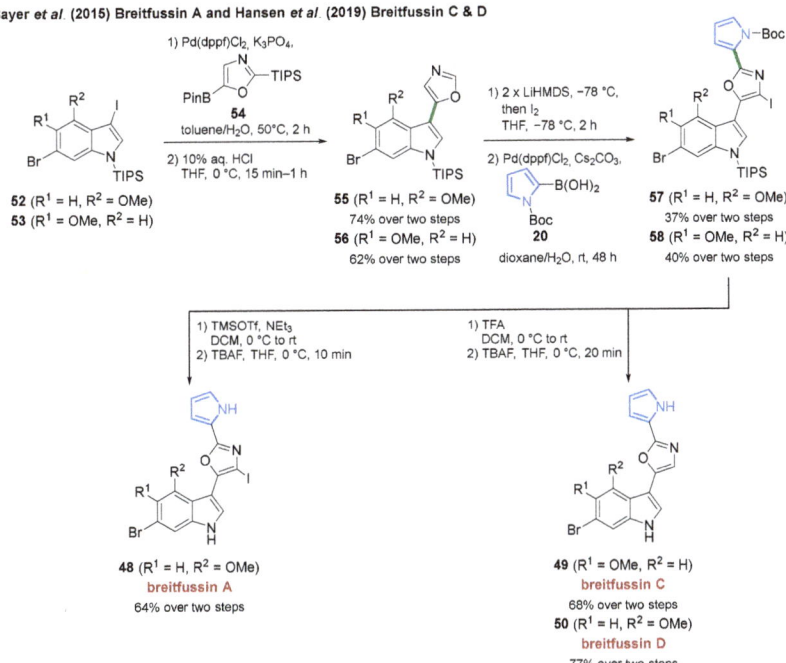

Scheme 4. Total synthesis of the three breitfussins A (**48**), C (**49**), and D (**50**) by introducing the oxazole and pyrrole functionalities via two consecutive Suzuki coupling reactions.

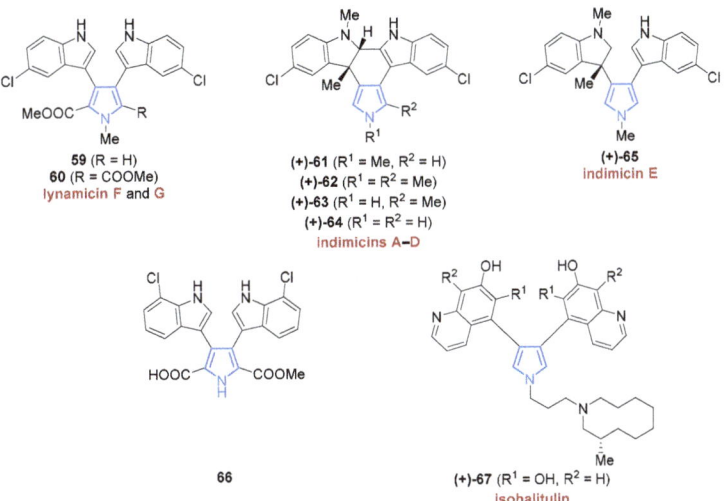

Figure 8. Structures of lynamicins F (**59**) and G (**60**), indimicins A–E (**61**–**65**), dichlorochromopyrrolic acid derivative **66**, and isohalitulin (**67**).

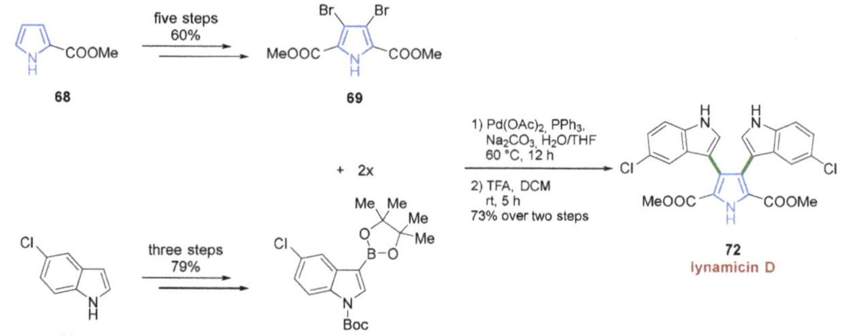

Scheme 5. Key step of the synthesis of lynamicin D (**72**) by a Suzuki coupling.

In addition to the alkaloids **59** and **60**, a new family of MNPs consisting of a unique 1,3-dimethyl-2-hydroindole motif, the indimicins (IDMs) A–E (**61**–**65**), were discovered in 2015 (Figure 8) [84]. Besides the usual spectroscopic data, an X-ray structure of indimicin A (**61**) could be obtained, which allowed determining the absolute configuration of the hydroindole moiety. Of compounds **61**–**65**, only indimicin B (**62**) was active against the breast cancer cell line MCF-7 (IC$_{50}$ value of 10.0 µM ± 0.3 µM), whereas all seven alkaloids **61**–**65** did not show any antimicrobial or cytotoxic activities against several indicator strains or cancer cell lines [84].

Very recently, the *Streptomyces* sp. SCSIO 11791 revealed another bisindolylpyrrole (**66**), displaying moderate cytotoxicity against a human breast cancer cell line (MDA-MB-435, IC$_{50}$ value of 19.4 µM), while no antibacterial properties could be observed (Figure 8) [87].

In isohalitulin (**67**), isolated from the marine sponge *haliclona tulearensis* in 2010, the structure is dominated by a bis-dihydroxyquinoline functionality (Figure 8) [88]. Compound **67** exhibits a detectable toxicity to brine shrimp (*Artemia salina*, LD$_{50}$ value of 0.9 mM). It is also worth mentioning that minute amounts and instability of isohalitulin (**67**) prevented the unequivocal determination of its structure. However, **67** shows very similar analytical data to its congener halitulin and should differ only in the position of the two phenolic OH groups (Figure 8). Although no experiments were performed to deduce the stereochemistry of **67**, the authors mentioned that, on the grounds of common biogenetic precursors, it most probably has the same absolute configuration as halitulin [88].

The total synthesis of lynamicin D (**72**) commenced with the synthesis of the coupling partners **69** and **71**, prepared from commercially available precursors **68** and **70**. Dibrominated pyrrole **69** was obtained by a Vilsmeier–Haack reaction, followed by oxidation, esterification, and final bromination. On the other side, 5-chloro-1*H*-indole (**70**) was first iodinated and Boc-protected and the introduction of the pinacol moiety on the basis of Pd-catalysis resulted in the formation of indole precursor **71**. Building blocks **69** and **71** were then subjected to the key Suzuki coupling. Final removal of the Boc-group gave lynamicin D (**72**) in 73% yield over two steps (Scheme 5) [86].

The suberitamides and denigrins constitute another family of highly substituted pyrrole alkaloids. The symmetrical, nearly planar suberitamide B (**73**) was isolated from the marine sponge *Pseudosuberties* sp. in 2020 and bears a fully substituted pyrrole core. This storniamide-related compound inhibits the enzymatic activity of Cb1-b (E3 ubiquitin ligase) with an IC$_{50}$ value of 11 µM, which, according to the authors, is caused by the rigid, highly substituted pyrrole scaffold (Figure 9) [89].

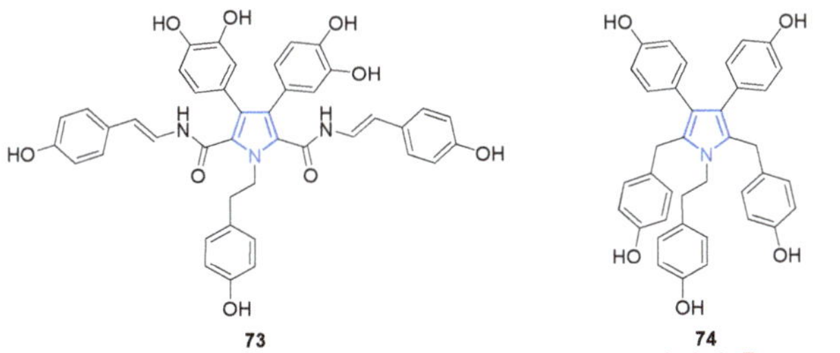

Figure 9. Highly substituted 3,4-diarylpyrroles suberitamide B (**73**) and denigrin E (**74**).

In 2020, denigrin E (**74**) was isolated from a new *Dactylia* sp. along with several members of the pyrrolone family. Unfortunately, no inhibitory activity against PAX3-FOXO1 luciferase expression was observed in biological assays (Figure 9) [90]. By considering the substitution pattern of these 3,4-diarylpyrroles **73** and **74**, a close relationship as potential precursors of lamellarins (see Section 2.4.1) in a biosynthetic context can be suggested.

Among the huge variety of marine alkaloids, aromatic polyketides (APK) represent another large class of MNPs and pyrrole-containing representatives have been described. The group of Zhang and co-workers isolated the decaketide pyrrole SEK43F (**75**) generated from pathway crosstalk of the host *Streptomyces albus* J1074 and the heterologous fls-gene cluster from *Micromonospora rosaria* SCSIO N160 (Figure 10) [91]. It should be mentioned that the configuration of the double bond in **75** could not be unequivocally determined. The same group also isolated another tri-methylated bis-pyrrole **76** (Figure 10) [91], which has only been known as a synthetic product before [92,93]. Both compounds **75** and **76** displayed negligible antibacterial activity, whereas the APK **75** showed weak to moderate cytotoxicity against four human cancer cell lines (SF-268, MCF-7, NCI-H460, and HePG-2, with IC$_{50}$ values of 56.46 μM ± 0.87 μM, 35.73 μM ± 1.45 μM, 44.62 μM ± 2.49 μM, and 39.22 μM ± 3.00 μM, respectively, Figure 10).

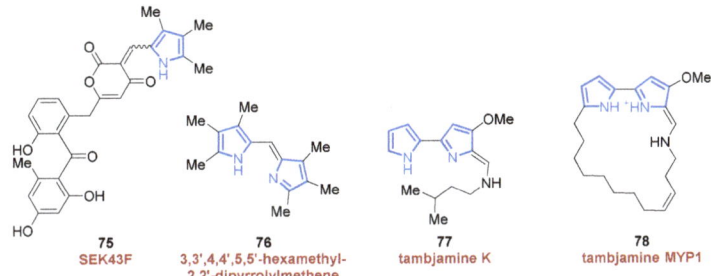

Figure 10. Representation of an APK (**75**) and three pyrroles **76**–**78** including the important class of tambjamines.

The family of tambjamines consisting of a central bi-pyrrole unit is counted among the 4-methoxypyrrolic natural products. In 2010, tambjamine K (**77**) was isolated as the main secondary metabolite from the Azorean nudibranch mollusk *Tambja ceutae* and in minute amounts from the bryozoan *Bugula dentata* (Figure 10) [94]. Just as its family members, tambjamine K (**77**) exhibited remarkable to moderate antiproliferative activity against tumor and non-tumor mammalian cells with IC$_{50}$ values between 3.5 nM and 19 μM. It is suspected that the strong activity is caused by the bipyrrolic structure with its DNA-targeting properties and by the ability to form ion complexes [94].

The macrocyclic tambjamine MYP1 (**78**) is produced by the marine bacterium *Pseudoalteromonas citrea* and was isolated in 2019 (Figure 10) [95]. The authors highlighted the important differences of the α- and β-rotamers in the tambjamine conformations, which are thought to play an essential role in their bioactivity. Moreover, the group provides an X-ray structure by co-crystallization of **78** with formic acid, unequivocally confirming the proposed structure of compound **78** [95].

Based on the promising bioactivity of compound **77**, Lindsley et al. were prompted to publish their first three-step total synthesis of tambjamine K (**77**) four months after its initial isolation [96]. The first step involved a Vilsmeier–Haack haloformylation which generated enamine **80** in 59% yield. A Suzuki coupling with Boc-1H-pyrrol-2-ylboronic acid (**20**) followed by acid-mediated condensation of isopentylamine resulted in the formation of tambjamine K (**77**) in 31% over two steps (Scheme 6) [96]. In addition to the natural product synthesis, a series of unnatural derivatives were synthesized followed by biological assays to evaluate basic structure–activity relationships (SAR). However, the natural product **77** showed moderate activity (IC_{50} values of 13.7 µM and 15.3 µM against HCT116 and MBA231, respectively), whereas the unnatural analogs were more potent in inhibiting the viability, proliferation, and invasion of HCT116, MBA231, SW 620, and H520 NSCLC cancer cell lines (IC_{50} values between 146 nM and 10 µM) [96].

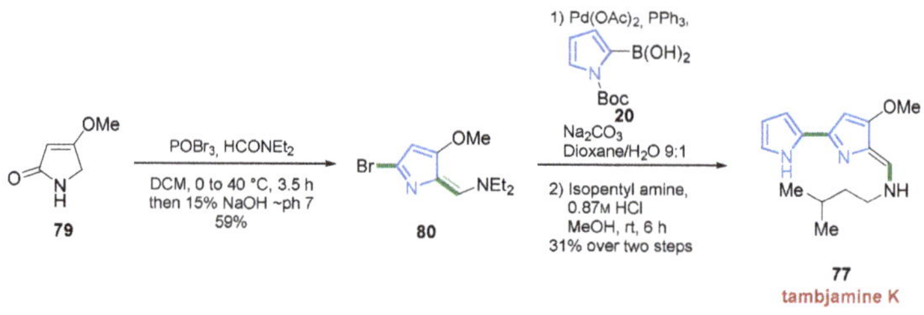

Scheme 6. A linear 3-step sequence to tambjamine K (**77**).

In addition to the tambjamines which consist of a bipyrrole core functionalized with various imines, the functionalization with an additional pyrrole moiety in the prodiginine structures represents another well-studied family. With the isolation of the marineosins A (**85a**) and B (**86**) in 2008, this prodiginine-related family opened up a new field of research with several new contributions being made in the last decade [97]. In 2014, the Reynolds laboratory focused on the final steps of the marineosin biosynthesis, by exploring the biosynthetic gene cluster *mar* which can produce marineosins by a heterologous expression in a *Streptomyces venezuelae* derived JND2 strain. They replaced the *marA* and *marG* gene with the spectinomycin resistance *aadA* gene which led to the isolation and elucidation of 16-ketopremarineosin A (**83**) and premarineosin A (**84**) as well as 23-hydroxyundecylprodiginine (HUPG) (**81**) and its oxidized derivative **82**, respectively (Figure 11). As marineosin production was not observed, the authors concluded that both genes, *marA* and *marG*, are essential for the biosynthesis of marineosins [98]. Three years later, the Reynolds group reported another gene (*marH*) from the same cluster which has the ability to catalyze the condensation of a methoxybipyrrole carbaldehyde (MBC) and 2-undecylpyrrole (UP) to generate undecylprodiginine (UPG). The gene also hydroxylates the C-23 position of UPG to construct HUPG (**81**) and hence is essential for the biosynthetic pathway of marineosins [99].

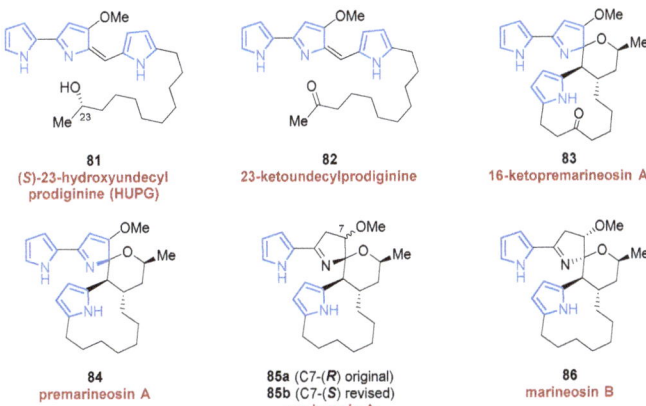

Figure 11. Different prodiginine-based pyrrole alkaloids **81** and **82** together with marineosin-type spiroaminals **83–86**.

Not only the biosynthetic pathway but also the stereoselective synthesis of marineosins, their substructures, and derivatives have attracted much attention. In 2014, the Reynolds laboratory followed up on their previous publications regarding marineosins and reported the first total synthesis of HUPG (**81**) and premarineosin A (**84**). To this end, a divergent synthetic approach of nine steps in total stereospecifically provided 23-hydroxyundecylprodiginine (**81**). The final cyclization forming the spiro-tetrahydropyran-aminal unit of the premarineosin A (**84**) was then achieved by a biosynthetic approach via the Rieske oxygenase MarG (Scheme 7) [100]. This strategy yields several other prodiginine derivatives and premarineosin analogs that show promising cytotoxic and antimalarial activities [100].

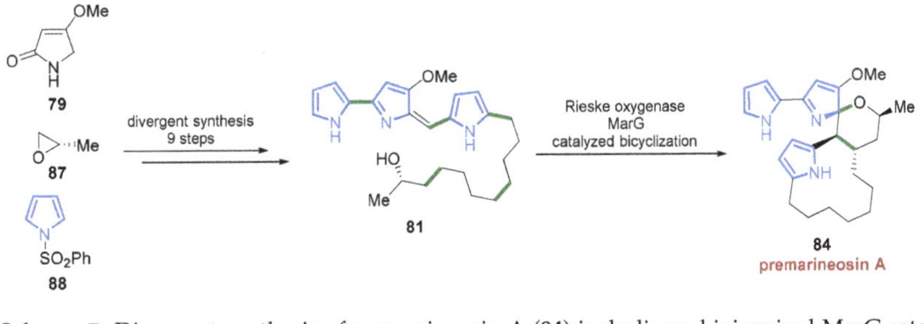

Scheme 7. Divergent synthesis of premarineosin A (**84**) including a bioinspired MarG catalyzed spirocyclization as the final step.

Based on unsuccessful synthetic attempts (with the exception of individual key motifs) of several research groups [101–106], Shi and co-workers presented the first total synthesis of marineosin A (**85a**) in 2016 [107]. The synthesis commenced with the commercially available (S)-pyrone **89**, which was converted into key fragment **90** in 10% yield over 14 steps. Lewis acid-mediated spirocyclization and ring-closing metathesis followed by hydrogenation furnished spiro lactam **91** in 37% yield over three steps. The last two steps consisted of a Paal–Knorr reaction and a Vilsmeier–Haack reaction, not only allowing for the preparation of the sensitive pyrrole moieties in a late-stage procedure but also directly giving access to marineosin A′ (Scheme 8). It is also worth mentioning that five X-ray structures of important intermediates could be obtained, underpinning the validity of the synthesis. However, the NMR spectra, appearance, and optical rotation of the resulting marineosin A′ (**85a**) exhibited some deviations when compared to the isolated natural product, suggesting that the natural and synthetic compounds likely differ in their stereochemistry [107].

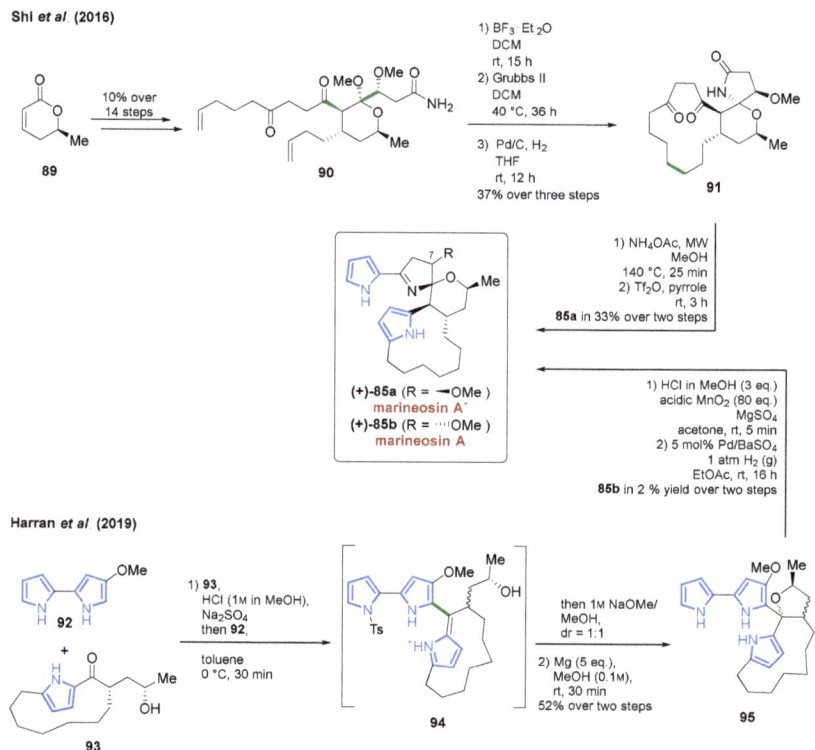

Scheme 8. The first total synthesis of 7-*epi*-marineosin A (**85a**) by Shi and co-workers in a linear 19 step sequence and the structural reassignment of C7-OMe from (*R*) to (*S*) by the Harran laboratory using a chromophore disruption approach.

It was however not until 2019, that the Harran group solved the puzzle by a total synthesis and concomitant reassignment of C7-(*R*) in **85a** to C7-(*S*) resulting in the structure **85b** for (+)-marineosin A [108]. To this end, a bioinspired approach with reversed fragment polarity was applied, starting from the previously prepared bipyrrole **92** and cyclic ketone **93**. Condensation product **94** was stabilized by quenching with NaOMe, generating a novel but still unstable premarineosin **95**. After exposure to acidic conditions, a prodiginine chromophore was formed, which, after 6-*exo* trig cyclization mediated by acidic MnO$_2$, was converted to a premarineosin derivative. The formed vinylogous imidate was hydrogenated from the less hindered face, resulting in the formation of (+)-marineosin A (**85b**), whose spectroscopic data are in full agreement with those reported for the isolated natural product **85b** (Scheme 8) [108].

2.2. Formylpyrroles

In addition to the acyl-, carboxy-, and carboxamido-pyrroles (**1–3**, **23–25** and **26–34**) shown in the previous Section (cf. Section 2.1), the formylpyrroles constitute another distinct family of the marine pyrrole alkaloids [109].

In the course of an investigation of the South China Sea sponge *Mycale lissochela* in 2017, two new formylpyrroles **96** and **97** bearing an aliphatic side chain with a terminal nitrile group were isolated (Figure 12) [110]. Both mycalenitrile-15 (**96**) and mycalenitrile-16 (**97**) showed excellent and good inhibition effects against PTP1B (protein-tyrosine phosphatase 1B, a recognized target for diabetes and obesity) with IC$_{50}$ values of 8.6 µmol/L and 3.1 µmol/L, respectively, resulting from the unsaturated side chain [110].

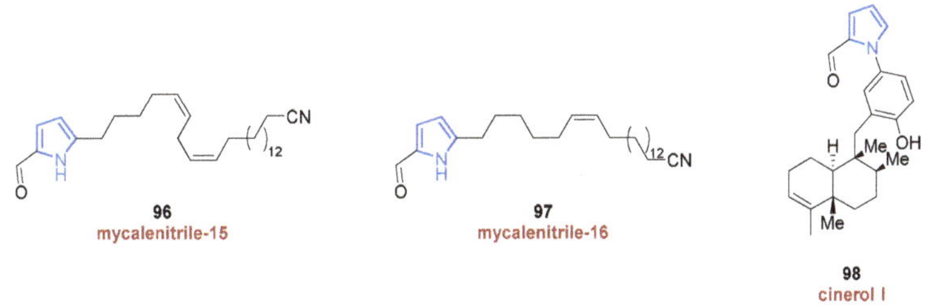

Figure 12. Mycalenitrile **96** and **97** as well as the pyrrole-terpenoid **98**.

An additional formylpyrrole, cinerol I (**98**), was isolated from the sponge *Dysidea cinerea* and belongs to the meroterpenoid family (Figure 12) [111]. Cinerol I (**98**), which lacks the unsaturated side chain present in compounds **96** and **97**, showed no inhibitory activity against PTP1B, ATP-citrate lyase (ACL), or SH2 domain-containing phosphatase-1 (SHP-1) [111].

Five new formylpyrroles **99–103** were isolated from the marine cyanobacterium *Moorea producens* in 2017 (Figure 13) [112]. Biosynthetically, they are suggested to originate from the amino acid tryptophan, the indole moiety of which is partly reduced to forge the annellated tetramethylenepyrrole framework. Further annellated pyrroles are depicted in Section 2.4. All pyrroles described herein feature a 3-formyl group, and compound **103** additionally carries a purine unit. The five isolated pyrroles **99–103** showed no noteworthy cytotoxicity or antibacterial properties [112].

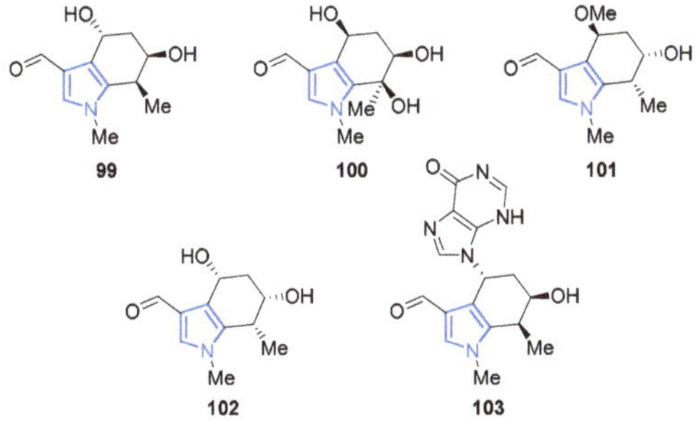

Figure 13. Representation of five tetrahydroindoles **99–103** isolated from *Moorea producens*.

2.3. Nitropyrroles

A new subclass of pyrroleterpene MNPs is represented by 2-nitro-substituted pyrroles carrying a diversely functionalized farnesyl chain attached to the 4-position of the pyrrole core. The nitropyrrolin and heronapyrrole families known to date are formed biosynthetically by means of an electrophilic aromatic substitution of the pyrrole core by a farnesyl pyrophosphate. Subsequent nitration, oxidation to epoxides and alcohols, as well as cascade cyclization reactions then produce a variety of different substituted metabolites.

The first MNP from this subclass was isolated back in 2006, however, the structural characterization appears to be incomplete and no information about the stereochemistry was given [113]. In 2010, the group of Fenical reported the isolation of five farnesyl-2-nitropyrroles **104–108** from the marine actinomycete strain CNQ-509 and referred to them as nitropyrrolins A–E (**104–108**) (Figure 14) [114]. The authors performed several chemical modifications, including an acetonide formation from epoxide **105**, and the Mosher method was applied to unequivocally identify the full stereochemistry of nitropyrrolins A–E (**104**–**108**). Among compounds **104**–**108**, nitropyrrolin D (**107**) displayed the most promising IC$_{50}$ value of 5.7 µM in biological assays against HCT-116 colon carcinoma cells, whereas a lower antibacterial activity against MRSA was observed for all nitropyrrolins **104**–**108** (MIC values >20 µg/mL). Some of the synthetic derivatives synthesized in the course of the structure elucidation process showed strong to moderate cytotoxic (IC$_{50}$ values between 9.2 µM and 24.4 µM) and promising antibacterial properties (MIC value of 2.8 µg/mL) [114].

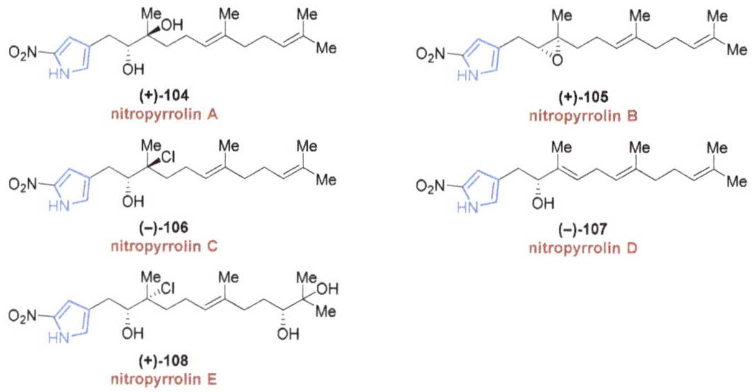

Figure 14. Nitropyrrolins A–E (**104**–**108**) represent the family of 4-farnesylated 2-nitropyrroles.

In 2016, the Morimoto group reported the first total synthesis of nitropyrrolins A (**104**), B (**105**), and D (**107**) in a sequential fashion (Scheme 9) [115]. As a key step, the authors performed a lithium–halogen exchange on bromopyrrole **109** and reacted the intermediary lithium species with epoxybromide **110**, which was prepared from a known epoxy alcohol. Subsequent deprotection and α-nitration of the pyrrole core then furnished nitropyrrolin B (**105**) in 7% over two steps. Treatment of the epoxide **105** with BF$_3$·OEt$_2$ and acetone produced the *cis*-acetonide, the stereochemistry of which could be investigated by NOE spectroscopy. Cleavage of the acetonide under acidic conditions then generated nitropyrrolin A (**104**) in 76% over two steps. When nitropyrrolin B (**105**) was reacted with TMSOTf, a regio- and stereoselective epoxide ring-opening occurred. In a one-pot approach, the intermediary allylic TMS-ether was cleaved under the addition of TBAF producing nitropyrrolin D (**107**) in 90% yield (Scheme 9) [115].

Only a few days after disclosure of nitropyrrolins A–E (**104**–**108**) as natural products, the group of Capon reported the extraction of three further 2-nitropyrroles, the heronapyrroles A–C (**111**–**113**) (Figure 15) [116]. These compounds share the same 4-farnesyl-2-nitropyrrole scaffold and are closely related to the nitropyrrolins **104**–**108** (Figure 14). The heronapyrroles **111**–**113** were isolated from a microbial culture of *Streptomyces* sp. strain CMB-M0423 in only minor quantities, which prevented a meaningful analysis of the full stereochemistries. However, on the basis of biosynthetic considerations, the absolute configurations were tentatively assigned as 7*S* and 15*R*. Although heronapyrroles A–C (**111**–**113**) neither displayed cytotoxicity against several cell lines (HeLa, HT-29, AGS) nor showed any activity towards Gram-negative bacteria such as *Pseudomonas aeruginosa* (ATCC 10145) and *Escherichia coli* (ATCC 11775), promising activity against Gram-positive bacteria such as *Staphylococcus aureus* (ATCC 9144, IC$_{50}$ values between 0.6 µM and 0.8 µM) and *Bacillus subtilis* (ATCC 6633, IC$_{50}$ values between 0.8 µM and 4.2 µM) could be observed [116].

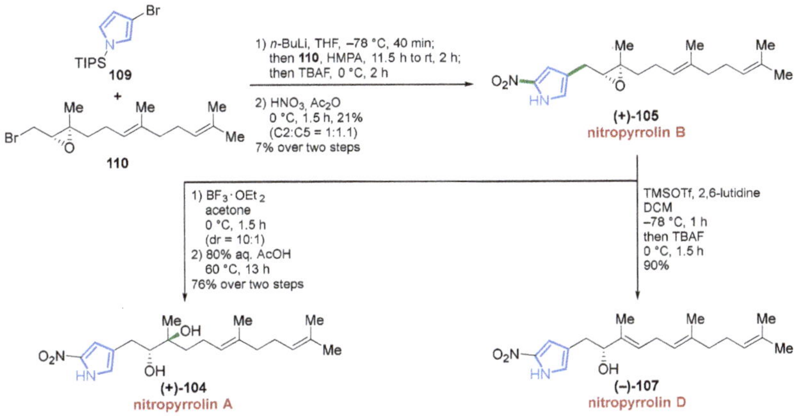

Scheme 9. Total synthesis of nitropyrrolins **104** and **105** via the key intermediate nitropyrrolin B (**105**) that is also suggested to be a biosynthetic precursor of nitropyrrolins A (**104**) and D (**107**).

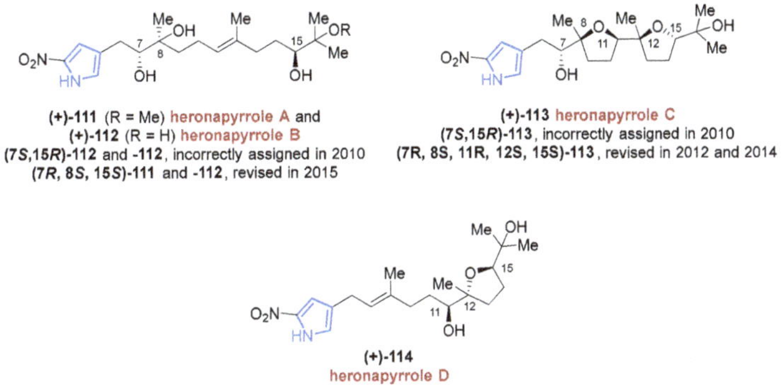

(+)-**111** (R = Me) heronapyrrole A and
(+)-**112** (R = H) heronapyrrole B
(7S,15R)-**112** and -**112**, incorrectly assigned in 2010
(7R, 8S, 15S)-**111** and -**112**, revised in 2015

(+)-**113** heronapyrrole C
(7S,15R)-**113**, incorrectly assigned in 2010
(7R, 8S, 11R, 12S, 15S)-**113**, revised in 2012 and 2014

(+)-**114** heronapyrrole D

Figure 15. The heronapyrroles A–D (**111**–**114**) only differ in their oxidation state in the farnesyl side chain.

Since the stereochemistries of heronapyrroles A–C (**111**–**113**) were only based on a biosynthetic assumption, several total syntheses of members belonging to the heronapyrrole family have been undertaken in the last decade. In 2012, Stark and co-workers focused on biosynthetic considerations and published a bioinspired synthesis attempting to synthesize heronapyrrole C (**113**) [117]. Starting with a lithium–halogen exchange-mediated coupling of 3-bromopyrrole **109** and farnesyl bromide **115** followed by nitration of the pyrrole core and Boc-protection, farnesylpyrrole **116** was generated in 13% over five steps. Asymmetric dihydroxylation of compound **116**, followed by a key double organocatalytic epoxidation using the (+)-Shi catalyst enabled a biomimetic polyepoxide cyclization cascade under acidic conditions, yielding pyrrole ent-**113b**. However, the product ent-**113b** showed an opposite optical rotation compared to the isolated natural product, prompting the authors to propose the corresponding enantiomer (+)-**113a** to be the true natural structure (Scheme 10) [117].

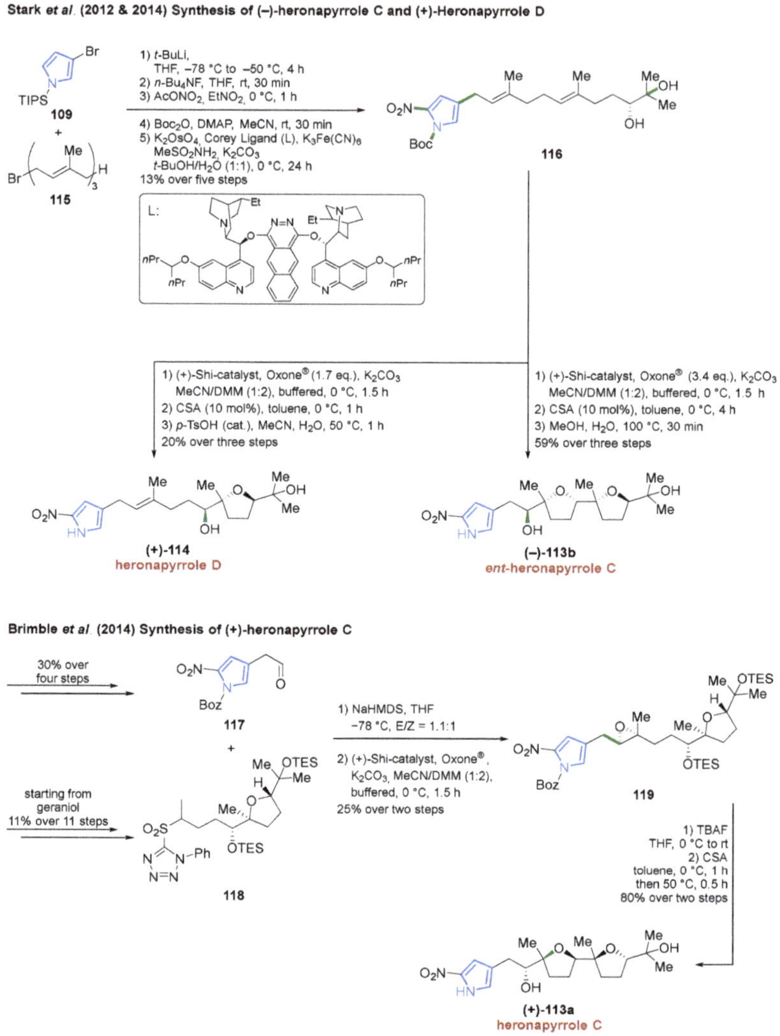

Scheme 10. First total synthesis of (+)-heronapyrrole C (**113a**) by Brimble in 2014 and its enantiomer (−)-heronapyrrole C (*ent*-**113b**) by Stark.

Just as heronapyrroles A–C (**111**–**113**), heronapyrrole D (**114**) could be isolated by Stark and co-workers from a microbial culture of *Streptomyces* sp. (strain CMB-M0423) in 2014 and showed significant inhibition of Gram-positive bacteria *Staphylococcus aureus* subsp. (ATCC 25923, IC_{50} value 1.8 µM), *Staphylococcus epidermis* (ATCC 12228, IC_{50} value 0.9 µM) and *Bacillus subtilis* (ATCC 6633, IC_{50} value 1.8 µM), but was inactive against Gram-negative bacteria *Pseudomonas aeruginosa* (ATCC 10145), *Escherichia coli* (ATCC 25922) and *Candida albicans* (ATCC 90028) [118]. Along with its isolation, the authors also published the total synthesis of (+)-heronapyrrole D (**114**), using the same strategy as in their previous synthesis of 2012. The only exception is represented by the Shi-epoxidation, in which substoichiometric amounts of the oxidant (Oxone®) were applied to generate *mono*-epoxides. Cyclization furnished the desired (+)-heronapyrrole D (**114**) (Scheme 10) [118].

Although the Stark laboratory further elaborated their studies on the nitration step and improved the entire synthesis in 2014 [119], the group of Brimble published the first total synthesis of the naturally occurring (+)-heronapyrrole C (**113a**) almost at the same time [120]. Based on their key intermediates **117** and **118**, synthesized in 4 and 11 steps, respectively, a Julia–Kocienski olefination merged the pyrrole subunit and the terpenoid side chain. A subsequent Shi-epoxidation then furnished compound **119** in 25% over two steps. The authors mentioned that the use of *N*-benzoyloxymethyl (Boz) as a protecting group was crucial to perform the final cyclization and deprotection under mild conditions. In this way, (+)-heronapyrrole C (**113a**) could be obtained in 80% yield over two steps (Scheme 10) [120]. The spectroscopic data of the (+)-isomer **113a** match those of the natural product and confirm the proposed reassignment by Stark et al. in 2012.

In 2015, the Morimoto group published the total synthesis of the remaining (+)-heronapyrroles A (**111**) and B (**112**) [121]. Taking into account the reported syntheses of (−)-heronapyrrole C (*ent*-**113b**) by Stark (2012) and (+)-heronapyrrole C (**113a**) by Brimble (2014) together with the biogenetic relationship of heronapyrroles A–C (**111**–**113**), a stereochemical reassignment of pyrroles **111** and **112** was proposed. Morimoto's group established a strategy similar to the approaches published by Stark and Brimble by installing the farnesylated chain through alkylation of pyrrole **109** with epoxy bromides **120** or **121**. In the case of (+)-heronapyrrole A **111**, the generated epoxide **122** was opened regioselectively by BF$_3$·OEt$_2$, yielding a masked C7–C8 *anti*-diol, which, after sodium-mediated ring-opening of the THF moiety and several further transformations, led to the formation (+)-heronapyrrole A (**111**) in 3% yield over seven steps (Scheme 11). Just as (+)-**111**, (+)-heronapyrrole B (**112**) was synthesized in a corresponding manner by opening the epoxide **123** via the same sequence to give a *cis*-acetonide, which, after nitration and acid-mediated cleavage of the acetonide functional groups, gave (+)-heronapyrrole B (**112**) in 18% yield over five steps (Scheme 11). In both cases, the absolute configuration was determined by the Mosher method which confirmed the proposed structure. As a consequence, the initially proposed stereochemistries for heronapyrroles A (**111**) and B (**112**) from the Stark laboratory in 2012 were reassigned [121].

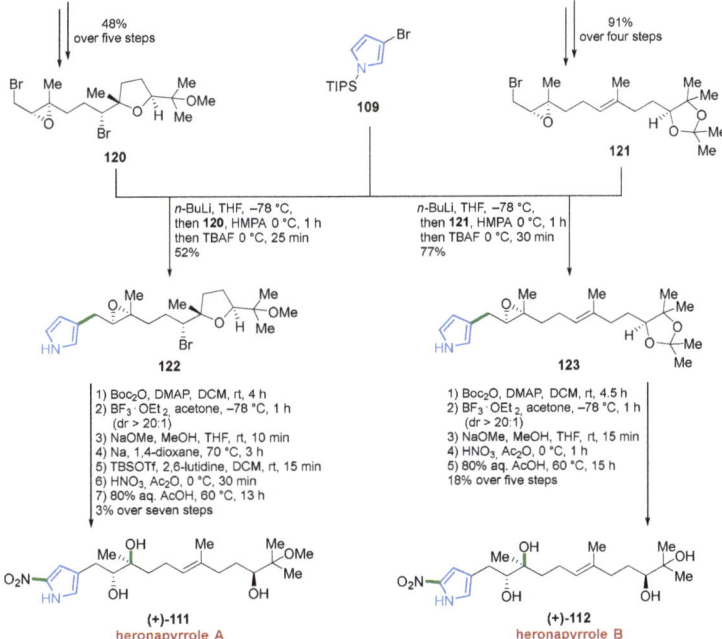

Scheme 11. Total synthesis of (+)-heronapyrrole A (**111**) and (+)-heronapyrrole B (**112**) by a convergent approach leading to stereochemical reassignments.

This rare class of nitropyrroles has attracted some attention from synthetic chemists in recent years. Not least because of previous synthetic work and the promising effects against Gram-positive bacteria, nitropyrroles may represent interesting targets for further drug design [115,117,118,120–123].

2.4. Annellated Pyrroles

In contrast to simple substituted pyrrole alkaloids, another structural class comprises compounds with an annellated pyrrole core. The position of fusion thereby can differ between 1,2-, 2,3- or 3,4-, with the fused ring being 6- or 7-membered. Additionally, these alkaloids often share a carbonyl moiety in α-position to the bridgehead atom.

From a series of nemoechines isolated in 2017 (see Figure 5, **31** and **32**), nemoechine B (**124**) stands out with its 1,2-condensed pyrrole unit [69]. The synthetically known compound **124** [124] was originally isolated in racemic form from *Agelas* aff. *nemoechinata* and the enantiomers were separated by chiral HPLC. Like its family members **31** and **32**, a lack of cytotoxicity against HL-60, HeLa, P388, and K562 cell lines was reported for both enantiomers (Figure 16) [69].

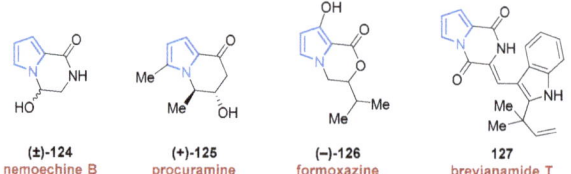

Figure 16. Structures of 1,2-annellated marine pyrrole alkaloids **124**–**127**.

In 2016, procuramine (**125**) was identified as a co-metabolite during the initial isolation and investigation of the biosynthetic pathway of curindolizine (**414**) from *Curvularia* sp. IFB-Z10 (see Figure 58). Structure elucidation was performed by spectroscopic methods and X-ray crystallography (Figure 16) [125].

A new pyrrolooxazine (**126**) was isolated from the marine mudflat fungus *Paecilomyces formosus*, yet the absolute configuration could not be determined because of decomposition during the isolation process. Formoxazine (**126**) showed potential as a radical scavenger in the DPPH assay with an IC$_{50}$ value of 0.1 µM and antibacterial activity against MDRSA and MRSA (MIC values of 6.25 µg/mL for both) (Figure 16) [126].

In the course of an investigation of marine-derived *Aspergillus versicolor* and in search for new Bacille Calmette-Guérin-inhibiting antibiotics against tuberculosis, the unknown brevianamide T (**127**) could be isolated in 2012 (Figure 16) [127]. Unfortunately, diketopiperazine **127**, isolated along with other members of the brevianamide family, showed no antibacterial properties against *Staphylococcus aureus* (ATCC 6538), *Bacillus subtilis* (ATCC 6633) (Gram-positive bacteria) or *Pseudomonas aeruginosa* (PAO1), *Escherichia coli* (ATCC 25922) (Gram-negative bacteria) or *Candida albicans* (SC 5314, yeast) [127].

A 2,3-fused pyrrole alkaloid, microindolinone A (**128**), was isolated from the actinomycete *Microbacterium* sp. MCCC 1A12207 from the deep sea in 2017 [128]. This tetrahydroindole represents one of two known saturated indoles of natural origin [129]. The absolute configuration at C5-OH was deduced with CD spectroscopy as 5R. No potent inhibition was found in anti-allergic bioactivity tests against RBL-2H3 cells (Figure 17) [128].

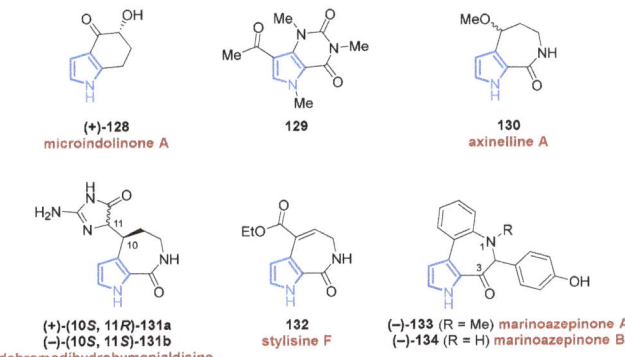

Figure 17. Various 2,3-fused pyrrole alkaloids **128–134** isolated between 2010 and 2020.

The natural product **129** was isolated from the gorgonian coral *Verrucella umbraculum* in 2012 and features a pyrrolopyrimidin scaffold. According to the authors, the biosynthesis of this purine alkaloid is similar to that of caffeine, which was also isolated from the same source (Figure 17) [130].

Another important class of MNPs is comprised of the pyrrolactams, which most probably derive from pyrrole-2-carboxamides. Axinelline A (**130**) was isolated alongside its brominated analog **353** (see Figure 51) from the marine sponge *Axinella* sp. in 2017, however, the absolute stereochemistry was not determined (Figure 17) [131].

The two diastereomers (11*R*)- and (11*S*)-debromodihydrohymenialdisine **131a** and **131b** were isolated from the sponge *Cymbastela cantharella* by the Debitus laboratory in 2011 (Figure 17) [132]. The authors assumed that compounds **131a** and **131b** biogenetically arise from dispacamide derivates. Because of their close relationship to the strong kinase inhibitor hymenialdisine, (11*R*)- and (11*S*)-debromodihydrohymenialdisine **131a** and **131b** were tested for Polo-Like-Kinase-1 (PLK-1) inhibition. Unfortunately, but in analogy to the bromo derivatives **386a** and **386b** (see Figure 55), a complete lack of activity was observed, demonstrating the importance of the conjugation at C-10 and C-11 of the unique cyclic system of hymenialdisine [132].

In 2018, the structurally related seven-membered pyrroloazepine stylisine F (**132**) was isolated alongside several other MNPs from the marine sponge *Stylissa massa*. However, the authors mentioned that stylisine F (**132**) most probably occurred as an artifact generated from the corresponding acid upon EtOH extraction. In basic biological investigations, weak or no inhibition against a variety of bacteria was detected (MIC $\geq$ 128 µg/mL, Figure 17) [133].

In 2015, Fenical and co-workers reported a culture-dependent technique in a nutrient-poor medium combined with long incubation times, which facilitated the cultivation of several marine bacteria able to produce secondary metabolites. The organic extract from strain CNX-216^T of a cultivated bacterium belonging to the Mooreiaceae family showed activity against *Pontibacillus* sp. and the authors were able to isolate the alkaloids marinoazepinones A (**133**) and B (**134**) from this extract [134]. Besides the incorporation of the unusual amino acid 4-hydroxyphenylglycine, the marinoazepinones **133** and **134** represent the first natural products featuring a rare azepin-3-one framework. CD spectroscopy, X-ray crystallography, and optical rotation were used to elucidate the absolute stereochemistry at C2, but no definite conclusions could be drawn. In bioactivity assays, marinoazepinone B (**134**) exhibited antibacterial activity against the Gram-positive *Pontibacillus* strain CNJ-912 (16 mm inhibition zone), whereas no activity was observed against the Gram-negative *Vibrio shiloi* strain CUA-364 (Figure 17) [134].

The rigidins represent another prominent class of 2,3-fused pyrrole alkaloids, sharing a pyrrolo [2,3-*d*]pyrimidine scaffold [135]. With the first rigidin isolated back in 1990 by Kobayashi and co-workers [136], many MNPs belonging to this family have been isolated until today [137,138]. Although several total syntheses of rigidins are known [139–143], we want to mention the one-pot multicomponent reaction reported by the Magedov laboratory in 2011, which provides synthetical access to tetrasubstituted 2-aminopyrroles in only four steps and includes the first total syntheses of rigidins B–D (**147**–**149**) [144]. In a first step, *N*-(methanesulfonamido)acetophenones **140** and **141** were prepared from starting materials **135** and **136**, respectively. The multicomponent reaction was then realized by combining either **140** or **141** with aldehydes **138** or **139** under the addition of cyanoacetamide (**137**). The resulting 2-aminopyrroles **142**–**145**, isolated in 83–86% yield, were then converted into pyrimidinediones and after final deprotection, the rigidins A–D (**146**–**149**) could be obtained in four steps at an overall yield of 53–61% (Scheme 12) [144].

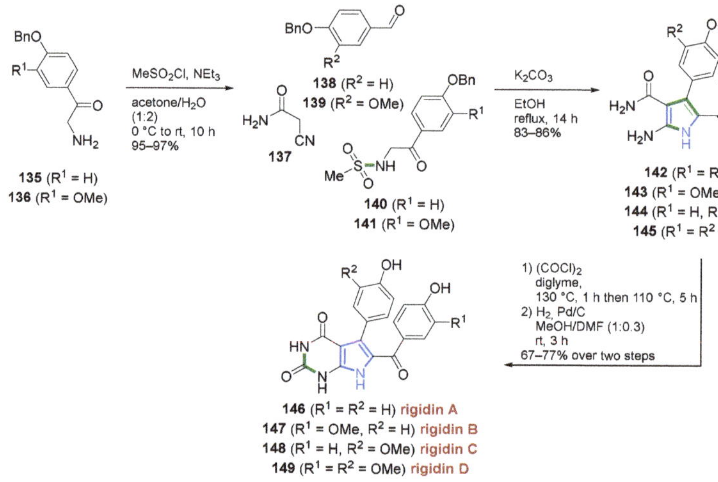

Scheme 12. The so-far shortest synthetic approach towards rigidin A (**146**), including the first syntheses of rigidins B–D (**147**–**149**) in a one-pot multicomponent reaction.

The annellated pyrrole alkaloids shown so far largely consist of a fused lactone or lactam structure, whereas 3,4-fused pyrroles often share a quinone system. This motif can be found in albumycin (**150**), a novel MNP isolated by heterologous expression from *Micromonospora rosaria* SCSIO N160 genes in *Streptomyces albus* J1074 (Figure 18). In antibacterial tests, only weak activities against several indicator strains were encountered (MIC values >64 µg/mL) [145].

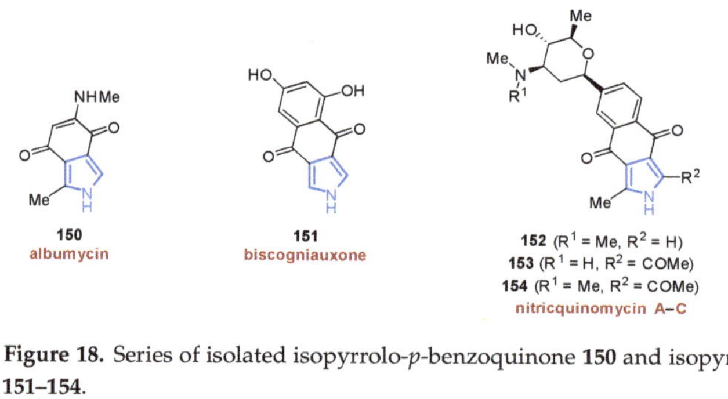

Figure 18. Series of isolated isopyrrolo-*p*-benzoquinone **150** and isopyrrolo-1,4-naphthoquinones **151**–**154**.

In 2016, another fused *p*-quinone, biscogniauxone (**151**), was isolated from the marine fungus *Biscogniauxia mediterranea* and belongs to the rare family of isopyrrolonaphthoquinones (Figure 18) [146]. It should be mentioned that the authors assumed the existence of further derivatives of compound **151**, as metabolites with similar UV spectra were detected in the extracts, albeit without isolation. Significant inhibition of glycogen synthase kinase (GSK-3β, IC_{50} value 8.04 µM ± 0.28 µM) was observed for biscogniauxone (**151**), while weak inhibition of *Staphylococcus epidermidis* and *Staphylococcus aureus* was found (IC_{50} values in the range of 100 µM) [146]. The nitricquinomycins A–C (**152–154**), isolated from *Streptomyces* sp. ZS-A45, complete the selection of isopyrrolonaphthoquinones (Figure 18) [147]. By comparing the spectroscopic data with those of previously reported naphthoquinones bearing a pyrrole core and using NOE experiments for the determination of the relative configuration, as well as ECD spectroscopy for the determination of the absolute configuration, the structure could be determined as indicated. Of compounds **152–154**, nitricquinomycin C (**154**) exhibited significant cytotoxicity against the human ovarian cancer cell line A2780 (IC_{50} value 4.77 µM ± 0.03 µM) but weak antibacterial potential against *Escherichia coli*, *Staphylococcus aureus*, and *Candida albicans* (MIC values > 40 µM) [147].

Another 3,4-fused pyrrole family are the spiroindimicins (SPMs), which contain a remarkable spirocyclic bisindole framework and are highly related congeners of the bisindole pyrroles **59–66** (cf. Figure 8). Spiroindimicins A–D (**155–158**) were isolated from *Streptomyces* sp. SCSIO 03032 in 2012 [148]. The molecular structures were resolved by spectroscopic methods, with the 3D structures of spiroindimicin A (**155**) and B (**156**) being unambiguously confirmed by X-ray crystallography (Figure 19). Spiroindimicin A (**155**) consists of a [5.6] spirocyclic core, whereas congeners B–D **156–158** contain a [5.5] spirocyclic core. This structural difference also influences the bioactivity, which in the case of [5.5] spirocyclic pyrroles **156–158** results in good to moderate antitumor activities against various cancer cell lines with IC_{50} values ranging between 5 µg/mL and 22 µg/mL. Biosynthetic studies suggest the formation of spiroindimicins are proposed to derive from lynamicin by an aryl-aryl coupling of C-3′ and C-5″ or by an aryl-aryl coupling of C-3′ and C-2″, furnishing the [5.6] or [5.5] spiro-cyclic alkaloids, respectively [148].

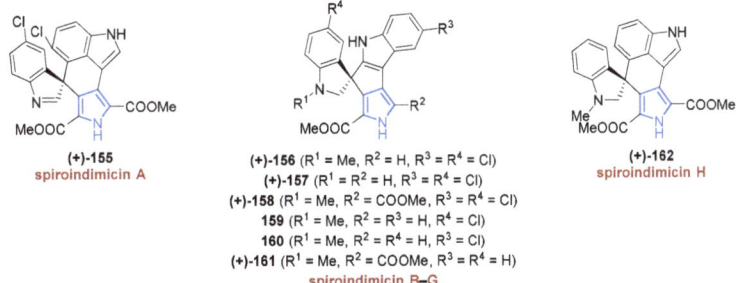

Figure 19. Structures of spiroindimicins A–H (**155–162**) isolated from marine actinobacteria.

The family of spiroindimicins was extended in 2017 by the monochlorinated compounds **159** and **160**, which were isolated from *Streptomyces* sp. MP131-18 (Figure 19) [149]. Spiroindimicins E (**159**) and F (**160**) did not show any activity against Gram-negative test cultures, being in line with the biological properties of their biosynthetic lynamicin-type precursors. In both cases, the antibacterial activity appears to increase with an increasing degree of chlorination on the bisindole backbone [149]. In addition to studies on the biosynthetic gene cluster of *Streptomyces* SCSIO 03032 [150], the group of Zhang, responsible for the isolation of spiroindimicins A–D (**155–158**), discovered the halogenase SpmH involved in the biosynthesis of SPMs and IDMs.

In 2019, inactivation of the encoding gene *spmH* then led to the isolation of spiroindimicins G (**161**) and H (**162**), which displayed moderate cytotoxicity against four cancer cell lines (IC_{50} values between 10.28 µM and 33.02 µM), comparable to their chlorinated congeners **155–160** (Figure 19) [151].

The first syntheses of these compounds were achieved by Sperry and co-workers in 2016 [152]. Starting with the alkylation of aniline **163** with bromide **164**, a subsequent Heck reaction and hydrogenation furnished the spirocyclic pentanone **165**. One key step is represented by the Fischer indolization, followed by Boc-protection and radical bromination. After hydrolysis and oxidation, ketone **166** was formed in 50% over five steps. Sequentially, a thioketal and then a vinylsulfone **167** were prepared which allowed for a Montforts pyrrole synthesis. After the final deprotection, (±)-spiroindimicin C (**157**) could be obtained. Additionally, reductive amination furnished (±)-spiroindimicin B (**156**) (Scheme 13) [152].

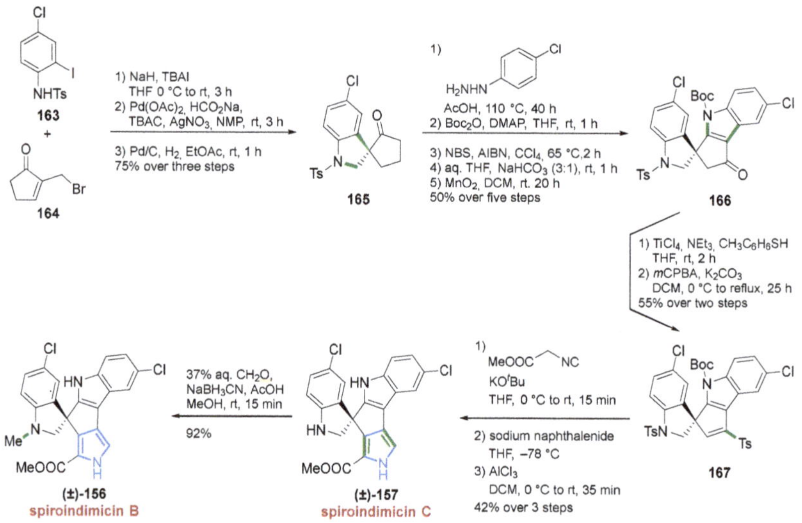

Scheme 13. Total synthesis of spiroindimicins **156**, **157** using the Fischer indolization and Montforts pyrrole synthesis.

Further studies and recent publications highlight the importance of these bisindole alkaloids as promising bioactive compounds and potential new lead structures [153,154].

The structurally remarkable subtipyrrolines A–C (**168–170**) incorporating a pyrrole-pyrrole-dihydropyridine framework, were isolated from the *Bacillus subtilis* SY2101 strain, derived from sediment samples of the Mariana Trench collected at a depth of 11,000 m (Figure 20) [155]. The structural elucidation was investigated by spectroscopic analysis and supported by X-ray crystallography. Bioactivity assays revealed moderate antiproliferative activities (human glioma U251 and U87MG cells, IC_{50} values of 36.3 µM and 26.1 µM) as well as moderate antimicrobial potential (*Escherichia coli* and *Candida albicans*, IC_{50} values between 34 µM and 46 µM, respectively) [155].

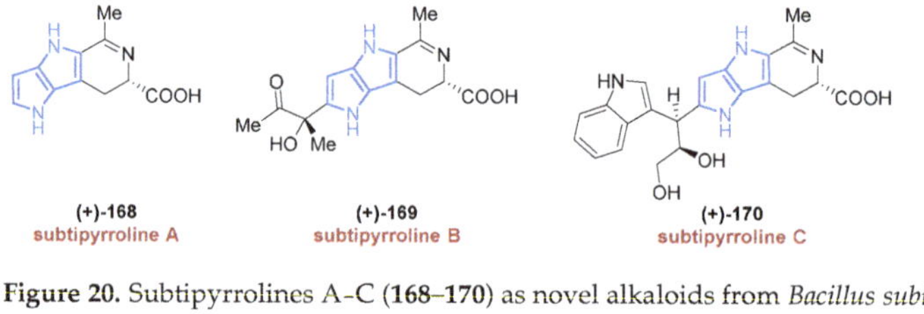

Figure 20. Subtipyrrolines A–C (**168–170**) as novel alkaloids from *Bacillus subtilis* SY2101.

2.4.1. Lamellarins and Related Natural Congeners

To date, more than 65 lamellarins have been discovered since the first isolation of a member of this class by Faulkner et al. in 1985 [156,157]. Divided into type I (with subsections a and b, comprising compounds with a saturated or unsaturated C-5–C-6 unit, respectively) containing a doubly annellated 2,3,4-triarylpyrrole core in form of a 1-aryl-6H-chromeno-[4′,3′:4,5]pyrrolo-[2,1-a]isoquinolin-6-one or type II with a simple 3,4-diarylpyrrol-2-carboxylate ring system, the lamellarins comprise a large and prominent class of marine alkaloids. These compounds, derived from sponges, tunicates, and mollusks, exhibit a broad range of often highly potent biological activities, making them interesting targets for synthetic chemists [157,158].

In 2012, Capon and co-workers investigated *Didemnum* sp. and isolated five new lamellarins A1–A5 (**171–175**) from the strain CMB-01656 and one further member (A6, **176**) from the strain CMB-02127 (Figure 21) [159]. Together with eight known derivatives, a structure–activity relationship (SAR) study was performed regarding the reversal of multidrug resistance. In the SAR study, the P-glycoprotein (P-gp) inhibition activity was proposed to increase with a higher degree of O-methylation. The synthesis of a permethylated derivative, featuring potential non-cytotoxic P-gp inhibitory activities then confirmed this assumption [159].

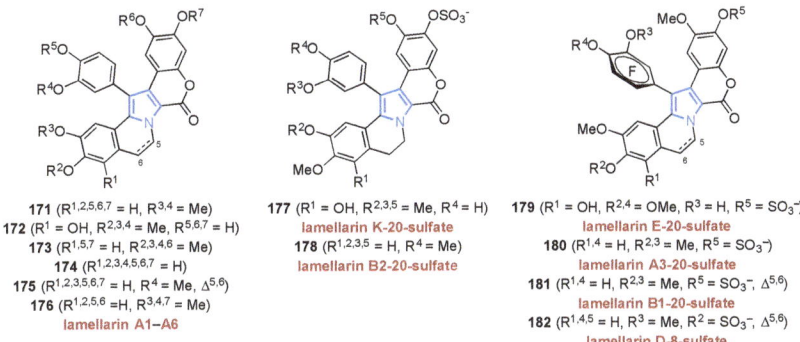

Figure 21. Members of the lamellarins **171–182** (type I) isolated from *Didemnum* sp. in 2012 and 2019.

The lamellarin sulfates represent a small subclass within the lamellarin family. In 2019, the group of Keyzers isolated six new lamellarin sulfates (**177–182**) from *Didemnum ternerratum*, a pacific tunicate (Figure 21) [160]. All of them showed similar analytical data to previously reported lamellarins except for the sulfate functional group. The substantial majority of naturally occurring lamellarins show no optical rotation with the exception of lamellarin S (half-life of racemization ≈ 90 days). Surprisingly, the newly isolated sulfates **179–182** showed optical activity in ECD analysis, which is due to the hindered rotation of ring F resulting in an axial chirality (atropisomerism). The bioactivity of lamellarins **177–182** against human colon carcinoma HCT-116 was investigated, with D-8-sulfate (**182**) showing appreciable cytotoxicity (IC$_{50}$ = 9.7 µM) [160].

In addition to the representative group of lamellarins [32,156,161–166], further related pyrroles like the polycitons, polycitrins [167], storniamides [168], and denigrins [90,169] as well as the fused alkaloids lukianols [170], dictyodendrins [171], purpurone [172], ningalins [173] and baculiferins can also be included, which extend the family of 3,4-diarylpyrroles. In the molecular backbone, structural variations from fused maleiimide units to highly conjugated carbazole-2,7-diones can be found.

The Capon laboratory isolated the new ningalins E (**183**) and F (**184**) from the species *Didemnum* (CMB-02127), which, according to the authors, share a biosynthetic pathway similar to that of the lamellarins by merging a tyrosine with a defined number of catechols (Figure 22). Only low cytotoxicities against human, bacterial, and fungal cell lines were observed, whereas the ningalins **183** and **184** showed moderate inhibition of the kinases CK1δ, CDK5, and GSK3β, potential targets for the treatment of neurodegenerative diseases (IC$_{50}$ values between 1.6 µM and 10.9 µM) [174].

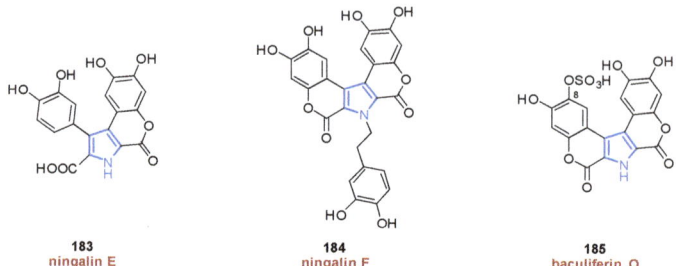

Figure 22. Related congeners **183**–**185** of the lamellarins sharing the central fused pyrrole core.

The class of the baculiferins was established by Lin and Bringmann in 2010, yielding pyrrole **185** alongside 14 other new members bearing a carbazole-2,7-dione central core (Figure 22). Baculiferin O (**185**) as a C8 sulfate representative inhibits several tumor cell lines with moderate activity around 33 µM [175].

Because of their promising biological activities such as antiproliferative, multidrug resistance reversal activity, cytotoxicity, and anti-HIV-1 activity, the lamellarin core has served as a potential lead structure for synthetic and medicinal chemists in the past decade [157,158]. The published syntheses of the lamellarins and derivates in the past decade, summarized in Table 1, provide an update of the existing summary by Opatz et al. in 2014 [158] and concentrate the recent review by Iwao et al. in 2020 [157].

Table 1. Summary of published synthesis of lamellarins and related analogs in the decade of 2010–2020.

Year	Author	Lamellarin and Related Congeners	Linear Steps [i]	Overall Yield
2010	Iwao [176]	Lamellarin α 20-sulfate	15	6%
		Lamellarin α 13-sulfate	15	4%
		Lamellarin α 13,20-disulfate	14	9%
2011	Banwell [177]	G trimethyl ether	10	3%
		Lamellarin S	11	6%
	Jia [178]	Lamellarin D	10	13%
		Lamellarin H	10	13%
		Lamellarin R	5	53%
		Ningalin B	8	14%
2012	Vazquez [179]	Lamellarin Q	6	28%
		Lamellarin O	7	25%
	Banwell [180]	Lamellarin K	9	57%
		Lamellarin T	9	43%
		Lamellarin U	8	44%
		Lamellarin W	9	45%
2013	Opatz [181]	(Dihydro-)/lamellarin η	8/9	62%/57%
		Lamellarin G trimethyl ether	7	69%
	Iwao [182]	Lukianol A/B	6/11	36%/11%

Table 1. Cont.

Year	Author	Lamellarin and Related Congeners	Linear Steps [i]	Overall Yield
2014	Yamaguchi [183]	Lamellarin C	9	3%
		Lamellarin I	9	3%
	Iwao [184]	Lamellarin N	11;13	42%;34%
		Lamellarin L	13	29%
2015	Iwao [185]	Lamellarin L	10	14%
		Lamellarin N	10	12%
	Opatz [186]	Lamellarin D trimethyl ether	9	43%
		Lamellarin H	10	41%
	Ruchirawat [187]	Aza/lamellarin D	13/13	12%/9%
		Aza/lamellarin N	13/13	28%/15%
	Tan and Yoshikai [188]	Lamellarin G trimethyl ether	5	20%
2016	Iwao [189]	Lamellarin U	12	5%
	Yang [190]	Lamellarin D trimethyl ether	3	8%
		Lamellarin H	4	7%
2017	Iwao [191]	Lamellarin N analogues	–	–
		Azalamellarin N analogues	–	–
	Iwao [192]	Lamellarin α	12	22%
		Lamellarin η	10	19%
	Chandrasekhar [193]	Lamellarin D trimethyl ether	6	44%
		Lamellarin D	7	29%
		Lamellarin H	7	37%
	Wu [194]	Lamellarin G trimethyl ether	3	51%
	Yang [195]	Lamellarin D trimethyl ether	2	37%
		Lamellarin H	3	31%
		Lamellarin D	6;8	12–14%
		Lamellarin χ	6;8	12–14%
	Ackermann [196]	Lamellarin D	10	30%
		Lamellarin H	10	29%
2018	Opatz [197]	Lamellarin G trimethyl ether	7;8	19–42%
	Chiu and Tonks [198]	Lamellarin R	5	18%
2019	Donohoe [199]	Lamellarin D	7	22%
		Lamellarin Q	7	20%
	Opatz and Michael [200]	Lamellarin G trimethyl ether	6;7	56–73%
	Khan [201]	Lamellarin G trimethyl ether	5	18%
		Lamellarin D trimethyl ether	6	16%
		Lamellarins H, U	7/6	11%/11%
		Dihydro/lamellarin η	7/6	9%/10%

Table 1. Cont.

Year	Author	Lamellarin and Related Congeners	Linear Steps [i]	Overall Yield
2020	Saito [202]	Lamellarin G trimethyl ether	6	26%
		Lamellarin H	8	17%
	Tsay [203]	Lamellarin R	3	50%
	Liou [204]	Lamellarin R	5	26%
		Lamellarin O	5	10%
		Lukianol A	6	38%
	Khan [205]	Lamellarins	6/6/6	21%/21%/21%
		S,Z,G,L,N,D	6/7/7	21%/19%/16%

[i] The longest linear sequence in the synthesis was counted.

This astounding number of syntheses highlights the importance of these pyrrole members of marine origin to many areas of life science. In addition to the constantly increasing number of total syntheses of lamellarins and their natural congeners, the number of synthetic derivatives and biological activity assays has increased similarly [206–214].

3. Halogenated Marine Pyrrole Alkaloids

This chapter presents the occurrence of halogenated pyrroles which constitute a highly diverse and structurally complex subclass of marine alkaloids. It is considered that at least 25% of organohalogen natural products are halogenated alkaloids, mostly featuring pyrrole, indole, carboline, and other N-heteroaromatic core structures [215,216]. This observation is not too surprising as the marine environment provides both chloride and bromide in virtually unlimited quantities as well as a variety of halogenase enzymes from different organisms, resulting in an excellent environment for biohalogenation of these electron-rich substrates [30,217,218]. From a medicinal point of view, the resulting structures are associated with numerous different pharmacological activities such as selective anti-histamine [219–221], anti-serotonergic [222], immunosuppressive [223], antibacterial [224], anti-malarial [225], and antiproliferative properties [226]. Therefore, halogenated pyrrole alkaloids can be viewed as potential lead compounds for the development of new, even more potent drugs [15,227].

Given the enormous dimensions and (bio)chemical diversity of marine life and its underexplored nature, it is not surprising that the number of isolated halogenated marine pyrroles is constantly increasing and that countless further halopyrroles are yet to be discovered.

3.1. Simple Pyrroles

Ethyl 3,4-dibromo-1H-pyrrole-2-carboxylate (**186**) was first isolated from the sponge *Stylissa massa* in 2014 and shows a weak antiproliferative activity against mouse lymphoma cells (L5178Y growth in 27.2% at 10 µg/mL, Figure 23) [228].

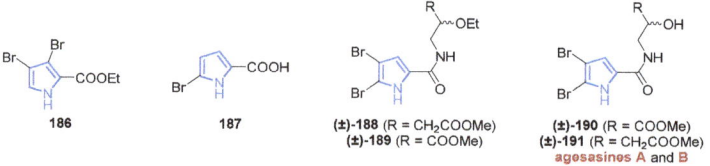

Figure 23. Simple bromopyrrole alkaloids **186**–**191** isolated from different marine sponges.

A related bromopyrrole **187** was isolated from another sponge (*Agelas cerebrum*) in 2011 and subjected to several antiproliferative tests (Figure 23) [229]. Here, compound **187** and other isolated bromopyrroles did not show any activity against cancer cells (A549 lung cancer cells, HT29 colonic cancer cells, and MDA-MB-231 breast cancer cells). However, when the crude mixture, from which **187** and further bromopyrroles were isolated, was subjected to biological tests, a strong cytotoxic activity (IC$_{50}$ values around 1 µg/mL) against all three human tumor cell lines could be observed. The authors attributed this effect to the yet underexplored synergism of natural product mixtures containing bromopyrroles [229]. Both compounds **186** and **187** were previously only known as synthetic products [230,231].

Two further simple substituted halopyrroles, **188** and **189**, could be isolated from the South China Sea sponge *Agelas* sp. in 2016. The enantiomers (+)-**188**, (−)-**188**, (+)-**189** and (−)-**189** did not appear to have any antifungal activities using the *Caenorhabditis elegans* candidiasis model (Figure 23) [66]. However, the racemic mixtures of (±)-**188** and (±)-**189** showed effective antifungal activity. Unfortunately, the authors did not provide any values or an explanation of this observation. Despite these results, the authors found out that the corresponding intramolecularly cyclized pyrroloketopiperazine natural products (see Figure 49, **342**–**344**) exhibited significant antifungal activities with survival rates around 50% [66].

Very recently, the corresponding agesasines A (**190**) and B (**191**) featuring the free alcohol functional groups, were isolated from Okinawan marine sponges *Agelas* spp. (Figure 23) [232]. Both compounds were isolated as racemates and, according to the authors, might be artifacts from the extraction process under acidic conditions. In basic antiproliferative tests against human cancer cell lines (HeLa, A549, and MCF7), no cytotoxicity could be observed [232].

In 2012, a new bromopyrrole, 4-bromo-*N*-(butoxymethyl)-1*H*-pyrrole-2-carboxamide (**192**), featuring an unusual ether group in its side chain, could be isolated from the marine sponge *Agelas mauritiana* (Figure 24) [233].

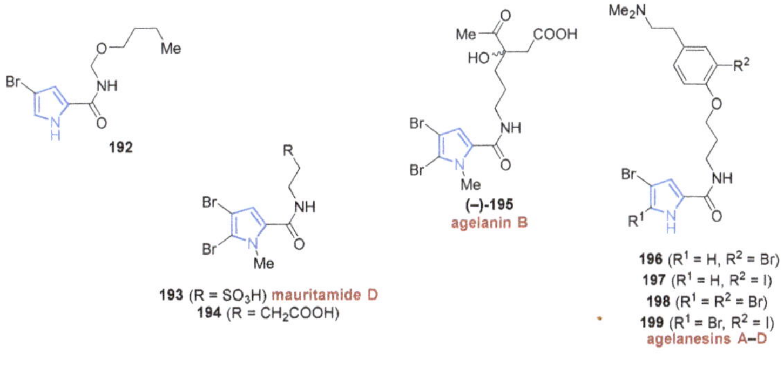

Figure 24. Simple bromopyrrole alkaloids **192**–**195** and structural similar agelanesins A–D (**196**–**199**).

Further structurally similar halopyrroles **193**–**199** possessing different substituents at their amide side chains were isolated from the Indonesian marine sponges *Agelas linnaei* (Figure 24) [234]. While mauritamide D (**193**), 4-(4,5-dibromo-1-methylpyrrole-2-carboxamido)-butanoic acid (**194**), and agelanin B (**195**) were inactive against L1578Y mouse lymphoma cell lines, the tyramine-unit bearing agelanesins A–D (**196**–**199**) showed prominent to good activity with IC$_{50}$ values between 9.25 µM and 16.76 µM in this assay. The authors mentioned that the cytotoxicity of the agelanesins **196**–**199** is interconnected with the degree of bromination of the pyrrole ring, resulting in an increased reactivity for the monobrominated agelanesins A (**196**) and B (**197**) compared to **198** and **199** [234].

The tribrominated pyrrole 4′-((3,4,5-tribromo-1*H*-pyrrol-2-yl)methyl)phenol (**200**) was isolated from the surface of the coralline alga *Neogoniolithon fosliei* in 2014 and exhibited broad-spectrum antibacterial activity against several *Pseudoalteromonas*, *Vibrio*, and *Staphylo-*

coccus spp. (inhibition zones > 10 mm, Figure 25). However, no antifungal or antiprotozoal activity was observed by investigating compound **200** [235].

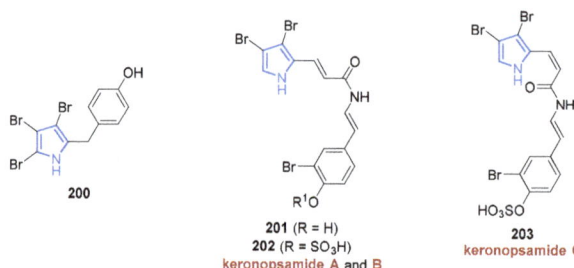

Figure 25. Structure of compound **200** and the bromotyrosine-based keronopsamides A–C (**201–203**).

A new class of bromopyrrole pigments derived from bromotyrosine were isolated from the marine ciliate *Pseudokeronopsis riccii* in 2010 and were named keronopsamides A–C (**201–203**) (Figure 25) [236].

In 2020, pyrrolosine (**204**), a tetrabrominated alkaloid symmetrically dimerized via two amide functionalities, was isolated from *Agelas oroides* [237] and should not be confused with another natural product named pyrrolosine (**206**), the structure of which had been identified as **205** and revised **206** during the 1990s (Figure 26) [238].

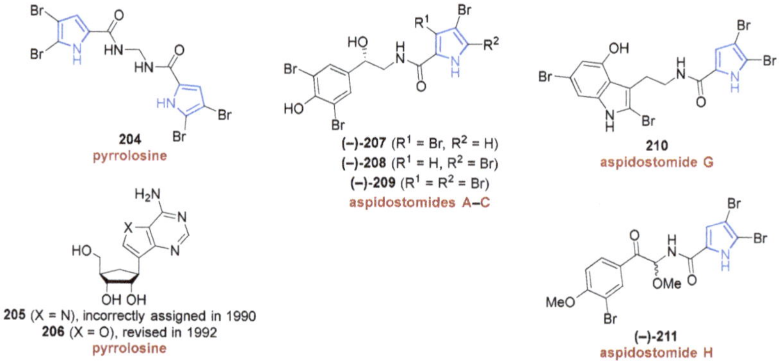

Figure 26. Molecular structures of bromopyrroles **204–211** isolated from sponges and bryozoans.

Further marine bromopyrrole alkaloids **207–211** substituted via amide groups were isolated from the Patagonian bryozoan *Aspidostoma giganteum* (Figure 26) [239]. The aspidostomides A–C (**207–209**), G (**210**) and H (**211**) bear the well-known bromotyrosine and bromotryptophan structural motifs frequently found in marine natural products [240]. While for aspidostomide A (**207**) the absolute configuration was determined as *R* by a modified Mosher method [241], the configurations of aspidostomides B (**208**) and C (**209**) were assumed to be the same as in compound **207**. The absolute configuration of aspidostomide H (**211**) could not yet be established [239].

In 2019, the first total syntheses of the enantiomeric aspidostomides B (**208**) and C (**209**) were realized by Khan and co-workers (Scheme 14) [242].

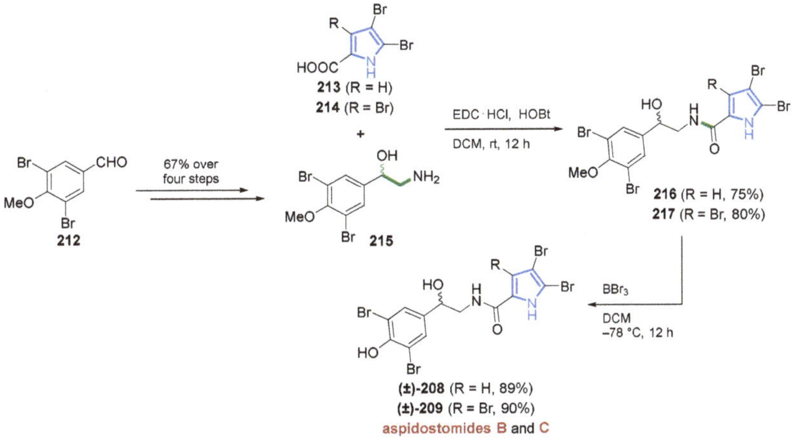

Scheme 14. First total syntheses of aspidostomides B (**208**) and C (**209**) starting from compound **212**.

Here, compound **212** was reacted in a Wittig olefination and then subjected to bromohydroxylation. Substitution of the bromine with NaN$_3$ followed by reduction furnished amine (±)-**215** in 67% yield over four steps. Amidation of (±)-**215** with either 4,5-dibromopyrrole carboxylic acid (**213**) or 3,4,5-tribromopyrrole carboxylic acid (**214**) delivered products **216** and **217**, respectively. Final demethylation by applying BBr$_3$ then gave the natural products aspidostomides B (**208**) in 67% and C (**209**) in 72% over two steps (Scheme 14) [242].

In 2018, nine new pseudoceratidines (**218–226**), of which the tedamides A–D (**223–226**) possess an unprecedented 4-bromo-4-methoxy-5-oxo-4,5-dihydro-1*H*-pyrrole-2-carboxamide moiety, were isolated from the marine sponge *Tedania brasiliensis* (Figure 27) [243]. It is important to mention that 3-debromopseudoceratidine (**218**) and 20-debromopseudoceratidine (**219**), 4-bromopseudoceratidine (**220**), and 19-bromopseudoceratidine (**221**), tedamides A and B (**223** and **225**), and tedamides C and D (**224** and **226**) have been isolated as pairs of inseparable structural isomers differing in their sites of bromination and oxidation. The inseparable mixture of compounds **218** and **219** showed antiparasitic activity on *Plasmodium falciparum* (EC$_{50}$ value of 5.8 µM ± 0.5 µM) and displayed weak cytotoxicity in the human liver cancer HepG2 cell line (MDL$_{50}$ ≥ 400 µM), but with excellent selectivity, as reflected by a dramatically reduced toxicity to healthy cells. The authors also synthesized a number of derivatives that were assayed against several protozoan parasite species, evidencing that the bromine substituents in the pyrrole unit of pseudoceratidine derivatives are inevitable for antiplasmodial activity [243].

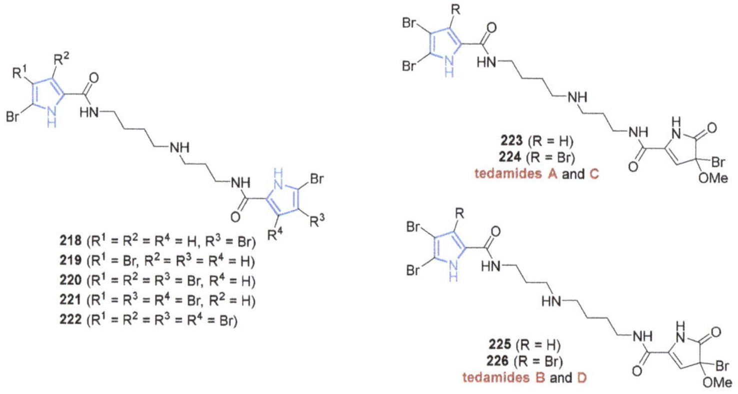

Figure 27. Nine new pseudoceratidines **218–226** from the marine sponge *Tedania brasiliensis*.

Another bromopyrrole alkaloid, clathrirole A (**227**), was isolated from the Myanmarese marine sponge *Clathria prolifera* in 2018 (Figure 28) [73]. It should be noted that the stereogenic centers of the tetrahydropyrimidinium ring of **227** were only assumed to have *R* configuration by comparison of its optical rotation with the enantiomeric *N*-methylmanzadicin C (**228**) which had been isolated and synthesized several years earlier [35,244,245].

Figure 28. New bromopyrrole alkaloid **227**. *N*-Methylmanzacidin C (**228**) is shown for comparison.

In this context, the correction of the stereoconfiguration of manzacidin B (**232a**) should also be mentioned. This MNP was synthesized by the Ohfune group in 2007 and its configuration was erroneously determined to match compound **232b** [246]. Three years later, the same group published an alternative synthetic route (Scheme 15) and with the aid of X-ray crystallography, the revised structure of manzacidin B (**232a**) was unambiguously confirmed [247]. Here, aldehyde **229** was transformed into compound **230** using Oppolzer's sultam as a chiral auxiliary, and subsequently generated the *N*-formyl lactone **231** already featuring the stereochemistry of natural manzacidin B (**232a**). Several further steps, including the installation of the pyrrole unit, then delivered the natural product **232a** [247]. Unfortunately, the correction did not provide any information about the experimental section, including reaction conditions and yields.

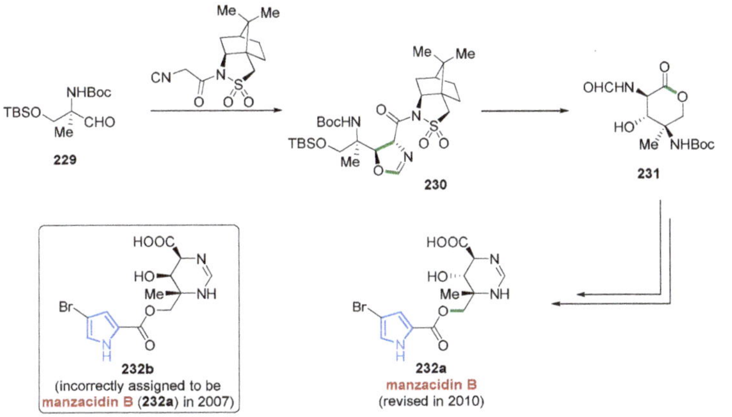

Scheme 15. An alternative synthetic route towards manzacidin B (**232a**) in 2010 revealed that it was incorrectly assigned as compound **232b** in 2007.

In 2015, the group of Köck isolated *N*-methylagelongine (**233**) from the Caribbean sponge *Agelas citrina* (Figure 29) [63].

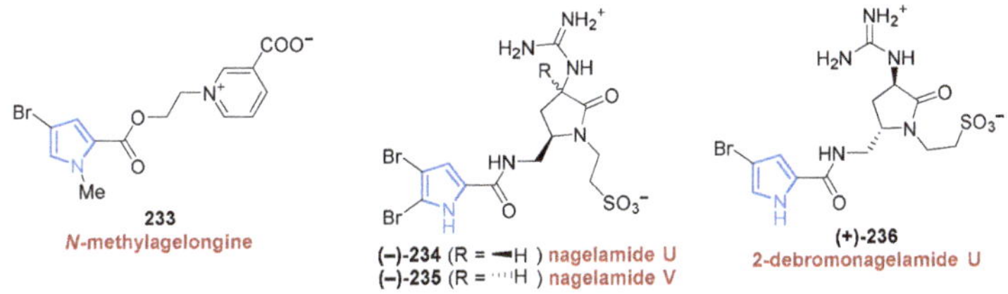

Figure 29. Simple bromopyrrole alkaloids **233**–**236** isolated from the *Agelas* sp.

Two new halopyrroles, nagelamide U and V (**234** and **235**) were isolated from a marine sponge *Agelas* sp. in 2013 and possess a γ-lactam ring with a taurine unit (Figure 29). Here, the relative stereochemistry was examined by ROESY correlations [65].

A related compound, 2-debromonagelamide U (**236**) was isolated from the Okinawan marine sponge *Agelas* sp. two years later. Compound **236** could inhibit the growth of *Trichophyton mentagrophytes* (IC_{50} value 16 μg/mL), a common fungus causing ringworm in companion animals (Figure 29) [248].

In 2019, three new pyoluteorin analogs, mindapyrroles A–C (**237**–**239**) were isolated from *Pseudomonas aeruginosa* strain 1682U.R.oa.27, a bacterium from the tissue homogenate of the giant shipworm *Kuphus polythalamius* (Figure 30) [249]. The chlorinated pyrrole alkaloids **237** and **239** inhibit the growth of multiple clinically relevant microbial pathogens (MIC values between 2 μg/mL and >32 μg/mL), with mindapyrrole B (**238**) showing the most potent antimicrobial activity (MIC values between 2 μg/mL and 8 μg/mL) and widest selectivity index over mammalian cells [249].

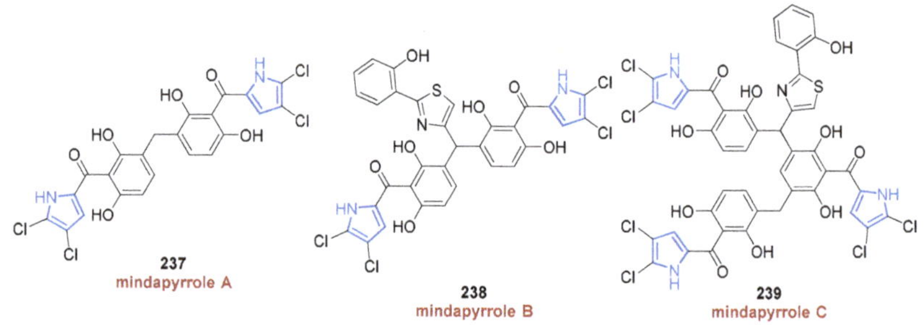

Figure 30. Mindapyrroles A–C (**237–239**) featuring several central resorcinol-cores.

New diterpene alkaloids, the agelasines O–R (**240–243**) bearing a bromopyrrole core, were isolated from the Okinawan marine sponge *Agelas* sp. in 2012 (Figure 31) [61]. The relative stereochemistries of compounds **240–243** were elucidated via ROESY-correlations. The agelasines O–R (**240–243**) showed good to moderate antimicrobial activities (IC$_{50}$ values ranging between 8 µg/mL and >32 µg/mL) against a wide range of bacteria, including strains of *Escherichia coli*, *Staphylococcus aureus*, and *Bacillus subtilis*. However, no cytotoxicity against murine leukemia L1210 and human epidermoid carcinoma KB cells was observed [61].

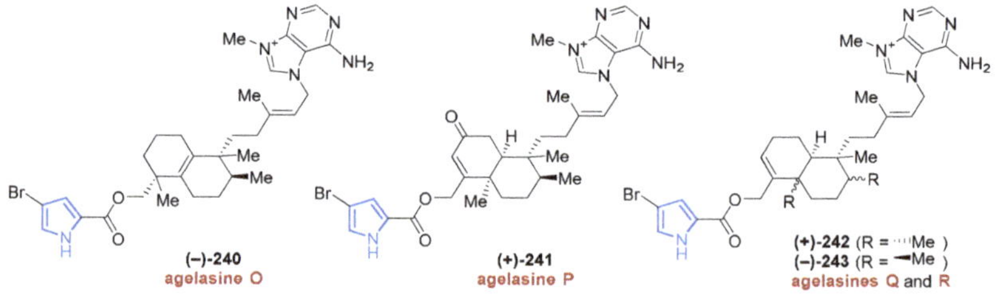

Figure 31. Agelasines O–R (**240–243**) with a 9-*N*-methyladenine unit from a marine sponge *Agelas* sp.

In 2010, Fenical and co-workers isolated marinopyrroles C–E (**244–246**) from the deep ocean actinomycete strain CNQ-418 [250], thereby extending the interesting class of biologically active marinopyrroles, of which marinopyrroles A (**250**) and B (**253**) had been isolated before (Figure 32) [251]. These metabolites contain an unprecedented, highly halogenated 1,3'-bipyrrole core which gives them an axis of chirality that, for marinopyrroles A and B as well as C–E (**244–246**), results in a stable *M*-configuration at room temperature. Marinopyrrole C (**244**) displayed significant activity against methicillin-resistant *Staphylococcus aureus* with MIC$_{90}$ values of less than 1 µg/mL. With derivatization experiments, the authors could also show that the presence of the hydrogen-bonding capacity of the salicyloyl hydroxyl groups, the free N–H functionality and the C-5' chlorine substituent were indispensable for the biological activity [250].

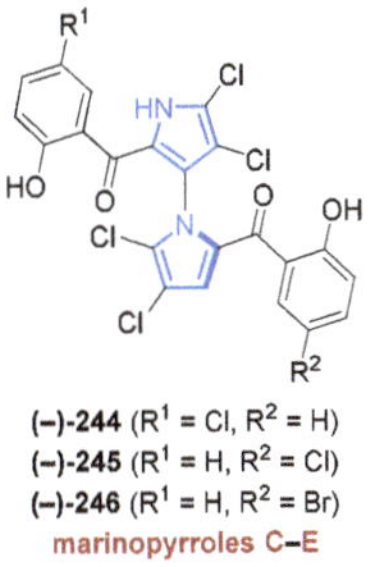

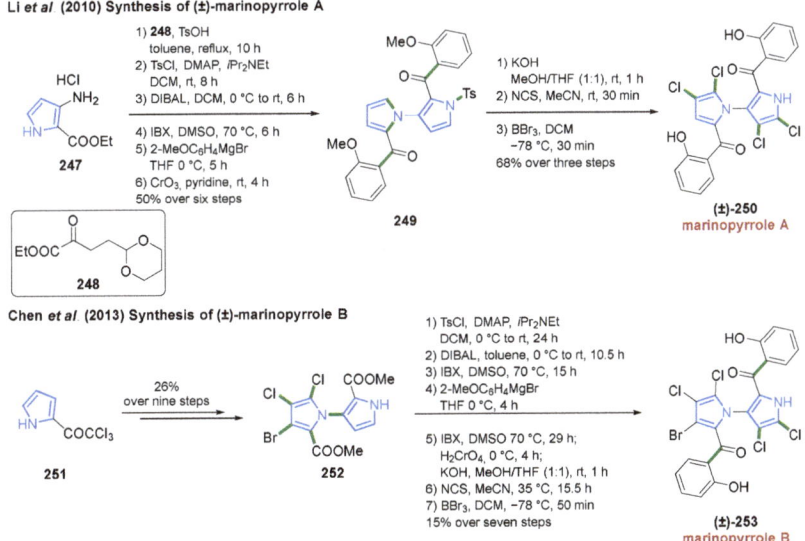

(−)-244 (R¹ = Cl, R² = H)
(−)-245 (R¹ = H, R² = Cl)
(−)-246 (R¹ = H, R² = Br)
marinopyrroles C–E

Figure 32. The unusual structure of marinopyrroles C–E (**244**–**246**) contain a rare 1,3′-bispyrrole functionality.

The first total synthesis of a member of the marinopyrrole family was realized by the Li laboratory in 2010 (Scheme 16) [252]. Starting with a TsOH-catalyzed condensation and cyclization of aminopyrrole **247** with α-ketoester **248** furnished an intermediary bi-pyrrole skeleton. After N-protection and transforming the diester to the dialdehyde via a reduction/oxidation sequence, the addition of 2-methoxyphenylmagnesium bromide followed by CrO_3 oxidation furnished the diketone **249** in 50% over six steps. After deprotection and chlorination of the pyrrole units with NCS, a final demethylation involving BBr_3 gave the natural product, (±)-marinopyrrole A (**250**) in 68% yield over three steps. Unfortunately, selective bromination towards (±)-marinopyrrole B (**253**) under various conditions was unsuccessful [252].

Scheme 16. First total synthesis of (±)-marinopyrrole A (**250**) by Li in 2010 and its congener marinopyrrole B (**253**) by Chen in 2013.

Three years later, the Chen laboratory synthesized (±)-marinopyrrole B (**253**) using a similar approach (Scheme 16) [253]. Here, the brominated chloropyrrole **252** was generated over nine steps starting from commercially available pyrrole **251**. The next seven steps were performed almost in the same manner as in the synthesis of marinopyrrole A reported by Li and co-workers, although some reaction conditions were improved. In this way, (±)-marinopyrrole B (**253**) could be obtained in 15% over seven steps [253].

Between 2012 and 2019, several pyrrolyloxazoles belonging to the phorbazole series were isolated from marine organisms. The first study of the Indo-Pacific dorid nudibranch *Aldisa andersoni* resulted in the isolation of 9-chloro-phorbazole D (**254**) and *N*1-methyl-phorbazole A (Figure 33) (**255**). Both compounds exhibit similar in vitro inhibitory activity against several human cancer lines with IC$_{50}$ values ranging between 18 µM and 34 µM [254].

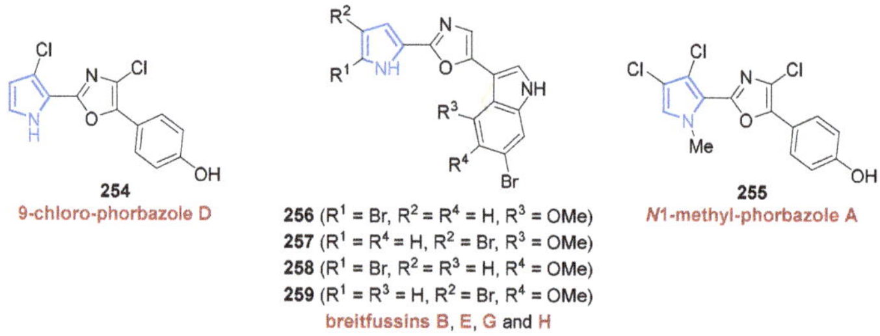

Figure 33. Phorbazol-based marine bromopyrrole alkaloids **254–259**.

A related class of natural bromopyrroles containing the pyrrolyloxazole functionality is the breitfussins. In analogy to breitfussin B (**256**), isolated from the hydrozoan *Thuiaria breitfussi* in 2012 [80], six new breitfussins C–H were discovered in the same producing organism as breitfussins E (**257**), G (**258**), and H (**259**) feature a brominated pyrrole core (Figure 33, for non-halogenated congeners see Figure 7) [81]. Compounds **258** and **259** were isolated as a mixture and thus not evaluated in cytotoxic activity assays, whereas breitfussins **256** and **257** did not show any cytotoxic activity against several tested cancer cell lines [81].

In 2015, breitfussin B (**256**) was synthesized by the Bayer group in the same manner as breitfussin A (**48**) (compare Scheme 4) [83]. In analogy to breitfussin A (**48**), the synthesis commenced with the readily available phenol **260**. After forming the indole building block **261**, iodination and TIPS-protection furnished compound **52**. The oxazole core **54** was installed and carefully iodinated with iodine to get access to compound **262**. Coupling with Boc-protected pyrrole boronic acid **20** then delivered intermediate **57** possessing the right indole-pyrrolyloxazole functionality. Bromination, protodeiodination, and removal of all protecting groups then furnished breitfussin B (**256**) in 4.3% overall yield (Scheme 17) [83].

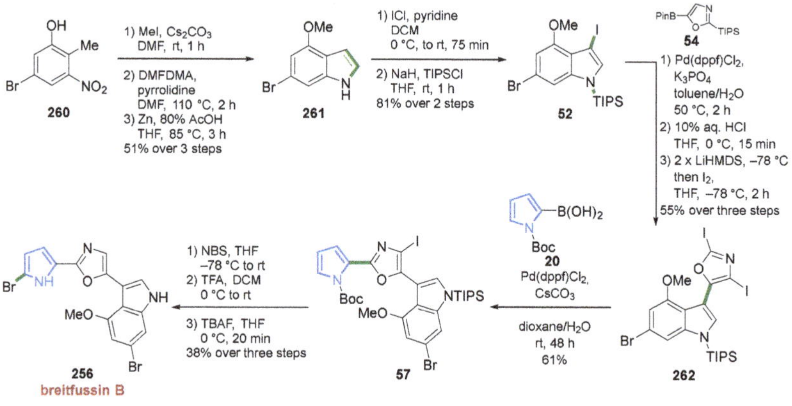

Scheme 17. Total synthesis of breitfussin B (**256**) starting from phenol **260**.

Simple Pyrrole (Amino)-Imidazole Alkaloids

The pyrrole-imidazole alkaloid (PIA) family comprises a myriad of simple to structurally complex molecules originating from marine organisms. The simplest PIA, oroidin, is believed to be the biogenetic precursor of any natural products belonging to this family and it is considered to be biosynthesized from the fundamental amino acids proline, ornithine, lysine, and/or histidine [13,38,255–257]. However, numerous further considerations on the biogenetical origin of PIAs can be found in the literature so that the biosynthesis of most of these alkaloids still lies in the realm of speculations. Many PIAs are reported to exhibit significant biological activities resulting in a great interest among synthetic chemists to provide solutions to finally get access to potent pharmaceutically relevant substances.

In 9-oxethyl-mukanadin F (**263**), isolated in 2016 by the Lin group from a not fully identified sponge *Agelas* sp., the oroidin 2-aminoimidazole moiety is replaced by a hydantoin ring (Figure 34) [66]. Compound **263** was isolated as a racemic mixture and displayed no antifungal activity against *Candida albicans* [66].

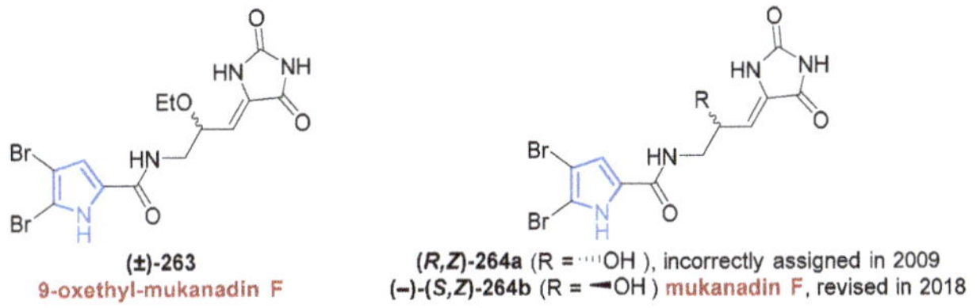

Figure 34. C-9 functionalized ene-hydantion marine pyrrole alkaloids **263** and **264**.

In 2018, the Barker group published a comprehensive work addressing stereochemical issues of related mukanadin-based alkaloids substituted at C-9 [79]. The publication also describes the total synthesis of (+)- and (−)-mukanadin F (**264a** and **264b**), which finally resulted in the reassignment of its absolute stereochemical configuration and shed light upon many inconsistencies concerning the stereochemistry of C-9-functionalized enehydantoin/imidazole marine natural products published as racemic or scalemic mixtures before (Figure 34 and Scheme 18) [220,258–261].

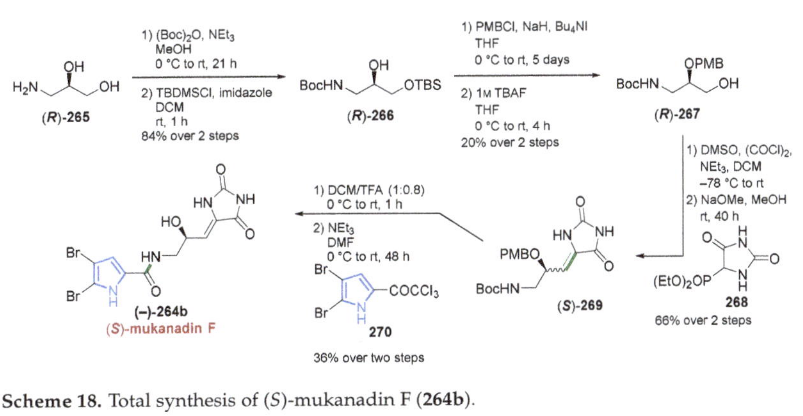

Scheme 18. Total synthesis of (*S*)-mukanadin F (**264b**).

The authors began the synthesis with a selective protection/deprotection sequence of aminodiol (*R*)-**265** producing alcohols (*R*)-**266** and (*R*)-**267**, sequentially. After Swern oxidation and HWE reaction with hydantoin phosphonate **268**, compound (*S*)-**269** could be obtained as a mixture of *E*/*Z* isomers (1:2) in 66% yield over two steps. Simultaneous Boc and PMB deprotection followed by a final C−N coupling step involving trichloroacetyl dibromopyrrole **270** gave (*S*)-mukanadin F ((*S*)-**264b**) as a mixture of *E*/*Z* isomers (1:1.3). The same procedure starting from (S)-**265** delivered (R)-mukanadin F ((R)-**264a**) as a mixture of E/Z isomers (1:2) (Scheme 18) [79].

Successful separation of the E/Z isomers of ((S)-**264b**) and ((R)-**246a**) and comparison of NMR spectroscopic data of the synthetic Z-configured enantiomers of mukanadin F (**264**) with those reported for the natural product were a match, confirming the alkene geometry [258]. However, new optical rotation measurements revealed that (S)-mukanadin F ((S)-**264b**) corresponds to the natural product, which is opposite to that proposed for the isolated sample in 2009 [258]. As a last point, the Baker group found out that C-9 functionalized ene-hydantoin/imidazole marine alkaloids are prone to isomerization and racemization with both effects occurring upon light irradiation or under acidic or basic conditions and therefore is likely to occur upon extraction [79]. These findings reveal that compounds of this class most likely exist in nature as pure enantiomers and that other publications concerning their isolation and stereochemical elucidation should be checked carefully.

Recently, E-dispacamide (**271**) and slagenin D (**272**) were isolated from the sponge *Agelas oroides* in 2020 (Figure 35). The absolute configuration of compound **272** was established by comparison of its specific rotation with that of synthetic *ent*-slagenin A, indicating its stereogenic centers to be 9S, 11S, 15S configured [237].

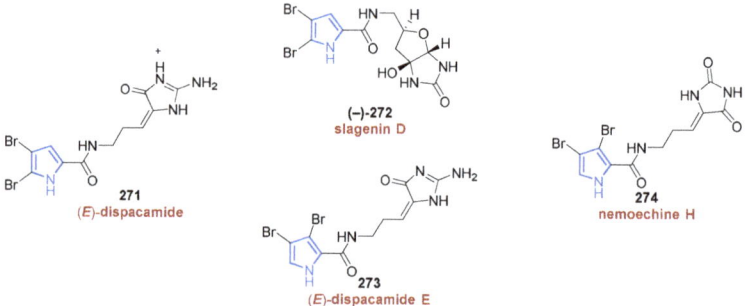

Figure 35. Related bromopyrrole alkaloids **271**–**274** bearing hydantoin.

A bromopyrrole marine alkaloid **273**, very similar to compound **271**, was isolated from the sponge *Stylissa massa* in 2014 and was given the name dispacamide E (**273**) (Figure 35) [228]. It showed significant inhibitory activities against the kinases GSK-3, DYRK1A, and CK-1 with IC_{50} values below 19 μM [228]. The reader is advised that careful reading is required to distinguish between the (E/Z) dispacamides, as the original trivial names relate to the Z-configured natural compounds [219,220]. However, new dispacamides possessing E-configuration are not consistently given either new trivial names or E/Z-designated former trivial names.

In nemoechine H (**274**), isolated from the sea sponge *Agelas nemoechinata* in 2019, only the hydantoin core is different compared to compound **273** (Figure 35). Compound **274** exhibited good to moderate cytotoxic activity against K562 and L-02 cell lines with IC_{50} values of 6.1 μM and 12.3 μM, respectively [262].

Very recently, three new related congeners, 9-hydroxydihydrodispacamide (**275**), 9-hydroxydihydrooroidin (**276**), and 9E-keramadine (**277**) were isolated from two different marine sponges *Agelas* spp. (Figure 36). Compounds **275** and **276** were isolated as racemates with the relative configuration of compound **275** still to be deduced [232]. Compound **277** was already known as a synthetic product but was isolated the first time from a natural source [263]. All three compounds **275**–**277** did not show any promising cytotoxicity against human cancer cell lines (HeLa, A549, MCF7) in basic antiproliferative tests [232].

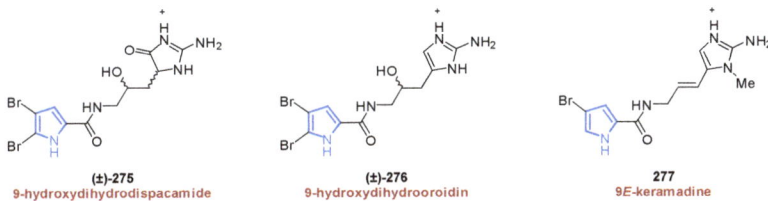

Figure 36. Three new PIAs **275**–**277** isolated from the sponge *Agelas* spp. in 2020.

The Berlinck group isolated debromooroidin **278** from a sponge identified as *Dictyonella* sp. in 2018, which displayed proteasome inhibition activity with IC_{50} values of 27 µM ± 6 µM (Figure 37) [264]. The authors also mentioned that the proteasome inhibitory activity is strongly influenced by the position of the bromine substituent in the pyrrole ring thereby confirming the findings of previous investigations [265,266].

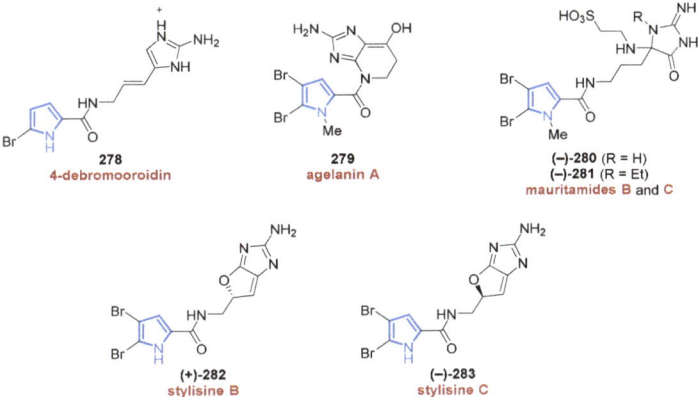

Figure 37. Oroidin-derived bromopyrrole alkaloids **278**–**283** bearing imidazole moieties.

In 2009, the acetone/methanol extract of the sponge *Agelas linnaei* permitted the isolation of agelanin A (**279**) and mauritamides B (**280**) and C (**281**) (Figure 37) [234]. The sulfonic acid congeners **280** and **281** contain a taurine unit which is quite a rare structural motif in marine sponge metabolites when combined with a bromopyrrole unit.

Further oroidin-derived pyrrole alkaloids, stylisines B (**282**) and C (**283**), were isolated in 2018 from the sponge *Stylissa massa* (Figure 37). Here, the stereogenic centers could be unambiguously determined via electronic circular dichroism experiments. Unfortunately, compounds **279**–**283** have not shown any promising biological activities so far [133].

In 2010, another new set of halopyrroles, the stylissazoles A–C (**284**–**286**), were isolated from species from the *Stylissa* genus (Figure 38) [267]. No absolute configuration could be determined for the dimeric pyrrole-2-aminoimidazoles **285** and **286** as no optical activity was observed. The authors mentioned that the interconversion of the configurationally unstable chiral carbons C6 and C7 might be the reason for this issue. However, the relative configuration of both stereogenic centers in stylissazole C (**286**) could be determined by NOESY experiments [267].

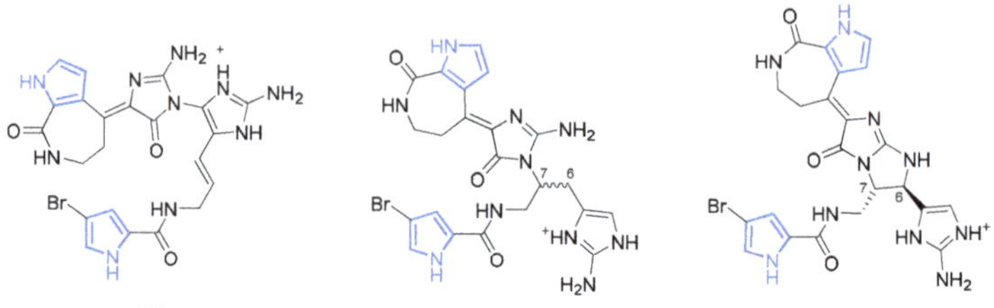

284 stylissazole A
285 stylissazole B
286 stylissazole C

Figure 38. Stylissazoles A–C (**284**–**286**) isolated from the marine sponge *Stylissa carteri*.

The unique bromopyrrole alkaloids agelamadin F (**287**) and tauroacidin E (**288**) were isolated from an Okinawan marine sponge of the genus *Agelas* in 2015 (Figure 39) [64]. Compound **287** is the first example of a bromopyrrole alkaloid bearing an aminoimidazole moiety connected to a pyridinium ring. Tauroacidin E (**288**), possessing an uncommon taurine unit, was isolated as a racemic structure. Both halopyrroles **287** and **288** showed moderate activities against KB and human leukemia K562 cells with IC$_{50}$ values in the range of 10 µg/mL [64].

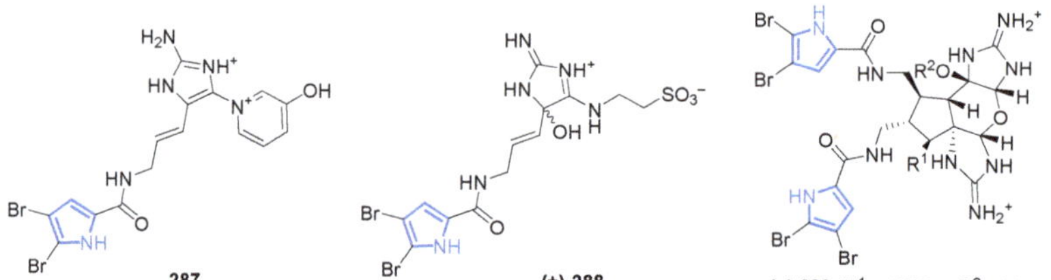

287 agelamadin F
(±)-**288** tauroacidin E
(−)-**289** (R^1 = OSO$_3^-$, R^2 = H) 14-O-sulfate massadine
(−)-**290** (R^1 = OMe, R^2 = H) 14-O-methyl massadine
(−)-**291** (R^1 = Cl, R^2 = Me) 3-O-methyl massadine chloride

Figure 39. Unusual aminoimidazole pyrrole alkaloids **287**–**291** with compounds **289**–**291** incorporating a complex contiguous imidazole ring system.

The complex class of massadines was extended by the isolation of three new compounds **289**–**291** from a deep-water sponge of the genus *Axinella* in 2012 (Figure 39) [268]. The eight stereogenic centers of 14-O-sulfate massadine (**289**), 14-O-methyl massadine (**290**), and 3-O-methyl massadine chloride (**94**) were determined by NMR spectroscopy and optical rotation measurements. The generated data confirmed the absolute stereochemistry earlier defined by Köck [269] and Fusetani [270] for related massadines and was also consistent with the data from its enantioselective total synthesis [271]. While compounds **289**–**291** did not show any inhibitory activity against the neurodegenerative disease kinase targets CDK5/p25, CK1δ, and GSK3β, 3-O-methyl massadine chloride (**291**) exhibited antibacterial activity against several Gram-positive and -negative bacteria with IC$_{50}$ values below 5 µM [268].

Three structurally similar alkaloids (**292**–**294**), possessing two or more contiguous ring systems were isolated from the sponge *Stylissa* aff. *carteri* in 2020 (Figure 40) [272]. The absolute stereochemistry of the two new hexacyclic analogs of palau'amine and styloguanidine, debromokonbu'acidin (**292**) and didebromocarteramine (**293**), was determined by comparison of experimental and theoretical ECD spectra. While compound **293** did not show any neuroprotective activity, compound **292** could reduce reactive oxygen species in neuroblastoma SY-SY5Y cells by 35% over a wide range of concentrations [272]. The stereochemistry of futunamine (**294**), featuring a new pyrrolo[1,2-c]imidazole core, was also deduced by ECD analyses. Furthermore, futunamine (**294**) showed neuroprotective effects at 10 µM. Unfortunately, none of the three new compounds **292**–**294** showed any cytotoxic activity [272].

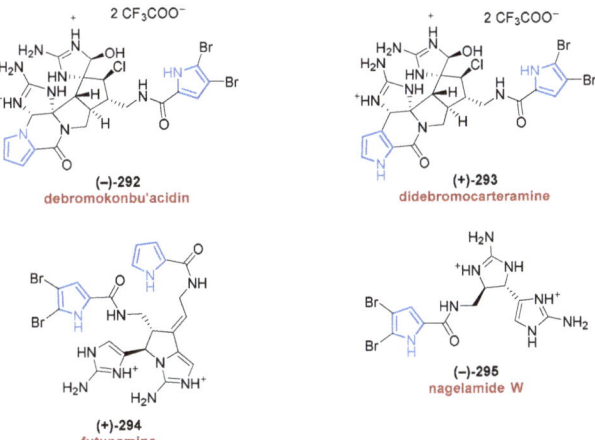

Figure 40. Biologically active bromopyrrole imidazole alkaloids **292**–**295** possessing unique structural motifs.

Nagelamide W (**295**), the first monomeric bromopyrrole alkaloid bearing two aminoimidazole moieties, was isolated from a marine sponge *Agelas* sp. by the Kobayashi group in 2013 (Figure 40) [65]. The relative stereochemistry of **295** was elucidated by ROESY correlations and the natural product **295** exhibited inhibitory activity against *Candida albicans* with an IC$_{50}$ value of 4 µg/mL [65].

In 2014, five new bromopyrrole alkaloids (**296**–**300**) were isolated from an Okinawan marine sponge of the genus *Agelas* (Figure 41) [273]. Tauroacidin C (**298**), tauroacidin D (**299**), and mukanadin G (**300**) were isolated as racemic mixtures. However, the relative stereochemistry of mukanadin G (**300**) was established by ROESY and computational experiments. While compounds **296**–**298** did not show any antimicrobial activity, mukanadin G (**300**) exhibited good to moderate antifungal activity against the human-pathogenic yeast *Candida albicans* and the invasive pathogenic fungus *Cryptococcus neoformans* with IC$_{50}$ values between 8 and 16 µM [273].

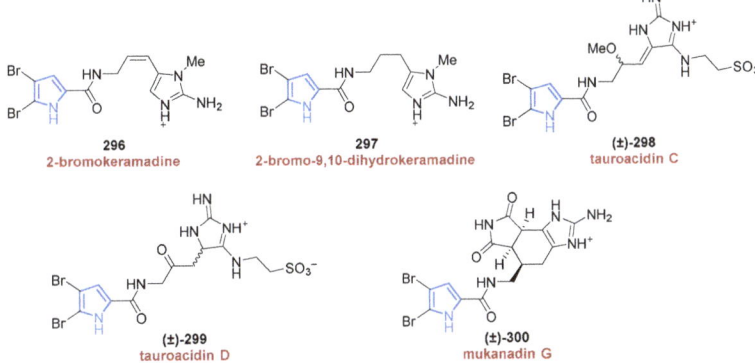

Figure 41. Related bromopyrrole alkaloids **296**–**300** and the antifungal mukanadin G (**300**) isolated from *Agelas* sp.

In decarboxyagelamadin C (**301**), isolated from the sponge *Agelas sceptrum* in 2016, a rare morpholine core is located between the pyrrole and imidazole moiety with the relative and absolute stereochemistry being established by NMR and ECD spectroscopy (Figure 42) [274]. Unfortunately, compound **301** did not show any activity in cytotoxicity tests and in antimicrobial assays.

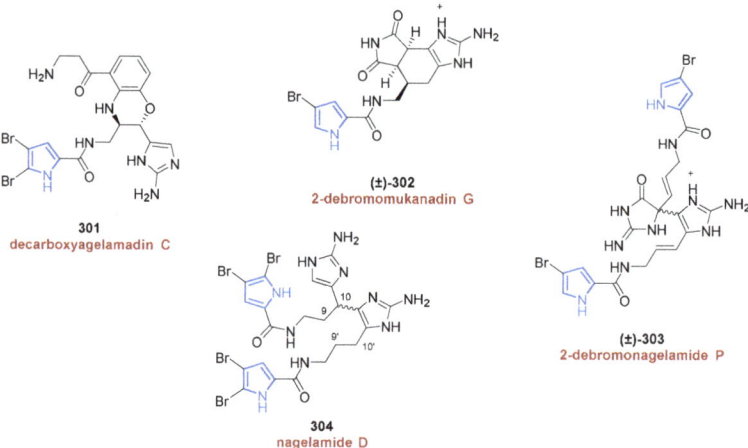

Figure 42. Oroidin-based bromopyrrole alkaloids **301–303** with nagelamide D (**304**) underwent a reevaluation in 2020.

A new bromopyrrole alkaloid also incorporating a fused 6-membered ring, 2-debromomukanadin G (**302**), was isolated from another *Agelas* sp. alongside 2-debromonagelamide P (**303**) (Figure 42) [248]. While both substances **302** and **303** were isolated as racemates, the relative configuration of compound **302** could be deduced by comparison of its coupling constants with those from mukanadin G (**300**). Compound **303** showed moderate antimicrobial activity against *Trichophyton mentagrophytes* (IC$_{50}$ value 32 µg/mL), whereas compound **302** exhibited moderate activity against *Cryptococcus neoformans* (IC$_{50}$ value 32 µg/mL). However, no cytotoxicity was observed against human epidermoid carcinoma KB and murine lymphoma L1210 cells [248].

We also want to mention an inconsistency in the assigned structure for the structurally related nagelamide D (**304**), which was originally isolated in 2004 as a racemate by the Kobayashi group (Figure 42) [275]. Five years later, a total synthesis by the Lovely group [276] revealed that either the assigned structure or the reported NMR data of Kobayashi's work was in error. However, no final evidence was given at this point. A recently published synthetical approach [277] of the same laboratory towards alkaloids belonging to the nagelamide class then corroborated the correctly proposed but incorrectly assigned structure by Kobayashi. In this case, crystallographic measurements [277] unequivocally demonstrated that the assignments for C9, C9', C10' as well as H9'a and H9'b were inadvertently switched in the original literature [275].

The Lovely group commenced their synthesis with the iodoimidazoles **305** and **306**, which were transformed into the corresponding coupling partners **307** and **308** over several steps, respectively. A Stille cross-coupling then delivered compound **309**. A reaction sequence involving several protection and deprotection reactions as well as the installation of the azide group via TsN$_3$ furnished diol **310**. Replacing the alcohol functional groups by a pyrrole hydantoin **311**, hydrolysis, and deprotection of the corresponding urea followed by azide hydrogenation finally furnished nagelamide D (**304**) in 32% over four steps (Scheme 19) [277].

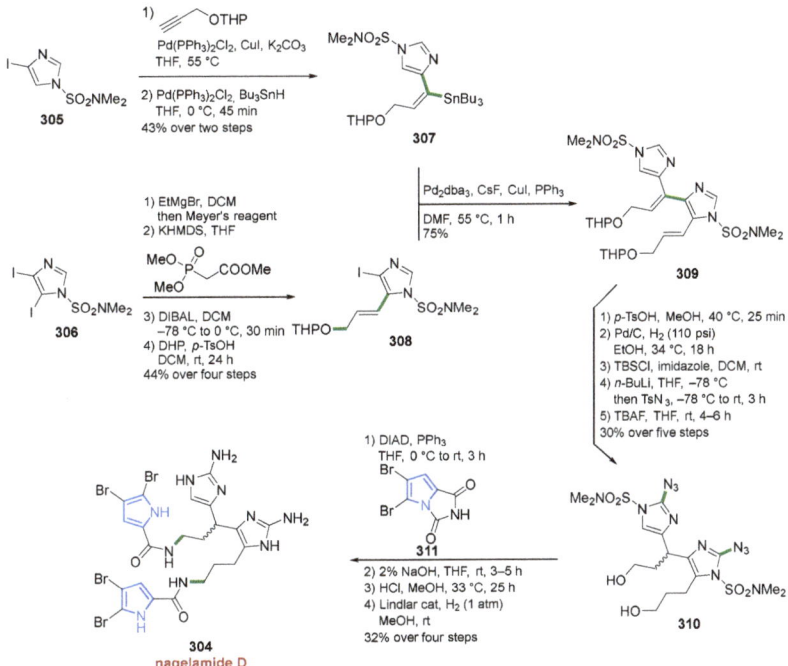

Scheme 19. A total synthesis of nagelamide D published by the Lovely group led to the correct assignment of nagelamide D (**304**).

A very similar class of compounds, the citrinamines A–D (**312**–**315**), were isolated from the Caribbean sponge *Agelas citrina* in 2015 by the Köck group (Figure 43) [63]. All four compounds **312**–**315** were isolated as racemic mixtures, with the relative configuration of citrinamine C (**314**) being elucidated with the aid of NOESY correlations and comparison of its NMR data with those of nagelamide B, a related congener isolated back in 2004 [275]. It should be mentioned that the same group isolated citrinamines C (**314**) and D (**315**) as a mixture, the separation of which by preparative chromatography failed. Citrinamines B–D (**313**–**315**) showed "considerable" inhibition zones in agar diffusion assays with *Mycobacterium phlei* (no values for the size of the inhibition zones were given). However, all compounds **312**–**315** exhibited no inhibition of cell proliferation of mouse fibroblasts [63]. Here, we would like to mention that the only structural difference between citrinamine A (**312**) and 2-debromonagelamide P (**303**) lies in the additional proton present in compound **303** (Figure 43). As the NMR spectra of both compounds **303** and **312** also appear to be identical, it is highly likely that both compounds **303** and **312** are in fact the same substance, although compound **303** was isolated as a salt and compound **312** as the free base.

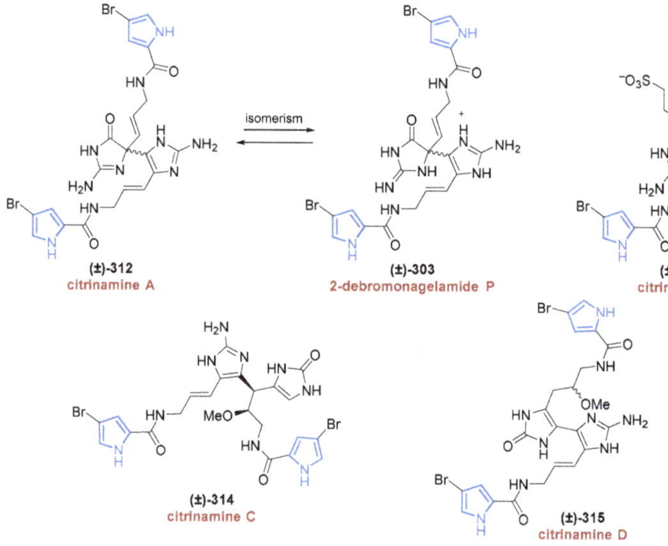

Figure 43. The dimeric bromopyrrole alkaloids citrinamines A–D (**312**–**315**).

The known class of nagelamides was extended by nagelamides I (**316**) and 2,2′-didebromonagelamide B (**317**), isolated from a marine sponge *Agelas* sp. (Figure 44) [278]. The relative configuration of compound **317** could be deduced by extensive NMR-spectroscopic analysis but the absolute configuration remains unknown. Both compounds **316** and **317** did not show cytotoxicity against murine lymphoma L1210 and human epidermoid carcinoma KB cells in vitro [278].

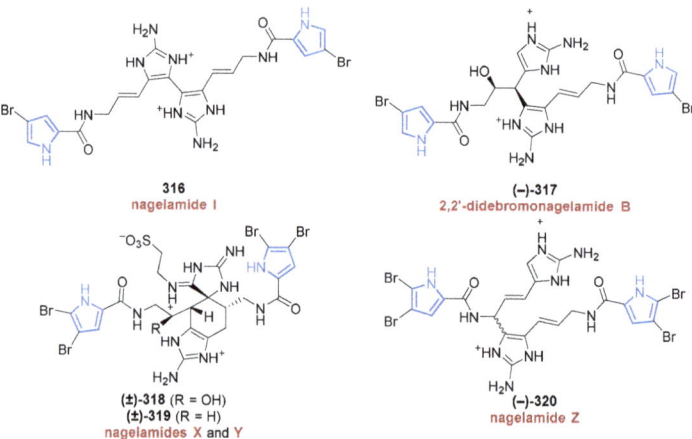

Figure 44. Five new family members (**316**–**320**) of the nagelamides from *Agelas* sp.

Nagelamides X–Z (**318**–**320**) were isolated from a marine sponge of the genus *Agelas* in 2013 (Figure 44) [279]. Here, the nagelamides X (**318**) and Y (**319**) incorporate a unique tricyclic skeleton consisting of spiro-connected tetrahydrobenzaminoimidazole and aminoimidazolidine moieties. Compounds **318** and **319** were isolated as racemic mixtures with the relative configuration being determined by 2D NMR spectroscopy. Nagelamide Z (**320**) was isolated as an optically active molecule, but its absolute configuration remains unsolved. Nagelamides X–Z (**318–320**) displayed antimicrobial activities against several bacteria and fungi, with IC$_{50}$ values partly being below 5 µg/mL [279].

In 2012, a new pair of dimeric pyrrole-aminoimidazole alkaloids, (−)-donnazoles A (**321**) and B (**322**), was isolated from the marine sponge *Axinella donnani* (Figure 45). The absolute configurations of **321** and **322** were determined via NOE correlations and ECD measurements [280].

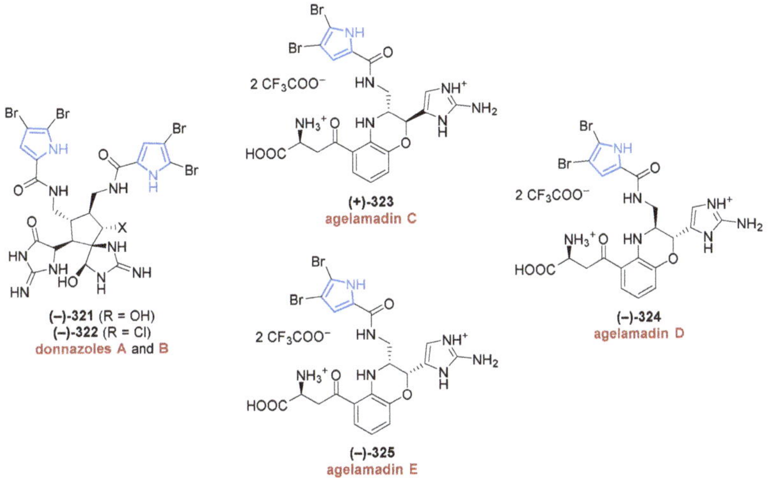

Figure 45. Donnazoles A (**321**) and B (**322**) from a marine sponge *Axinella donnani* and further agelamadins C–E (**323–325**).

The agelamadins C–E (**323–325**), isolated from a marine sponge of the genus *Agelas* in 2014, share the same flat structure but differ in their stereochemistries (Figure 45) [281]. The configurations of compounds **323–325** were elucidated by 2D NMR spectroscopy, ECD calculations, and by a phenylglycine methyl ester (PGME) method. To this end, (*R*)- and (*S*)-PGME are condensed with a carboxylic acid functionality, to generate amides enabling the determination of the absolute configuration by means of the diamagnetic anisotropic effect [282]. While agelamadin D (**324**) did not show any antimicrobial activity, agelamadins C (**323**) and E (**325**) displayed moderate inhibitory activity against the human pathogen *Cryptococcus neoformans* with IC$_{50}$ values of 32 µg/mL each [281].

3.2. Annellated Pyrroles

Annellated pyrroles are prevalent in nature. For example, many well-known biologically active alkaloid families, including the lamellarins and indolizidins, as well as many stemona alkaloids, feature annellated pyrrole moieties [283–285].

Between 2010 and 2012, the highly halogenated 5- and 8-ring annellated pyrroles **326–328** were isolated from marine bacteria (Figure 46). The *Pseudoalteromonas*-derived 2,3,5,7-tetrabromobenzofuro[3,2-*b*]pyrrole (**326**) displayed significant antimicrobial activity against methicillin-resistant *Staphylococcus aureus* (ATCC 43300, IC$_{50}$ value of 1.93 µM ± 0.05 µM) [286].

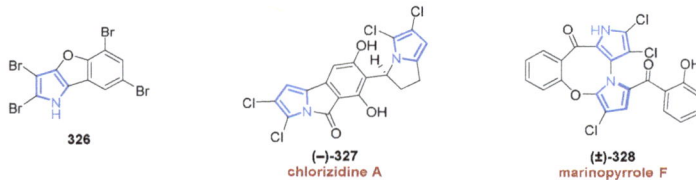

Figure 46. Annellated halopyrroles **326**–**328** derived from marine bacteria.

The biologically active (−)-chlorizidine A (**327**) was isolated from a marine *Streptomyces* sp. and exhibited noteworthy activity in a human colon cancer cytotoxicity bioassay with IC$_{50}$ values of 3.2–4.9 µM (Figure 46) [287]. Interestingly, the alkaloid **327** completely lost its activity when both phenolic functionalities were methylated. The authors also mentioned that a series of derivatives lacking the key 5*H*-pyrrolo[2,1-*a*]isoindol-5-one moiety led to inactivity, strongly suggesting its presence is indispensable for biological activity [287].

The structure of (±)-marinopyrrole F (**328**), isolated from a *Streptomyces* sp. in 2010, contains an unusual eight-membered ring (Figure 46) [250]. In contrast to its enantiopure metabolites, marinopyrroles C–E (**244**–**246**, see Figure 32), (±)-marinopyrrole F (**328**) was isolated in racemic form. With the help of chiral HPLC, the authors found out that enantioenriched **328** completely racemizes within 18 h, most probably caused by the fused ether ring lowering the barrier for atropisomerism. However, (±)-marinopyrrole F (**328**) was much less active against MRSA and HCT-116 (MIC$_{90}$ value 3.1 µg/mL) compared to (−)-marinopyrrole C (**244**, MIC$_{90}$ value 0.16 µg/mL) [250].

In 2018, 4-debromougibohlin (**329**) and 5-debromougibohlin (**330**) were isolated from a marine sponge *Dictyonella* sp. by the Berlinck group (Figure 47). Unfortunately, both compounds did not show any proteasome inhibitory activity in a respective assay [264].

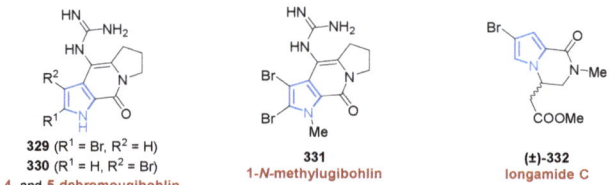

Figure 47. Structures of 2,3-annellated marine pyrrole alkaloids **329**–**332**.

In 2019, a related halopyrrole alkaloid incorporating the carbamoylpyrrole-like core structure, 1-*N*-methylugibohlin (**331**), was isolated from the sea sponge *Agelas nemoechinata*, but did not show cytotoxic activity against K562, A549, HeLa, or HCT-116 cells in vitro (Figure 47) [262].

Longamide C (**332**), obtained from an organic extract of *Agelas nakamurai* in 2010, was isolated as a racemic mixture (Figure 47). However, ROESY correlations indicated a half chair conformation of the six-membered ring. Compound **332** did not show any promising antimicrobial or cytotoxic activity [234].

In 2017, the Lin group isolated stylisines A–F (**333**, **282**, **283**, **334**, **335**, **132**) from the marine sponge *Stylissa massa*, of which stylisine A, D, and E (**333**–**335**) feature an annellated bromopyrrole moiety (Figure 48) [133]. The absolute stereochemistry of compounds **334** and **335** was deduced from ECD experiments. However, no antibacterial activity was observed for all three compounds **333**–**335** [133]. One year later, 5-debromougibohlin (**330**, Figure 47) was isolated and erroneously presented as a "new" bromo alkaloid [264], since it has the same structure as stylisine A (**333**).

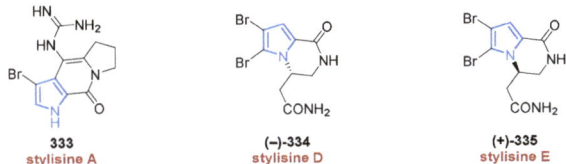

Figure 48. Stylisines A (**333**), D (**334**), and E (**335**) from the marine sponge *Stylissa massa*.

At this point, the stereoselective synthesis of (−)-stylisine D (**334**) reported by Petkovic and Savic in 2019 should be mentioned (Scheme 20) [288]. The synthesis commenced with an N-protection and propargylation followed by routine transformations to generate allene **337** in 55% yield over three steps. After installing Boc-L-proline (**338**) which furnished compound **339** possessing the right configuration, compound **340** was obtained over four steps under transfer of chirality. After bromination and hydrolysis, a final oxidation step delivered (−)-longamide B (**341**), another bromopyrrole isolated from the sponge *Stylissa massa*. (−)-Stylisine D (**334**) was obtained by amidation of the carboxylic group of (−)-longamide B (**341**).

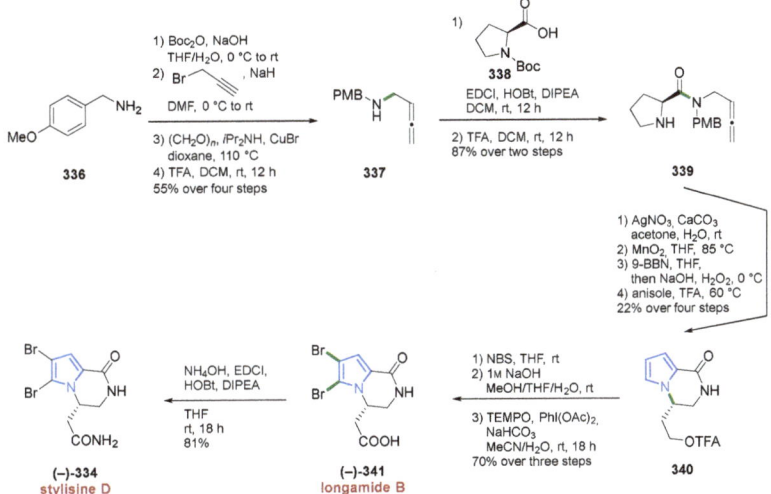

Scheme 20. Synthesis of stylisine D (**334**) and intermediate longamide B (**341**) via a metal-catalyzed cyclisation of allene **339** in a stereoselective manner.

In 2016, the family of longamides was extended by the isolation of longamides D–F (**342**–**344**) from a marine sponge *Agelas* sp. (Figure 49) [66]. Compounds **342**–**344** were isolated as racemic mixtures which were separated into pure enantiomers. The absolute stereochemistry of **342**–**344** was then determined by chiral HPLC and ECD spectroscopy. In the *Caenorhabditis elegans* candidiasis model, metabolites (+)-**342**, (−)-**343** and (+)-**344** exhibited significant antifungal activity with survival rates around 50%, whereas the corresponding enantiomers (−)-**342**, (+)-**343** and (−)-**344** did not show any activity, strongly suggesting the absolute configuration at C-9 to have an appreciable effect [66].

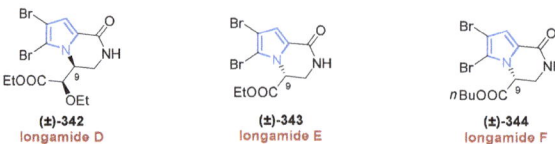

Figure 49. Longamides D–F (342–344) from the South China Sea sponge *Agelas* sp.

In 2014, several structurally unique annellated halopyrroles 345–348 were isolated from the Patagonian bryozoan *Aspidostoma giganteum* by Palermo and co-workers (Figure 50) [239]. The absolute configurations of bromotryptophan-derived aspidostomides D (345) and E (346) were determined by a modification of Mosher's method in combination with NOE correlations. While the elimination product of 345 and 346, aspidostomide F (347), the N–N-linked dimeric aspidazide A (348) and compound 345 only exhibited moderate to weak cytotoxic activity against the 786-O human renal carcinoma cell line (IC$_{50}$ values between 27.0 µM and >100 µM), aspidostomide E (346) proved active with an IC$_{50}$ value of 7.8 µM [239].

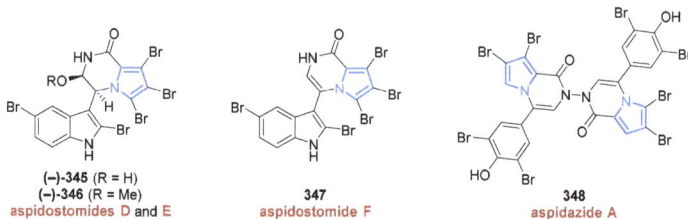

Figure 50. New aspidostomides D–F (345–347) and aspidazide A (348) from the patagonian bryozoan *Aspidostoma giganteum*.

In 2017, a new family of annellated halopyrroles, the callyspongisines, were isolated from the Great Australian Bight marine sponge *Callyspongia* sp. (CMB-01152) (Figure 51) [289]. In callyspongisines A (349), a very rare imino-oxazoline core is spirocyclic to a seven-membered ring contiguous to a pyrrole unit. Due to insufficient quantities of 349–352, the stereochemistry could not be determined and the authors also mentioned that callyspongisines B–D (350–352) could be storage and handling artifacts of 349 instead of being of natural origin [289]. The potent kinase inhibitory activity observed in *Callyspongia* sp. was attributed to hymenialdisine, while compounds 349–352 did not show any cytotoxic activity against a range of prokaryotic, eukaryotic, and mammalian cell lines [289].

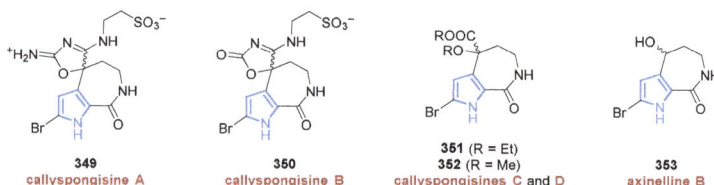

Figure 51. Callyspongisines A–D (349–352) and pyrrololactam 353 of which only compound 349 is speculated to be of natural origin.

A related pyrrolactam alkaloid, axinelline B (353), was isolated from the *n*-BuOH extract of a marine sponge of the genus *Axinella* in 2017 (Figure 51). Unfortunately, the authors did not give any information about the stereochemistry or biological activity of compound 353 [131].

Annellated Pyrrole (Amino)-Imidazole Alkaloids

Several contiguous tetracyclic brominated pyrrole-imidazole alkaloids **354–356** were isolated or synthesized between 2016 and 2019.

In 5-bromophakelline (**354**), isolated from an Indonesian marine sponge of the genus *Agelas*, the relative and absolute configuration was deduced with the help of NOESY correlations and X-ray crystallography (Figure 52). However, no antimicrobial activity against *Mycobacterium smegmatis* (NBRC 3207), a model organism for tuberculosis was observed [290].

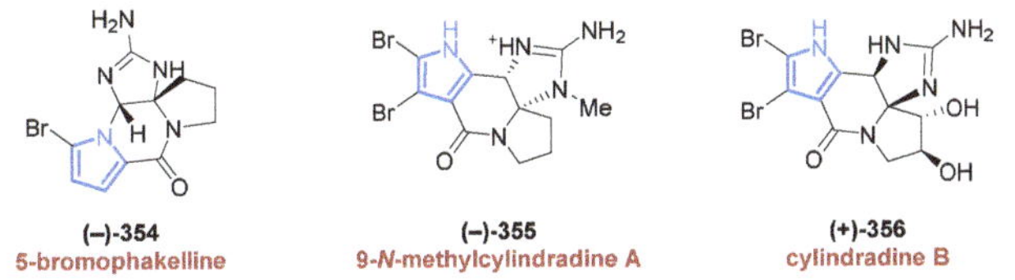

Figure 52. Brominated pyrrole-imidazole alkaloids **354–356** bearing guanidine units.

Compound **355** was isolated from the sponge *Agelas nemoechinata* in 2019 (Figure 52). The relative and absolute configuration of 9-*N*-methylcylindradine A (**355**) was determined by NOESY correlations and by the comparison of its optical rotation with the known (+)-cylindradine A. Unfortunately, no cytotoxic activity against K562 and L-02 cell lines could be observed [262].

At this point, we would also like to mention the first total synthesis of (+)-cylindradine B (**356**) (Scheme 21) [291], which was isolated from the marine sponge *Axinella cylindratus* back in 2008 [292].

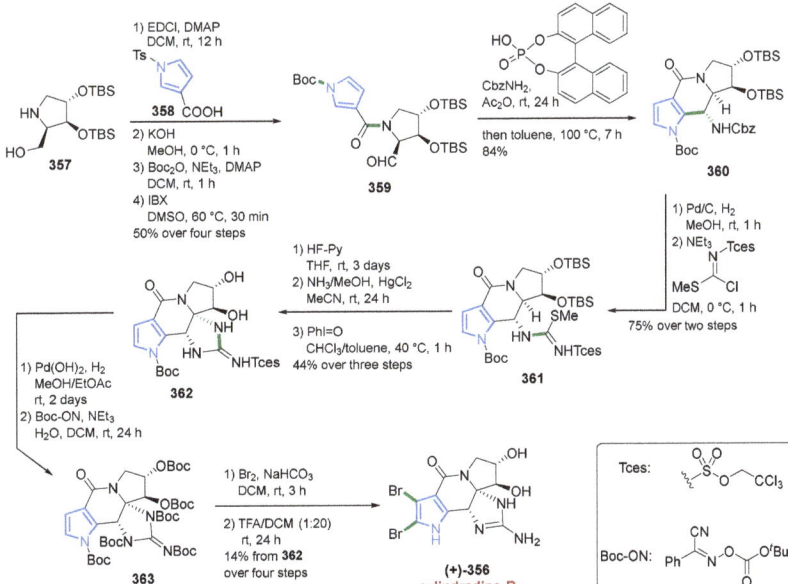

Scheme 21. First total synthesis of (+)-cylindradine B (**356**) via key Pictet–Spengler reaction.

The authors commenced their synthesis with prolinol derivative **357** which was transformed with pyrrole **358** into the Pictet–Spengler precursor **359** over several steps. The Pictet–Spengler reaction then selectively gave compound **360** under addition of (±)-

1,1′-binaphthyl-2,2′-diyl hydrogen phosphate. In the next steps, the guanidine group was attached via an isothiourea intermediate **361**, which reacted with NH$_3$/MeOH furnishing compound **362**. After changing the protective groups, the Boc-protected pyrrole **363** was brominated by using bromine and a final deprotection by applying TFA furnished (+)-cylindradine B (**356**) in 14% yield over four steps (Scheme 21) [291].

In 2010, a compound very similar to **354**, dibromohydroxyphakellin (**364**), was isolated from *Agelas linnaei* and represents the first described 12-OH analog of the phakellin family (Figure 53) [234]. By comparison of its optical rotation data with those of related compounds, it was assumed that dibromohydroxyphakellin (**364**) was isolated as a scalemic mixture. No cytotoxicity was observed against the murine L1578Y mouse lymphoma cell line [234].

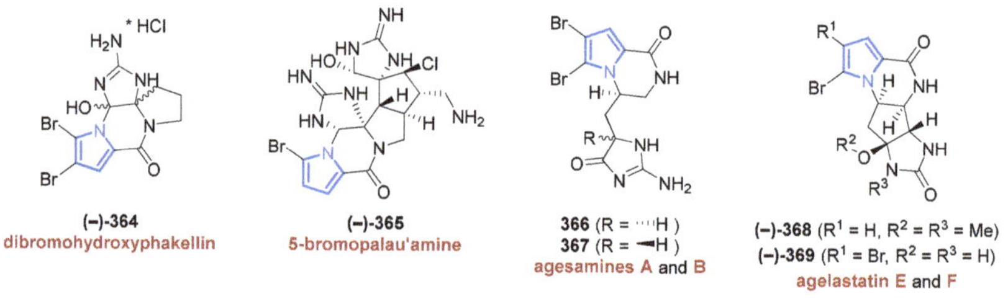

Figure 53. Structurally complex annellated bromopyrroles **364–369** isolated from *Dyctionella* sp. or *Agelas* sp.

In 5-bromopalau'amine (**365**), isolated from *Dictyonella* sp. (marine sponge), the relative configuration of the eight stereogenic centers was determined by ROESY correlations [264] and was in accordance with the data reported for the revised structure of palau'amine (Figure 53) [293]. Compound **365** displayed proteasome inhibition activity with an IC$_{50}$ value of 9.2 µM ± 3.2 µM, whereas the debrominated analog, palau'amine, was fourfold more active. Due to these data, the authors mentioned that both, bromination and the position of the bromine substituent in the pyrrole moiety seem to significantly influence the ability to inhibit the 20S yeast proteasome [264].

In 2019, a new class of annellated bromopyrroles, the agesamines A (**366**) and B (**367**), were isolated as an inseparable epimeric mixture from an Indonesian sponge of the genus *Agelas* (Figure 53). The absolute configuration of both compounds **366** and **367** was elucidated by ECD measurements [294].

The related agelastatins E (**368**) and F (**369**) were isolated from the marine sponge *Agelas dendromorpha* in 2010 (Figure 53) [295]. The relative configuration of both compounds **368** and **369** was determined by NOESY correlations and by comparison to the known congener agelastatin A. As agelastatin A is a highly cytotoxic compound, agelastatins E (**368**) and F (**369**) were screened for cytotoxicity against the human KB cell line. Unfortunately, both compounds **368** and **369** lacked significant activity [295].

Concerning the agelastatin family, the total synthesis of agelastatins A–F (**375–378, 368, 369**), published by the Movassaghi group in 2010, should be mentioned (Scheme 22) [296]. The synthesis commenced with the known pyrrole **370**, which was converted into the annellated pyrrole **371** in 62% yield over four steps. After the addition of a stannylmethylurea in the presence of Liebeskind's CuTC reagent and treatment with methanolic HCl, (+)-*O*-Me-pre-agelastatin A (**372**) was obtained. Subsequent heating in aqueous methanesulfonic acid then furnished the natural product agelastatin A (**375**) in 49% yield as well as a side product (**374**). Bromination or OH-methylation of agelastatin A (**375**) gave agelastatin B (**376**) or E (**368**), respectively. Moreover, (−)-*O*-Me-di-*epi*-agelastatin A (**374**) could be further converted to agelastatin C (**377**) by an elimination/epoxidation/aqueous epimerization sequence. By reacting the former intermediate **371** with a stannylurea, agelastatins D and F (**369**) could be synthesized in a similar way (Scheme 22) [296].

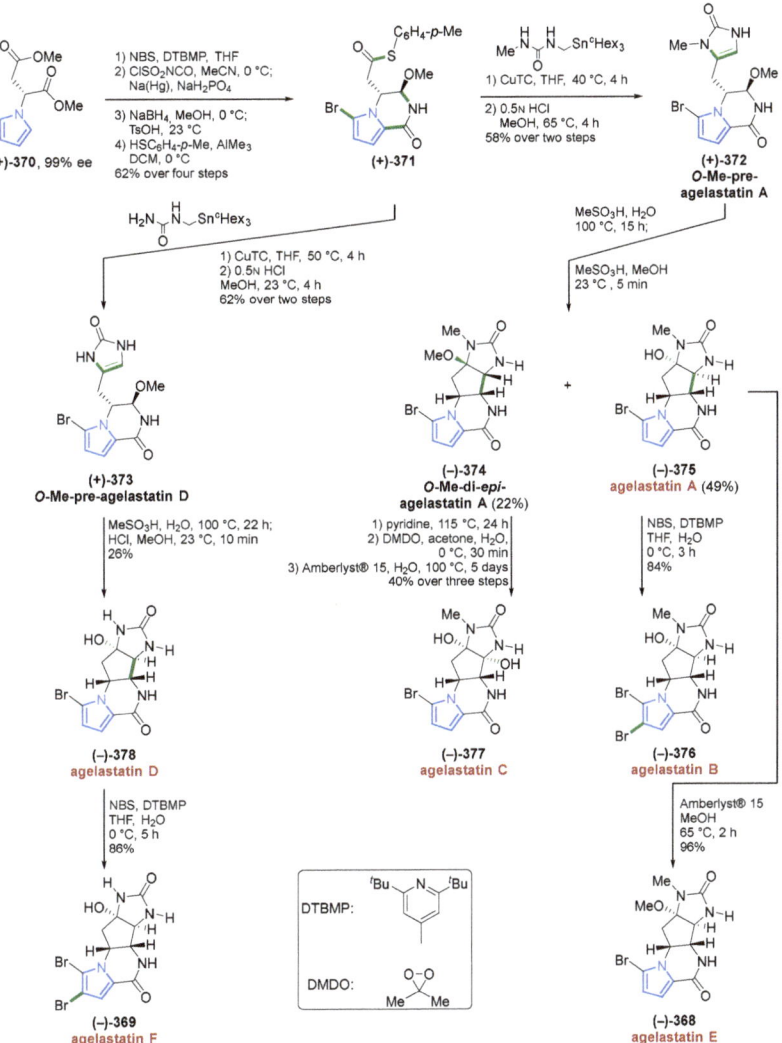

Scheme 22. Enantioselective synthesis of all known (−)-agelastatins, including the first total synthesis of agelastatins C–F (**377**, **378**, **368**, **369**).

In 2020, a new member of the agesamine family, agesamine C (**379**), could be isolated from the sea sponge *Agelas oroides* collected off the Tel Aviv coast (Figure 54). The relative and absolute configuration of the bicyclic moiety in **379** was deduced by comparison of its *J*-values with those of agesamines A (**366**) and B (**367**) [237].

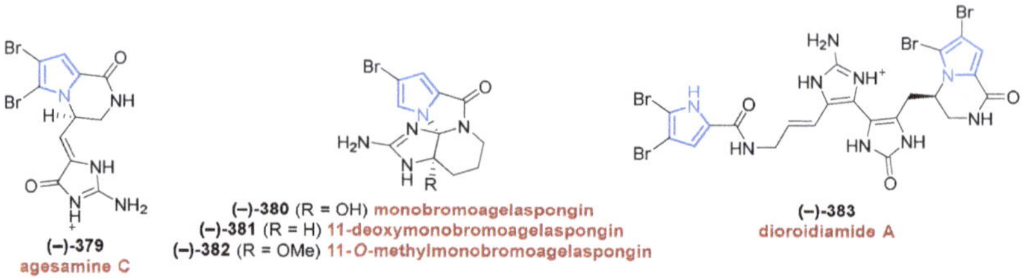

Figure 54. Structurally diverse bromopyrrole alkaloids **379–383** isolated from *Agelas oroides*.

Monobromoagelaspongin (**380**) was first isolated from the sponge *Agelas oroides* as a racemic mixture in 2017 and no information was given on the relative configuration or its biological activities [297]. However, in 2020, the relative and absolute configuration could be determined alongside the isolation of further bromopyrroles (Figure 54) [237].

The same sponge also delivered the agelaspongin analogs **381** and **382**, the relative and absolute configurations of which were either determined by NOESY data combined with ECD spectroscopy or by comparison of its chiroptical properties with those of model compounds (Figure 54) [237]. The sponge also was the source of a new compound, named dioroidamide A (**383**). Compound **383** presents a negative specific rotation value which is also the case for many other structurally related marine alkaloids, and based on their shared biosynthesis, the authors assumed that **383** should possess the same absolute configuration as depicted in Figure 54 [237]. With the isolated natural products **379–383** itself, no biological tests were performed. However, as the antimicrobial and antibacterial activity of the sponge extract was attributed to other natural products contained, compounds **379–383** have not been found to show any promising activities so far [237].

In 2014, two structurally unique dimeric bromopyrroles, named agelamadins A (**384**) and B (**385**), were isolated from a sponge of the genus *Agelas* by the Kobayashi group [298]. Both compounds **384** and **385** were isolated as racemic mixtures, with their relative configurations determined by ROESY correlations (Figure 55). Agelamadins A (**384**) and B (**385**) showed antimicrobial activity against several Gram-positive species with IC$_{50}$ values ranging between 4 µM and 16 µM. However, no cytotoxicity was observed against human murine lymphoma L1210 cells and human epidermoid carcinoma cells in vitro [298].

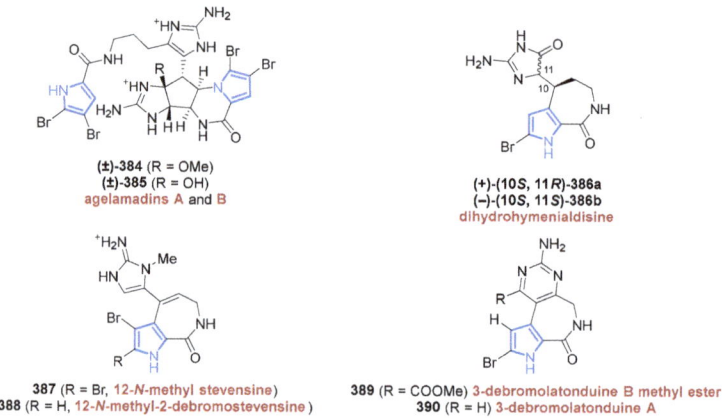

Figure 55. Annellated bromopyrroles **384–390** from different marine sponges.

Two new bromopyrroles **368a** and **368b**, annellated by a seven-membered ring and structurally related to hymenialdisine, were isolated from the marine sponge *Cymbastela cantharella* in 2011 (Figure 55) [132]. The absolute structure of (+)-dihydrohymenialdisine (**368a**) was unequivocally determined by X-ray crystallography, whereas the absolute configuration of (−)-dihydrohymenialdisine (**368b**) could not be deduced. Since the corresponding lead structure, hymenialdisine, is active against the kinase PLK-1, both substances **368a** and **368b** were also tested for PLK-1 inhibition but did not show any activity. Apparently, the conjugation of hymenialdisine through the C-10/C-11 double bond (which is saturated in **368a** and **368b**) is indispensable for its strong activity on a wide range of cyclin-dependent kinases [132].

The structurally similar compounds **387–390** were isolated from a marine sponge of the genus *Stylissa* in 2012 (Figure 55) [299]. While 12-*N*-methylstevensine (**387**) displayed strong cytotoxic activity against L5178Y mouse lymphoma cells with an EC$_{50}$ value of 3.5 µg/mL, 12-*N*-methyl-2-debromostevensine (**388**), 3-debromolatonduine B methyl ester (**389**), and 3-debromolatonduine A (**390**) only exhibited weak activity (no values given). These data suggest that the presence or absence of bromine atoms significantly influences the antiproliferative activity [299].

At this stage, it should also be mentioned the recently published total synthesis of the related pyrroloazepinone-containing alkaloid 2-debromohymenin (**396**) (Scheme 23) [300]. First, the commercially available 4-iodoimidazole **305** was transformed into alkyne **391** by a Sonogashira reaction. Subsequent deprotection and reaction with pyrrolecarbonyl chloride **392** furnished compound **393**. An intramolecular gold-catalyzed alkyne hydroarylation then resulted in the formation of the core pyrroloazepinone moiety in **394**. Subsequent hydrogenation followed by the installation of an azide group generated azido derivative **395**. Bromination using NBS, removal of the sulfonyl urea, and final conversion of the azide to an amine group as well as removing the N-OMe group at the same time using Mo(CO)$_6$, furnished 2-debromohymenin (**396**) [300].

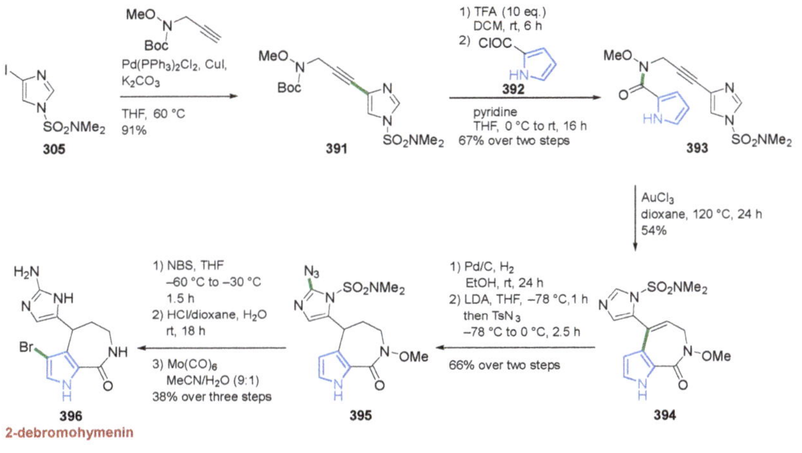

Scheme 23. Total synthesis of 2-debromohymenin (**396**) via a key gold-catalyzed alkyne hydroarylation.

3.3. Sceptrins

The members of the exceptional family of the sceptrin alkaloids are characterized by their cyclobutane ring which is constructed by the dimerization of oroidin and its derivatives [301]. They are known to exhibit a broad range of biological activities, such as anticancer, antifungal, antibacterial, and anti-inflammatory [226,302–304]. Sceptrin was isolated and fully elucidated in 1981 by Faulkner and co-workers who also established its absolute configuration [224]. Many sceptrin derivatives have been isolated since.

In 2017, agelestes A (**397**) and B (**398**) were isolated from a South China sponge of the genus *Agelas* (Figure 56) [305]. Although nakamuric acid (**400**) was already isolated in 1999 [306], the authors revealed its absolute configuration for the first time (Figure 56) [306]. The same sponge *Agelas* sp. also led to the isolation of hexazosceptrin (**401**), bearing a rare cyclohexane-fused-cyclobutane skeleton. All relative and absolute configurations were determined by extensive spectroscopic analyses and ECD. All four compounds **397**, **398**, **400**, and **401** displayed moderate antimicrobial activity (MIC values ranging between 16 µg/mL and 32 µg/mL) [305].

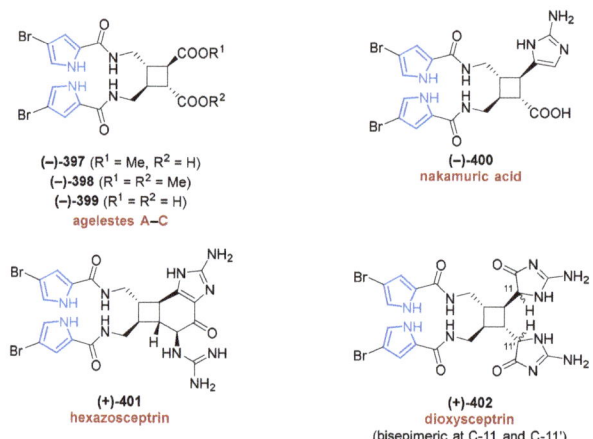

Figure 56. Several different substituted bromopyrroles **397**–**402** belonging to the sceptrin-family.

One year later, two sceptrin derivatives, ageleste C (**399**) and dioxysceptrin (**402**) were isolated from the marine sponge *Agelas Kosrae* (Figure 56) [307]. The relative and absolute configurations of compounds **399** and **402** were determined by ROESY correlations and by ECD spectroscopy. However, due to the absence of reliable ROESY correlations, the configuration at C-11 and C-11′ could not be determined. Ageleste C (**399**) and the bisepimeric dioxysceptrin (**402**) showed good to moderate anti-proliferative activity against six cancer cell lines (IC$_{50}$ values ranging between 7.92 µM and > 50 µM), however, only compound **399** displayed moderate inhibition of *Candida albicans*-derived isocitrate lyase (IC$_{50}$ value 22.09 µM), a key enzyme in microbial metabolism [307].

In 2010, the New Caledonian sponge *Agelas dendromorpha* led to the isolation of benzosceptrin C (**403**) featuring a rare benzocyclobutane moiety (Figure 57). Unfortunately, no cytotoxicity against the KB cell line was observed [295].

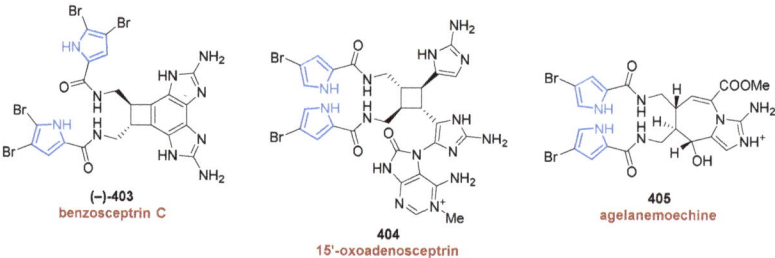

Figure 57. Further sceptrins **403** and **404** together with the congener agelanemoechine (**405**).

In 2016, the Köck group investigated the tropical sponge *Agelas sceptrum* which led to the isolation of 15′-oxoadenosceptrin (**404**), a hybrid PIA incorporating an adenine moiety. Unfortunately, no cytotoxic or antimicrobial activity was observed for compound **404** (Figure 57) [274].

In 2019, a unique alkaloid **405** bearing an imidazo [1,5-*a*] azepine nucleus was isolated from the marine sponge *Agelas nemoechinata*, with its relative and absolute configuration being determined by NOESY correlations and ECD spectroscopy, respectively. Agelanemoechine (**405**) showed potent pro-angiogenic activity in zebrafish (effect equivalent to the established Danhong injection as a positive control, Figure 57) [308].

At this point, the very recently published total synthesis of the dimeric PIA sceptrin (**411**) should be mentioned, which enables direct entry to this class of biologically active metabolites (Scheme 24) [309]. Astonishingly, sceptrin (**411**) was synthesized in only four steps by applying a photochemical intermolecular [2+2] dimerization of compound **408**. The authors synthesized building block **408** by initial hydroboration of protected propargylamine **406** to give pinacol ester **407** which then underwent a Suzuki–Miyaura cross-coupling with 3-bromoimidazopyrimidine. The key dimerization was carried out with blue LEDs in the presence of an iridium catalyst and provided the *all-trans* dimer **409** in 41% yield. Completion of the synthesis included acid-promoted deprotection, installation of the bromopyrrole unit **410**, and hydrazine-based conversion of the guanidine unit to an imidazole moiety in one pot [309].

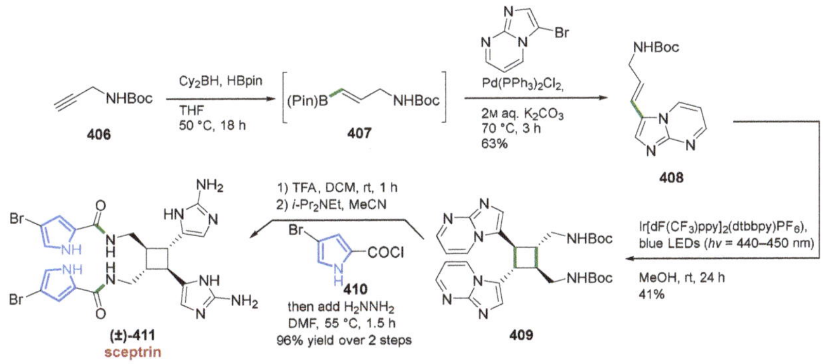

Scheme 24. A four-step synthesis of sceptrin (**411**), including a photochemical intermolecular [2 + 2] dimerization as the key step.

Although there have been successful approaches towards sceptrin (**411**) since 2004, this new approach gives synthetic access to the sceptrin family in a minimum number of steps compared to the 11–25 steps required before [310–312]. It should also be mentioned that the synthetic work of the Chen laboratory in 2014 led to the revision of the absolute stereochemistry of many sceptrin-based natural products and of sceptrin (**411**) itself [312]. For more than 30 years, many groups have based their stereochemical results on the comparison with the incorrectly determined absolute configuration of sceptrin (**411**) from a publication of 1981 [224]. Hence, careful reading and checking are strongly recommended to avoid confusion.

4. Miscellaneous

Among the known marine pyrroles, there are also complex architectural frameworks containing macrocyclic ring systems, not only one or more sugar residues, but also multiple amide bonds forming peptides or even cyclopeptides. Therefore, in the following section, structures and classes are presented that could not be classified in the previous chapters due to their mostly complex and intriguing scaffolds.

In 2019, a scalarane sesterterpenoid featuring a 6/6/6/6/5-pentacyclic core was isolated from the sponge *Scalarispongia* sp. The fused pyrrole **412** represents the first pyrrole derivative in the rare class of N-heterocyclic scalaranes (Figure 35). MNP **412** was found to show moderate inhibition against six human cancer cell lines in bioactivity assays (GI_{50} values ranging between 14.9 µM and 26.2 µM) [313].

The bispyrrole curvulamine (**413**) originates from the fungus *Curvularia* sp. IFB-Z10, produced in a symbiontic way with the host, the White Croaker (*Argyrosomus argentatus*)

(Figure 58) [314]. In the course of structure elucidation and determining the crystal structure of the unprecedented framework of curvulamine A, the authors also made efforts to elucidate the biosynthetic pathway using NMR-based ^{13}C labeling experiments. Curvulamine (**413**) possesses antibacterial activity in the sub-micromolar range [314], whereas the biogenetic related trispyrrole curindolizine (**414**) lacks these bioactivities. However, anti-inflammatory activities in lipopolyssacharide (LPS)-stimulated RAW 264.7 macrophages (IC$_{50}$ = 5.31 µM ± 0.21 µM) could be observed. Surprisingly, as a by-product of reisolating curvulamine (**413**), curindolizine (**414**) was discovered in 2016, two years after the initial isolation of curvulamine (**413**) from the same fungus (Figure 58). On this basis, it is also assumed that curindolizine (**414**) represents the product of an in vivo Michael addition of the metabolites curvulamine (**413**) and the elimination product derived from procuramine (**125**) (cf. Figure 16 [125]).

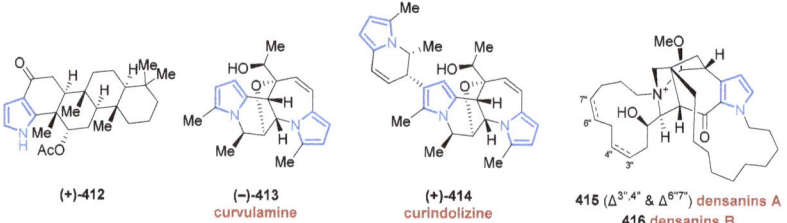

Figure 58. Polycyclic, complex molecular frameworks of condensed pyrrole MNPs **412**–**416**.

Another complex polycyclic scaffold is displayed by the densanins A (**415**) and B (**416**) (Figure 58) [315]. After extensive NMR studies, including the application of the Mosher ester method, the 3D structure featuring seven stereogenic centers and a 1-azabicyclo[3.2.1] octane core was determined to be biosynthetically derived from 3-alkylpyridines. The hexacyclic diamines **415** and **416**, isolated from the sponge *Haliclona densaspicula* in 2012, showed no cytotoxicity but promising inhibition of the NO production in LPS-induced BV2 microglial cells (IC$_{50}$ values of 1.05 µM and 2.14 µM, respectively) [315].

Their promising bioactivity and challenging structures have inspired organic chemists ever since to develop a successful total synthesis of these MNPs [316–318]. The group of Maimone published the first successful synthesis of (−)-curvulamine (**413a**) in 2012, which was only feasible after extensive reconnaissance and several failures (Scheme 25) [319,320]. Starting from commercially available chemicals, they employed a feasible 10 step sequence to (−)-curvulamine (**413a**). The first key step was the coupling of racemic cyanohydrin **417**, as a masked acyl anion, with pyrroloazepinone **418**. This regioselective process was mediated by NaHMDS, followed by quenching the resulting enolate with NIS. After extensive investigation, the iodide was found to undergo cyclization under simple irradiation conditions in MeOH.

In this way, compound **419** was prepared in a 30% yield over two steps. After addition of lithiated ethyl vinyl ether, subsequent epimerization to the favored diastereomer **421**, and activation of the secondary alcohol with ClCSOPh, the thiocarbonate epimers (1R/1S)-**422** could be separated. The desired isomer **422** was reduced by deoxygenation and hydrolysis of the enol ether. The final step involves a diastereoselective reduction of the racemic ketone under CBS reduction conditions, yielding a 1:1 epimeric mixture of alcohols **413a** and **413b** that was readily separated into the enantiopure MNPs (Scheme 25) [319].

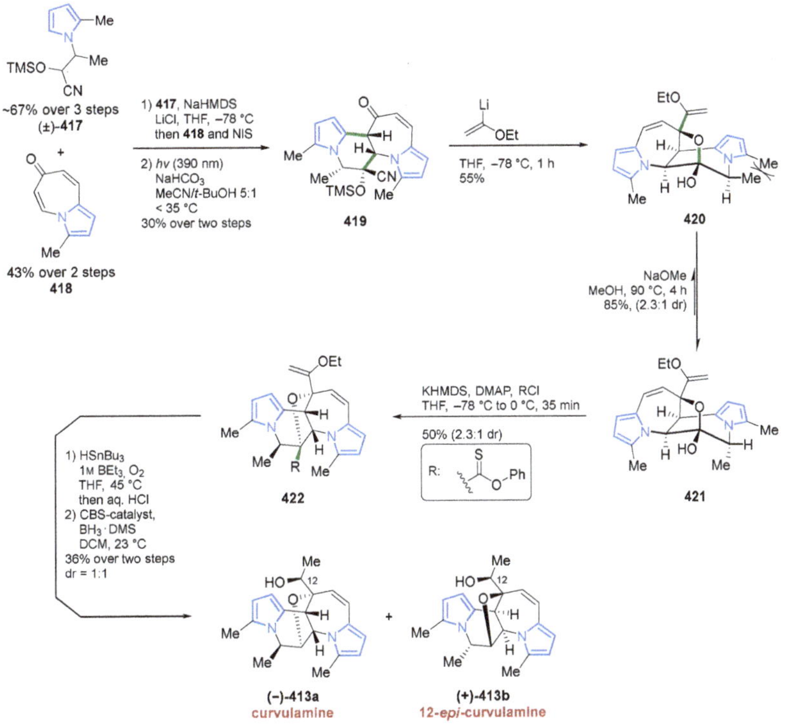

Scheme 25. A linear ten-step sequence yielding the natural bispyrrole (−)-curvulamine **413a**.

Syntheses such as the one shown by Maimone et al. play a significant in the development of potential active pharmaceutical ingredients as marine organisms often cannot be easily cultivated for mass production [319]. Further synthetic attempts, e.g., to prepare densanins, were undertaken by Yang and co-workers in 2016, whereas only the BCD tricyclic core could be achieved [321].

4.1. Pyrroloiminoquinone and Related Analogs

The pyrroloiminoquinones feature a central core in a broad variety of MNPs, divided into subclasses of iso-/batzellins, damirons, discorhabdins, epinardins, makaluvamines, prianosins, tsitsikammamins, wakayins, and veiutamines [322–324]. Among them, a new subclass of the heteroatom-rich macrophilones was established in 2017. Macrophilone A (**423**), isolated from the *Macrorhynchia philippina*, represents a rare example of the underexplored group of hydroids (Figure 59) [325]. Macrophilone A (**423**), together with a synthetic derivative prepared in the same study, was able to block the conjugation cascade of small ubiquitin-like modifier (SUMO). The SUMO conjugation to protein substrates occurs through an enzymatic cascade and is critical for the regulation of various cellular processes. It is often disrupted in diseases, including cancer, resulting in the disturbance of the protein balance [325].

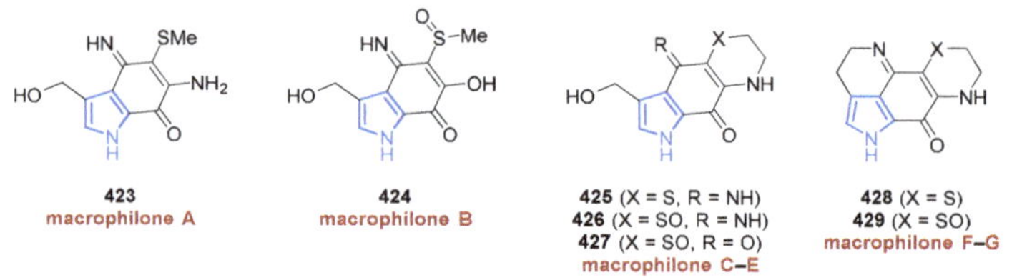

Figure 59. Members of the macrophilones group **423–429**.

Once more, the group of Gustafson and co-workers published the isolation of six further macrophilones B–G (**424–429**) from the same source one year later (Figure 59) [326]. Just as its related congener macrophilone A (**423**), compounds **424–429** showed moderate to weak inhibition effects of SUMO conjugation cascade (IC$_{50}$ values ranging between 11.9 μM and >100 μM). Furthermore, they exhibited significant toxicity against several cancer cell lines (no values given) [326].

To investigate their bioactivity potential, the first isolation of macrophilone A (**423**) was accompanied by its synthesis [325]. The authors started their ingeniously short approach from commercial formylindole **430**, which was nitrated and the aldehyde functionality reduced subsequently to furnish compound **431**. Oxidation by Fremy's salt yielded the iminoquinone, which, after the introduction of the thioether group by sodium methanethiolate, furnished the natural product **423** in just 4% yield over three steps (Scheme 26) [325].

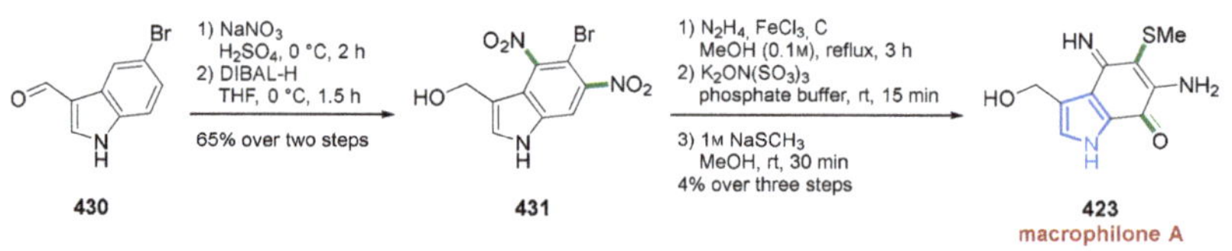

Scheme 26. Synthesis of macrophilone A (**423**) in a linear sequence of 5 total steps.

In 2019, makaluvamine Q (**432**) was discovered, marking the first time a makaluvamine derivative was isolated from a marine *Tsitsikamma* sponge within the Latrunculiidae family (Figure 60). Besides the shown DNA intercalation and topoisomerase I inhibition (27% inhibition of DNA nicking), makaluvamine Q (**432**) was found to be most active against HeLa cells in cell viability assays (14.7% ± 0.5% metabolic activity at 10 μM). In addition, the authors showed possible biosynthetic relationships between the isolated subclasses [327].

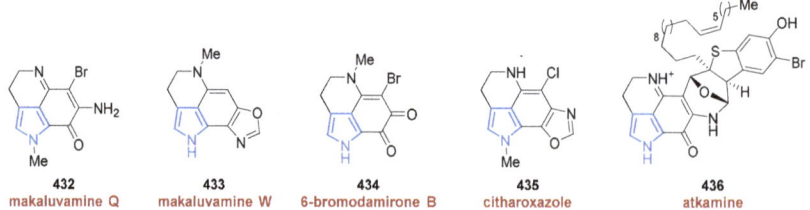

Figure 60. Pyrroloiminoquinones and related derivatives **432–436** isolated from natural sources, which share a similar biosynthetic pathway.

Only a few months later, the Keyzers lab isolated makaluvamine W (**433**) and 6-bromodamirone B (**434**) from the sponge *Strongylodesma tongaensis* (Figure 60). Both isolated pyrrole derivatives **433** and **434** lacked cytotoxic activity against the leukemia cell line HL-60, highlighting the importance of an iminoquinone scaffold in bioactivity considerations [328].

The benzoxazole moiety in makaluvamine W (**433**) is also found in citharoxazole (**435**), isolated from the sponge *Latrunculia (Biannulata) citharistae* in 2011 (Figure 60). The latter compound represented the first oxazole derivative in this family at that time [329].

In 2013, the Hamann laboratory isolated a complex heptacyclic pyrroloiminoquinone **436** containing seven stereogenic centers together with five different heterocycles (Figure 60). The TFA salt of atkamine (**436**) was isolated from the sponge *Latrunculia* sp. The structure elucidation of this complex framework was guided by spectroscopic methods, including ECD spectroscopy to analyze the absolute configuration. Furthermore, preparative olefin metathesis was used to localize the (*E*)-configured double bond [330].

Due to their promising bioactivity, a large number of synthetic studies have been conducted on these pyrrole alkaloids (e.g., makaluvamines [331,332], damirones [333,334], batzellines [335,336]). The first synthesis of makaluvone was completed by the Tokuyama group in 2012 [337]. Starting with 4-methoxy-2-nitroaniline and using a procedure reported by the Buchwald group [338], the 4-iodoindoline **437** was prepared in a 22% yield over nine steps. Subsequent construction of the quinoline scaffold using a benzyne intermediate generated by LiTMP and trapping of the carbanion by a bromine donor resulted in the formation of tricyclic system **438**. DDQ-oxidation to form the indole, removal of the N-protecting groups, and oxidation of the aromatic core yielded the iminoquinone **439**. The last two steps included the methylation of the pyrrole nitrogen, methyl ether cleavage, and isomerization to makaluvone **442** (Scheme 27) [337].

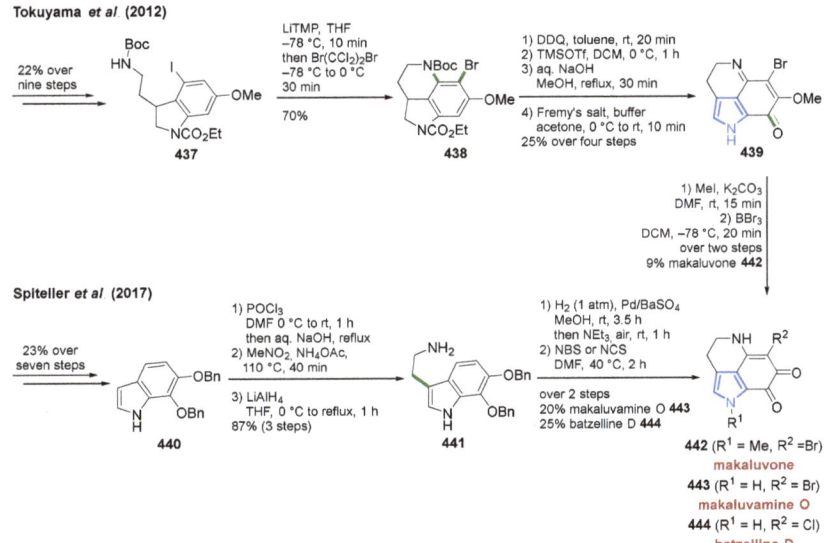

Scheme 27. Two different routes which target pyrroloquinolines **442**, **443**, and **444**. The first route favors the formation of the quinoline followed by pyrrole aromatization, while the second one uses a biomimetic approach with a late-stage quinoline ring closure.

A shorter and more efficient synthetic sequence to several aminoquinolines was reported five years later by the Spiteller group (Scheme 27) [339]. Using vanillin as starting material, the indole **440** was prepared in 23% yield over seven steps. Vilsmeier formylation, Henry reaction, and LiAlH$_4$ reduction of the nitroolefin then furnished the tryptamine **441**. Removal of the benzylic protecting groups under hydrogenolytic conditions, oxidation of the prepared hydroquinone followed by biomimetic intramolecular Michael addition and aerobic reoxidation then gave the targeted pyrroloquinoline. The last step involved halogenation to obtain makaluvamine O (**443**) and batzelline D (**444**), respectively [339].

A new member of the tsitsikammamines, namely 16,17-dehydrotsitsikammamine A (**445**), was identified from the Antarctic sponge *Latrunculia biformis* in 2018 (Figure 61). The crude extract of bis-pyrroloiminoquinone **445** showed promising anticancer activity against seven cancer cell lines (inhibition percentage >90% each at 200 µg/mL) [340].

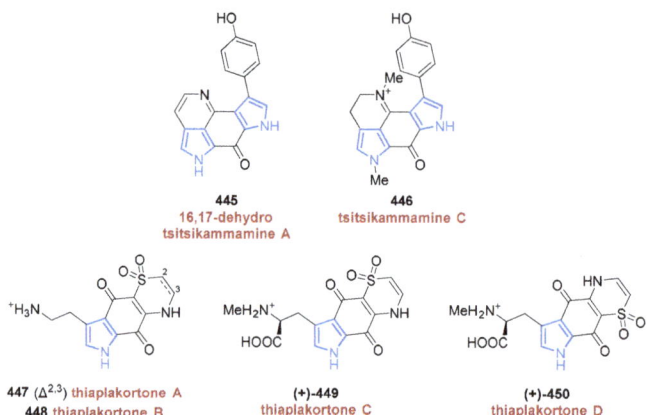

Figure 61. Pyrroloiminoquinones **445** and **446** as well as pyrroloquinones **447–450**.

The new tsitsikammamine C (**446**) was isolated as the TFA-salt from *Zyzzya* sp. in 2012 and represents the 18-methyl derivative of tsitsikammamine B (Figure 61). In biological assays, a potent growth inhibition of *Plasmodium falciparum* chloroquine-sensitive (3D7, IC$_{50}$ value of 13 nM) and chloroquine-resistant (Dd2, IC$_{50}$ value of 18 nM) cell lines was observed [341].

Thiazine-derived metabolites were discovered in the Australian marine sponge *Plakortis lita* in 2013 and given the names thiaplakortones A–D (**447–450**) (Figure 61) [342]. The structures were determined by using NMR and MS analytics as well as comparing chiroptical data to literature values to confirm the absolute configuration of the 2-methylaminopropanoic acid side chain of thiaplakortone C (**449**) and D (**450**). This substituent also suggests the biosynthesis from L-tryptophan and cysteine to yield the tricyclic framework. As the aforementioned tsitsikammamine C (**446**), all tested thiaplakortones **447–450** display significant antimalarial activity against chloroquine-sensitive (3D7, IC$_{50}$ values ranging between 51 nM and 650 nM) and chloroquine-resistant (Dd2, IC$_{50}$ values ranging between 6.6 nM and 171 nM) *Plasmodium falciparum* cell lines [342].

In 2014, the first synthesis of thiaplakortone A (**447**) was realized by the Quinn laboratory (Scheme 28) [343]. Starting from commercially available 4-hydroxyindole (**451**), indole **452** was obtained in 54% yield over five steps. Benzyl-deprotection, oxidation, and treatment with 2-aminoethanesulfinic acid, generated an intermediary dihydrothiazine, which, upon saponification and final deprotection, led to the formation of thiaplakortone A (**447**) (Scheme 28) [343].

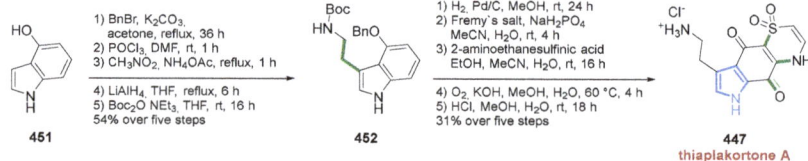

Scheme 28. Facile total synthesis of thiaplakortone A (**447**) in a nine-step approach.

Another subclass of biologically active pyrrole alkaloids is the zyzzyanones, merging the *bis*-pyrrolo functionality together with a pyrroloquinone scaffold. The known zyzzyanones A–D (**457–460**), isolated in 1996, were synthesized for the first time by Velu and co-workers in 2013 (Scheme 29) [344]. The authors developed a modular approach that provides access to all four zyzzyanones A–D (**457–460**). Starting with the known tosyl-protected indole-4,7-dione (**453**) [345], treatment with benzylamine resulted in amination. The bispyrroloquinone framework was constructed by ring-closing procedure with diethyl acetal **454** and Mn(OAc)$_3$. After methylation with MeI, the expected monomethylated amine **455** was obtained alongside the unexpected demethylated amine **456**. Both intermediates **455** and **456** were converted in a series of deprotection and/or formylation reactions to generate the zyzzyanones A–D (**457–460**) [344].

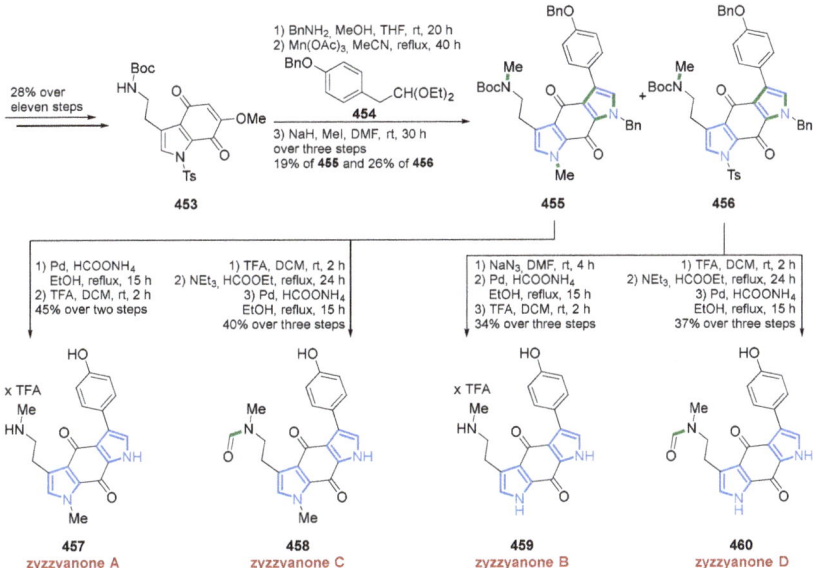

Scheme 29. A divergent modular approach providing access to known zyzzyanones A–D (**457–460**).

The discorhabdin journey started with the isolation of the first member of the class, discorhabdin C (its congeners A and B were reported later), in 1986 [346]. In the following years, a dozen more family members were isolated, biologically evaluated, and synthesized. In the decade 2010–2020, 12 further members were identified (Figures 62 and 63). The representatives of this diverse subclass featuring promising bioactivities contain a tetracyclic pyrroloiminoquinone core with a spirocyclic cyclohexadienone moiety. The discorhabdins are thought to be biosynthetically derived from makaluvamines, formed by the coupling of tyramine derivatives with the biosynthetic key precursor of simple pyrroloiminoquinones. In addition, these intermediates also give access to many further subclasses already mentioned [323].

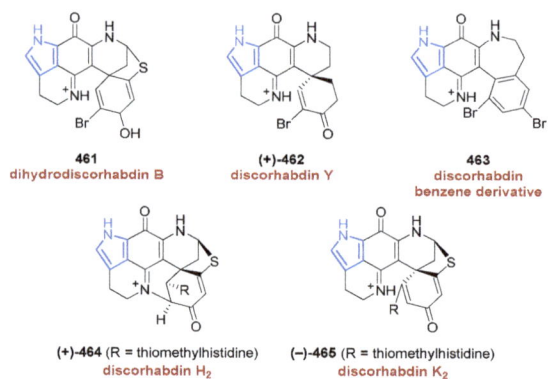

Figure 62. Discorhabdins **461**–**465** resulted from the sponge *Latrunculia* sp. collected in Alaskan and New Zealandian oceans.

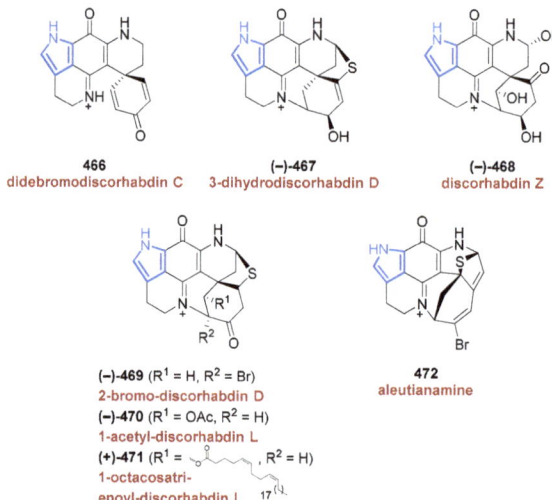

Figure 63. Further discorhabdins **466**–**471**, including a new complex pyrroloiminoquinone **472**.

An interesting and at the same time cautionary discovery was made in 2010 when discorhabdin A was isolated for the first time from *Latrunculia oparinae*. In addition to the strong dependence of the color of the solution on the solvent when ethanol (red) and methanol (green) were used, the optical rotation also changed its sign in this solvent switch [347].

Similarly, the Hamann laboratory published the isolation of two new compounds, dihydrodiscorhabdin B (**461**) and discorhabdin Y (**462**) from the Alaskan sponge *Latrunculia* sp. (Figure 62) [348]. Upon structure elucidation using CD and optical rotation, pyrrole **461** showed decomposition, therefore only the absolute stereoinformation of discorhabdin Y (**462**) could be assigned. The azepine derivative **463** was also identified in the same sponge for the first time as a natural product (Figure 62) [348]. Previously, it was only known as a semisynthetic compound, prepared by reduction of natural discorhabdin C and treatment of the resulting dienol with sulfuric acid, initiating an alkenyl (C-20) migration to form discorhabdin benzene derivative (**463**) [349].

Two new diastereomers of discorhabdin H and K, namely discorhabdin H$_2$ (**464**) and K$_2$ (**465**) were isolated from different sponge populations of *Latrunculia* sp. in 2010

(Figure 62) [350]. Combined structure elucidation was performed by NMR, MS, and extensive ECD-spectroscopy, allowing the assignment of the absolute configuration of the known discorhabdins 2-hydroxy-D, D, H, N, and Q by comparing the recorded with experimental ECD spectra. Furthermore, natural (+)-(6S,8S)-discorhabdin B was used as a starting point for semi-synthesis to establish the absolute configurations of discorhabdins S, T, and U [350].

The synthetically known didebromodiscorhabdin C (**466**) [351], along with two new discorhabdin derivatives **467** and **468** were isolated for the first time from the sponge *Sceptrella* sp. (Figure 63) [352]. Following previous studies, the absolute configuration was solved by a combination of optical rotation and ECD spectroscopy. In bioactivity studies, average to striking effects were observed against Gram-positive and Gram-negative bacteria (MIC values ranging between 25 µg/mL and >100 µg/mL), as well as against the K562 leukemia cell line and sortase A (IC_{50} values ranging between 2.1 µM and 127.4 µM), with the hemiaminal **468** remarkably showing a more than tenfold higher inhibition than *p*-(hydroxymercury)benzoic acid sodium salt as a positive control [352].

Promising anticancer activity against six cell lines was observed by bioactivity-guided isolation (IC_{50} values of crude extract ranging between 4.0 and 56.2 µg/mL) of three new discorhabdins **469**–**471** from *Latrunculia biformis* (Figure 63) [353]. Discorhabdins **470** and **471** are the first derivatives bearing an ester moiety, containing a simple acetyl group or a C_{28}-fatty acid. In the publication, the binding affinity of discorhabdins to anticancer targets (topoisomerase I–II, indoleamine 2,3-dioxygenase) was also determined [353].

Aleutianamine (**472**), the first member of a new class of pyrroloiminoquinone alkaloids, is characterized by a highly fused and multiply bridged heptacyclic ring system and was isolated from the North Pacific sponge *Latrunculia austini* Samaai (Figure 63) [354]. The elucidation of the structure required the combination of preparative spectroscopic methods and advanced computational approaches. It has been supposed that this complex molecular framework is derived from two proteinogenic amino acids, tryptophan, and tyrosine. The authors mentioned that makaluvamine F or discorhabdin A might be the precursors of aleutianamine (**472**), which exhibits promising activity against pancreatic cancer cell lines (IC_{50} values between 25 nM and 1 µM) [354].

4.2. Glycosylated Pyrroles

In 2016, the known synthetic product jaspamycin (**473**) [355], which is used as a tool compound for the investigation of Parkinson's disease, was isolated from a marine sponge *Jaspis splendens* and was therefore reported for the first time as a naturally occurring metabolite (Figure 64) [356]. The full stereochemistry of the attached sugar was identical to that of the synthetic product.

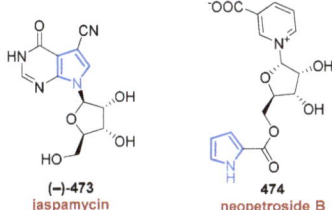

Figure 64. Sugar-substituted marine pyrrole alkaloids **473**–**474**.

Another marine pyrrole alkaloid, neopetroside B (**474**), contains a rare *N*-glycosylpyridinium moiety and was isolated from a *Neopetrosia* sp. sponge in 2015 (Figure 64) [357]. The absolute configuration of compound **474** was determined by comparison with a similar congener from the same work, the sugar unit of which was cleaved off, followed by the synthesis of acetylated (+)-2-octyl glycosides. Comparison of these compounds with authentic samples according to the procedure of Leontein then revealed the D-configuration of the sugar unit [357,358].

In 2016, two new pyrrole oligoglycosides, plancipyrrosides A (**475**) and B (**476**) were isolated from the Vietnamese starfish *Acanthaster planci* (Figure 65) [359]. The absolute configuration was determined by comparison with the previously confirmed absolute configurations of the hydrolyzed sugar moieties. Plancipyrroside B (**476**) exhibits a stronger inhibitory effect on lipopolysaccharide-induced nitric oxide production in RAW 264.7 cells (5.94 µM ± 0.34 µM) than plancipyrroside A (16.61 µM ± 1.85 µM) [359].

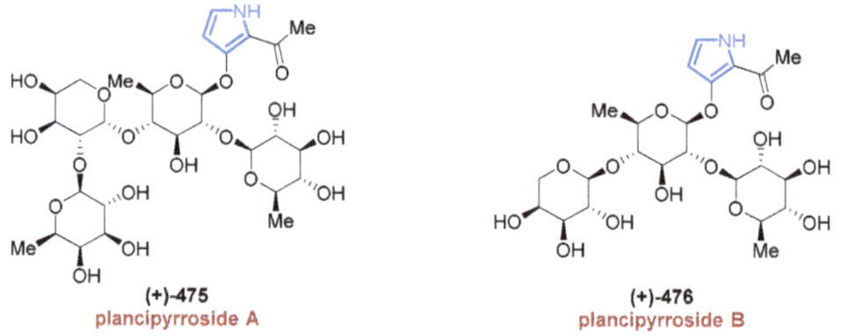

Figure 65. Oligosaccharide-substituted pyrroles **475** and **476** from a marine starfish *Acanthaster planci*.

The sugar-containing pyrrole alkaloids, phallusialides A–E (**477–481**) were discovered in a marine bacterium of the genus *Micromonospora* in 2019 (Figure 66) [360]. The relative and absolute configurations of compounds **477–481** were determined by ROESY correlations and ECD spectroscopy. While phallusialide A (**477**) and B (**478**) displayed moderate to weak antibacterial activity (MIC values between 32 µg/mL and 64 µg/mL), phallusialides C–E (**479–481**) failed to show any detectable activity in the same assay (MIC values > 256 µg/mL). The authors speculated that the lack of halogenation at the pyrrole core of compound **479** and the additional sugar moieties in compounds **480** and **481** were responsible for the inactivity [360].

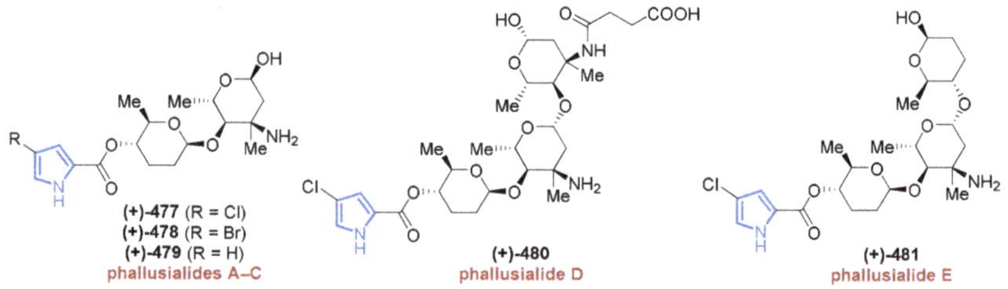

Figure 66. A new group of phallusialides A–D (**477–481**) discovered from a marine bacterium.

4.3. Peptides

Recently, two new unique bromopyrrole peptides, seribunamide A (**482**) and haloirciniamide A (**483**), have been extracted from an Indonesian marine sponge of the genus *Ircinia* (Figure 67) [361]. Their relative and absolute stereochemistries were determined by ROESY correlations and on the basis of derivatization [362] with Marfey's reagent, 1-fluoro-2,4-dinitrophenyl-5-L-alanine amide. Compounds **482** and **483** did not show any cytotoxicity against several human tumor cell lines [361].

(−)-482
seribunamide A

(−)-483
haloirciniamide A

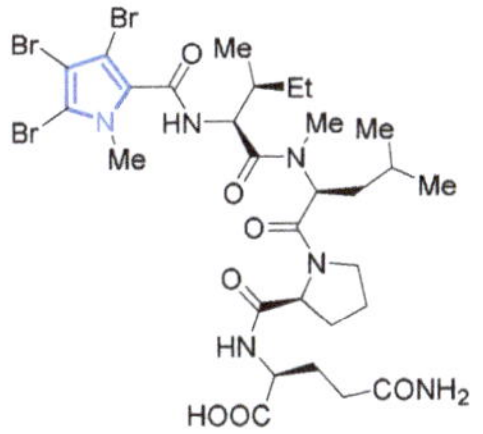

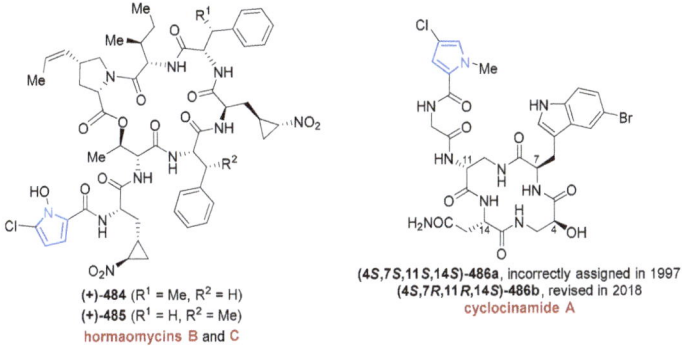

Figure 67. Bromopyrrole peptides **482**–**483** isolated from marine sponges.

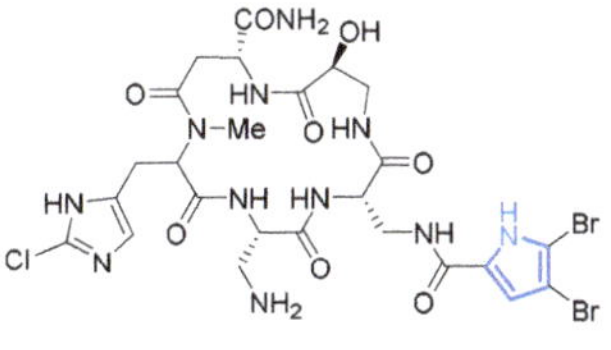

In 2015, the structurally unique cyclopeptides hormaomycins B (**484**) and C (**485**) were discovered from a mudflat-derived *Streptomyces* sp. [363] (Figure 68). Both compounds **484** and **485** possess very rare 3-(2-nitrocyclopropyl)alanine units and their absolute configurations were determined by comparing their CD spectra with that of a related hormaomycin. Hormaomycins B (**484**) and C (**485**) showed significant inhibitory effects against various Gram-positive bacteria (MIC values ranging between 0.23 μM and 56 μM), whereas, for Gram-negative bacteria, MIC values between 0.9 μM and 115 μM were determined [363].

(+)-484 (R^1 = Me, R^2 = H)
(+)-485 (R^1 = H, R^2 = Me)
hormaomycins B and C

(4*S*,7*S*,11*S*,14*S*)-486a, incorrectly assigned in 1997
(4*S*,7*R*,11*R*,14*S*)-486b, revised in 2018
cyclocinamide A

Figure 68. Macrocyclic peptides **484**–**486** containing a pyrrole motif on their N-termini.

At this point, the cyclopeptidic and highly antitumor active pyrrole alkaloid cyclocinamide A (**486b**) should also be mentioned, which was isolated from a sponge of the genus *Psammocinia* by Crews and co-workers back in 1997 [364]. Roughly twenty years later, a total synthesis of **486b** by the Konopelsky group led to the revision of its absolute stereoconfiguration from **486a** to **486b** (Figure 68) [365].

5. Conclusions

Pyrrole alkaloids, a very rich family of secondary metabolites widespread among marine organisms, have fascinated the chemical community for many decades. Their large structural variety not only endows them with unique biological activities but also prompts questions concerning the biochemistry of marine life which still require a thorough examination. On the other hand, the seemingly endless number of architectural complex pyrrole alkaloids discovered so far has also led to a considerable number of structural revisions, and the literature is riddled with unknown stereochemistries and inconsistencies in their naming. Synthetic chemists are animated to find new solutions concerning the total syntheses of marine pyrrole alkaloids, thereby providing a larger availability of these compounds which is crucial for the development of derivatives with improved biological activities. New and improved analytical techniques are needed to allow the unambiguous elucidation of relative and absolute configurations of the often-minute quantities of marine natural products available from their producers.

Author Contributions: Conceptualization, T.O., K.S. and L.G.; writing—original draft preparation, K.S. and L.G.; writing—review and editing, T.O., K.S. and L.G.; visualization, K.S. and L.G.; supervision, T.O. All authors have read and agreed to the published version of the manuscript.

Funding: This research received no external funding.

Conflicts of Interest: The authors declare no conflict of interest.

References

1. Tasdemir, D. Naturstoffe aus dem Meer für Medizin und Landwirtschaft. In *Biodiversität im Meer und an Land. Vom Wert Biologischer Vielfalt*; Deutsches GeoForschungsZentrum GFZ: Potsdam, Germany, 2020; pp. 47–49.
2. Jiménez, C. Marine Natural Products in Medicinal Chemistry. *ACS Med. Chem. Lett.* **2018**, *9*, 959–961. [CrossRef]
3. Blessie, E.J.; Wruck, W.; Abbey, B.A.; Ncube, A.; Graffmann, N.; Amarh, V.; Arthur, P.A.; Adjaye, J. Transcriptomic Analysis of Marine Endophytic Fungi Extract Identifies Highly Enriched Anti-Fungal Fractions Targeting Cancer Pathways in HepG2 Cell Lines. *BMC Genom.* **2020**, *21*, 265. [CrossRef]
4. Delgado-Roche, L.; González, K.; Mesta, F.; Couder, B.; Tavarez, Z.; Zavala, R.; Hernandez, I.; Garrido, G.; Rodeiro, I.; Vanden Berghe, W. Polyphenolic Fraction Obtained from *Thalassia testudinum* Marine Plant and Thalassiolin B Exert Cytotoxic Effects in Colorectal Cancer Cells and Arrest Tumor Progression in a Xenograft Mouse Model. *Front. Pharmacol.* **2020**, *11*, 592985. [CrossRef]
5. Barreca, M.; Stathis, A.; Barraja, P.; Bertoni, F. An Overview on Anti-Tubulin Agents for the Treatment of Lymphoma Patients. *Pharmacol. Ther.* **2020**, *211*, 107552. [CrossRef] [PubMed]
6. Dario, M.; Karlo, W.; Nela, M.; Sylvain, L.; Maris, T.; Maria Kolympadi, M.; Gabriela, A.; Dean, M. Marine Natural Products with High Anticancer Activities. *Curr. Med. Chem.* **2020**, *27*, 1243–1307.
7. Lu, W.-Y.; Li, H.-J.; Li, Q.-Y.; Wu, Y.-C. Application of Marine Natural Products in Drug Research. *Bioorg. Med. Chem.* **2021**, *35*, 116058. [CrossRef] [PubMed]
8. Vizetto-Duarte, C.; Castelo-Branco, P.; Custódio, L. Marine Natural Products as a Promising Source of Therapeutic Compounds to Target Cancer Stem Cells. *Curr. Med. Chem.* **2021**, *28*, 4343–4355. [CrossRef]
9. Sun, T.-T.; Zhu, H.-J.; Cao, F. Marine Natural Products as a Source of Drug Leads Against Respiratory Viruses: Structural and Bioactive Diversity. *Curr. Med. Chem.* **2021**, *28*, 3568–3594. [CrossRef] [PubMed]
10. Ren, X.; Xie, X.; Chen, B.; Liu, L.; Jiang, C.; Qian, Q. Marine Natural Products: A Potential Source of Anti-Hepatocellular Carcinoma Drugs. *J. Med. Chem.* **2021**, *64*, 7879–7899. [CrossRef]
11. Stonik, V.A. Marine Natural Products: A Way to New Drugs. *Acta Nat.* **2009**, *1*, 15–25. [CrossRef]
12. Barreca, M.; Spanò, V.; Montalbano, A.; Cueto, M.; Díaz Marrero, A.R.; Deniz, I.; Erdogan, A.; Lukic Bilela, L.; Moulin, C.; Taffin-de-Givenchy, E.; et al. Marine Anticancer Agents: An Overview with a Particular Focus on Their Chemical Classes. *Mar. Drugs* **2020**, *18*, 619. [CrossRef] [PubMed]
13. Lindel, T. Chapter Three – Chemistry and Biology of the Pyrrole-Imidazole Alkaloids. In *The Alkaloids: Chemistry and Biology*, 1st ed.; Elsevier: Cambridge, MA, USA; San Diego, CA, USA; London, UK; Oxford, UK, 2017; Volume 77, pp. 117–219.
14. Singh, K.S.; Majik, M.S. Pyrrole-Derived Alkaloids of Marine Sponges and their Biological Properties. In *Studies in Natural Products Chemistry*, 1st ed.; Atta-ur-Rahman, Ed.; Elsevier: Amsterdam, The Netherlands; Oxford, UK; Cambridge, MA, USA, 2019; Volume 62, pp. 377–409.
15. Gholap, S.S. Pyrrole: An Emerging Scaffold for Construction of Valuable Therapeutic agents. *Eur. J. Med. Chem.* **2016**, *110*, 13–31. [CrossRef] [PubMed]
16. Spanò, V.; Rocca, R.; Barreca, M.; Giallombardo, D.; Montalbano, A.; Carbone, A.; Raimondi, M.V.; Gaudio, E.; Bortolozzi, R.; Bai, R.; et al. Pyrrolo[2′,3′:3,4]cyclohepta[1,2-d][1,2]oxazoles, a New Class of Antimitotic Agents Active Against Multiple Malignant Cell Types. *J. Med. Chem.* **2020**, *63*, 12023–12042. [CrossRef] [PubMed]
17. Zheng, L.; Gao, T.; Ge, Z.; Ma, Z.; Xu, J.; Ding, W.; Shen, L. Design, Synthesis and Structure-Activity Relationship Studies of Glycosylated Derivatives of Marine Natural Product Lamellarin D. *Eur. J. Med. Chem.* **2021**, *214*, 113226. [CrossRef]
18. Rdwan, M.; Alrugaie, O.; Al Abdulmonem, W.; Alfaifi, M.; Elbehairi, S.E. Synthesis and Antiproliferative Activity of 2,4-Bis(indol-3-yl)pyrrole Derivatives: Marine Nortopsentin Analogs. *Egypt. J. Chem.* **2021**, *64*, 4697–4706.
19. Singh, N.; Singh, S.; Kohli, S.; Singh, A.; Asiki, H.; Rathee, G.; Chandra, R.; Anderson, E.A. Recent Progress in the Total Synthesis of Pyrrole-Containing Natural Products (2011–2020). *Org. Chem. Front.* **2021**. [CrossRef]
20. Netz, N.; Opatz, T. Marine Indole Alkaloids. *Mar. Drugs* **2015**, *13*, 4814–4914. [CrossRef] [PubMed]
21. Islam, M.T.; Mubarak, M.S. Pyrrolidine Alkaloids and their Promises in Pharmacotherapy. *Adv. Tradit. Med.* **2020**, *20*, 13–22. [CrossRef]
22. Moreira, R.; Pereira, D.M.; Valentão, P.; Andrade, P.B. Pyrrolizidine Alkaloids: Chemistry, Pharmacology, Toxicology and Food Safety. *Int. J. Mol. Sci.* **2018**, *19*, 1668. [CrossRef]
23. Huang, R.; Zhou, X.; Xu, T.; Yang, X.; Liu, Y. Diketopiperazines from Marine Organisms. *Chem. Biodivers.* **2010**, *7*, 2809–2829. [CrossRef]

24. Huang, R.-M.; Yi, X.-X.; Zhou, Y.; Su, X.; Peng, Y.; Gao, C.-H. An Update on 2,5-Diketopiperazines from Marine Organisms. *Mar. Drugs* **2014**, *12*, 6213–6235. [CrossRef]
25. Willems, T.; De Mol, M.L.; De Bruycker, A.; De Maeseneire, S.L.; Soetaert, W.K. Alkaloids from Marine Fungi: Promising Antimicrobials. *Antibiotics* **2020**, *9*, 340. [CrossRef] [PubMed]
26. Rajesh, R.; Niteshkumar, S.; Chetan, S.; Rajshekhar, K. Marine Bromopyrrole Alkaloids: Synthesis and Diverse Medicinal Applications. *Curr. Top. Med. Chem.* **2014**, *14*, 253–273.
27. Tanaka, N.; Kusama, T.; Kashiwada, Y.; Kobayashi, J.I. Bromopyrrole Alkaloids from Okinawan Marine Sponges *Agelas* spp. *Chem. Pharm. Bull.* **2016**, *64*, 691–694. [CrossRef]
28. Jin, Z. Muscarine, Imidazole, Oxazole and Thiazole Alkaloids. *Nat. Prod. Rep.* **2016**, *33*, 1268–1317. [CrossRef] [PubMed]
29. Jordan, P.M. Biosynthesis of Tetrapyrroles. In *New Comprehensive Biochemistry*; Elsevier/North-Holland Biomedical Press: Amsterdam, The Netherlands, 1991; Volume 19, pp. 1–309.
30. Walsh, C.T.; Garneau-Tsodikova, S.; Howard-Jones, A.R. Biological Formation of Pyrroles: Nature's Logic and Enzymatic Machinery. *Nat. Prod. Rep.* **2006**, *23*, 517–531. [CrossRef] [PubMed]
31. Kashman, Y.; Koren-Goldshlager, G.; Gravalos, M.D.G.; Schleyer, M. Halitulin, A New Cytotoxic Alkaloid from The Marine Sponge *Haliclona tulearensis*. *Tetrahedron Lett.* **1999**, *40*, 997–1000. [CrossRef]
32. Malla Reddy, S.; Srinivasulu, M.; Satyanarayana, N.; Kondapi, A.K.; Venkateswarlu, Y. New Potent Cytotoxic Lamellarin Alkaloids from Indian Ascidian *Didemnum obscurum*. *Tetrahedron* **2005**, *61*, 9242–9247. [CrossRef]
33. Cafieri, F.; Fattorusso, E.; Taglialatela-Scafati, O. Novel Bromopyrrole Alkaloids from the Sponge *Agelas dispar*. *J. Nat. Prod.* **1998**, *61*, 122–125. [CrossRef]
34. Marina, G.; Lucija Peterlin, M.; Danijel, K. Antibacterial and Antibiofilm Potentials of Marine Pyrrole-2-Aminoimidazole Alkaloids and their Synthetic Analogs. *Mini-Rev. Med. Chem.* **2018**, *18*, 1640–1658.
35. Tsukamoto, S.; Tane, K.; Ohta, T.; Matsunaga, S.; Fusetani, N.; van Soest, R.W.M. Four New Bioactive Pyrrole-Derived Alkaloids from the Marine Sponge *Axinella brevistyla*. *J. Nat. Prod.* **2001**, *64*, 1576–1578. [CrossRef] [PubMed]
36. Liu, R.; Liu, Y.; Zhou, Y.-D.; Nagle, D.G. Molecular-Targeted Antitumor Agents. 15. Neolamellarins from the Marine Sponge *Dendrilla nigra* Inhibit Hypoxia-Inducible Factor-1 Activation and Secreted Vascular Endothelial Growth Factor Production in Breast Tumor Cells. *J. Nat. Prod.* **2007**, *70*, 1741–1745. [CrossRef]
37. Christian, B. Lamellarins, from A to Z: A Family of Anticancer Marine Pyrrole Alkaloids. *Anti-Cancer Agents Med. Chem.* **2004**, *4*, 363–378.
38. Al-Mourabit, A.; Zancanella, M.A.; Tilvi, S.; Romo, D. Biosynthesis, Asymmetric Synthesis, and Pharmacology, Including Cellular Targets, of the Pyrrole-2-aminoimidazole Marine Alkaloids. *Nat. Prod. Rep.* **2011**, *28*, 1229–1260. [CrossRef] [PubMed]
39. Thapa, H.R.; Robbins, J.M.; Moore, B.S.; Agarwal, V. Insights into Thiotemplated Pyrrole Biosynthesis Gained from the Crystal Structure of Flavin-Dependent Oxidase in Complex with Carrier Protein. *Biochemistry* **2019**, *58*, 918–929. [CrossRef] [PubMed]
40. Bao, J.; Wang, J.; Zhang, X.-Y.; Nong, X.-H.; Qi, S.-H. New Furanone Derivatives and Alkaloids from the Co-Culture of Marine-Derived Fungi *Aspergillus sclerotiorum* and *Penicillium citrinum*. *Chem. Biodivers.* **2017**, *14*, e1600327. [CrossRef]
41. Ding, L.; Dahse, H.-M.; Hertweck, C. Cytotoxic Alkaloids from *Fusarium incarnatum* Associated with the Mangrove Tree *Aegiceras corniculatum*. *J. Nat. Prod.* **2012**, *75*, 617–621. [CrossRef]
42. Han, X.; Liu, Z.; Zhang, Z.; Zhang, X.; Zhu, T.; Gu, Q.; Li, W.; Che, Q.; Li, D. Geranylpyrrol A and Piericidin F from *Streptomyces* sp. CHQ-64 $\Delta rdmF$. *J. Nat. Prod.* **2017**, *80*, 1684–1687. [CrossRef]
43. Macherla, V.R.; Liu, J.; Bellows, C.; Teisan, S.; Nicholson, B.; Lam, K.S.; Potts, B.C.M. Glaciapyrroles A, B, and C, Pyrrolosesquiterpenes from a *Streptomyces* sp. Isolated from an Alaskan Marine Sediment. *J. Nat. Prod.* **2005**, *68*, 780–783. [CrossRef]
44. Riclea, R.; Dickschat, J.S. The Absolute Configuration of the Pyrrolosesquiterpenoid Glaciapyrrol A. *Chem. Eur. J.* **2011**, *17*, 11930–11934. [CrossRef]
45. Chen, M.; Yan, Y.; Ge, H.; Jiao, W.-H.; Zhang, Z.; Lin, H.-W. Pseudoceroximes A–E and Pseudocerolides A–E—Bromotyrosine Derivatives from a *Pseudoceratina* sp. Marine Sponge Collected in the South China Sea. *Eur. J. Org. Chem.* **2020**, *2020*, 2583–2591. [CrossRef]
46. Zhu, F.; Lin, Y. Marinamide, a Novel Alkaloid and its Methyl Ester Produced by the Application of Mixed Fermentation Technique to Two Mangrove Endophytic Fungi from the South China Sea. *Chin. Sci. Bull.* **2006**, *51*, 1426. [CrossRef]
47. Elsebai, M.F.; Rempel, V.; Schnakenburg, G.; Kehraus, S.; Müller, C.E.; König, G.M. Identification of a Potent and Selective Cannabinoid CB1 Receptor Antagonist from *Auxarthron reticulatum*. *ACS Med. Chem. Lett.* **2011**, *2*, 866–869. [CrossRef]
48. Zhu, F.; Chen, G.; Wu, J.; Pan, J. Structure Revision and Cytotoxic Activity of Marinamide and its Methyl Ester, Novel Alkaloids Produced by Co-cultures of Two Marine-derived Mangrove Endophytic Fungi. *Nat. Prod. Res.* **2013**, *27*, 1960–1964. [CrossRef] [PubMed]
49. Shao, C.-L.; Wang, C.-Y.; Gu, Y.-C.; Wei, M.-Y.; Pan, J.-H.; Deng, D.-S.; She, Z.-G.; Lin, Y.-C. Penicinoline, a New Pyrrolyl 4-Quinolinone Alkaloid with an Unprecedented Ring System from an Endophytic Fungus *Penicillium* sp. *Bioorg. Med. Chem. Lett.* **2010**, *20*, 3284–3286. [CrossRef] [PubMed]
50. Abe, M.; Imai, T.; Ishii, N.; Usui, M.; Okuda, T.; Oki, T. Quinolactacide, a New Quinolone Insecticide from *Penicillium citrinum* Thom F 1539. *Biosci. Biotechnol. Biochem.* **2005**, *69*, 1202–1205. [CrossRef] [PubMed]
51. Gao, H.; Zhang, L.; Zhu, T.; Gu, Q.; Li, D. Unusual Pyrrolyl 4-Quinolinone Alkaloids from the Marine-Derived Fungus *Penicillium* sp. ghq208. *Chem. Pharm. Bull.* **2012**, *60*, 1458–1460. [CrossRef]

52. Naveen, B.; Ommi, N.B.; Mudiraj, A.; Mallikarjuna, T.; Babu, P.P.; Nagarajan, R. Total Synthesis of Penicinoline E, Marinamide, Methyl Marinamide and their Antimalarial Activity. *ChemistrySelect* **2017**, *2*, 3256–3261. [CrossRef]
53. Liu, C.-M.; Hermann Theron, E.; Liu, M.; Bull Daniel, N.; Palleroni Norberto, J.; Prosser Barbara La, T.; Westley Ohn, W.; Miller Philip, A. X-14547A, a New Ionophorous Antibiotic Produced by *Streptomyces antibioticus* NRRL 8167. Discovery, Fermentation, Biological Properties and Taxonomy of the Producing Culture. *J. Antibiot.* **1979**, *32*, 95–99. [CrossRef] [PubMed]
54. Zhang, D.; Nair, M.; Murry, M.; Zhang, Z. Insecticidal Activity of Indanomycin. *J. Antibiot.* **1997**, *50*, 617–620. [CrossRef]
55. Larsen, S.; Boeck, L.A.; Mertz, F.; Paschal, J.; Occolowitz, J. 16-Deethylindanomycin (A83094A), a Novel Pyrrole-ether Antibiotic Produced by a Strain of *Streptomyces setonii*. Taxonomy, Fermentation, Isolation and Characterization. *J. Antibiot.* **1988**, *41*, 1170–1177. [CrossRef] [PubMed]
56. Rommel, K.R.; Li, C.; Kelly, W.L. Identification of a Tetraene-Containing Product of the Indanomycin Biosynthetic Pathway. *Org. Lett.* **2011**, *13*, 2536–2539. [CrossRef]
57. Lian, X.-Y.; Zhang, Z. Indanomycin-related Antibiotics from Marine *Streptomyces antibioticus* PTZ0016. *Nat. Prod. Res.* **2013**, *27*, 2161–2167. [CrossRef] [PubMed]
58. Costantino, V.; Fattorusso, E.; Imperatore, C.; Mangoni, A. Glycolipids from Sponges. Part 17. Clathrosides and Isoclathrosides, Unique Glycolipids from the Caribbean Sponge *Agelas clathrodes*. *J. Nat. Prod.* **2006**, *69*, 73–78. [CrossRef]
59. Costantino, V.; Fattorusso, E.; Mangoni, A.; Rosa, M.D.; Ianaro, A.; Maffia, P. Glycolipids from Sponges. IV. Immunomodulating Glycosyl Ceramides from the Marine Sponge *agelas dispar*. *Tetrahedron* **1996**, *52*, 1573–1578. [CrossRef]
60. Abdjul, D.B.; Yamazaki, H.; Kanno, S.-i.; Takahashi, O.; Kirikoshi, R.; Ukai, K.; Namikoshi, M. Structures and Biological Evaluations of Agelasines Isolated from the Okinawan Marine Sponge *Agelas nakamurai*. *J. Nat. Prod.* **2015**, *78*, 1428–1433. [CrossRef]
61. Kubota, T.; Iwai, T.; Takahashi-Nakaguchi, A.; Fromont, J.; Gonoi, T.; Kobayashi, J.i. Agelasines O–U, New Diterpene Alkaloids with a 9-N-methyladenine Unit from a Marine Sponge *Agelas* sp. *Tetrahedron* **2012**, *68*, 9738–9744. [CrossRef]
62. Appenzeller, J.; Mihci, G.; Martin, M.-T.; Gallard, J.-F.; Menou, J.-L.; Boury-Esnault, N.; Hooper, J.; Petek, S.; Chevalley, S.; Valentin, A.; et al. Agelasines J, K, and L from the Solomon Islands Marine Sponge *Agelas cf. mauritiana*. *J. Nat. Prod.* **2008**, *71*, 1451–1454. [CrossRef] [PubMed]
63. Cychon, C.; Lichte, E.; Köck, M. The Marine Sponge *Agelas citrina* as a Source of the New Pyrrole-imidazole Alkaloids Citrinamines A–D and N-methylagelongine. *Beilstein J. Org. Chem.* **2015**, *11*, 2029–2037. [CrossRef]
64. Kusama, T.; Tanaka, N.; Kashiwada, Y.; Kobayashi, J.i. Agelamadin F and Tauroacidin E, Bromopyrrole Alkaloids from an Okinawan Marine Sponge *Agelas* sp. *Tetrahedron Lett.* **2015**, *56*, 4502–4504. [CrossRef]
65. Tanaka, N.; Kusama, T.; Takahashi-Nakaguchi, A.; Gonoi, T.; Fromont, J.; Kobayashi, J.i. Nagelamides U–W, Bromopyrrole Alkaloids from a Marine Sponge *Agelas* sp. *Tetrahedron Lett.* **2013**, *54*, 3794–3796. [CrossRef]
66. Zhu, Y.; Wang, Y.; Gu, B.-B.; Yang, F.; Jiao, W.-H.; Hu, G.-H.; Yu, H.-B.; Han, B.-N.; Zhang, W.; Shen, Y.; et al. Antifungal Bromopyrrole Alkaloids from the South China Sea Sponge *Agelas* sp. *Tetrahedron* **2016**, *72*, 2964–2971. [CrossRef]
67. Chu, M.-J.; Tang, X.-L.; Qin, G.-F.; de Voogd, N.J.; Li, P.-L.; Li, G.-Q. Three New Non-brominated Pyrrole Alkaloids from the South China Sea sponge *Agelas nakamurai*. *Chin. Chem. Lett.* **2017**, *28*, 1210–1213. [CrossRef]
68. Chu, M.-J.; Tang, X.-L.; Qin, G.-F.; Sun, Y.-T.; Li, L.; de Voogd, N.J.; Li, P.-L.; Li, G.-Q. Pyrrole Derivatives and Diterpene Alkaloids from the South China Sea Sponge *Agelas nakamurai*. *Chem. Biodivers.* **2017**, *14*, e1600446. [CrossRef] [PubMed]
69. An, L.; Song, W.; Tang, X.; de Voogd, N.J.; Wang, Q.; Chu, M.; Li, P.; Li, G. Alkaloids and Polyketides from the South China Sea Sponge *Agelas* aff. *nemoechinata*. *RSC Adv.* **2017**, *7*, 14323–14329. [CrossRef]
70. Nakamura, H.; Ohizumi, Y.; Kobayashi, J.i.; Hirata, Y. Keramadine, a Novel Antagonist of Serotonergic Receptors Isolated from the Okinawan Sea Sponge *Agelas* sp. *Tetrahedron Lett.* **1984**, *25*, 2475–2478. [CrossRef]
71. Schroif-Grégoire, C.; Appenzeller, J.; Debitus, C.; Zaparucha, A.; Al-Mourabit, A. Debromokeramadine from the Marine Sponge *Agelas cf. mauritiana*: Isolation and Short Regioselective and Flexible Synthesis. *Tetrahedron* **2015**, *71*, 3609–3613. [CrossRef]
72. Jahn, T.; König, G.M.; Wright, A.D.; Wörheide, G.; Reitner, J. Manzacidin D: An Unprecedented Secondary Metabolite from the "Living Fossil" Sponge *Astrosclera willeyana*. *Tetrahedron Lett.* **1997**, *38*, 3883–3884. [CrossRef]
73. Woo, S.-Y.; Win, N.N.; Wong, C.P.; Ito, T.; Hoshino, S.; Ngwe, H.; Aye, A.A.; Han, N.M.; Zhang, H.; Hayashi, F.; et al. Two New Pyrrolo-2-aminoimidazoles from a Myanmarese Marine Sponge, *Clathria prolifera*. *J. Nat. Med.* **2018**, *72*, 803–807. [CrossRef]
74. Annoura, H.; Tatsuoka, T. Total Syntheses of Hymenialdisine and Debromohymenialdisine: Stereospecific Construction of the 2-amino-4-oxo-2-imidazolin-5(Z)-disubstituted Y Ylidene Ring System. *Tetrahedron Lett.* **1995**, *36*, 413–416. [CrossRef]
75. Cho, H.; Matsuki, S.; Mizuno, A.; Annoura, H.; Tatsuoka, T. Synthesis of Pyrroloazepines. Facile Synthesis of 2-substituted Pyrrole Derivatives by the Phosgene Method. *J. Heterocycl. Chem.* **1997**, *34*, 87–91. [CrossRef]
76. Takale, B.S.; Desai, N.V.; Siddiki, A.A.; Chaudhari, H.K.; Telvekar, V.N. Synthesis and Biological Evaluation of Pyrrole-2-carboxamide Derivatives: Oroidin Analogues. *Med. Chem. Res.* **2014**, *23*, 1387–1396. [CrossRef]
77. Xu, Y.-z.; Yakushijin, K.; Horne, D.A. Synthesis of C11N5 Marine Sponge Alkaloids: (±)-Hymenin, Stevensine, Hymenialdisine, and Debromohymenialdisine. *J. Org. Chem.* **1997**, *62*, 456–464. [CrossRef]
78. Ermolenko, L.; Zhaoyu, H.; Lejeune, C.; Vergne, C.; Ratinaud, C.; Nguyen, T.B.; Al-Mourabit, A. Concise Synthesis of Didebromohamacanthin A and Demethylaplysinopsine: Addition of Ethylenediamine and Guanidine Derivatives to the Pyrrole-Amino Acid Diketopiperazines in Oxidative Conditions. *Org. Lett.* **2014**, *16*, 872–875. [CrossRef]

79. van Rensburg, M.; Copp, B.R.; Barker, D. Synthesis and Absolute Stereochemical Reassignment of Mukanadin F: A Study of Isomerization of Bromopyrrole Alkaloids with Implications on Marine Natural Product Isolation. *Eur. J. Org. Chem.* **2018**, *2018*, 3065–3074. [CrossRef]
80. Hanssen, K.Ø.; Schuler, B.; Williams, A.J.; Demissie, T.B.; Hansen, E.; Andersen, J.H.; Svenson, J.; Blinov, K.; Repisky, M.; Mohn, F.; et al. A Combined Atomic Force Microscopy and Computational Approach for the Structural Elucidation of Breitfussin A and B: Highly Modified Halogenated Dipeptides from Thuiaria breitfussi. *Angew. Chem. Int. Ed.* **2012**, *51*, 12238–12241. [CrossRef] [PubMed]
81. Hansen, K.Ø.; Andersen, J.H.; Bayer, A.; Pandey, S.K.; Lorentzen, M.; Jørgensen, K.B.; Sydnes, M.O.; Guttormsen, Y.; Baumann, M.; Koch, U.; et al. Kinase Chemodiversity from the Arctic: The Breitfussins. *J. Med. Chem.* **2019**, *62*, 10167–10181. [CrossRef] [PubMed]
82. Ndukwe, I.E.; Lam, Y.-h.; Pandey, S.K.; Haug, B.E.; Bayer, A.; Sherer, E.C.; Blinov, K.A.; Williamson, R.T.; Isaksson, J.; Reibarkh, M.; et al. Unequivocal Structure Confirmation of a Breitfussin Analog by Anisotropic NMR Measurements. *Chem. Sci.* **2020**, *11*, 12081–12088. [CrossRef] [PubMed]
83. Pandey, S.K.; Guttormsen, Y.; Haug, B.E.; Hedberg, C.; Bayer, A. A Concise Total Synthesis of Breitfussin A and B. *Org. Lett.* **2015**, *17*, 122–125. [CrossRef] [PubMed]
84. Zhang, W.; Ma, L.; Li, S.; Liu, Z.; Chen, Y.; Zhang, H.; Zhang, G.; Zhang, Q.; Tian, X.; Yuan, C.; et al. Indimicins A–E, Bisindole Alkaloids from the Deep-Sea-Derived *Streptomyces* sp. SCSIO 03032. *J. Nat. Prod.* **2014**, *77*, 1887–1892. [CrossRef]
85. McArthur, K.A.; Mitchell, S.S.; Tsueng, G.; Rheingold, A.; White, D.J.; Grodberg, J.; Lam, K.S.; Potts, B.C.M. Lynamicins A–E, Chlorinated Bisindole Pyrrole Antibiotics from a Novel Marine Actinomycete. *J. Nat. Prod.* **2008**, *71*, 1732–1737. [CrossRef]
86. Sigala, I.; Ganidis, G.; Thysiadis, S.; Zografos, A.L.; Giannakouros, T.; Sarli, V.; Nikolakaki, E. Lynamicin D an Antimicrobial Natural Product Affects Splicing by Inducing the Expression of SR Protein Kinase 1. *Bioorg. Med. Chem.* **2017**, *25*, 1622–1629. [CrossRef]
87. Song, Y.; Yang, J.; Yu, J.; Li, J.; Yuan, J.; Wong, N.-K.; Ju, J. Chlorinated Bis-indole Alkaloids from Deep-sea Derived *Streptomyces* sp. SCSIO 11791 with Antibacterial and Cytotoxic Activities. *J. Antibiot.* **2020**, *73*, 542–547. [CrossRef]
88. Sorek, H.; Rudi, A.; Aknin, M.; Gaydou, E.M.; Kashman, Y. Isohalitulin and Haliclorensins B and C, Three Marine Alkaloids from *Haliclona tulearensis*. *J. Nat. Prod.* **2010**, *73*, 456–458. [CrossRef] [PubMed]
89. Kim, C.-K.; Wang, D.; Wilson, B.A.P.; Saurí, J.; Voeller, D.; Lipkowitz, S.; O'Keefe, B.R.; Gustafson, K.R. Suberitamides A–C, Aryl Alkaloids from a *Pseudosuberites* sp. Marine Sponge that Inhibit Cbl-b Ubiquitin Ligase Activity. *Mar. Drugs* **2020**, *18*, 536. [CrossRef]
90. Kang, U.; Cartner, L.K.; Wang, D.; Kim, C.-K.; Thomas, C.L.; Woldemichael, G.M.; Gryder, B.E.; Shern, J.F.; Khan, J.; Castello-Branco, C.; et al. Denigrins and Dactylpyrroles, Arylpyrrole Alkaloids from a *Dactylia* sp. Marine Sponge. *J. Nat. Prod.* **2020**, *83*, 3464–3470. [CrossRef]
91. Huang, C.; Yang, C.; Zhu, Y.; Zhang, W.; Yuan, C.; Zhang, C. Marine Bacterial Aromatic Polyketides from Host-Dependent Heterologous Expression and Fungal Mode of Cyclization. *Front. Chem.* **2018**, *6*, 528. [CrossRef] [PubMed]
92. Guseva, G.B.; Antina, E.V.; V'yugin, A.I.; Loginova, A.E. Complex Formation of Cu(II), Ni(II), Zn(II), Co(II), and Cd(II) Acetates with 3,3′,4,4′,5,5′-hexamethyldipyrrolylmethene. *Russ. J. Coord. Chem.* **2008**, *34*, 599–605. [CrossRef]
93. Lund, K.-l.; Thompson, A. Synthesis of Symmetric meso-H-Dipyrrin Hydrobromides from 2-Formylpyrroles. *Synlett* **2014**, *25*, 1142–1144. [CrossRef]
94. Carbone, M.; Irace, C.; Costagliola, F.; Castelluccio, F.; Villani, G.; Calado, G.; Padula, V.; Cimino, G.; Lucas Cervera, J.; Santamaria, R.; et al. A New Cytotoxic Tambjamine Alkaloid from the Azorean Nudibranch *Tambja ceutae*. *Bioorg. Med. Chem. Lett.* **2010**, *20*, 2668–2670. [CrossRef]
95. Picott, K.J.; Deichert, J.A.; deKemp, E.M.; Schatte, G.; Sauriol, F.; Ross, A.C. Isolation and Characterization of Tambjamine MYP1, A Macrocyclic Tambjamine Analogue from Marine Bacterium *Pseudoalteromonas citrea*. *MedChemComm* **2019**, *10*, 478–483. [CrossRef] [PubMed]
96. Aldrich, L.N.; Stoops, S.L.; Crews, B.C.; Marnett, L.J.; Lindsley, C.W. Total Synthesis and Biological Evaluation of Tambjamine K and a Library of Unnatural Analogs. *Bioorg. Med. Chem. Lett.* **2010**, *20*, 5207–5211. [CrossRef] [PubMed]
97. Boonlarppradab, C.; Kauffman, C.A.; Jensen, P.R.; Fenical, W. Marineosins A and B, Cytotoxic Spiroaminals from a Marine-Derived Actinomycete. *Org. Lett.* **2008**, *10*, 5505–5508. [CrossRef] [PubMed]
98. Salem, S.M.; Kancharla, P.; Florova, G.; Gupta, S.; Lu, W.; Reynolds, K.A. Elucidation of Final Steps of the Marineosins Biosynthetic Pathway through Identification and Characterization of the Corresponding Gene Cluster. *J. Am. Chem. Soc.* **2014**, *136*, 4565–4574. [CrossRef]
99. Lu, W.; Kancharla, P.; Reynolds, K.A. MarH, a Bifunctional Enzyme Involved in the Condensation and Hydroxylation Steps of the Marineosin Biosynthetic Pathway. *Org. Lett.* **2017**, *19*, 1298–1301. [CrossRef]
100. Kancharla, P.; Lu, W.; Salem, S.M.; Kelly, J.X.; Reynolds, K.A. Stereospecific Synthesis of 23-Hydroxyundecylprodiginines and Analogues and Conversion to Antimalarial Premarineosins via a Rieske Oxygenase Catalyzed Bicyclization. *J. Org. Chem.* **2014**, *79*, 11674–11689. [CrossRef]
101. Aldrich, L.N.; Dawson, E.S.; Lindsley, C.W. Evaluation of the Biosynthetic Proposal for the Synthesis of Marineosins A and B. *Org. Lett.* **2010**, *12*, 1048–1051. [CrossRef]

102. Cai, X.-C.; Wu, X.; Snider, B.B. Synthesis of the Spiroiminal Moiety of Marineosins A and B. *Org. Lett.* **2010**, *12*, 1600–1603. [CrossRef]
103. Panarese, J.D.; Konkol, L.C.; Berry, C.B.; Bates, B.S.; Aldrich, L.N.; Lindsley, C.W. Spiroaminal Model Systems of the Marineosins with Final Step Pyrrole Incorporation. *Tetrahedron Lett.* **2013**, *54*, 2231–2234. [CrossRef]
104. Li, G.; Zhang, X.; Li, Q.; Feng, P.; Shi, Y. A Concise Approach to the Spiroiminal Fragment of Marineosins. *Org. Biomol. Chem.* **2013**, *11*, 2936–2938. [CrossRef]
105. Aldrich, L.N.; Berry, C.B.; Bates, B.S.; Konkol, L.C.; So, M.; Lindsley, C.W. Towards the Total Synthesis of Marineosin A: Construction of the Macrocyclic Pyrrole and an Advanced, Functionalized Spiroaminal Model. *Eur. J. Org. Chem.* **2013**, *2013*, 4215–4218. [CrossRef]
106. Cai, X.-C.; Snider, B.B. Synthesis of the Spiroiminal Moiety and Approaches to the Synthesis of Marineosins A and B. *J. Org. Chem.* **2013**, *78*, 12161–12175. [CrossRef]
107. Xu, B.; Li, G.; Li, J.; Shi, Y. Total Synthesis of the Proposed Structure of Marineosin A. *Org. Lett.* **2016**, *18*, 2028–2031. [CrossRef]
108. Feng, Z.; Allred, T.K.; Hurlow, E.E.; Harran, P.G. Anomalous Chromophore Disruption Enables an Eight-Step Synthesis and Stereochemical Reassignment of (+)-Marineosin A. *J. Am. Chem. Soc.* **2019**, *141*, 2274–2278. [CrossRef]
109. Wood, J.M.; Furkert, D.P.; Brimble, M.A. 2-Formylpyrrole Natural Products: Origin, Structural Diversity, Bioactivity and Synthesis. *Nat. Prod. Rep.* **2019**, *36*, 289–306. [CrossRef] [PubMed]
110. Xue, D.-Q.; Liu, H.-L.; Chen, S.-H.; Mollo, E.; Gavagnin, M.; Li, J.; Li, X.-W.; Guo, Y.-W. 5-Alkylpyrrole-2-carboxaldehyde Derivatives from the Chinese Sponge *Mycale lissochela* and their PTP1B Inhibitory Activities. *Chin. Chem. Lett.* **2017**, *28*, 1190–1193. [CrossRef]
111. Jiao, W.-H.; Li, J.; Wang, D.; Zhang, M.-M.; Liu, L.-Y.; Sun, F.; Li, J.-Y.; Capon, R.J.; Lin, H.-W. Cinerols, Nitrogenous Meroterpenoids from the Marine Sponge *Dysidea cinerea*. *J. Nat. Prod.* **2019**, *82*, 2586–2593. [CrossRef]
112. Jiang, W.; Bu, Y.; Kawaguchi, M.; Osada, H.; Fukuoka, M.; Uchida, H.; Watanabe, R.; Suzuki, T.; Nagai, H. Five New Indole Derivatives from the Cyanobacterium *Moorea producens*. *Phytochem. Lett.* **2017**, *22*, 163–166. [CrossRef]
113. Fenical, W.; Jensen, P.R. Developing a New Resource for Drug Discovery: Marine Actinomycete Bacteria. *Nat. Chem. Biol.* **2006**, *2*, 666–673. [CrossRef]
114. Kwon, H.C.; Espindola, A.P.D.M.; Park, J.-S.; Prieto-Davó, A.; Rose, M.; Jensen, P.R.; Fenical, W. Nitropyrrolins A−E, Cytotoxic Farnesyl-α-nitropyrroles from a Marine-Derived Bacterium within the Actinomycete Family *Streptomycetaceae*. *J. Nat. Prod.* **2010**, *73*, 2047–2052. [CrossRef]
115. Mitani, H.; Matsuo, T.; Kodama, T.; Nishikawa, K.; Tachi, Y.; Morimoto, Y. Total Synthesis of Nitropyrrolins A, B, and D. *Tetrahedron* **2016**, *72*, 7179–7184. [CrossRef]
116. Raju, R.; Piggott, A.M.; Barrientos Diaz, L.X.; Khalil, Z.; Capon, R.J. Heronapyrroles A−C: Farnesylated 2-Nitropyrroles from an Australian Marine-Derived *Streptomyces* sp. *Org. Lett.* **2010**, *12*, 5158–5161. [CrossRef] [PubMed]
117. Schmidt, J.; Stark, C.B.W. Biomimetic Synthesis and Proposal of Relative and Absolute Stereochemistry of Heronapyrrole C. *Org. Lett.* **2012**, *14*, 4042–4045. [CrossRef]
118. Schmidt, J.; Khalil, Z.; Capon, R.J.; Stark, C.B.W. Heronapyrrole D: A Case of Co-inspiration of Natural Product Biosynthesis, Total Synthesis and Biodiscovery. *Beilstein J. Org. Chem.* **2014**, *10*, 1228–1232. [CrossRef]
119. Schmidt, J.; Stark, C.B.W. Synthetic Endeavors toward 2-Nitro-4-Alkylpyrroles in the Context of the Total Synthesis of Heronapyrrole C and Preparation of a Carboxylate Natural Product Analogue. *J. Org. Chem.* **2014**, *79*, 1920–1928. [CrossRef]
120. Ding, X.-B.; Furkert, D.P.; Capon, R.J.; Brimble, M.A. Total Synthesis of Heronapyrrole C. *Org. Lett.* **2014**, *16*, 378–381. [CrossRef]
121. Matsuo, T.; Hashimoto, S.; Nishikawa, K.; Kodama, T.; Kikuchi, S.; Tachi, Y.; Morimoto, Y. Total Synthesis and Complete Stereochemical Assignment of Heronapyrroles A and B. *Tetrahedron Lett.* **2015**, *56*, 5345–5348. [CrossRef]
122. Ding, X.-B.; Brimble, M.A.; Furkert, D.P. Nitropyrrole Natural Products: Isolation, Biosynthesis and Total Synthesis. *Org. Biomol. Chem.* **2016**, *14*, 5390–5401. [CrossRef] [PubMed]
123. Ding, X.-B.; Furkert, D.P.; Brimble, M.A. General Synthesis of the Nitropyrrolin Family of Natural Products via Regioselective CO2-Mediated Alkyne Hydration. *Org. Lett.* **2017**, *19*, 5418–5421. [CrossRef]
124. Allmann, T.C.; Moldovan, R.-P.; Jones, P.G.; Lindel, T. Synthesis of Hydroxypyrrolone Carboxamides Employing Selectfluor. *Chem. Eur. J.* **2016**, *22*, 111–115. [CrossRef] [PubMed]
125. Han, W.B.; Zhang, A.H.; Deng, X.Z.; Lei, X.; Tan, R.X. Curindolizine, an Anti-Inflammatory Agent Assembled via Michael Addition of Pyrrole Alkaloids Inside Fungal Cells. *Org. Lett.* **2016**, *18*, 1816–1819. [CrossRef]
126. Yun, K.; Leutou, A.S.; Rho, J.-R.; Son, B.W. Formoxazine, a New Pyrrolooxazine, and Two Amines from the Marine–Mudflat-Derived Fungus *Paecilomyces formosus*. *Bull. Korean Chem. Soc.* **2016**, *37*, 103–104. [CrossRef]
127. Song, F.; Liu, X.; Guo, H.; Ren, B.; Chen, C.; Piggott, A.M.; Yu, K.; Gao, H.; Wang, Q.; Liu, M.; et al. Brevianamides with Antitubercular Potential from a Marine-Derived Isolate of *Aspergillus versicolor*. *Org. Lett.* **2012**, *14*, 4770–4773. [CrossRef]
128. Niu, S.; Zhou, T.-T.; Xie, C.-L.; Zhang, G.-Y.; Yang, X.-W. Microindolinone A, a Novel 4,5,6,7-Tetrahydroindole, from the Deep-Sea-Derived Actinomycete *Microbacterium* sp. MCCC 1A11207. *Mar. Drugs* **2017**, *15*, 230. [CrossRef]
129. Henne, P.; Zeeck, A.; Grabley, S.; Thiericke, R. Secondary Metabolites by Chemical Screening. 35.1 6,7-Dihydroxy-4,5,6,7-Tetrahydroindole-4-one, A New Type of Indole-Derivative from Nocardia SP. *Nat. Prod. Rep.* **1997**, *10*, 43–47.
130. Huang, R.; Peng, Y.; Zhou, X.; Fu, M.; Tian, S.; Liu, Y. A New Pyrimidinedione Derivative from the Gorgonian Coral *Verrucella umbraculum*. *Nat. Prod. Res.* **2013**, *27*, 319–322. [CrossRef]

131. Xu, W.-G.; Xu, J.-J.; Wang, J.; Xing, G.-S.; Qiao, W.; Duan, H.-Q.; Zhao, C.; Tang, S.-A. Axinellin A and B: Two New Pyrrolactam Alkaloids from *Axinella* sp. *Chem. Nat. Compd.* **2017**, *53*, 325–327. [CrossRef]
132. Sauleau, P.; Retailleau, P.; Nogues, S.; Carletti, I.; Marcourt, L.; Raux, R.; Mourabit, A.A.; Debitus, C. Dihydrohymenialdisines, New Pyrrole-2-aminoimidazole Alkaloids from the Marine Sponge *Cymbastela cantharella*. *Tetrahedron Lett.* **2011**, *52*, 2676–2678. [CrossRef]
133. Sun, J.; Wu, J.; An, B.; Voogd, N.J.d.; Cheng, W.; Lin, W. Bromopyrrole Alkaloids with the Inhibitory Effects against the Biofilm Formation of Gram Negative Bacteria. *Mar. Drugs* **2018**, *16*, 9. [CrossRef]
134. Choi, E.J.; Nam, S.J.; Paul, L.; Beatty, D.; Kauffman, C.A.; Jensen, P.R.; Fenical, W. Previously Uncultured Marine Bacteria Linked to Novel Alkaloid Production. *Chem. Biol.* **2015**, *22*, 1270–1279. [CrossRef]
135. van der Westhuyzen, A.E.; Frolova, L.V.; Kornienko, A.; van Otterlo, W.A.L. Chapter Four – The Rigidins: Isolation, Bioactivity, and Total Synthesis–Novel Pyrrolo[2,3-d]Pyrimidine Analogues Using Multicomponent Reactions. In *The Alkaloids: Chemistry and Biology*, 1st ed.; Elsevier: Cambridge, MA, USA; San Diego, CA, USA; London, UK; Oxford, UK, 2018; Volume 79, pp. 191–220.
136. Kobayashi, J.i.; Cheng, J.-f.; Kikuchi, Y.; Ishibashi, M.; Yamamura, S.; Ohizumi, Y.; Ohtac, T.; Nozoec, S. Rigidin, a Novel Alkaloid with Calmodulin Antagonistic Activity from the Okinawan Marine Tunicate *Eudistoma cf. rigida*. *Tetrahedron Lett.* **1990**, *31*, 4617–4620. [CrossRef]
137. Tsuda, M.; Nozawa, K.; Shimbo, K.; Kobayashi, J.i. Rigidins B−D, New Pyrrolopyrimidine Alkaloids from a Tunicate *Cystodytes* Species. *J. Nat. Prod.* **2003**, *66*, 292–294. [CrossRef]
138. Davis, R.A.; Christensen, L.V.; Richardson, A.D.; Da Rocha, R.M.; Ireland, C.M. Rigidin E, a New Pyrrolopyrimidine Alkaloid from a Papua New Guinea Tunicate Eudistoma Species. *Mar. Drugs* **2003**, *1*, 27–33. [CrossRef]
139. Edstrom, E.D.; Wei, Y. Synthesis of a Novel pyrrolo[2,3-d]pyrimidine Alkaloid, Rigidin. *J. Org. Chem.* **1993**, *58*, 403–407. [CrossRef]
140. Sakamoto, T.; Kondo, Y.; Sato, S.; Yamanaka, H. Total Synthesis of a Marine Alkaloid, Rigidin. *Tetrahedron Lett.* **1994**, *35*, 2919–2920. [CrossRef]
141. Gupton, J.T.; Banner, E.J.; Scharf, A.B.; Norwood, B.K.; Kanters, R.P.F.; Dominey, R.N.; Hempel, J.E.; Kharlamova, A.; Bluhn-Chertudi, I.; Hickenboth, C.R.; et al. The Application of Vinylogous Iminium Salt Derivatives to an Efficient Synthesis of the Pyrrole Containing Alkaloids Rigidin and Rigidin E. *Tetrahedron* **2006**, *62*, 8243–8255. [CrossRef]
142. Cao, B.; Ding, H.; Yang, R.; Wang, X.; Xiao, Q. Total Synthesis of a Marine Alkaloid—Rigidin E. *Mar. Drugs* **2012**, *10*, 1412–1421. [CrossRef]
143. Frolova, L.V.; Magedov, I.V.; Romero, A.E.; Karki, M.; Otero, I.; Hayden, K.; Evdokimov, N.M.; Banuls, L.M.Y.; Rastogi, S.K.; Smith, W.R.; et al. Exploring Natural Product Chemistry and Biology with Multicomponent Reactions. 5. Discovery of a Novel Tubulin-Targeting Scaffold Derived from the Rigidin Family of Marine Alkaloids. *J. Med. Chem.* **2013**, *56*, 6886–6900. [CrossRef]
144. Frolova, L.V.; Evdokimov, N.M.; Hayden, K.; Malik, I.; Rogelj, S.; Kornienko, A.; Magedov, I.V. One-Pot Multicomponent Synthesis of Diversely Substituted 2-Aminopyrroles. A Short General Synthesis of Rigidins A, B, C, and D. *Org. Lett.* **2011**, *13*, 1118–1121. [CrossRef]
145. Huang, C.; Yang, C.; Zhang, W.; Zhu, Y.; Ma, L.; Fang, Z.; Zhang, C. Albumycin, a New Isoindolequinone from *Streptomyces albus* J1074 Harboring the Fluostatin Biosynthetic Gene Cluster. *J. Antibiot.* **2019**, *72*, 311–315. [CrossRef]
146. Wu, B.; Wiese, J.; Schmaljohann, R.; Imhoff, J.F. Biscogniauxone, a New Isopyrrolonaphthoquinone Compound from the Fungus Biscogniauxia mediterranea Isolated from Deep-Sea Sediments. *Mar. Drugs* **2016**, *14*, 204. [CrossRef] [PubMed]
147. Zhou, B.; Huang, Y.; Zhang, H.-J.; Li, J.-Q.; Ding, W.-j. Nitricquinomycins A-C, Uncommon Naphthopyrroledione from the *Streptomyces* sp. ZS-A45. *Tetrahedron* **2019**, *75*, 3958–3961. [CrossRef]
148. Zhang, W.; Liu, Z.; Li, S.; Yang, T.; Zhang, Q.; Ma, L.; Tian, X.; Zhang, H.; Huang, C.; Zhang, S.; et al. Spiroindimicins A–D: New Bisindole Alkaloids from a Deep-Sea-Derived Actinomycete. *Org. Lett.* **2012**, *14*, 3364–3367. [CrossRef]
149. Paulus, C.; Rebets, Y.; Tokovenko, B.; Nadmid, S.; Terekhova, L.P.; Myronovskyi, M.; Zotchev, S.B.; Rückert, C.; Braig, S.; Zahler, S.; et al. New Natural Products Identified by Combined Genomics-metabolomics Profiling of Marine *Streptomyces* sp. MP131-18. *Sci. Rep.* **2017**, *7*, 42382. [CrossRef] [PubMed]
150. Ma, L.; Zhang, W.; Zhu, Y.; Zhang, G.; Zhang, H.; Zhang, Q.; Zhang, L.; Yuan, C.; Zhang, C. Identification and Characterization of a Biosynthetic Gene Cluster for Tryptophan Dimers in Deep Sea-derived *Streptomyces* sp. SCSIO 03032. *Appl. Microbiol. Biotechnol.* **2017**, *101*, 6123–6136. [CrossRef] [PubMed]
151. Liu, Z.; Ma, L.; Zhang, L.; Zhang, W.; Zhu, Y.; Chen, Y.; Zhang, W.; Zhang, C. Functional Characterization of the Halogenase SpmH and Discovery of New Deschloro-tryptophan Dimers. *Org. Biomol. Chem.* **2019**, *17*, 1053–1057. [CrossRef]
152. Blair, L.M.; Sperry, J. Total Syntheses of (±)-Spiroindimicins B and C Enabled by a Late-stage Schöllkopf–Magnus–Barton–Zard (SMBZ) reaction. *Chem. Commun.* **2016**, *52*, 800–802. [CrossRef]
153. Zhang, Z.; Ray, S.; Imlay, L.; Callaghan, L.T.; Niederstrasser, H.; Mallipeddi, P.L.; Posner, B.A.; Wetzel, D.M.; Phillips, M.A.; Smith, M.W. Total Synthesis of (+)-Spiroindimicin A and Congeners Unveils their Antiparasitic Activity. *Chem. Sci.* **2021**, *12*, 10388–10394. [CrossRef]
154. Ma, L.; Zhang, W.; Liu, Z.; Huang, Y.; Zhang, Q.; Tian, X.; Zhang, C.; Zhu, Y. Complete Genome Sequence of *Streptomyces* sp. SCSIO 03032 Isolated from Indian Ocean Sediment, Producing Diverse Bioactive Natural Products. *Mar. Genom.* **2021**, *55*, 100803. [CrossRef]
155. Qin, L.; Yi, W.; Lian, X.-Y.; Wang, N.; Zhang, Z. Subtipyrrolines A–C, Novel Bioactive Alkaloids from the Mariana Trench-associated Bacterium *Bacillus subtilis* SY2101. *Tetrahedron* **2020**, *76*, 131516. [CrossRef]

156. Andersen, R.J.; Faulkner, D.J.; He, C.H.; Van Duyne, G.D.; Clardy, J. Metabolites of the Marine Prosobranch Mollusk *Lamellaria* sp. *J. Am. Chem. Soc.* **1985**, *107*, 5492–5495. [CrossRef]
157. Fukuda, T.; Ishibashi, F.; Iwao, M. Chapter One—Lamellarin Alkaloids: Isolation, Synthesis, and Biological Activity. In *The Alkaloids: Chemistry and Biology*, 1st ed.; Elsevier: Cambridge, MA, USA; San Diego, CA, USA; London, UK; Oxford, UK, 2020; Volume 83, pp. 1–112.
158. Imbri, D.; Tauber, J.; Opatz, T. Synthetic Approaches to the Lamellarins—A Comprehensive Review. *Mar. Drugs* **2014**, *12*, 6142–6177. [CrossRef] [PubMed]
159. Plisson, F.; Huang, X.-C.; Zhang, H.; Khalil, Z.; Capon, R.J. Lamellarins as Inhibitors of P-Glycoprotein-Mediated Multidrug Resistance in a Human Colon Cancer Cell Line. *Chem. Asian J.* **2012**, *7*, 1616–1623. [CrossRef] [PubMed]
160. Bracegirdle, J.; Robertson, L.P.; Hume, P.A.; Page, M.J.; Sharrock, A.V.; Ackerley, D.F.; Carroll, A.R.; Keyzers, R.A. Lamellarin Sulfates from the Pacific Tunicate *Didemnum ternerratum*. *J. Nat. Prod.* **2019**, *82*, 2000–2008. [CrossRef] [PubMed]
161. Lindquist, N.; Fenical, W.; Van Duyne, G.D.; Clardy, J. New Alkaloids of the Lamellarin Class from the Marine Ascidian *Didemnum chartaceum* (Sluiter, 1909). *J. Org. Chem.* **1988**, *53*, 4570–4574. [CrossRef]
162. Urban, S.; Butler, M.; Capon, R. Lamellarins O and P: New Aromatic Metabolites From the Australian Marine Sponge *Dendrilla cactos*. *Aust. J. Chem.* **1994**, *47*, 1919–1924. [CrossRef]
163. Urban, S.; Hobbs, L.; Hooper, J.; Capon, R. Lamellarins Q and R: New Aromatic Metabolites From an Australian Marine Sponge, *Dendrilla cactos*. *Aust. J. Chem.* **1995**, *48*, 1491–1494. [CrossRef]
164. Urban, S.; Capon, R. Lamellarin-S: A New Aromatic Metabolite From an Australian Tunicate, *Didemnum* sp. *Aust. J. Chem.* **1996**, *49*, 711–713. [CrossRef]
165. Reddy, M.V.R.; Faulkner, D.J.; Venkateswarlu, Y.; Rao, M.R. New Lamellarin Alkaloids from an Unidentified Ascidian from the Arabian Sea. *Tetrahedron* **1997**, *53*, 3457–3466. [CrossRef]
166. Cantrell, C.L.; Groweiss, A.; Gustafson, K.R.; Boyd, M.R. A New Staurosporine Analog from the Prosobranch Mollusk *Coriocella Nigra*. *Nat. Prod. Lett.* **1999**, *14*, 39–46. [CrossRef]
167. Rudi, A.; Goldberg, I.; Stein, Z.; Frolow, F.; Benayahu, Y.; Schleyer, M.; Kashman, Y. Polycitone A and Polycitrins A and B: New Alkaloids from the Marine Ascidian *Polycitor* sp. *J. Org. Chem.* **1994**, *59*, 999–1003. [CrossRef]
168. Palermo, J.A.; Rodríguez Brasco, M.F.; Seldes, A.M. Storniamides A–D: Alkaloids from a Patagonian sponge *Cliona* sp. *Tetrahedron* **1996**, *52*, 2727–2734. [CrossRef]
169. Murali Krishna Kumar, M.; Devilal Naik, J.; Satyavathi, K.; Ramana, H.; Raghuveer Varma, P.; Purna Nagasree, K.; Smitha, D.; Venkata Rao, D. Denigrins A–C: New Antitubercular 3,4-diarylpyrrole Alkaloids from *Dendrilla nigra*. *Nat. Prod. Res.* **2014**, *28*, 888–894. [CrossRef]
170. Yoshida, W.Y.; Lee, K.K.; Carroll, A.R.; Scheuer, P.J. A Complex Pyrrolo-oxazinone and Its Iodo Derivative Isolated from a Tunicate. *Helv. Chim. Acta* **1992**, *75*, 1721–1725. [CrossRef]
171. Zhang, W.; Ready, J.M. Total Synthesis of the Dictyodendrins as an Arena to Highlight Emerging Synthetic Technologies. *Nat. Prod. Rep.* **2017**, *34*, 1010–1034. [CrossRef]
172. Chan, G.W.; Francis, T.; Thureen, D.R.; Offen, P.H.; Pierce, N.J.; Westley, J.W.; Johnson, R.K.; Faulkner, D.J. Purpurone, an Inhibitor of ATP-citrate Lyase: A Novel Alkaloid from the Marine Sponge *Iotrochota* sp. *J. Org. Chem.* **1993**, *58*, 2544–2546. [CrossRef]
173. Kang, H.; Fenical, W. Ningalins A−D: Novel Aromatic Alkaloids from a Western Australian Ascidian of the Genus *Didemnum*. *J. Org. Chem.* **1997**, *62*, 3254–3262. [CrossRef]
174. Plisson, F.; Conte, M.; Khalil, Z.; Huang, X.-C.; Piggott, A.M.; Capon, R.J. Kinase Inhibitor Scaffolds against Neurodegenerative Diseases from a Southern Australian Ascidian, *Didemnum* sp. *ChemMedChem* **2012**, *7*, 983–990. [CrossRef]
175. Fan, G.; Li, Z.; Shen, S.; Zeng, Y.; Yang, Y.; Xu, M.; Bruhn, T.; Bruhn, H.; Morschhäuser, J.; Bringmann, G.; et al. Baculiferins A–O, O-sulfated Pyrrole Alkaloids with Anti-HIV-1 Activity, from the Chinese Marine Sponge *Iotrochota baculifera*. *Bioorg. Med. Chem.* **2010**, *18*, 5466–5474. [CrossRef]
176. Iwao, M.; Fukuda, T.; Saeki, S.; Ohta, T. Divergent Synthesis of Lamellarin α 13-Sulfate, 20-Sulfate, and 13,20-Disulfate. *Heterocycles* **2010**, *80*, 841–846. [CrossRef]
177. Hasse, K.; Willis, A.C.; Banwell, M.G. Modular Total Syntheses of Lamellarin G Trimethyl Ether and Lamellarin S. *Eur. J. Org. Chem.* **2011**, *2011*, 88–99. [CrossRef]
178. Li, Q.; Jiang, J.; Fan, A.; Cui, Y.; Jia, Y. Total Synthesis of Lamellarins D, H, and R and Ningalin B. *Org. Lett.* **2011**, *13*, 312–315. [CrossRef]
179. Ramírez-Rodríguez, A.; Méndez, J.M.; Jiménez, C.C.; León, F.; Vazquez, A. A Paal–Knorr Approach to 3,4-Diaryl-Substituted Pyrroles: Facile Synthesis of Lamellarins O and Q. *Synthesis* **2012**, *44*, 3321–3326. [CrossRef]
180. Flynn, B.; Banwell, M. Convergent Total Syntheses of the Pentacyclic Lamellarins K, T, U and W via the Addition of Azomethine Ylides to Tethered Tolans. *Heterocycles* **2012**, *84*, 1141–1170. [CrossRef]
181. Imbri, D.; Tauber, J.; Opatz, T. A High-Yielding Modular Access to the Lamellarins: Synthesis of Lamellarin G Trimethyl Ether, Lamellarin η and Dihydrolamellarin η. *Chem. Eur. J.* **2013**, *19*, 15080–15083. [CrossRef]
182. Takamura, K.; Matsuo, H.; Tanaka, A.; Tanaka, J.; Fukuda, T.; Ishibashi, F.; Iwao, M. Total Synthesis of the Marine Natural Products Lukianols A and B. *Tetrahedron* **2013**, *69*, 2782–2788. [CrossRef]
183. Ueda, K.; Amaike, K.; Maceiczyk, R.M.; Itami, K.; Yamaguchi, J. β-Selective C–H Arylation of Pyrroles Leading to Concise Syntheses of Lamellarins C and I. *J. Am. Chem. Soc.* **2014**, *136*, 13226–13232. [CrossRef]

184. Komatsubara, M.; Umeki, T.; Fukuda, T.; Iwao, M. Modular Synthesis of Lamellarins via Regioselective Assembly of 3,4,5-Differentially Arylated Pyrrole-2-carboxylates. *J. Org. Chem.* **2014**, *79*, 529–537. [CrossRef]
185. Iwao, M.; Fukuda, T.; Sato, D. A Synthesis of Lamellarins via Regioselective Assembly of 1,2,3-Differentially Substituted 5,6-Dihydropyrrolo[2,1-a]Isoquinoline Core. *Heterocycles* **2015**, *91*, 782. [CrossRef]
186. Dialer, C.; Imbri, D.; Hansen, S.P.; Opatz, T. Synthesis of Lamellarin D Trimethyl Ether and Lamellarin H via 6π-Electrocyclization. *J. Org. Chem.* **2015**, *80*, 11605–11610. [CrossRef]
187. Theppawong, A.; Ploypradith, P.; Chuawong, P.; Ruchirawat, S.; Chittchang, M. Facile and Divergent Synthesis of Lamellarins and Lactam-Containing Derivatives with Improved Drug Likeness and Biological Activities. *Chem. Asian J.* **2015**, *10*, 2631–2650. [CrossRef] [PubMed]
188. Tan, W.W.; Yoshikai, N. Copper-catalyzed Condensation of Imines and α-Diazo-β-dicarbonyl Compounds: Modular and Regiocontrolled Synthesis of Multisubstituted Pyrroles. *Chem. Sci.* **2015**, *6*, 6448–6455. [CrossRef] [PubMed]
189. Iwao, M.; Fukuda, T.; Anzai, M. Regioselective Synthesis of 2,4-Differentially Arylated Pyrroles and Its Application to The Synthesis of Lamellarins. *Heterocycles* **2016**, *93*, 593. [CrossRef]
190. Manjappa, K.B.; Syu, J.-R.; Yang, D.-Y. Visible-Light-Promoted and Yb(OTf)3-Catalyzed Constructions of Coumarin-Pyrrole-(Iso)quinoline-Fused Pentacycles: Synthesis of Lamellarin Core, Lamellarin D Trimethyl Ether, and Lamellarin H. *Org. Lett.* **2016**, *18*, 332–335. [CrossRef]
191. Fukuda, T.; Umeki, T.; Tokushima, K.; Xiang, G.; Yoshida, Y.; Ishibashi, F.; Oku, Y.; Nishiya, N.; Uehara, Y.; Iwao, M. Design, Synthesis, and Evaluation of A-ring-modified Lamellarin N Analogues as Noncovalent Inhibitors of the EGFR T790M/L858R Mutant. *Bioorg. Med. Chem.* **2017**, *25*, 6563–6580. [CrossRef]
192. Fukuda, T.; Katae, T.; Harada, I.; Iwao, M. Synthesis of Lamellarins via Regioselective Assembly of 1,2-Diarylated [1]Benzopyrano[3,4-b]pyrrol-4(3H)-one Core. *Heterocycles* **2017**, *95*, 950–971. [CrossRef]
193. Lade, D.M.; Pawar, A.B.; Mainkar, P.S.; Chandrasekhar, S. Total Synthesis of Lamellarin D Trimethyl Ether, Lamellarin D, and Lamellarin H. *J. Org. Chem.* **2017**, *82*, 4998–5004. [CrossRef]
194. Zheng, K.-L.; You, M.-Q.; Shu, W.-M.; Wu, Y.-D.; Wu, A.-X. Acid-Mediated Intermolecular [3 + 2] Cycloaddition toward Pyrrolo[2,1-a]isoquinolines: Total Synthesis of the Lamellarin Core and Lamellarin G Trimethyl Ether. *Org. Lett.* **2017**, *19*, 2262–2265. [CrossRef]
195. Manjappa, K.B.; Lin, J.-M.; Yang, D.-Y. Construction of Pentacyclic Lamellarin Skeleton via Grob Reaction: Application to Total Synthesis of Lamellarins H and D. *J. Org. Chem.* **2017**, *82*, 7648–7656. [CrossRef]
196. Mei, R.; Zhang, S.-K.; Ackermann, L. Concise Synthesis of Lamellarin Alkaloids by C–H/N–H Activation: Evaluation of Metal Catalysts in Oxidative Alkyne Annulation. *Synlett* **2017**, *28*, 1715–1718. [CrossRef]
197. Colligs, V.C.; Dialer, C.; Opatz, T. Synthesis of Lamellarin G Trimethyl Ether by von Miller–Plöchl-Type Cyclocondensation. *Eur. J. Org. Chem.* **2018**, *2018*, 4064–4070. [CrossRef]
198. Chiu, H.-C.; Tonks, I.A. Trimethylsilyl-Protected Alkynes as Selective Cross-Coupling Partners in Titanium-Catalyzed [2+2+1] Pyrrole Synthesis. *Angew. Chem. Int. Ed.* **2018**, *57*, 6090–6094. [CrossRef]
199. Shirley, H.J.; Koyioni, M.; Muncan, F.; Donohoe, T.J. Synthesis of Lamellarin Alkaloids Using Orthoester-masked α-Keto Acids. *Chem. Sci.* **2019**, *10*, 4334–4338. [CrossRef] [PubMed]
200. Klintworth, R.; de Koning, C.B.; Opatz, T.; Michael, J.P. A Xylochemically Inspired Synthesis of Lamellarin G Trimethyl Ether via an Enaminone Intermediate. *J. Org. Chem.* **2019**, *84*, 11025–11031. [CrossRef]
201. Kumar, V.; Awasthi, A.; Salam, A.; Khan, T. Scalable Total Syntheses of Some Natural and Unnatural Lamellarins: Application of a One-Pot Domino Process for Regioselective Access to the Central 1,2,4-Trisubstituted Pyrrole Core. *J. Org. Chem.* **2019**, *84*, 11596–11603. [CrossRef]
202. Watanabe, T.; Mutoh, Y.; Saito, S. Synthesis of Lactone-fused Pyrroles by Ruthenium-catalyzed 1,2-Carbon Migration-cycloisomerization. *Org. Biomol. Chem.* **2020**, *18*, 81–85. [CrossRef]
203. Hwu, J.R.; Roy, A.; Panja, A.; Huang, W.-C.; Hu, Y.-C.; Tan, K.-T.; Lin, C.-C.; Hwang, K.-C.; Hsu, M.-H.; Tsay, S.-C. Domino Reaction for the Synthesis of Polysubstituted Pyrroles and Lamellarin R. *J. Org. Chem.* **2020**, *85*, 9835–9843. [CrossRef]
204. Satyanarayana, I.; Yang, D.-Y.; Liou, T.-J. Synthesis of lamellarin R, lukianol A, lamellarin O and their analogues. *RSC Adv.* **2020**, *10*, 43168–43174. [CrossRef]
205. Kumar, V.; Salam, A.; Kumar, D.; Khan, T. Concise and Scalable Total Syntheses of Lamellarin Z and other Natural Lamellarins. *ChemistrySelect* **2020**, *5*, 14510–14514. [CrossRef]
206. Boonya-udtayan, S.; Yotapan, N.; Woo, C.; Bruns, C.J.; Ruchirawat, S.; Thasana, N. Synthesis and Biological Activities of Azalamellarins. *Chem. Asian J.* **2010**, *5*, 2113–2123. [CrossRef] [PubMed]
207. Kamiyama, H.; Kubo, Y.; Sato, H.; Yamamoto, N.; Fukuda, T.; Ishibashi, F.; Iwao, M. Synthesis, Structure–activity Relationships, and Mechanism of Action of Anti-HIV-1 Lamellarin α 20-Sulfate Analogues. *Bioorg. Med. Chem.* **2011**, *19*, 7541–7550. [CrossRef] [PubMed]
208. Korotaev, V.Y.; Sosnovskikh, V.Y.; Barkov, A.Y.; Slepukhin, P.A.; Ezhikova, M.A.; Kodess, M.I.; Shklyaev, Y.V. A Simple Synthesis of the Pentacyclic Lamellarin Skeleton from 3-Nitro-2-(trifluoromethyl)-2H-chromenes and 1-Methyl(benzyl)-3,4-dihydroisoquinolines. *Tetrahedron* **2011**, *67*, 8685–8698. [CrossRef]

209. Neagoie, C.; Vedrenne, E.; Buron, F.; Mérour, J.-Y.; Rosca, S.; Bourg, S.; Lozach, O.; Meijer, L.; Baldeyrou, B.; Lansiaux, A.; et al. Synthesis of Chromeno[3,4-b]indoles as Lamellarin D Analogues: A Novel DYRK1A Inhibitor Class. *Eur. J. Med. Chem.* **2012**, *49*, 379–396. [CrossRef]
210. Shen, L.; Xie, N.; Yang, B.; Hu, Y.; Zhang, Y. Design and Total Synthesis of Mannich Derivatives of Marine Natural Product Lamellarin D as Cytotoxic Agents. *Eur. J. Med. Chem.* **2014**, *85*, 807–817. [CrossRef] [PubMed]
211. Kumar, K.S.; Meesa, S.R.; Rajesham, B.; Bhasker, B.; Ashfaq, M.A.; Khan, A.A.; Rao, S.S.; Pal, M. AlCl3-mediated Heteroarylation-cyclization Strategy: One-pot Synthesis of Dused Quinoxalines Containing the Central Core of Lamellarin D. *RSC Adv.* **2016**, *6*, 48324–48328. [CrossRef]
212. Colligs, V.; Hansen, S.P.; Imbri, D.; Seo, E.-J.; Kadioglu, O.; Efferth, T.; Opatz, T. Synthesis and Biological Evaluation of a D-ring-Contracted Analogue of lamellarin D. *Bioorg. Med. Chem.* **2017**, *25*, 6137–6148. [CrossRef]
213. Vyasamudri, S.; Yang, D.-Y. Application of Differential Eeactivity Towards Synthesis of Lamellarin and 8-Oxoprotoberberine Derivatives: Study of Photochemical Properties of Aryl-substituted Benzofuran-8-oxoprotoberberines. *Tetrahedron* **2018**, *74*, 1092–1100. [CrossRef]
214. Praud-Tabariès, A.; Bottzeck, O.; Blache, Y. Synthesis of Lamellarin Q Analogues as Potential Antibiofilm Compounds. *J. Heterocycl. Chem.* **2019**, *56*, 1458–1463. [CrossRef]
215. Scheurer, P.J. *Marine Natural Products*; Chemical and Biological Perspectives; Academic Press: New York, NY, USA, 1983; Volume 5.
216. Gribble, G.W. Chapter 1—Occurrence of Halogenated Alkaloids. In *The Alkaloids: Chemistry and Biology*, 1st ed.; Elsevier: San Diego, CA, USA; Waltham, MA, USA; London, UK; Oxford, UK; Amsterdam, The Netherlands, 2012; Volume 71, pp. 1–165.
217. Wagner, C.; El Omari, M.; König, G.M. Biohalogenation: Nature's Way to Synthesize Halogenated Metabolites. *J. Nat. Prod.* **2009**, *72*, 540–553. [CrossRef]
218. Schnepel, C.; Sewald, N. Enzymatic Halogenation: A Timely Strategy for Regioselective C−H Activation. *Chem. Eur. J.* **2017**, *23*, 12064–12086. [CrossRef]
219. Cafieri, F.; Fattorusso, E.; Mangoni, A.; Taglialatela-Scafati, O. Dispacamides, Anti-histamine Alkaloids from Caribbean *Agelas* Sponges. *Tetrahedron Lett.* **1996**, *37*, 3587–3590. [CrossRef]
220. Cafieri, F.; Carnuccio, R.; Fattorusso, E.; Taglialatela-Scafati, O.; Vallefuoco, T. Anti-histaminic Activity of Bromopyrrole Alkaloids Isolated from Caribbean *Agelas* Sponges. *Bioorg. Med. Chem. Lett.* **1997**, *7*, 2283–2288. [CrossRef]
221. Rane, R.A.; Nandave, M.; Nayak, S.; Naik, A.; Shah, D.; Alwan, W.S.; Sahu, N.U.; Naphade, S.S.; Palkar, M.B.; Karunanidhi, S.; et al. Synthesis and Pharmacological Evaluation of Marine Bromopyrrole Alkaloid-based Hybrids with Anti-inflammatory Activity. *Arab. J. Chem.* **2017**, *10*, 458–464. [CrossRef]
222. Cafieri, F.; Fattorusso, E.; Mangoni, A.; Taglialatela-Scafati, O.; Carnuccio, R. A Novel Bromopyrrole Alkaloid from the Sponge *Agelas* Longissima with Antiserotonergic Activity. *Bioorg. Med. Chem. Lett.* **1995**, *5*, 799–804. [CrossRef]
223. Kinnel, R.B.; Gehrken, H.P.; Scheuer, P.J. Palau'amine: A Cytotoxic and Immunosuppressive Hexacyclic Bisguanidine Antibiotic from the Sponge *Stylotella agminata*. *J. Am. Chem. Soc.* **1993**, *115*, 3376–3377. [CrossRef]
224. Walker, R.P.; Faulkner, D.J.; Van Engen, D.; Clardy, J. Sceptrin, An Antimicrobial Agent from the Sponge *Agelas sceptrum*. *J. Am. Chem. Soc.* **1981**, *103*, 6772–6773. [CrossRef]
225. Scala, F.; Fattorusso, E.; Menna, M.; Taglialatela-Scafati, O.; Tierney, M.; Kaiser, M.; Tasdemir, D. Bromopyrrole Alkaloids as Lead Compounds Against Protozoan Parasites. *Mar. Drugs* **2010**, *8*, 2162–2174. [CrossRef]
226. Cipres, A.; O'Malley, D.P.; Li, K.; Finlay, D.; Baran, P.S.; Vuori, K. Sceptrin, a Marine Natural Compound, Inhibits Cell Motility in a Variety of Cancer Cell Lines. *ACS Chem. Biol.* **2010**, *5*, 195–202. [CrossRef]
227. Bhardwaj, V.; Gumber, D.; Abbot, V.; Dhiman, S.; Sharma, P. Pyrrole: A Resourceful Small Molecule in Key Medicinal Hetero-aromatics. *RSC Adv.* **2015**, *5*, 15233–15266. [CrossRef]
228. Ebada, S.S.; Linh, M.H.; Longeon, A.; de Voogd, N.J.; Durieu, E.; Meijer, L.; Bourguet-Kondracki, M.-L.; Singab, A.N.B.; Müller, W.E.G.; Proksch, P. Dispacamide E and Other Bioactive Bromopyrrole Alkaloids from Two Indonesian Marine Sponges of the Genus *Stylissa*. *Nat. Prod. Commun.* **2014**, *29*, 231–238. [CrossRef]
229. Regalado, E.; Laguna, A.; Mendiola Martínez, J.; Thomas, O.; Nogueiras, C. Bromopyrrole Alkaloids from the Caribbean Sponge *Agelas cerebrum*. *Quim. Nova* **2011**, *34*, 289–291. [CrossRef]
230. Handy, S.T.; Sabatini, J.J.; Zhang, Y.; Vulfova, I. Protection of Poorly Nucleophilic Pyrroles. *Tetrahedron Lett.* **2004**, *45*, 5057–5060. [CrossRef]
231. Assmann, M.; Lichte, E.; Pawlik, J.; Koeck, M. Chemical Defenses of the Caribbean Sponges *Agelas wiedenmayeri* and *Agelas conifera*. *Mar. Ecol. Prog. Ser.* **2000**, *207*, 255–262. [CrossRef]
232. Lee, S.; Tanaka, N.; Takahashi, S.; Tsuji, D.; Kim, S.-Y.; Kojoma, M.; Itoh, K.; Kobayashi, J.i.; Kashiwada, Y. Agesasines A and B, Bromopyrrole Alkaloids from Marine Sponges *Agelas* spp. *Mar. Drugs* **2020**, *18*, 455. [CrossRef]
233. Yang, F.; Hamann, M.T.; Zou, Y.; Zhang, M.-Y.; Gong, X.-B.; Xiao, J.-R.; Chen, W.-S.; Lin, H.-W. Antimicrobial Metabolites from the Paracel Islands Sponge *Agelas mauritiana*. *J. Nat. Prod.* **2012**, *75*, 774–778. [CrossRef] [PubMed]
234. Hertiani, T.; Edrada-Ebel, R.; Ortlepp, S.; van Soest, R.W.M.; de Voogd, N.J.; Wray, V.; Hentschel, U.; Kozytska, S.; Müller, W.E.G.; Proksch, P. From Anti-fouling to Biofilm Inhibition: New Cytotoxic Secondary Metabolites from two Indonesian *Agelas* Sponges. *Bioorg. Med. Chem.* **2010**, *18*, 1297–1311. [CrossRef] [PubMed]

235. Tebben, J.; Motti, C.; Tapiolas, D.; Thomas-Hall, P.; Harder, T. A Coralline Algal-associated Bacterium, *pseudoalteromonas* Strain J010, Yields Five New Korormicins and a Bromopyrrole. *Mar. Drugs* **2014**, *12*, 2802–2815. [CrossRef] [PubMed]
236. Guella, G.; Frassanito, R.; Mancini, I.; Sandron, T.; Modeo, L.; Verni, F.; Dini, F.; Petroni, G. Keronopsamides, a New Class of Pigments from Marine Ciliates. *Eur. J. Org. Chem.* **2010**, *2010*, 427–434. [CrossRef]
237. Kovalerchik, D.; Singh, R.P.; Schlesinger, P.; Mahajni, A.; Shefer, S.; Fridman, M.; Ilan, M.; Carmeli, S. Bromopyrrole Alkaloids of the Sponge *Agelas oroides* Collected Near the Israeli Mediterranean Coastline. *J. Nat. Prod.* **2020**, *83*, 374–384. [CrossRef] [PubMed]
238. Otter, B.A.; Patil, S.A.; Klein, R.S.; Ealick, S.E. A Corrected Structure for Pyrrolosine. *J. Am. Chem. Soc.* **1992**, *114*, 668–671. [CrossRef]
239. Patiño C, L.P.; Muniain, C.; Knott, M.E.; Puricelli, L.; Palermo, J.A. Bromopyrrole Alkaloids Isolated from the Patagonian Bryozoan *Aspidostoma giganteum*. *J. Nat. Prod.* **2014**, *77*, 1170–1178. [CrossRef] [PubMed]
240. Peng, J.; Li, J.; Hamann, M.T. The Marine Bromotyrosine Derivatives. In *The Alkaloids: Chemistry and Biology*, 1st ed.; Elsevier: Cambridge, MA, USA; San Diego, CA, USA; London, UK; Oxford, UK, 2005; Volume 61, pp. 59–262.
241. Ohtani, I.; Kusumi, T.; Kashman, Y.; Kakisawa, H. High-field FT NMR Application of Mosher's Method. The Absolute Configurations of Marine Terpenoids. *J. Am. Chem. Soc.* **1991**, *113*, 4092–4096. [CrossRef]
242. Hussain, M.A.; Khan, F.A. Total Synthesis of (±) Aspidostomide B, C, Regioisomeric N-methyl Aspidostomide D and their Derivatives. *Tetrahedron Lett.* **2019**, *60*, 151040. [CrossRef]
243. Parra, L.L.L.; Bertonha, A.F.; Severo, I.R.M.; Aguiar, A.C.C.; de Souza, G.E.; Oliva, G.; Guido, R.V.C.; Grazzia, N.; Costa, T.R.; Miguel, D.C.; et al. Isolation, Derivative Synthesis, and Structure–Activity Relationships of Antiparasitic Bromopyrrole Alkaloids from the Marine Sponge Tedania brasiliensis. *J. Nat. Prod.* **2018**, *81*, 188–202. [CrossRef]
244. Kobayashi, J.; Kanda, F.; Ishibashi, M.; Shigemori, H. Manzacidins A-C, Novel Tetrahydropyrimidine Alkaloids from the Okinawan Marine Sponge *Hymeniacidon* sp. *J. Org. Chem.* **1991**, *56*, 4574–4576. [CrossRef]
245. Namba, K.; Shinada, T.; Teramoto, T.; Ohfune, Y. Total Synthesis and Absolute Structure of Manzacidin A and C. *J. Am. Chem. Soc.* **2000**, *122*, 10708–10709. [CrossRef]
246. Shinada, T.; Ikebe, E.; Oe, K.; Namba, K.; Kawasaki, M.; Ohfune, Y. Synthesis and Absolute Structure of Manzacidin B. *Org. Lett.* **2007**, *9*, 1765–1767, Erratum in **2010**, *12*, 2170. [CrossRef] [PubMed]
247. Shinada, T.; Ikebe, E.; Oe, K.; Namba, K.; Kawasaki, M.; Ohfune, Y. Synthesis and Absolute Structure of Manzacidin B. *Org. Lett.* **2010**, *12*, 2170. [CrossRef]
248. Kobayashi, J.i.; Nakamura, K.; Kusama, T.; Tanaka, N.; Sakai, K.; Gonoi, T.; Fromont, J. 2-Debromonagelamide U, 2-Debromomukanadin G, and 2-Debromonagelamide P from Marine Sponge *Agelas* sp. *Heterocycles* **2015**, *90*, 425. [CrossRef]
249. Lacerna, N.M.; Miller, B.W.; Lim, A.L.; Tun, J.O.; Robes, J.M.D.; Cleofas, M.J.B.; Lin, Z.; Salvador-Reyes, L.A.; Haygood, M.G.; Schmidt, E.W.; et al. Mindapyrroles A–C, Pyoluteorin Analogues from a Shipworm-Associated Bacterium. *J. Nat. Prod.* **2019**, *82*, 1024–1028. [CrossRef]
250. Hughes, C.C.; Kauffman, C.A.; Jensen, P.R.; Fenical, W. Structures, Reactivities, and Antibiotic Properties of the Marinopyrroles A−F. *J. Org. Chem.* **2010**, *75*, 3240–3250. [CrossRef]
251. Hughes, C.C.; Prieto-Davo, A.; Jensen, P.R.; Fenical, W. The Marinopyrroles, Antibiotics of an Unprecedented Structure Class from a Marine *Streptomyces* sp. *Org. Lett.* **2008**, *10*, 629–631. [CrossRef]
252. Cheng, C.; Pan, L.; Chen, Y.; Song, H.; Qin, Y.; Li, R. Total Synthesis of (±)-Marinopyrrole A and Its Library as Potential Antibiotic and Anticancer Agents. *J. Comb. Chem.* **2010**, *12*, 541–547. [CrossRef]
253. Cheng, P.; Clive, D.L.J.; Fernandopulle, S.; Chen, Z. Racemic Marinopyrrole B by Total Synthesis. *Chem. Commun.* **2013**, *49*, 558–560. [CrossRef]
254. Nuzzo, G.; Ciavatta, M.L.; Kiss, R.; Mathieu, V.; Leclercqz, H.; Manzo, E.; Villani, G.; Mollo, E.; Lefranc, F.; D'Souza, L.; et al. Chemistry of the Nudibranch *Aldisa andersoni*: Structure and Biological Activity of Phorbazole Metabolites. *Mar. Drugs* **2012**, *10*, 1799–1811. [CrossRef]
255. Forte, B.; Malgesini, B.; Piutti, C.; Quartieri, F.; Scolaro, A.; Papeo, G. A Submarine Journey: The Pyrrole-imidazole Alkaloids. *Mar. Drugs* **2009**, *7*, 705–753. [CrossRef] [PubMed]
256. Stout, E.P.; Wang, Y.-G.; Romo, D.; Molinski, T.F. Pyrrole Aminoimidazole Alkaloid Metabiosynthesis with Marine Sponges *Agelas conifera* and *Stylissa caribica*. *Angew. Chem. Int. Ed.* **2012**, *51*, 4877–4881. [CrossRef] [PubMed]
257. Wang, X.; Ma, Z.; Wang, X.; De, S.; Ma, Y.; Chen, C. Dimeric Pyrrole–imidazole Alkaloids: Synthetic Approaches and Biosynthetic Hypotheses. *Chem. Commun.* **2014**, *50*, 8628–8639. [CrossRef]
258. Yasuda, T.; Araki, A.; Kubota, T.; Ito, J.; Mikami, Y.; Fromont, J.; Kobayashi, J.i. Bromopyrrole Alkaloids from Marine Sponges of the Genus *Agelas*. *J. Nat. Prod.* **2009**, *72*, 488–491. [CrossRef]
259. Uemoto, H.; Tsuda, M.; Kobayashi, J.i. Mukanadins A−C, New Bromopyrrole Alkaloids from Marine Sponge *Agelas nakamurai*. *J. Nat. Prod.* **1999**, *62*, 1581–1583. [CrossRef]
260. Vergne, C.; Appenzeller, J.; Ratinaud, C.; Martin, M.-T.; Debitus, C.; Zaparucha, A.; Al-Mourabit, A. Debromodispacamides B and D: Isolation from the Marine Sponge *Agelas mauritiana* and Stereoselective Synthesis Using a Biomimetic Proline Route. *Org. Lett.* **2008**, *10*, 493–496. [CrossRef]
261. Aiello, A.; D'Esposito, M.; Fattorusso, E.; Menna, M.; Müller, W.E.G.; Perović-Ottstadt, S.; Schröder, H.C. Novel Bioactive Bromopyrrole Alkaloids from the Mediterranean Sponge *Axinella verrucosa*. *Bioorg. Med. Chem.* **2006**, *14*, 17–24. [CrossRef]

262. Li, T.; Li, P.-L.; Luo, X.-C.; Tang, X.-L.; Li, G.-Q. Three New Dibromopyrrole Alkaloids from the South China Sea Sponge *Agelas nemoechinata*. *Tetrahedron Lett.* **2019**, *60*, 1996–1998. [CrossRef]
263. Daninos-Zeghal, S.; Al Mourabit, A.; Ahond, A.; Poupat, C.; Potier, P. Synthèse de Métabolites Marins 2-aminoimidazoliques: Hyménidine, Oroïdine et Kéramadine. *Tetrahedron* **1997**, *53*, 7605–7614. [CrossRef]
264. de Souza, R.T.M.P.; Freire, V.F.; Gubiani, J.R.; Ferreira, R.O.; Trivella, D.B.B.; Moraes, F.C.; Paradas, W.C.; Salgado, L.T.; Pereira, R.C.; Amado Filho, G.M.; et al. Bromopyrrole Alkaloid Inhibitors of the Proteasome Isolated from a *Dictyonella* sp. Marine Sponge Collected at the Amazon River Mouth. *J. Nat. Prod.* **2018**, *81*, 2296–2300. [CrossRef]
265. Beck, P.; Lansdell, T.A.; Hewlett, N.M.; Tepe, J.J.; Groll, M. Indolo-Phakellins as β5-Specific Noncovalent Proteasome Inhibitors. *Angew. Chem. Int. Ed.* **2015**, *54*, 2830–2833. [CrossRef]
266. Lansdell, T.A.; Hewlett, N.M.; Skoumbourdis, A.P.; Fodor, M.D.; Seiple, I.B.; Su, S.; Baran, P.S.; Feldman, K.S.; Tepe, J.J. Palau'amine and Related Oroidin Alkaloids Dibromophakellin and Dibromophakellstatin Inhibit the Human 20S Proteasome. *J. Nat. Prod.* **2012**, *75*, 980–985. [CrossRef]
267. Patel, K.; Laville, R.; Martin, M.-T.; Tilvi, S.; Moriou, C.; Gallard, J.-F.; Ermolenko, L.; Debitus, C.; Al-Mourabit, A. Unprecedented Stylissazoles A–C from *Stylissa carteri*: Another Dimension for Marine Pyrrole-2-aminoimidazole Metabolite Diversity. *Angew. Chem. Int. Ed.* **2010**, *49*, 4775–4779. [CrossRef]
268. Zhang, H.; Khalil, Z.; Conte, M.M.; Plisson, F.; Capon, R.J. A Search for Kinase Inhibitors and Antibacterial Agents: Bromopyrrolo-2-aminoimidazoles from a Deep-water Great Australian Bight sponge, *Axinella* sp. *Tetrahedron Lett.* **2012**, *53*, 3784–3787. [CrossRef]
269. Grube, A.; Immel, S.; Baran, P.S.; Köck, M. Massadine Chloride: A Biosynthetic Precursor of Massadine and Stylissadine. *Angew. Chem. Int. Ed.* **2007**, *46*, 6721–6724. [CrossRef]
270. Nishimura, S.; Matsunaga, S.; Shibazaki, M.; Suzuki, K.; Furihata, K.; van Soest, R.W.M.; Fusetani, N. Massadine, a Novel Geranylgeranyltransferase Type I Inhibitor from the Marine Sponge *Stylissa* aff. *massa*. *Org. Lett.* **2003**, *5*, 2255–2257. [CrossRef]
271. Seiple, I.B.; Su, S.; Young, I.S.; Nakamura, A.; Yamaguchi, J.; Jørgensen, L.; Rodriguez, R.A.; O'Malley, D.P.; Gaich, T.; Köck, M.; et al. Enantioselective Total Syntheses of (−)-Palau'amine, (−)-Axinellamines, and (−)-Massadines. *J. Am. Chem. Soc.* **2011**, *133*, 14710–14726. [CrossRef]
272. Miguel-Gordo, M.; Gegunde, S.; Jennings, L.K.; Genta-Jouve, G.; Calabro, K.; Alfonso, A.; Botana, L.M.; Thomas, O.P. Futunamine, a Pyrrole–Imidazole Alkaloid from the Sponge *Stylissa* aff. *carteri* Collected off the Futuna Islands. *J. Nat. Prod.* **2020**, *83*, 2299–2304. [CrossRef]
273. Kusama, T.; Tanaka, N.; Takahashi-Nakaguchi, A.; Gonoi, T.; Fromont, J.; Kobayashi, J.i. Bromopyrrole Alkaloids from a Marine Sponge *Agelas* sp. *Chem. Pharm. Bull.* **2014**, *62*, 499–503. [CrossRef]
274. Muñoz, J.; Köck, M. Hybrid Pyrrole–Imidazole Alkaloids from the Sponge *Agelas sceptrum*1. *J. Nat. Prod.* **2016**, *79*, 434–437. [CrossRef]
275. Endo, T.; Tsuda, M.; Okada, T.; Mitsuhashi, S.; Shima, H.; Kikuchi, K.; Mikami, Y.; Fromont, J.; Kobayashi, J.i. Nagelamides A−H, New Dimeric Bromopyrrole Alkaloids from Marine Sponge *Agelas* Species. *J. Nat. Prod.* **2004**, *67*, 1262–1267. [CrossRef]
276. Bhandari, M.R.; Sivappa, R.; Lovely, C.J. Total Synthesis of the Putative Structure of Nagelamide D. *Org. Lett.* **2009**, *11*, 1535–1538. [CrossRef]
277. Bhandari, M.R.; Herath, A.K.; Rasapalli, S.; Yousufuddin, M.; Lovely, C.J. Total Synthesis of the Nagelamides – Synthetic Studies toward the Reported Structure of Nagelamide D and Nagelamide E Framework. *J. Org. Chem.* **2020**, *85*, 12971–12987. [CrossRef]
278. Iwai, T.; Kubota, T.; Fromont, J.; Kobayashi, J.i. Nagelamide I and 2,2′-Didebromonagelamide B, New Dimeric Bromopyrrole–Imidazole Alkaloids from a Marine Sponge *Agelas* sp. *Chem. Pharm. Bull.* **2014**, *62*, 213–216. [CrossRef] [PubMed]
279. Tanaka, N.; Kusama, T.; Takahashi-Nakaguchi, A.; Gonoi, T.; Fromont, J.; Kobayashi, J.i. Nagelamides X–Z, Dimeric Bromopyrrole Alkaloids from a Marine Sponge *Agelas* sp. *Org. Lett.* **2013**, *15*, 3262–3265. [CrossRef] [PubMed]
280. Muñoz, J.; Moriou, C.; Gallard, J.-F.; Marie, P.D.; Al-Mourabit, A. Donnazoles A and B from *Axinella donnani* Sponge: Very Close Derivatives from the Postulated Intermediate 'Pre-axinellamine'. *Tetrahedron Lett.* **2012**, *53*, 5828–5832. [CrossRef]
281. Kusama, T.; Tanaka, N.; Sakai, K.; Gonoi, T.; Fromont, J.; Kashiwada, Y.; Kobayashi, J.I. Agelamadins C–E, Bromopyrrole Alkaloids Comprising Oroidin and 3-Hydroxykynurenine from a Marine Sponge *Agelas* sp. *Org. Lett.* **2014**, *16*, 5176–5179. [CrossRef]
282. Yabuuchi, T.; Kusumi, T. Phenylglycine Methyl Ester, a Useful Tool for Absolute Configuration Determination of Various Chiral Carboxylic Acids. *J. Org. Chem.* **2000**, *65*, 397–404. [CrossRef]
283. Bailly, C. Lamellarins: A Tribe of Bioactive Marine Natural Products. In *Outstanding Marine Molecules*; La Barre, S., Kornprobst, J.-M., Eds.; Wiley-VCH: Weinheim, Germany, 2014; pp. 377–386.
284. Sharma, V.; Kumar, V. Indolizine: A Biologically Active Moiety. *Med. Chem. Res.* **2014**, *23*, 3593–3606. [CrossRef]
285. Greger, H. Structural Classification and Biological Activities of *Stemona* Alkaloids. *Phytochem. Rev.* **2019**, *18*, 463–493. [CrossRef]
286. Fehér, D.; Barlow, R.; McAtee, J.; Hemscheidt, T.K. Highly Brominated Antimicrobial Metabolites from a Marine *Pseudoalteromonas* sp. *J. Nat. Prod.* **2010**, *73*, 1963–1966. [CrossRef] [PubMed]
287. Alvarez-Mico, X.; Jensen, P.R.; Fenical, W.; Hughes, C.C. Chlorizidine, a Cytotoxic 5H-Pyrrolo[2,1-a]isoindol-5-one-Containing Alkaloid from a Marine *Streptomyces* sp. *Org. Lett.* **2013**, *15*, 988–991. [CrossRef] [PubMed]
288. Jovanovic, M.; Petkovic, M.; Jovanovic, P.; Simic, M.; Tasic, G.; Eric, S.; Savic, V. Proline Derived Bicyclic Derivatives Through Metal Catalysed Cyclisations of Allenes: Synthesis of Longamide B, Stylisine D and their Derivatives. *Eur. J. Org. Chem.* **2020**, *2020*, 295–305. [CrossRef]

289. Plisson, F.; Prasad, P.; Xiao, X.; Piggott, A.M.; Huang, X.-c.; Khalil, Z.; Capon, R.J. Callyspongisines A–D: Bromopyrrole Alkaloids from an Australian Marine Sponge, *Callyspongia* sp. *Org. Biomol. Chem.* **2014**, *12*, 1579–1584. [CrossRef]
290. Abdjul, D.; Yamazaki, H.; Kanno, S.-I.; Tomizawa, A.; Rotinsulu, H.; Wewengkang, D.; Sumilat, D.; Ukai, K.; Kapojos, M.; Namikoshi, M. An Anti-mycobacterial Bisfunctionalized Sphingolipid and New Bromopyrrole Alkaloid from the Indonesian Marine Sponge *Agelas* sp. *J. Nat. Med.* **2017**, *71*, 531–536. [CrossRef] [PubMed]
291. Iwata, M.; Kamijoh, Y.; Yamamoto, E.; Yamanaka, M.; Nagasawa, K. Total Synthesis of Pyrrole–Imidazole Alkaloid (+)-Cylindradine B. *Org. Lett.* **2017**, *19*, 420–423. [CrossRef] [PubMed]
292. Kuramoto, M.; Miyake, N.; Ishimaru, Y.; Ono, N.; Uno, H. Cylindradines A and B: Novel Bromopyrrole Alkaloids from the Marine Sponge *Axinella cylindratus*. *Org. Lett.* **2008**, *10*, 5465–5468. [CrossRef]
293. Buchanan, M.S.; Carroll, A.R.; Quinn, R.J. Revised Structure of Palau'amine. *Tetrahedron Lett.* **2007**, *48*, 4573–4574. [CrossRef]
294. Tsukamoto, S.; Katsuki, A.; Kato, H.; Ise, Y.; Losung, F.; Mangindaan, R. Agesamines A and B, New Dibromopyrrole Alkaloids from the Sponge *Agelas* sp. *Heterocycles* **2019**, *98*, 558. [CrossRef]
295. Tilvi, S.; Moriou, C.; Martin, M.-T.; Gallard, J.-F.; Sorres, J.; Patel, K.; Petek, S.; Debitus, C.; Ermolenko, L.; Al-Mourabit, A. Agelastatin E, Agelastatin F, and Benzosceptrin C from the Marine Sponge *Agelas dendromorpha*. *J. Nat. Prod.* **2010**, *73*, 720–723. [CrossRef] [PubMed]
296. Movassaghi, M.; Siegel, D.S.; Han, S. Total Synthesis of All (−)-Agelastatin Alkaloids. *Chem. Sci.* **2010**, *1*, 561–566. [CrossRef]
297. Sauleau, P.; Moriou, C.; Al Mourabit, A. Metabolomics Approach to Chemical Diversity of the Mediterranean Marine Sponge *Agelas oroides*. *Nat. Prod. Res.* **2017**, *31*, 1625–1632. [CrossRef]
298. Kusama, T.; Tanaka, N.; Sakai, K.; Gonoi, T.; Fromont, J.; Kashiwada, Y.; Kobayashi, J.i. Agelamadins A and B, Dimeric Bromopyrrole Alkaloids from a Marine Sponge *Agelas* sp. *Org. Lett.* **2014**, *16*, 3916–3918. [CrossRef]
299. Fouad, M.A.; Debbab, A.; Wray, V.; Müller, W.E.G.; Proksch, P. New Bioactive Alkaloids from the Marine Sponge *Stylissa* sp. *Tetrahedron* **2012**, *68*, 10176–10179. [CrossRef]
300. Singh, R.P.; Bhandari, M.R.; Torres, F.M.; Doundoulakis, T.; Gout, D.; Lovely, C.J. Total Synthesis of (±)-2-Debromohymenin via Gold-Catalyzed Intramolecular Alkyne Hydroarylation. *Org. Lett.* **2020**, *22*, 3412–3417. [CrossRef]
301. Beniddir, M.A.; Evanno, L.; Joseph, D.; Skiredj, A.; Poupon, E. Emergence of Diversity and Stereochemical Outcomes in the Biosynthetic Pathways of Cyclobutane-centered Marine Alkaloid Dimers. *Nat. Prod. Rep.* **2016**, *33*, 820–842. [CrossRef]
302. Bernan, V.S.; Roll, D.M.; Ireland, C.M.; Greenstein, M.; Maiese, W.M.; Steinberg, D.A. A Study on the Mechanism of Action of Sceptrin, an Antimicrobial Agent Isolated from the South Pacific Sponge *Agelas mauritiana*. *J. Antimicrob. Chemother.* **1993**, *32*, 539–550. [CrossRef]
303. Bickmeyer, U.; Drechsler, C.; Köck, M.; Assmann, M. Brominated Pyrrole Alkaloids from Marine *Agelas* Sponges Reduce Depolarization-induced Cellular Calcium Elevation. *Toxicon* **2004**, *44*, 45–51. [CrossRef] [PubMed]
304. Mohammed, R.; Peng, J.; Kelly, M.; Hamann, M.T. Cyclic Heptapeptides from the Jamaican Sponge *Stylissa caribica*. *J. Nat. Prod.* **2006**, *69*, 1739–1744. [CrossRef]
305. Sun, Y.-T.; Lin, B.; Li, S.-G.; Liu, M.; Zhou, Y.-J.; Xu, Y.; Hua, H.-M.; Lin, H.-W. New Bromopyrrole Alkaloids from the Marine Sponge *Agelas* sp. *Tetrahedron* **2017**, *73*, 2786–2792. [CrossRef]
306. Eder, C.; Proksch, P.; Wray, V.; van Soest, R.W.M.; Ferdinandus, E.; Pattisina, L.A. Sudarsono New Bromopyrrole Alkaloids from the Indopacific Sponge *Agelas nakamurai*. *J. Nat. Prod.* **1999**, *62*, 1295–1297. [CrossRef] [PubMed]
307. Kwon, O.-S.; Kim, D.; Kim, H.; Lee, Y.-J.; Lee, H.-S.; Sim, C.J.; Oh, D.-C.; Lee, S.K.; Oh, K.-B.; Shin, J. Bromopyrrole Alkaloids from the Sponge *Agelas kosrae*. *Mar. Drugs* **2018**, *16*, 513. [CrossRef] [PubMed]
308. Li, T.; Tang, X.; Luo, X.; Wang, Q.; Liu, K.; Zhang, Y.; de Voogd, N.J.; Yang, J.; Li, P.; Li, G. Agelanemoechine, a Dimeric Bromopyrrole Alkaloid with a Pro-Angiogenic Effect from the South China Sea Sponge *Agelas nemoechinata*. *Org. Lett.* **2019**, *21*, 9483–9486. [CrossRef]
309. Nguyen, L.V.; Jamison, T.F. Total Synthesis of (±)-Sceptrin. *Org. Lett.* **2020**, *22*, 6698–6702. [CrossRef]
310. Baran, P.S.; Zografos, A.L.; O'Malley, D.P. Short Total Synthesis of (±)-Sceptrin. *J. Am. Chem. Soc.* **2004**, *126*, 3726–3727. [CrossRef]
311. Birman, V.B.; Jiang, X.-T. Synthesis of Sceptrin Alkaloids. *Org. Lett.* **2004**, *6*, 2369–2371. [CrossRef] [PubMed]
312. Ma, Z.; Wang, X.; Wang, X.; Rodriguez, R.A.; Moore, C.E.; Gao, S.; Tan, X.; Ma, Y.; Rheingold, A.L.; Baran, P.S.; et al. Asymmetric Syntheses of Sceptrin and Massadine and Evidence for Biosynthetic Enantiodivergence. *Science* **2014**, *346*, 219–224. [CrossRef]
313. Lee, Y.-J.; Kim, S.H.; Choi, H.; Lee, H.-S.; Lee, J.S.; Shin, H.J.; Lee, J. Cytotoxic Furan- and Pyrrole-Containing Scalarane Sesterterpenoids Isolated from the Sponge *Scalarispongia* sp. *Molecules* **2019**, *24*, 840. [CrossRef]
314. Han, W.B.; Lu, Y.H.; Zhang, A.H.; Zhang, G.F.; Mei, Y.N.; Jiang, N.; Lei, X.; Song, Y.C.; Ng, S.W.; Tan, R.X. Curvulamine, a New Antibacterial Alkaloid Incorporating Two Undescribed Units from a *Curvularia* Species. *Org. Lett.* **2014**, *16*, 5366–5369. [CrossRef] [PubMed]
315. Hwang, B.S.; Oh, J.S.; Jeong, E.J.; Sim, C.J.; Rho, J.-R. Densanins A and B, New Macrocyclic Pyrrole Alkaloids Isolated from the Marine Sponge *Haliclona densaspicula*. *Org. Lett.* **2012**, *14*, 6154–6157. [CrossRef] [PubMed]
316. Garg, N.K.; Hiebert, S.; Overman, L.E. Total Synthesis of (−)-Sarain A. *Angew. Chem. Int. Ed.* **2006**, *45*, 2912–2915. [CrossRef]
317. Toma, T.; Kita, Y.; Fukuyama, T. Total Synthesis of (+)-Manzamine A. *J. Am. Chem. Soc.* **2010**, *132*, 10233–10235. [CrossRef]
318. Defant, A.; Mancini, I.; Raspor, L.; Guella, G.; Turk, T.; Sepčić, K. New Structural Insights into Saraines A, B, and C, Macrocyclic Alkaloids from the Mediterranean Sponge *Reniera* (*Haliclona*) *sarai*. *Eur. J. Org. Chem.* **2011**, *2011*, 3761–3767. [CrossRef]
319. Haelsig, K.T.; Xuan, J.; Maimone, T.J. Total Synthesis of (−)-Curvulamine. *J. Am. Chem. Soc.* **2020**, *142*, 1206–1210. [CrossRef]

320. Xuan, J.; Haelsig, K.T.; Sheremet, M.; Machicao, P.A.; Maimone, T.J. Evolution of a Synthetic Strategy for Complex Polypyrrole Alkaloids: Total Syntheses of Curvulamine and Curindolizine. *J. Am. Chem. Soc.* **2021**, *143*, 2970–2983. [CrossRef] [PubMed]
321. Shi, S.; Shi, H.; Li, J.; Li, F.; Chen, L.; Zhang, C.; Huang, Z.; Zhao, N.; Li, N.; Yang, J. Synthesis of the BCD Tricyclic Core of Densanins A and B. *Org. Lett.* **2016**, *18*, 1949–1951. [CrossRef]
322. Yu, H.; Yasuyuki, K. Pyrroloiminoquinone Alkaloids: Discorhabdins and Makaluvamines. *Curr. Org. Chem.* **2005**, *9*, 1567–1588.
323. Hu, J.-F.; Fan, H.; Xiong, J.; Wu, S.-B. Discorhabdins and Pyrroloiminoquinone-Related Alkaloids. *Chem. Rev.* **2011**, *111*, 5465–5491. [CrossRef]
324. Wada, Y.; Harayama, Y.; Kamimura, D.; Yoshida, M.; Shibata, T.; Fujiwara, K.; Morimoto, K.; Fujioka, H.; Kita, Y. The Synthetic and Biological Studies of Discorhabdins and Related Compounds. *Org. Biomol. Chem.* **2011**, *9*, 4959–4976. [CrossRef]
325. Zlotkowski, K.; Hewitt, W.M.; Yan, P.; Bokesch, H.R.; Peach, M.L.; Nicklaus, M.C.; O'Keefe, B.R.; McMahon, J.B.; Gustafson, K.R.; Schneekloth, J.S. Macrophilone A: Structure Elucidation, Total Synthesis, and Functional Evaluation of a Biologically Active Iminoquinone from the Marine Hydroid *Macrorhynchia philippina*. *Org. Lett.* **2017**, *19*, 1726–1729. [CrossRef]
326. Yan, P.; Ritt, D.A.; Zlotkowski, K.; Bokesch, H.R.; Reinhold, W.C.; Schneekloth, J.S.; Morrison, D.K.; Gustafson, K.R. Macrophilones from the Marine Hydroid Macrorhynchia philippina Can Inhibit ERK Cascade Signaling. *J. Nat. Prod.* **2018**, *81*, 1666–1672. [CrossRef]
327. Kalinski, J.-C.J.; Waterworth, S.C.; Siwe Noundou, X.; Jiwaji, M.; Parker-Nance, S.; Krause, R.W.M.; McPhail, K.L.; Dorrington, R.A. Molecular Networking Reveals Two Distinct Chemotypes in Pyrroloiminoquinone-Producing *Tsitsikamma favus* Sponges. *Mar. Drugs* **2019**, *17*, 60. [CrossRef]
328. Taufa, T.; Gordon, R.M.A.; Hashmi, M.A.; Hira, K.; Miller, J.H.; Lein, M.; Fromont, J.; Northcote, P.T.; Keyzers, R.A. Pyrroloquinoline Derivatives from a Tongan Specimen of the Marine Sponge *Strongylodesma tongaensis*. *Tetrahedron Lett.* **2019**, *60*, 1825–1829. [CrossRef]
329. Genta-Jouve, G.; Francezon, N.; Puissant, A.; Auberger, P.; Vacelet, J.; Pérez, T.; Fontana, A.; Mourabit, A.A.; Thomas, O.P. Structure Elucidation of the New Citharoxazole from the Mediterranean Deep-sea Sponge *Latrunculia (Biannulata) citharistae*. *Magn. Reson. Chem.* **2011**, *49*, 533–536. [CrossRef] [PubMed]
330. Zou, Y.; Hamann, M.T. Atkamine: A New Pyrroloiminoquinone Scaffold from the Cold Water Aleutian Islands Latrunculia Sponge. *Org. Lett.* **2013**, *15*, 1516–1519. [CrossRef] [PubMed]
331. Iwao, M.; Motoi, O.; Fukuda, T.; Ishibashi, F. New Synthetic Approach to Pyrroloiminoquinone Marine Alkaloids. Total Synthesis of Makaluvamines A, D, I, and K. *Tetrahedron* **1998**, *54*, 8999–9010. [CrossRef]
332. Kraus, G.A.; Selvakumar, N. Synthetic Routes to Pyrroloiminoquinone Alkaloids. A Direct Synthesis of Makaluvamine C. *J. Org. Chem.* **1998**, *63*, 9846–9849. [CrossRef]
333. Sadanandan, E.V.; Cava, M.P. Total Syntheses of Damirone A and Damirone B. *Tetrahedron Lett.* **1993**, *34*, 2405–2408. [CrossRef]
334. Roberts, D.; Joule, J.A.; Bros, M.A.; Alvarez, M. Synthesis of Pyrrolo[4,3,2-de]quinolines from 6,7-Dimethoxy-4-methylquinoline. Formal Total Syntheses of Damirones A and B, Batzelline C, Isobatzelline C, Discorhabdin C, and Makaluvamines A−D. *J. Org. Chem.* **1997**, *62*, 568–577. [CrossRef]
335. Liang Tao, X.; Cheng, J.-F.; Nishiyama, S.; Yamamura, S. Synthetic Studies on Tetrahydropyrroloquinoline-containing Natural Products: Syntheses of Discorhabdin C, Batzelline C and Isobatzelline C. *Tetrahedron* **1994**, *50*, 2017–2028. [CrossRef]
336. Alvarez, M.; Bros, M.A.; Gras, G.; Ajana, W.; Joule, J.A. Syntheses of Batzelline A, Batzeline B, Isobatzelline A, and Isobatzelline B. *Eur. J. Org. Chem.* **1999**, *1999*, 1173–1183. [CrossRef]
337. Oshiyama, T.; Satoh, T.; Okano, K.; Tokuyama, H. Total Synthesis of Makaluvamine A/D, Damirone B, Batzelline C, Makaluvone, and Isobatzelline C Featuring One-pot Benzyne-mediated Cyclization–functionalization. *Tetrahedron* **2012**, *68*, 9376–9383. [CrossRef]
338. Tidwell, J.H.; Buchwald, S.L. Synthesis of Polysubstituted Indoles and Indolines by Means of Zirconocene-Stabilized Benzyne Complexes. *J. Am. Chem. Soc.* **1994**, *116*, 11797–11810. [CrossRef]
339. Backenköhler, J.; Spindler, S.; Spiteller, P. Total Synthesis of Damirone C, Makaluvamine O, Makaluvone, Batzelline C and Batzelline D. *ChemistrySelect* **2017**, *2*, 2589–2592. [CrossRef]
340. Li, F.; Janussen, D.; Peifer, C.; Pérez-Victoria, I.; Tasdemir, D. Targeted Isolation of Tsitsikammamines from the Antarctic Deep-Sea Sponge *Latrunculia biformis* by Molecular Networking and Anticancer Activity. *Mar. Drugs* **2018**, *16*, 268. [CrossRef] [PubMed]
341. Davis, R.A.; Buchanan, M.S.; Duffy, S.; Avery, V.M.; Charman, S.A.; Charman, W.N.; White, K.L.; Shackleford, D.M.; Edstein, M.D.; Andrews, K.T.; et al. Antimalarial Activity of Pyrroloiminoquinones from the Australian Marine Sponge *Zyzzya* sp. *J. Med. Chem.* **2012**, *55*, 5851–5858. [CrossRef] [PubMed]
342. Davis, R.A.; Duffy, S.; Fletcher, S.; Avery, V.M.; Quinn, R.J. Thiaplakortones A–D: Antimalarial Thiazine Alkaloids from the Australian Marine Sponge *Plakortis lita*. *J. Org. Chem.* **2013**, *78*, 9608–9613. [CrossRef] [PubMed]
343. Pouwer, R.H.; Deydier, S.M.; Le, P.V.; Schwartz, B.D.; Franken, N.C.; Davis, R.A.; Coster, M.J.; Charman, S.A.; Edstein, M.D.; Skinner-Adams, T.S.; et al. Total Synthesis of Thiaplakortone A: Derivatives as Metabolically Stable Leads for the Treatment of Malaria. *ACS Med. Chem. Lett.* **2014**, *5*, 178–182. [CrossRef] [PubMed]
344. Nadkarni, D.H.; Murugesan, S.; Velu, S.E. Total Synthesis of Zyzzyanones A–D. *Tetrahedron* **2013**, *69*, 4105–4113. [CrossRef]
345. Sadanandan, E.V.; Pillai, S.K.; Lakshmikantham, M.V.; Billimoria, A.D.; Culpepper, J.S.; Cava, M.P. Efficient Syntheses of the Marine Alkaloids Makaluvamine D and Discorhabdin C: The 4,6,7-Trimethoxyindole Approach. *J. Org. Chem.* **1995**, *60*, 1800–1805. [CrossRef]

346. Perry, N.B.; Blunt, J.W.; McCombs, J.D.; Munro, M.H.G. Discorhabdin C, a Highly Cytotoxic Pigment from a Sponge of the Genus *Latrunculia*. *J. Org. Chem.* **1986**, *51*, 5476–5478. [CrossRef]
347. Makar'eva, T.N.; Krasokhin, V.B.; Guzii, A.G.; Stonik, V.A. Strong Ethanol Solvate of Discorhabdin, Isolated from the Far-east Sponge *Latruculia oparinae*. *Chem. Nat. Compd.* **2010**, *46*, 152–153. [CrossRef]
348. Na, M.; Ding, Y.; Wang, B.; Tekwani, B.L.; Schinazi, R.F.; Franzblau, S.; Kelly, M.; Stone, R.; Li, X.-C.; Ferreira, D.; et al. Anti-infective Discorhabdins from a Deep-Water Alaskan Sponge of the Genus *Latrunculia*. *J. Nat. Prod.* **2010**, *73*, 383–387. [CrossRef]
349. Copp, B.R.; Fulton, K.F.; Perry, N.B.; Blunt, J.W.; Munro, M.H.G. Natural and Synthetic Derivatives of Discorhabdin C, a Cytotoxic Pigment from the New Zealand Sponge *Latrunculia cf. bocagei*. *J. Org. Chem.* **1994**, *59*, 8233–8238. [CrossRef]
350. Grkovic, T.; Pearce, A.N.; Munro, M.H.G.; Blunt, J.W.; Davies-Coleman, M.T.; Copp, B.R. Isolation and Characterization of Diastereomers of Discorhabdins H and K and Assignment of Absolute Configuration to Discorhabdins D, N, Q, S, T, and U. *J. Nat. Prod.* **2010**, *73*, 1686–1693. [CrossRef]
351. Aubart, K.M.; Heathcock, C.H. A Biomimetic Approach to the Discorhabdin Alkaloids: Total Syntheses of Discorhabdins C and E and Dethiadiscorhabdin D. *J. Org. Chem.* **1999**, *64*, 16–22. [CrossRef]
352. Jeon, J.-e.; Na, Z.; Jung, M.; Lee, H.-S.; Sim, C.J.; Nahm, K.; Oh, K.-B.; Shin, J. Discorhabdins from the Korean Marine Sponge *Sceptrella* sp. *J. Nat. Prod.* **2010**, *73*, 258–262. [CrossRef]
353. Li, F.; Peifer, C.; Janussen, D.; Tasdemir, D. New Discorhabdin Alkaloids from the Antarctic Deep-Sea Sponge *Latrunculia biformis*. *Mar. Drugs* **2019**, *17*, 439. [CrossRef] [PubMed]
354. Zou, Y.; Wang, X.; Sims, J.; Wang, B.; Pandey, P.; Welsh, C.L.; Stone, R.P.; Avery, M.A.; Doerksen, R.J.; Ferreira, D.; et al. Computationally Assisted Discovery and Assignment of a Highly Strained and PANC-1 Selective Alkaloid from Alaska's Deep Ocean. *J. Am. Chem. Soc.* **2019**, *141*, 4338–4344. [CrossRef]
355. Hinshaw, B.C.; Gerster, J.F.; Robins, R.K.; Townsend, L.B. Pyrrolopyrimidine nucleosides. V. Relative Chemical Reactivity of the 5-Cyano Group of the Nucleoside Antibiotic Toyocamycin and Desaminotoyocamycin. Synthesis of Analogs of Sangivamycin. *J. Org. Chem.* **1970**, *35*, 236–241. [CrossRef]
356. Wang, D.; Feng, Y.; Murtaza, M.; Wood, S.; Mellick, G.; Hooper, J.N.A.; Quinn, R.J. A Grand Challenge: Unbiased Phenotypic Function of Metabolites from *Jaspis splendens* against Parkinson's Disease. *J. Nat. Prod.* **2016**, *79*, 353–361. [CrossRef]
357. Shubina, L.K.; Makarieva, T.N.; Yashunsky, D.V.; Nifantiev, N.E.; Denisenko, V.A.; Dmitrenok, P.S.; Dyshlovoy, S.A.; Fedorov, S.N.; Krasokhin, V.B.; Jeong, S.H.; et al. Pyridine Nucleosides Neopetrosides A and B from a Marine *Neopetrosia* sp. Sponge. Synthesis of Neopetroside A and Its β-Riboside Analogue. *J. Nat. Prod.* **2015**, *78*, 1383–1389. [CrossRef]
358. Leontein, K.; Lindberg, B.; Lönngren, J. Assignment of Absolute Configuration of Sugars by g.l.c. of their Acetylated Glycosides formed from Chiral Alcohols. *Carbohydr. Res.* **1978**, *62*, 359–362. [CrossRef]
359. Vien, L.T.; Hanh, T.T.H.; Huong, P.T.T.; Dang, N.H.; Thanh, N.V.; Lyakhova, E.; Cuong, N.X.; Nam, N.H.; Kiem, P.V.; Kicha, A.; et al. Pyrrole Oligoglycosides from the Starfish *Acanthaster planci* Suppress Lipopolysaccharide-Induced Nitric Oxide Production in RAW264.7 Macrophages. *Chem. Pharm. Bull.* **2016**, *64*, 1654–1657. [CrossRef]
360. Zhang, F.; Braun, D.R.; Chanana, S.; Rajski, S.R.; Bugni, T.S. Phallusialides A–E, Pyrrole-Derived Alkaloids Discovered from a Marine-Derived *Micromonospora* sp. Bacterium Using MS-Based Metabolomics Approaches. *J. Nat. Prod.* **2019**, *82*, 3432–3439. [CrossRef]
361. Fernández, R.; Bayu, A.; Aryono Hadi, T.; Bueno, S.; Pérez, M.; Cuevas, C.; Yunovilsa Putra, M. Unique Polyhalogenated Peptides from the Marine Sponge *Ircinia* sp. *Mar. Drugs* **2020**, *18*, 396. [CrossRef]
362. Marfey, P. Determination of D-amino acids. II. Use of a Bifunctional Reagent, 1,5-Difluoro-2,4-dinitrobenzene. *Carlsberg Res. Commun.* **1984**, *49*, 591. [CrossRef]
363. Bae, M.; Chung, B.; Oh, K.-B.; Shin, J.; Oh, D.-C. Hormaomycins B and C: New Antibiotic Cyclic Depsipeptides from a Marine Mudflat-Derived *Streptomyces* sp. *Mar. Drugs* **2015**, *13*, 5187–5200. [CrossRef] [PubMed]
364. Clark, W.D.; Corbett, T.; Valeriote, F.; Crews, P. Cyclocinamide A. An Unusual Cytotoxic Halogenated Hexapeptide from the Marine Sponge *Psammocinia*. *J. Am. Chem. Soc.* **1997**, *119*, 9285–9286. [CrossRef]
365. Cooper, J.K.; Li, K.; Aubé, J.; Coppage, D.A.; Konopelski, J.P. Application of the DP4 Probability Method to Flexible Cyclic Peptides with Multiple Independent Stereocenters: The True Structure of Cyclocinamide A. *Org. Lett.* **2018**, *20*, 4314–4317. [CrossRef] [PubMed]

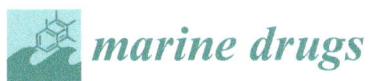

Article

New Prenylated Indole Homodimeric and Pteridine Alkaloids from the Marine-Derived Fungus *Aspergillus austroafricanus* Y32-2

Peihai Li [1,2,3,†], Mengqi Zhang [1,2,3,†], Haonan Li [1], Rongchun Wang [1,3], Hairong Hou [1,3], Xiaobin Li [1,3,*], Kechun Liu [1,3,*] and Hao Chen [4,*]

1. Engineering Research Center of Zebrafish Models for Human Diseases and Drug Screening of Shandong Province, Shandong Provincial Engineering Laboratory for Biological Testing Technology, Biology Institute, Qilu University of Technology (Shandong Academy of Sciences), Jinan 250103, China; liph@sdas.org (P.L.); mengqi@sdas.org (M.Z.); 17862958363@163.com (H.L.); wangrc@sdas.org (R.W.); houhr@sdas.org (H.H.)
2. State Key Laboratory of Biobased Material and Green Papermaking, Qilu University of Technology (Shandong Academy of Sciences), Jinan 250353, China
3. Key Laboratory for Biosensor of Shandong Province, Biology Institute, Qilu University of Technology (Shandong Academy of Sciences), Jinan 250103, China
4. Key Laboratory of Marine Bioactive Substances, First Institute of Oceanography, Ministry of Natural Resources, Qingdao 266061, China
* Correspondence: lixb@sdas.org (X.L.); hliukch@sdas.org (K.L.); hchen@fio.org.cn (H.C.); Tel./Fax: +86-531-82605352 (X.L.); +86-531-82605331 (K.L.); +86-532-88963855 (H.C.)
† These authors contributed equally to this work.

Citation: Li, P.; Zhang, M.; Li, H.; Wang, R.; Hou, H.; Li, X.; Liu, K.; Chen, H. New Prenylated Indole Homodimeric and Pteridine Alkaloids from the Marine-Derived Fungus *Aspergillus austroafricanus* Y32-2. *Mar. Drugs* **2021**, *19*, 98. https://doi.org/10.3390/md19020098

Academic Editor: Asunción Barbero

Received: 16 January 2021
Accepted: 5 February 2021
Published: 9 February 2021

Publisher's Note: MDPI stays neutral with regard to jurisdictional claims in published maps and institutional affiliations.

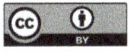

Copyright: © 2021 by the authors. Licensee MDPI, Basel, Switzerland. This article is an open access article distributed under the terms and conditions of the Creative Commons Attribution (CC BY) license (https://creativecommons.org/licenses/by/4.0/).

Abstract: Chemical investigation of secondary metabolites from the marine-derived fungus *Aspergillus austroafricanus* Y32-2 resulted in the isolation of two new prenylated indole alkaloid homodimers, di-6-hydroxydeoxybrevianamide E (**1**) and dinotoamide J (**2**), one new pteridine alkaloid asperpteridinate A (**3**), with eleven known compounds (**4–14**). Their structures were elucidated by various spectroscopic methods including HRESIMS and NMR, while their absolute configurations were determined by ECD calculations. Each compound was evaluated for pro-angiogenic, anti-inflammatory effects in zebrafish models and cytotoxicity for HepG2 human liver carcinoma cells. As a result, compounds **2**, **4**, **5**, **7**, **10** exhibited pro-angiogenic activity in a PTK787-induced vascular injury zebrafish model in a dose-dependent manner, compounds **7**, **8**, **10**, **11** displayed anti-inflammatory activity in a CuSO$_4$-induced zebrafish inflammation model, and compound **6** showed significant cytotoxicity against HepG2 cells with an IC$_{50}$ value of 30 μg/mL.

Keywords: marine-derived fungus; *Aspergillus austroafricanus*; novel bioactive metabolites; pro-angiogenesis; anti-inflammatory effects

1. Introduction

The ocean has the characteristics of high salinity, high pressure, low temperature, low oxygen content, and oligotrophic environment, which enables microorganisms to have unique metabolic adaptation mechanisms and produce natural products with novel structures and diverse bioactivities [1]. Marine-derived fungi have been found to be a rich source of natural products due to their complex genetic background and abundant metabolites [2]. In recent years, a large number of novel secondary metabolites, such as polyketides, alkaloids, terpenes, steroids, peptides, etc., have been discovered from marine-derived *Aspergillus* species [3], and showed diverse bioactivities like antibacterial, antitumor, antioxidant, and anti-inflammatory activities [4]. More than 80% natural products were directly or indirectly related to small molecule drugs for the treatment of various diseases in the last 30 years, and many marine alkaloids with bioactivities have been comprehensively studied for drug development [5,6].

In our previous study, a series of fungal secondary metabolites were isolated and characterized with antitumor or cardiovascular effects [7,8]. To discover more natural products with pharmacological activities from marine-derived fungi, the fungal strain *Aspergillus austroafricanus* Y32-2 has been isolated from a seawater sample collected from the Indian Ocean. Chemical investigation of the secondary metabolites of Y32-2 fermented on rice medium resulted in the isolation of fourteen compounds, including two new prenylated indole alkaloid homodimers and one new pteridine alkaloid, named di-6-hydroxydeoxybrevianamide E (**1**), dinotoamide J (**2**) and asperpteridinate A (**3**), along with eleven known compounds (**4–14**) [7,9–16] (Figure 1). Among them, compound **4** was isolated for the first time as a natural product.

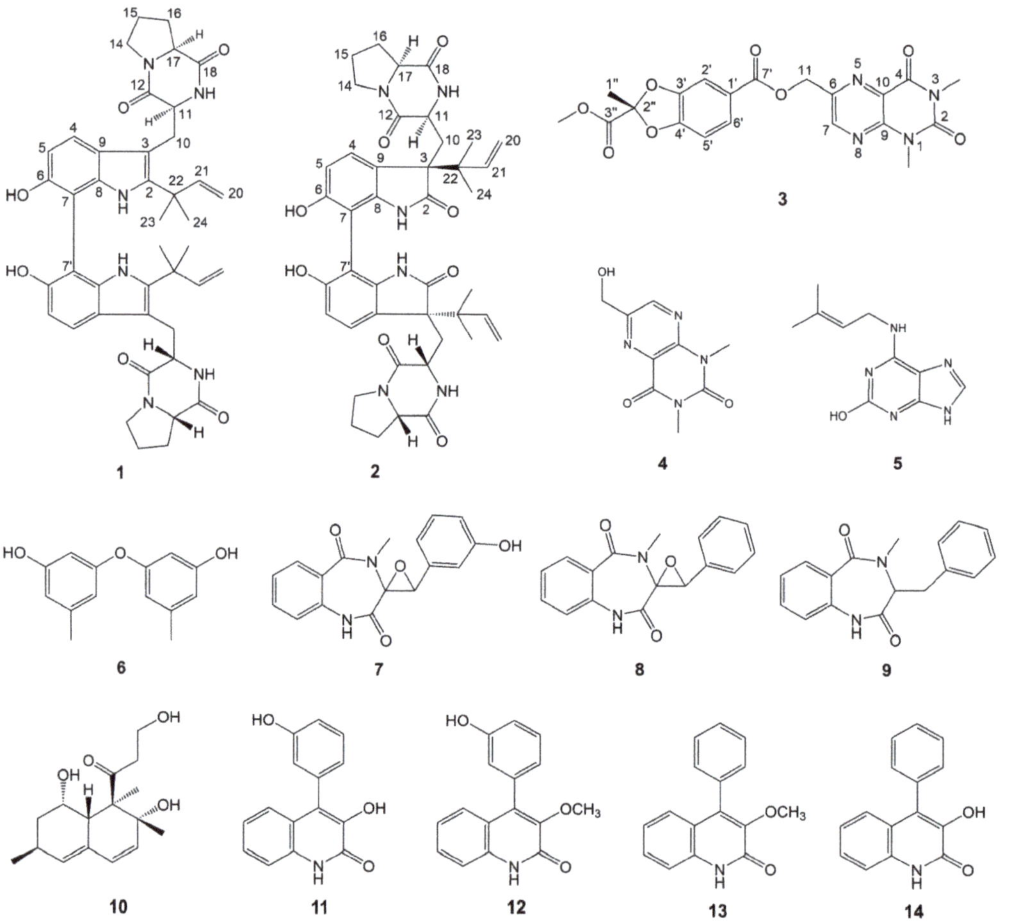

Figure 1. Structures of Compounds 1–14.

The prenylated indole alkaloids contain a bicyclo[2.2.2]diazaoctane or diketopiperazine ring, and has been reported to have antitumor, antibacterial, and insecticidal activities [17]. Here two new prenylated indole alkaloid homodimers and other isolated compounds were all tested for pro-angiogenic and anti-inflammatory effects in zebrafish models and cytotoxicity towards HepG2 human liver carcinoma cells. Compounds **2**, **4**, **5**, **7**, and **10** exhibited angiogenesis promoting activity in a dose-dependent manner. Compounds **7**, **8**, **10**, and **11** also displayed anti-inflammatory activity in a dose-dependent manner. In addition, compound **6** showed cytotoxicity against HepG2 cells. In this paper, the isolation, structure elucidation, and bioactivity of all isolated compounds are reported.

2. Results and Discussion

2.1. Structure Elucidation

Compound **1**, obtained as yellow amorphous powder, possessed a molecular formula of $C_{42}H_{48}N_6O_6$ by the negative HR-ESI-MS (m/z 731.3559 [M − H]$^-$, calculated 731.3557), requiring 22 unsaturations. The HPLC chromatographic behavior of **1** was unusual and existed always as a 1:1 inseparable mixture. Many of the NMR signals also appeared in pairs, hinting towards structural distinctiveness and complexity. The ^{1}H NMR spectrum (Table 1) in DMSO-d_6 of **1** showed two pairs of mutually coupled aromatic protons at δ_H 7.35, 7.37 (each H, d, J = 8.4 Hz) and 6.80, 6.81 (each H, d, J = 8.4 Hz), a set of vinyl proton signals at δ_H 6.15, 6.17 (each H, dd, J = 17.5, 10.7 Hz), 5.06 (2H, br d, J = 17.5 Hz) and 5.01 (2H, br d, J = 10.7 Hz), four methyl singlets at δ_H 1.42 (12H, s), as well as six active hydrogen signals at δ_H 9.09 (2H, br s), 8.45, 8.58 (each H, s) and 6.21, 6.30 (each H, s). The ^{13}C NMR spectrum (Table 1) showed four amidocarbonyl carbon signals at δ_C 169.3, 169.4 (C-18, 18′) and 165.6 (C-12, 12′, overlapped), twenty aromatic or olefinic carbon signals, containing four vinyl carbons at δ_C 146.4, 146.5 (C-21, 21′) and 111.29, 111.33 (C-20, 20′), and four nitrogen-bearing methine signals at δ_C 58.5 (C-17, 17′, overlapped) and 55.0, 55.3 (C-11, 11′). The above NMR features were similar to those of 6-hydroxydeoxybrevianamide E [18], a cyclic dipeptide produced by *Aspergillus* and *Penicillium* species, and a careful and rigorous analysis of the ^{1}H, ^{1}H-COSY and HMBC correlations (Figure 2) also supported this inference. However, there were two obvious differences in their NMR signals: (1) different substitution patterns on the indole ring; (2) most of the NMR signals in **1** appeared in pairs. Based on the HSQC and HMBC correlation, the C-7, 7′ (δ_C 104.0, 104.1) were aromatic quaternary carbon signals that were different from 6-hydroxydeoxybrevianamide E, confirmed that the positions C-7, 7′ of the indole ring were substituted. Considering its molecular formula, compound **1** was deduced as a dimer of 6-hydroxydeoxybrevianamide E via C-7 and C-7′. Due to a certain steric hindrance, the structure existed as a 1:1 mixture of inseparable rotamers. The relative configuration of the cyclic dipeptide moiety was determined by the NOESY correlation (Figure 2) of H-11 and H-17. Based on the relative configuration, two probable forms of its absolute configuration, 1a (11*S*, 17*S*, 11′*S*, 17′*S*) and 1b (11*R*, 17*R*, 11′*R*, 17′*R*), were respectively used for the ECD calculations, and the absolute configuration was assigned as 11*S*, 17*S*, 11′*S*, 17′*S* (Figure 3), which was in consistent with that of 6-hydroxydeoxybrevianamide E. Therefore, the structure of **1** was unequivocally established as shown in Figure 1 and named as di-6-hydroxydeoxybrevianamide E.

Table 1. 400 MHz ^{1}H and 150 MHz ^{13}C NMR data of compounds **1** and **2** in DMSO-d_6.

No.	1		2	
	δ_C Type	δ_H (Mult., J in Hz)	δ_C Type	δ_H (Mult., J in Hz)
2,2′	139.1, 139.2 C	—	180.1 C	—
3,3′	104.75, 104.82 C	—	55.9 C	—
4,4′	117.6, 117.8 CH	7.35, 7.37 (each H, d, 8.4)	126.0 CH	7.11 (2H, d, 8.2)
5,5′	109.9, 110.0 CH	6.80, 6.81 (each H, d, 8.4)	106.9 CH	6.39 (2H, d, 8.2)
6,6′	150.0, 150.1 C	—	155.7 C	—
7,7′	104.0, 104.1 C	—	104.0 C	—
8,8′	134.4, 134.5 C	—	143.4 C	—
9,9′	122.6, 122.7 C	—	118.4 C	—
10,10′	25.3, 25.4 CH$_2$	2.94, 3.52 (each 2H, m)	30.3 CH$_2$	2.03 (2H, dd, 14.7, 5.2) 2.80 (2H, dd, 14.7, 4.7)
11,11′	55.0, 55.3 CH	4.33, 4.38 (each H, dd, 9.2, 4.2)	52.6 CH	3.41 (2H, dd, 5.2, 4.7)

Table 1. Cont.

No.	1		2	
	δ_C Type	δ_H (Mult., J in Hz)	δ_C Type	δ_H (Mult., J in Hz)
12,12′	165.6 C	—	165.6 C	—
14,14′	44.8 CH$_2$	3.37, 3.47 (each 2H, m)	45.1 CH$_2$	3.23, 3.35 (each 2H, m)
15,15′	22.2 CH$_2$	1.75–1.91 (4H, m)	22.3 CH$_2$	1.67–1.79 (4H, m)
16,16′	27.6 CH$_2$	1.85, 2.12 (each 2H, m)	27.1 CH$_2$	1.77, 1.99 (each 2H, m)
17,17′	58.5 CH	4.22 (2H, t-like, 7.2)	58.3 CH	4.02 (2H, t-like, 7.6)
18,18′	169.3, 169.4 C	—	169.8 C	—
20,20′	111.29, 111.33 CH$_2$	5.01 (2H, br d, 10.7) 5.06 (2H, br d, 17.5)	112.6 CH$_2$	4.94 (2H, br d, 17.5) 5.00 (2H, br d, 10.9)
21,21′	146.4, 146.5 CH	6.15, 6.17 (each H, dd, 17.5, 10.7)	143.9 CH	6.15 (2H, dd, 17.5, 10.9)
22,22′	38.6, 38.7 C	—	42.2 C	—
23,23′	27.5, 27.6 CH$_3$	1.42 (6H, s)	21.1 CH$_3$	0.98 (6H, s)
24,24′	27.5, 27.6 CH$_3$	1.42 (6H, s)	22.6 CH$_3$	0.96 (6H, s)
1,1′-NH	—	8.45, 8.58 (each H, s)	—	9.31 (2H, s)
19,19′-NH	—	6.21, 6.30 (each H, s)	—	7.57 (2H, s)
6,6′-OH	—	9.09 (2H, br s)	—	9.28 (2H, br s)

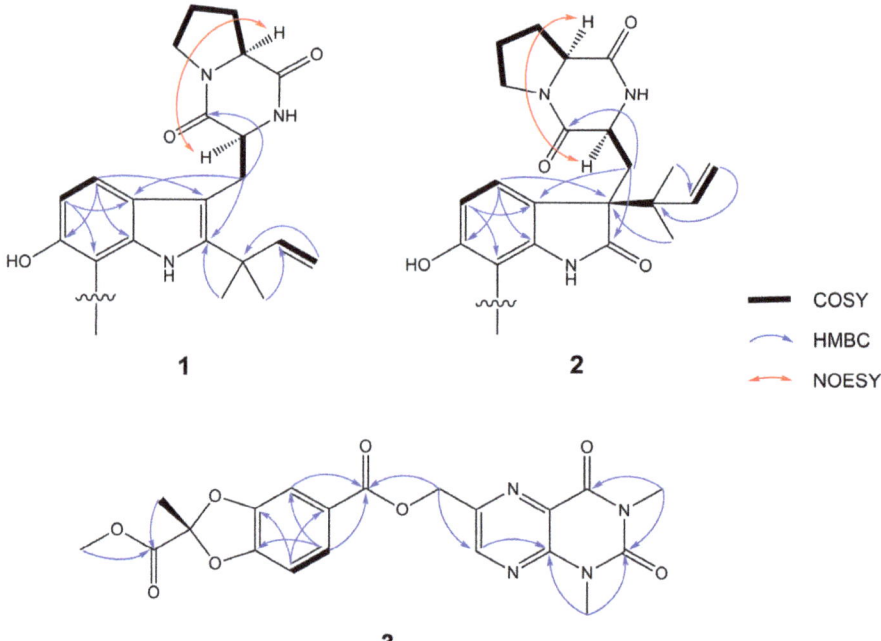

Figure 2. The ^{1}H, ^{1}H-correlation spectroscopy (^{1}H, ^{1}H-COSY), key heteronuclear multiple-bond correlation spectroscopy (HMBC) and nuclear overhauser effect spectroscopy (NOESY) correlations of compounds **1**, **2** (only half showed) and **3**.

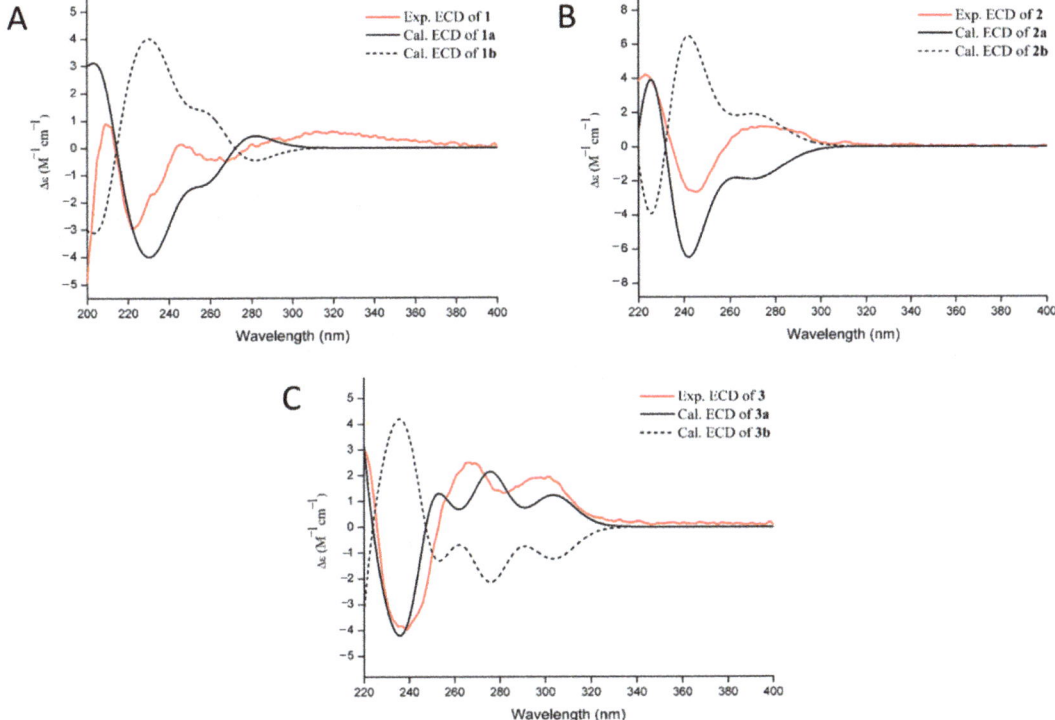

Figure 3. Measured CD and calculated equivalent circulating density (ECD) curves of compounds **1** (**A**), **2** (**B**) and **3** (**C**).

Compound **2** was obtained as a yellow amorphous powder. The molecular formula was determined to be $C_{42}H_{48}N_6O_8$ by the negative HRESIMS (m/z 763.3440 [M − H]$^-$, calculated 763.3456), indicating 22 degrees of unsaturation. The NMR spectra (Table 1) of **2** revealed 24 proton and 21 C-atom signals, suggesting **2** to be a symmetrical homodimer. The ^{1}H NMR spectrum for **2** showed two aromatic proton signals at δ_H 7.11 (1H, d, J = 8.2 Hz) and 6.39 (1H, d, J = 8.2 Hz), three vinyl proton signals at δ_H 4.94 (1H, br d, J = 17.5 Hz), 5.00 (1H, br d, J = 10.9 Hz) and 6.15 (1H, dd, J = 17.5, 10.9 Hz), two methyl singlets at δ_H 0.96 (3H, s), 0.98 (3H, s), as well as three active hydrogen signals at δ_H 7.57 (1H, s), 9.28 (1H, br s), and 9.31 (1H, s). The ^{13}C NMR data (Table 1) revealed the presence of three carbonyl carbon signals at δ_C 180.1 (C-2), 169.8 (C-18) and 165.6 (C-12), eight aromatic or olefinic carbon signals containing two vinyl carbons at δ_C 143.9 (C-21) and 112.6 (C-20), and two nitrogen-bearing methines at δ_C 58.3 (C-17) and 52.6 (C-11). Extensive comparison of the above NMR spectra with those of notoamide J [17] revealed that both structures were very similar, except for the substitution patterns on the C-7 position of indole ring. Considering its molecular formula, compound **2** was also identified as a homodimer of notoamide J via C-7 and C-7′. Due to one single signal set in the NMR spectrum, one single peak in the chiral column chromatography and less steric hindrance in the structure than compound **1**, it was deduced to be a freely rotating homologous dimer. With the aid of the ^{1}H, ^{1}H-COSY, HSQC and HMBC correlations, the planar structure of **2** was established as shown (Figure 1). The relative configuration of the cyclic dipeptide moiety was deduced by a NOESY correlation between H-11 and H-17, suggested that both protons had the same co-facial orientation. Because of the similar NMR data between **2** and notoamide J, the relative configuration of the positions C-3, C-11 and C-17 were determined to be similar to that of notoamide J [17]. By comparison of the experimental and calculated ECD spectra of **2**, the absolute configuration was tentatively assigned as 3R, 11S, 17S, 3′R, 11′S, and

17′S (Figure 3), which was also probably verified by the identical CD spectrum between **2** and notoamide J. So, the structure of **2** was tentatively assigned as shown in Figure 1 and named as dinotoamide J.

Asperpteridinate A was obtained as a yellow amorphous powder. The molecular formula $C_{20}H_{18}N_4O_8$ was assigned on the basis of the HRESIMS peak at m/z 465.1018 $[M + Na]^+$ (calcd. 465.1023), requiring 14 degrees of unsaturation. The ^{1}H NMR spectrum of **3** showed the signals for a 1,2,4-trisubstituted benzene ring system at δ_H 7.49 (1H, d, J = 1.4 Hz), 7.10 (1H, d, J = 8.3 Hz) and 7.65 (1H, dd, J = 8.3, 1.4 Hz), one vinyl proton at δ_H 8.94 (1H, s), three O-methyl or N-methyl at δ_H 3.74 (3H, s), 3.53 (3H, s), 3.31 (3H, s), one O-methylene at δ_H 5.49 (2H, s), one methyl at δ_H 1.90 (3H, s). The ^{13}C NMR data (Table 2) revealed the presence of four carbonyl at δ_C 150.6 (C-2), 159.7 (C-4), 164.8 (C-7′), 166.4 (C-3″), ten aromatic or olefinic carbons, containing four vinyl carbons at δ_C 145.8 (C-6), 147.2 (C-7), 147.7 (C-9), 127.2 (C-10), one O-methyl at δ_C 53.5 (O-CH3), one O-methylene at δ_C 64.7 (O-CH2-). ^{1}H and ^{13}C NMR (Table 2) spectra analysis revealed that some signals of **3** was similar to that of compound **4** [9] and 2, 2-dimethyl-1, 3-dioxa-benzo[d]pentane-6-carboxylic acid [19]. With the aid of the ^{1}H, ^{1}H-COSY, HSQC, and HMBC correlations, the structure of **3** was established as shown (Figures 1 and 2). The absolute configuration of **3** at C-2″ was also determined as 2″R by ECD calculations (Figure 3).

Table 2. 400 MHz ^{1}H and 150 MHz ^{13}C NMR data of compound **3** in DMSO-d_6.

No.	δ_C, Type	δ_H, (Mult., J Hz)
2	150.6 C	—
4	159.7 C	—
6	145.8 C	—
7	147.2 CH	8.94 (1H, s)
9	147.7 C	—
10	127.2 C	—
11	64.7 CH$_2$	5.49 (2H, s)
1′	123.6 C	—
2′	109.2 CH	7.49 (1H, d, 1.4)
3′	147.0 C	—
4′	150.9 C	—
5′	108.8 CH	7.10 (1H, d, 8.3)
6′	125.9 CH	7.65 (1H, dd, 8.3, 1.4)
7′	164.8 C	—
1″	21.7 CH$_3$	1.90 (3H, s)
2″	112.6 C	—
3″	166.4 C	—
N1-Me	29.2 CH$_3$	3.53 (3H, s)
N3-Me	28.7 CH$_3$	3.31 (3H, s)
3″-OMe	53.5 CH$_3$	3.74 (3H, s)

2.2. Biological Activity

In previous report, some alkaloids from marine-derived fungus showed pro-angiogenic activities in a zebrafish model [8]. We are also committed to find more marine natural products with angiogenesis related activity. In the present study, all isolated compounds were tested for the pro-angiogenic activities in a vatalanib (PTK787) induced vascular injury zebrafish model (Table S1). Compounds **5** and **7** (at concentrations of 30, 70 and 120 μg/mL) significantly promoted the angiogenesis, compounds **2** and **10** (70 and 120 μg/mL) also had effects, and compounds **4** (120 μg/mL) exhibited moderate effects (Figure 4). Compared to compound **7**, compounds **8** and **9** were inactive with respect to pro-angiogenesis, indicating that phenolic hydroxyl group is necessary for pro-angiogenic activity. All compounds were also evaluated for anti-inflammatory effects in $CuSO_4$-induced zebrafish inflammation model (Table S1). Compound **11** (30, 70, and 120 μg/mL) displayed potent anti-inflammatory activity, and compounds **7**, **8**, and **10** (70, and 120 μg/mL) had moderate effects (Figure 5). Compound **7** showed better anti-inflammatory activity than **8**, while **9** was ineffective, suggesting the phenolic hydroxyl group and the epoxide oxygen are important in the anti-inflammatory activity. Meanwhile, compared to compound **11**, compounds **12–14** displayed no anti-inflammatory activity, indicating that both phenolic and alcohol-hydroxyl groups are necessary for anti-inflammatory activity. In addition, all compounds were tested for cytotoxicity against human liver carcinoma cells HepG2 by MTT method (Table S1) [20], and compound **6** exhibit cytotoxicity with an IC_{50} value of 30 μg/mL (Figure S1). The pro-angiogenic, anti-inflammatory activities in zebrafish and cytotoxicity against HepG2 cells of these compounds were reported here for the first time.

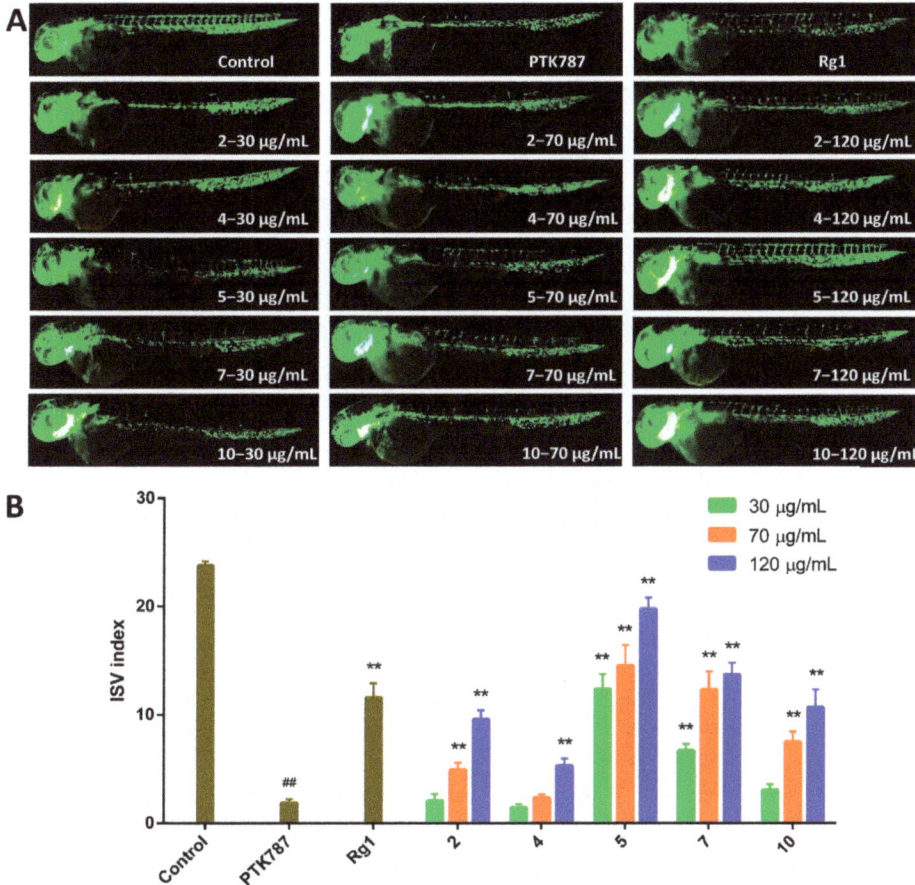

Figure 4. Results of pro-angiogenesis activities. (**A**) Typical images of intersomitic vessels (ISV) in transgenic fluorescent zebrafish (Tg (vegfr2: GFP)) treated with PTK787 and different concentrations (30, 70 and 120 μg/mL) of compounds **2**, **4**, **5**, **7**, and **10**, using ginsenoside Rg1 (120 μg/mL) as a positive control. (**B**) Quantitative analysis of the ISV index (number of intact vessels * 1+number of defective vessels * 0.5) in zebrafish treated with compounds **2**, **4**, **5**, **7**, and **10**. Data represented as mean ± SEM. ## $p < 0.01$ compared to the control group; ** $p < 0.01$ compared to the PTK787 group.

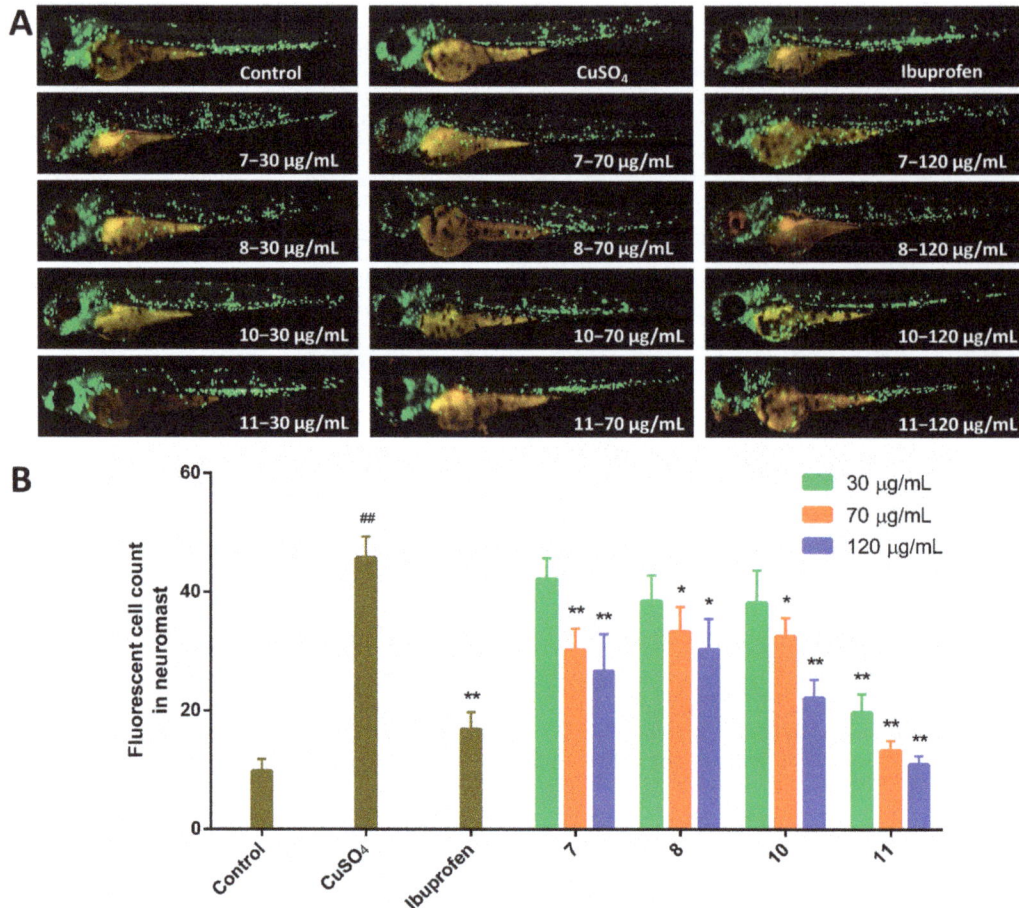

Figure 5. Results of anti-inflammatory activities. (**A**) Typical images on inflammatory sites in CuSO$_4$-induced transgenic macrophages fluorescent of compounds **7**, **8**, **10**, and **11**, using ibuprofen (10 μM) as a positive control. (**B**) Quantitative analysis of the number of fluorescent macrophages. The data are represented as the mean ± SEM. ## $p < 0.01$ compared to the control group; * $p < 0.05$ and ** $p < 0.01$ compared to the CuSO$_4$ group.

3. Materials and Methods

3.1. General Experimental Procedures

Optical rotations were measured on a JASCO P-2000 digital polarimeter (JASCO, Tokyo, Japan). UV spectra were performed on an Eppendorf BioSpectrometer Basic photometer. IR spectra were recorded on a JASCO FT/IR-4600 spectrometer in KBr discs. CD data were obtained on a JASCO J-810 spectropolarimeter. NMR spectra were collected using a JEOL JNM-ECP 600 spectrometer (JEOL, Tokyo, Japan). HRESIMS data were acquired on an Agilent 6210 ESI/TOF mass spectrometer (Agilent, Santa Clara, CA, USA). Analytical high performance liquid chromatography (HPLC) system (Waters, Milford, MA, USA) consisted of Waters e2695, UV Detector 2489, and software Empower using a C18 column (Diamonsil C18(2), 250 × 4.6 mm, 5 μM). Semipreparative HPLC was operated on the same system using a C18 column (Cosmosil 5C18-MS-II, 250 × 10 mm, 5 μM). Vacuum-liquid chromatography (VLC) used silica gel H (Qingdao Marine Chemical Factory, Qingdao, China). Thin layer chromatography (TLC) and column chromatography were performed on plates pre-coated with silica gel GF254 (10–40 μm) and Sephadex LH-20 (GE Healthcare Biosciences, Uppsala, Sweden), respectively.

3.2. Fungal Material

The fungus Y32-2 was isolated from the seawater sample collected from a depth of about 30 m in the Indian Ocean (88°59′51″ E, 2°59′54″ S) in 2013. It was identified as *Aspergillus austroafricanus* (GenBank access No. MK267449) by rDNA amplification and sequence analysis of the ITS region. The producing strain was prepared on potato dextrose agar medium stored at 4 °C.

3.3. Fermentation and Extraction

The fungus was cultured in 500 mL Erlenmeyer flasks with fermentation media containing 80 g of rice and 120 mL of sea water at 28 °C for 40 days. The whole fermented material was extracted exhaustively with EtOAc. Then the EtOAc extract was dried under reduced pressure to obtain residue (30.1 g).

3.4. Purification and Identification

The EtOAc extract was subjected to silica gel chromatography with a vacuum liquid chromatography (VLC) column, using a stepwise gradient solvent system of petroleum ether (PE)-CH_2Cl_2 (7:3, 3:7 and 0:1), then of CH_2Cl_2-MeOH (99:1, 49:1, 19:1, 9:1, 4:1, 1:1, and 0:1) to obtain thirteen primary fractions (Fr.1–Fr.13). Fr.6–Fr.11 were individually subjected to Sephadex LH-20 column (120 × 2 cm) chromatography with CH_2Cl_2-MeOH (1:1) as mobile phase, and then fractions were purified separately by semipreparative HPLC column (Cosmosil 5C18-MS-II, 250 × 10 mm, 5 μM) using different gradients of MeOH in H_2O. Fr.6 (3.5 g) afforded **6** (70% MeOH-H_2O, v/v; t_R = 23.5 min; 12.4 mg), **8** (60% MeOH-H_2O, v/v; t_R = 20.5 min; 91.2 mg), **9** (60% MeOH-H_2O, v/v; t_R = 21.9 min; 12.8 mg), **13** (65% MeOH-H_2O, v/v; t_R = 25.9 min; 8.6 mg), **14** (60% MeOH-H_2O, v/v; t_R = 24.8 min; 4.7 mg). Fr.7 (2.7 g) afforded **4** (40% MeOH-H_2O, v/v; t_R = 18.5 min; 4.4 mg). Fr.8 (1.5 g) afforded **1** (70% MeOH-H_2O, v/v; t_R = 10.4 min, 14.4min; 6.5 mg), **7** (60% MeOH-H_2O, v/v; t_R = 16.9 min; 21.4 mg), **11** (60% MeOH-H_2O, v/v; t_R = 22.8 min; 5.6 mg), **12** (65% MeOH-H_2O, v/v; t_R = 26.0 min; 14.3 mg). Fr.9 (0.5 g) afforded **3** (65% MeOH-H_2O, v/v; t_R = 28.5 min; 4.5 mg), **10** (60% MeOH-H_2O, v/v; t_R = 22.5 min; 5.5 mg). Fr.10 (1.1 g) afforded **2** (60% MeOH-H_2O, v/v; t_R = 15.0 min; 5.1 mg). Fr.11 (1.3 g) afforded **5** (50% MeOH-H_2O, v/v; t_R = 14.5 min; 3.0 mg).

Di-6-hydroxydeoxybrevianamide E (**1**): Yellow amorphous powder; $[\alpha]_D^{20}$ +24 (c 0.1, MeOH); UV (MeOH) λ_{max} 216, 299 nm; IR (KBr) ν_{max} 3460, 2973, 2925, 1667, 1440, 1306, 1192, 1108, 1001, 920, 809 cm^{-1}; ^1H and ^{13}C NMR data, see Table 1; HRESIMS m/z 731.3559 [M − H]$^-$ (calcd. for $C_{42}H_{48}N_6O_6$, 731.3557).

Dinotoamide J (**2**): Yellow amorphous powder; $[\alpha]_D^{20}$ +22 (c 0.1, MeOH); UV (MeOH) λ_{max} 210, 226 and 295 nm; IR (KBr) ν_{max} 3447, 1646, 1442, 1186, 1105, 618 cm^{-1}; ^1H and ^{13}C NMR data, see Table 1; HRESIMS m/z 763.3440 [M − H]$^-$ (calcd. for $C_{42}H_{48}N_6O_8$, 763.3456).

Asperpteridinate A: Yellow amorphous powder; $[\alpha]_D^{20}$ +63 (c 0.1, MeOH); UV (MeOH) λ_{max} 218, 239, 300, 334 nm; ^1H and ^{13}C NMR data, see Table 2; IR (KBr) ν_{max} 3465, 1633, 1263, 1192, 1105, 615 cm^{-1}; HRESIMS m/z 465.1018 [M + Na]$^+$ (calcd. for $C_{20}H_{18}N_4O_8$, 465.1023).

3.5. ECD Computational Calculation

The conformational analyses were carried out by random searching in the Sybyl-X 2.0 using the MMFF94S force field with an energy cutoff of 5.0 kcal/mol [21]. Subsequently, the conformers were re-optimized using DFT at the PBE0-D3/def2-SVP level in MeOH using the polarizable conductor calculation model (SMD) by the GAUSSIAN 09 program [22]. The energies, oscillator strengths, and rotational strengths (velocity) of the first 30 electronic excitations were calculated using the TDDFT methodology at the CAM-B3LYP-D3/def2-SVP level in MeOH. The ECD spectra were simulated by the overlapping Gaussian function (half the bandwidth at 1/e peak height, sigma = 0.30 for all) [23]. To get the final spectra, the simulated spectra of the conformers were averaged according to the Boltzmann distribution theory and their relative Gibbs free energy (ΔG).

3.6. Bioassay Protocols

3.6.1. Cell Culture and Cytotoxicity Assay

According to previous report [24], The HepG2 cells were cultured with DMEM medium, pH 7.0, supplemented with 10% FBS and 1% antibiotics (10,000 IU mL^{-1} of penicillin and 10 mg mL^{-1} of streptomycin), and the culture flasks were incubated under a humidified atmosphere of 37 °C and 5% CO_2. The cytotoxic activities of all compounds against HepG2 cells in vitro were determined by modified MTT assays as described previously [21]. Cells were seeded into a 96-well plate at a density 5×10^4 per well. After overnight incubation, the cells were treated with the chemicals for 24 h, and 10 µL MTT (5 mg/mL) was added to each well at 37 °C for 4 h, then 100 µL lysis buffer was added for the cell lysis. The OD value of each sample was detected at 560 nm using a microplate reader. The experiments were carried out in triplicate.

3.6.2. Zebrafish Maintenance

The zebrafish (*Danio rerio*) strains used in this assay were the AB wild-type, Tg (vegfr2-GFP) and Tg (zlyz-EGFP) transgenic lines [25,26]. They were maintained at 28.0 °C ± 0.5 °C in an automatic circulating tank system with light-dark cycle (14 h:10 h). The healthy adult zebrafish were placed in a breeding tank in the evening, and mated in the next morning. The fertilized eggs were collected, disinfected with methylene blue solution, and then raised in clean culture water including 5.0 mM NaCl, 0.17 mM KCl, 0.4 mM $CaCl_2$, and 0.16 mM $MgSO_4$ in a light-operated incubator.

3.6.3. Pro-Angiogenesis Assay

Vascular insufficiency in zebrafish was modeled by VEGFR tyrosine kinase inhibitor PTK787 to evaluate the effects of compounds on pro-angiogenesis according to previous report [8,26]. The healthy zebrafish larvae were separated into 24-well plates (ten embryos per well) in a 2 mL final volume of culture water at 24 h post fertilization (hpf). 0.2 µg/mL PTK787 was co-treated with each test compound (30, 70, 120 µg/mL) as test group. The control group was fresh culture water, the model group was 0.2 µg/mL PTK787, the positive drug group was 0.2 µg/mL PTK787 and 120 µg/mL ginsenoside Rg1. After 24 h incubation in a light-operated incubator at 28.0 °C ± 0.5 °C, the number of intersegmental blood vessels (ISVs) were captured by a fluorescent microscope (Olympus, SZX2-ILLTQ, Tokyo, Japan). Intact and defective vessels were counted separately and ISVs index was defined as follows: ISV index = number of intact vessels × 1 + number of defective vessels × 0.5 [27]. The zebrafish larvae without PTK787 in test group was used to evaluate the effects of compounds on anti-angiogenesis under the same conditions above described. All treatments were performed in triplicate.

3.6.4. Anti-Inflammatory Assay

The zebrafish inflammation model was induced by $CuSO_4$ to evaluate the effects of compounds on anti-inflammation [28]. In total, 72 hpf zebrafish larvae were distributed into 24-well plates (ten embryos per well) in a 2 mL final volume of culture water, and treated with different concentrations of each test compound (30, 70, 120 µg/mL) for 2 h as test group. Then $CuSO_4$ was added and incubated for 1 h. The control group was fresh culture water, the model group was 20 µM $CuSO_4$ and the positive drug group was 20 µM $CuSO_4$ and 10 µM ibuprofen. After 4 h incubation in a light-operated incubator at 28.0 °C ± 0.5 °C, the number of macrophages were imaged by a fluorescent microscope (Olympus, SZX2-ILLTQ, Tokyo, Japan). All treatments were performed in triplicate.

3.6.5. Statistical Analysis

Statistical analysis were processed by GraphPad Prism 6.0 software. All the experimental data were shown as mean ± SEM. The comparison between groups was performed by student's test. * $p < 0.05$ was considered as significant difference. ** $p < 0.01$ was a very significant difference.

4. Conclusions

To summarize, two new indole alkaloid dimers di-6-hydroxydeoxybrevianamide E (**1**), dinotoamide J (**2**) and one new pteridine alkaloid asperpteridinate A (**3**), together with eleven known compounds (**4–14**) were isolated from the marine-derived fungus *Aspergillus austroafricanus* Y32-2. Their structures including the absolute configurations were elucidated by various spectroscopic methods and ECD calculations. Among them, both di-6-hydroxydeoxybrevianamide E (**1**) and dinotoamide J (**2**) are homologous dimers that represent the novel examples of prenylated indole alkaloids. Asperpteridinate A is the first new alkaloid composed of pteridine and 1, 3-benzodioxole structures. All compounds were evaluated for pro-angiogenic, anti-inflammatory activities in the zebrafish models and cytotoxicity against HepG2 cells. Compounds **2**, **4**, **5**, **7**, and **10** exhibited pro-angiogenic activity, and compounds **7**, **8**, **10**, and **11** displayed anti-inflammatory activity in a dose-dependent manner, and compound **6** showed significant cytotoxicity against HepG2 cells with an IC$_{50}$ value of 30 µg/mL. The results suggested that these compounds could be promising candidates for further pharmacologic and biosynthetic research.

Supplementary Materials: The following are available online at https://www.mdpi.com/1660-3397/19/2/98/s1, HRESIMS, 1D and 2D NMR spectra of all new compounds **1–3**, biological activities of all isolated compounds and dose–response curves of compound **6**, the atom coordinates and energies of new compounds **1–3**.

Author Contributions: P.L. performed isolation, structure determination and bioassays of the compounds and wrote the manuscript. M.Z. performed the fermentation of the fungus, extraction of the culture broths and isolation of the compounds. H.L. and R.W. performed the bioassays. H.H. carried out taxonomic identification of the fungus. X.L. and K.L. designed the study and revised the manuscript. H.C. collected the samples from the Indian Ocean and revised the manuscript. All authors have read and agreed to the published version of the manuscript.

Funding: This work was supported by the National Key R&D Program of China (2018YFC1707300), the Project funded by China Postdoctoral Science Foundation (2019M662418), the International Science and Technology Cooperation Program of Shandong Academy of Sciences (No. 2019GHZD10), the Foundation of State Key Laboratory of Biobased Material and Green Papermaking, Qilu University of Technology, Shandong Academy of Sciences (No. ZZ20190402), the National Natural Science Foundation of China (81602982), the Taishan Scholar Project from Shandong Province (ts20190950), and the China Ocean Mineral Resources Research and Development Association (DY135-R2-1-06 and DY135-B2-11).

Institutional Review Board Statement: The experiments were performed in accordance with standard ethical guidelines. The procedures were approved by the Ethics Committee of the Biology Institute of Shandong Academy of Science (SYXK LU 2020 0015).

Conflicts of Interest: The authors declare no conflict of interest.

References

1. Barbosa, F.; Pinto, E.; Kijjoa, A.; Pinto, M.; Sousa, E. Targeting antimicrobial drug resistance with marine natural products. *Int. J. Antimicrob. Agents* **2020**, *56*, 106005. [CrossRef]
2. Ma, H.G.; Liu, Q.; Zhu, G.L.; Liu, H.S.; Zhu, W.M. Marine natural products sourced from marine-derived *Penicillium* fungi. *J. Asian Nat. Prod. Res.* **2016**, *18*, 92–115. [CrossRef] [PubMed]
3. Lee, Y.M.; Kim, M.J.; Li, H.; Zhang, P.; Bao, B.; Lee, K.J.; Jung, J.H. Marine-derived *Aspergillus* species as a source of bioactive secondary metabolites. *Mar. Biotechnol.* **2013**, *15*, 499–519. [CrossRef] [PubMed]
4. Wang, K.W.; Ding, P. New bioactive metabolites from the marine-derived fungi *Aspergillus*. *Mini-Rev. Med. Chem.* **2018**, *18*, 1072–1094. [CrossRef]

5. Carbone, D.; Parrino, B.; Cascioferro, S.; Pecoraro, C.; Giovannetti, E.; Sarno, V.D.; Musella, S.; Auriemma, G.; Cirrincione, G.; Diana, P. 1,2,4-oxadiazole topsentin analogs with antiproliferative activity against pancreatic cancer cells, targeting GSK3β kinase. *ChemMedChem* **2021**, *16*, 537–554. [CrossRef] [PubMed]
6. Parrino, B.; Carbone, D.; Cascioferro, S.; Pecoraro, C.; Giovannetti, E.; Deng, D.; Sarno, V.D.; Musella, S.; Auriemma, G.; Cusimano, M.G.; et al. 1,2,4-oxadiazole topsentin analogs as staphylococcal biofilm inhibitors targeting the bacterial transpeptidase Sortase A. *Eur. J. Med. Chem.* **2020**, *209*, 112892. [CrossRef]
7. Li, P.; Fan, Y.; Chen, H.; Chao, Y.; Du, N.; Chen, J. Phenylquinolinones with antitumor activity from the Indian ocean-derived fungus *Aspergillus versicolor* Y31–2. *Chin. J. Oceanol. Limnol.* **2016**, *34*, 1072–1075. [CrossRef]
8. Fan, Y.; Li, P.; Chao, Y.; Chen, H.; Du, N.; He, Q.; Liu, K. Alkaloids with cardiovascular effects from the marine-derived fungus *Penicillium expansum* Y32. *Mar. Drugs* **2015**, *13*, 6489–6504. [CrossRef] [PubMed]
9. Zuleta, I.A.; Vitelli, M.L.; Baggio, R.; Garland, M.T.; Seldes, A.M.; Palermo, J.A. Novel pteridine alkaloids from the sponge *Clathria* sp. *Tetrahedron* **2002**, *58*, 4481–4486. [CrossRef]
10. Gubiani, J.R.; Teles, H.L.; Silva, G.H.; Young, M.C.M.; Pereira, J.O.; Bolzani, V.S.; Araujo, A.R. Cyclo-(trp-phe) diketopiperazines from the endophytic fungus *Aspergillus versicolor* isolated from *Piper aduncum*. *Quim. Nova* **2017**, *40*, 138–142. [CrossRef]
11. Yurchenk, A.N.; Smetanina, O.F.; Kalinovsky, A.I.; Pivkin, M.V.; Dmitrenok, P.S.; Kuznetsova, T.A. A new meroterpenoid from the marine fungus *Aspergillus versicolor* (Vuill.) Tirab. *Russ. Chem. Bull.* **2010**, *59*, 852–856. [CrossRef]
12. Hodge, R.P.; Harris, C.M.; Harris, T.M. Verrucofortine, a major metabolite of *Penicillium verrucosum* var. *cyclopium*, the fungus that produces the mycotoxin verrucosidin. *J. Nat. Prod.* **1988**, *51*, 66–73. [CrossRef]
13. Xin, Z.; Fang, Y.; Zhu, T.; Duan, L.; Gu, Q.; Zhu, W. Antitumor components from sponge-derived fungus *Penicillium auratiogriseum* Sp-19. *Chin. J. Mar. Drugs* **2006**, *25*, 1–6.
14. Feng, Y.; Han, J.; Zhang, Y.; Su, X.; Essmann, F.; Grond, S. Study on the alkaloids from two great white sharks antitumor components from sponge-derived fungus *Penicillium auratiogriseum* Sp-19. *Chin. J. Mar. Drugs* **2016**, *35*, 16–22.
15. Fujiia, Y.; Asahara, M.; Ichinoec, M.; Nakajima, H. Fungal melanin inhibitor and related compounds from *Penicillium decumbens*. *Phytochemistry* **2002**, *60*, 703–708. [CrossRef]
16. Ma, Y.; Qiao, K.; Kong, Y.; Li, M.; Guo, L.; Miao, Z.; Fan, C. A new isoquinolone alkaloid from an endophytic fungus R22 of *Nerium indicum*. *Nat. Prod. Res.* **2016**, *31*, 1258556. [CrossRef]
17. Tsukamoto, S.; Kato, H.; Samizo, M.; Nojiri, Y.; Ohnuki, H.; Hirota, H.; Ohta, T. Notoamides F-K, Prenylated indole alkaloids isolated from a marine-derived *Aspergillus* sp. *J. Nat. Prod.* **2008**, *71*, 2064–2067. [CrossRef]
18. Jennifer, M.F.; David, H.S.; Sachiko, T.; Robert, M.W. Studies on the biosynthesis of the notoamides: Synthesis of an isotopomer of 6-hydroxydeoxybrevianamide E and biosynthetic incorporation into notoamide. *J. Org. Chem.* **2011**, *76*, 5954–5958.
19. Li, Y.; Teng, Y.; Cheng, Y.; Wu, L. Study on the chemical constituents of mulberry. *J. Shenyang Pharm. Univ.* **2003**, *6*, 422–424.
20. Qi, J.; Liu, S.; Liu, W.; Cai, G.; Liao, G. Identification of UAP1L1 as tumor promotor in gastric cancer through regulation of CDK6. *Aging* **2020**, *12*, 6904–6927. [CrossRef]
21. *Sybyl Software*, version X 2.0; Tripos Associates Inc.: St. Louis, MO, USA, 2013.
22. Frisch, M.J.; Trucks, G.W.; Schlegel, H.B.; Scuseria, G.E.; Robb, M.A.; Cheeseman, J.R.; Scalmani, G.; Barone, V.; Mennucci, B.; Petersson, G.A.; et al. *Gaussian 09*; revision C 01; Gaussian, Inc.: Wallingford, CT, USA, 2009.
23. Stephens, P.J.; Harada, N. ECD cotton effect approximated by the Gaussian curve and other methods. *Chirality* **2010**, *22*, 229–233. [CrossRef] [PubMed]
24. Ottoni, C.A.; Maria, D.A.; Gonçalves, P.J.R.O.; Araújo, W.L.; Souza, A.O. Biogenic *Aspergillus tubingensis* silver nanoparticles' in vitro effects on human umbilical vein endothelial cells, normal human fibroblasts, HEPG2, and *Galleria mellonella*. *Toxicol. Res.* **2019**, *8*, 789801. [CrossRef] [PubMed]
25. Li, T.; Tang, X.; Luo, X.; Wang, Q.; Liu, K.; Zhang, Y.; Voogd, N.J.; Yang, J.; Li, P.; Li, G. Agelanemoechine, a dimeric bromopyrrole alkaloid with a pro-angiogenic effect from the south China sea sponge *Agelas nemoechinata*. *Org. Lett.* **2019**, *21*, 9483–9486. [CrossRef] [PubMed]
26. Wang, Q.; Tang, X.; Liu, H.; Luo, X.; Sung, P.J.; Li, P.; Li, G. Clavukoellians G–K, new nardosinane and aristolane sesquiterpenoids with angiogenesis promoting activity from the marine soft coral *Lemnalia* sp. *Mar. Drugs* **2020**, *18*, 171. [CrossRef]
27. Zhou, Z.Y.; Huan, L.Y.; Zhao, W.R.; Tang, N.; Jin, Y.; Tang, J.Y. *Spatholobi caulis* extracts promote angiogenesis in HUVECs in vitro and in zebrafish embryos in vivo via up-regulation of VEGFRs. *J. Ethnopharmacol.* **2017**, *200*, 74–83. [CrossRef]
28. Gui, Y.H.; Liu, L.; Wu, W.; Zhang, Y.; Jia, Z.L.; Shi, Y.P.; Kong, H.T.; Liu, K.C.; Jiao, W.H.; Lin, H.W. Discovery of nitrogenous sesquiterpene quinone derivatives from sponge *Dysidea septosa* with anti-inflammatory activity in vivo zebrafish model. *Bioorg. Chem.* **2020**, *94*, 103435. [CrossRef] [PubMed]

MDPI
St. Alban-Anlage 66
4052 Basel
Switzerland
Tel. +41 61 683 77 34
Fax +41 61 302 89 18
www.mdpi.com

Marine Drugs Editorial Office
E-mail: marinedrugs@mdpi.com
www.mdpi.com/journal/marinedrugs

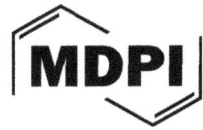

www.ingramcontent.com/pod-product-compliance
Lightning Source LLC
LaVergne TN
LVHW070504100526
838202LV00014B/1787